Clinical Andrology

Clinical Andrology

EAU/ESAU Course Guidelines

Edited by

Lars Björndahl, MD, PhD
Centre for Andrology and Sexual Medicine
Endocrinology Clinic, Department of Medicine, Huddinge
Karolinska University Hospital and Karolinska Institutet
Stockholm, Sweden

Aleksander Giwercman, MD, PhD
Reproductive Medicine Centre
Skåne University Hospital Malmö
Lund University
Malmö, Sweden

Herman Tournaye, MD, PhD
Centre for Reproductive Medicine
University Hospital of the Dutch-speaking Brussels Free University
Brussels, Belgium

Wolfgang Weidner, MD
Department of Urology, Pediatric Urology and Andrology
University of Giessen
Giessen, Germany

Published in association with the European Academy of Urology

informa
healthcare

New York London

Published in 2010 by Informa Healthcare, Telephone House, 69-77 Paul Street, London EC2A 4LQ, UK.
Simultaneously published in the USA by Informa Healthcare, 52 Vanderbilt Avenue, 7th floor, New York, NY 10017, USA.

A CIP record for this book is available from the British Library.

ISBN-13: 978-1-8418-4680-4

Orders may be sent to: Informa Healthcare, Sheepen Place, Colchester, Essex CO3 3LP, UK
Telephone: +44 (0)20 7017 5540
Email: CSDhealthcarebooks@informa.com
Website: http://informahealthcarebooks.com/

For corporate sales please contact: CorporateBooksIHC@informa.com
For foreign rights please contact: RightsIHC@informa.com
For reprint permissions please contact: PermissionsIHC@informa.com

Typeset by Aptara, Inc.
Printed and bound in the United Kingdom

Foreword

I am very honored to have the opportunity to include a few words in this edition of *Clinical Andrology*. At first glance one may think "Yet another book on andrology," albeit a very comprehensive one. But this is, in many ways, a truly unique publication: not only because it provides very comprehensive coverage of this difficult and multidisciplinary field, but also because it represents a unique collaboration between a scientific publisher and top experts from a number of societies operating in this challenging medical area. *Clinical Andrology* will be an important reference publication for our young colleagues taking part in a joint training program organized by the European Academy of Andrology (EAA), the European Federation of Endocrine Societies (EFES), the European Society of Human Reproduction and Embryology (ESHRE), and the European Association of Urology (EAU). Aside from this direct link to a specialization program, *Clinical Andrology* offers the state of the art in all aspects covered by what we nowadays consider to be in the realm of andrological urology, and it will surely prove a valuable reference document also for experienced colleagues.

Over the past decennia, a great progress has been made in the understanding of both the physiology and the pathophysiology of the male reproductive system, and it is generally recognized now that specialized training in clinical andrology is needed to keep pace with the emerging techniques for assisted reproduction. The curricula of the various medical specialties involved have been lagging behind. Sustainable high-quality structures to train professionals are needed and this first collaborative training effort is an enormous step forward and all collaborators consider it a solid foundation to further build on.

One only needs to look at the table of contents to understand the complexity of this field and the range of skills involved to appropriately treat the different patients groups. The most important attributes for a clinical andrologist would be the ability to take a clinical history and carry out a competent clinical examination. This may sound straightforward, but it clearly is not. A clinical andrologist will need to have a range of skills at his/her disposal, and the evaluation of many patients, more often than not, will involve a team of experts (reproductive endocrinologist, geneticists, gynecologists, sex therapists, oncologists, etc.). Also in oncology settings we see reproductive health problems, including sexual dysfunction and impaired fertility, which should be dealt with in a multidisciplinary setting.

The ability to coordinate all efforts to ensure centralized management and oversight to guarantee continuity of patient care requires a high level of competency.

We need to set, unify, and raise the standards in all areas of care, but andrology will definitely be a field that will be taxed heavily in the years to come. Changing demographics, with the first wave of the Baby Boomer generation approaching 60 years of age will greatly affect the demands on healthcare professionals. Additionally, changes in social patterns influence the demand on experts with particular andrological expertise: delayed parenthood, second marriages, a greater acceptance of diverse family units, and more openness about gender-related problems are just a few factors that will affect practice patterns.

The trend of further specialization is visible in most medical fields, and clear division lines between responsibilities relating to patient care seem to fade. Education of young colleagues should remain a central activity if we, as medical associations, fully commit to optimizing patient care.

I cannot commend the editors—Lars Björndahl, Aleksander Giwercman, Herman Tournaye, and Wolfgang Weidner—enough for bringing together this wealth of information and motivate and engage so many eminent experts in this area to provide high-quality contributions. I take the liberty to speak also on behalf of the all colleagues directly benefiting from all these efforts: it has most certainly paid off—my sincere congratulations.

Per-Anders Abrahamsson
Secretary-General, European Association of Urology

Preface

You are holding in your hands the first edition of *Clinical Andrology*. As editors, we would shortly explain the intentions behind this textbook and also ask for your help in improving the editions we are expecting to follow the opus one.

During the recent years, it has became more and more evident that diseases of male reproductive system represent a serious and common health problem. At least 15% of all couples experience infertility problems, the contribution of male-related factors assumed to be as frequent as the female ones. Together with sexual dysfunction, fertility problems represent one of the most common disorders in our society. Another issue receiving increasing attention is age-related androgen deficiency and the link between low testosterone levels and the risk of metabolic and cardiovascular disorders. However, proper and evidence-based management of these conditions is seriously hampered by lack of *clinical andrologists*—specialists in disorders of male reproductive system. During the past few years, collaboration between European Academy of Andrology (EAA) and European Association of Urology (EAU), aiming to establish a joint training program within the field of clinical andrology, has been established. Four different subareas of this clinical discipline have been defined: (a) infertility, (b) hypogonadism, (c) sexual dysfunction, and (d) male accessory sex gland infections.

The aim of this textbook is to cover all these four fields and to provide a comprehensive evidence based and clinically oriented tool for training clinical andrologists. However, it can also be used in teaching at the pregraduate level as well as an aid in the daily life of more experienced andrologists. According to these quite ambitious goals, we have approached some of the highest ranked experts within the field of clinical andrology to contribute to this book. The authors were asked to focus on the clinical aspects of andrology basing and documenting their recommendations by stating proper levels of evidence. We thank all the authors for their invaluable efforts.

We are aware of the fact that the first edition of a textbook will not be perfect. However, we hope that the readers, trainees, students will find it valuable in their work with clinical andrology. We would also appreciate constructive *feedback*—negative or positive—since this will be an important tool for improving the forthcoming editions. Therefore, do not hesitate to let us know your opinion about *Clinical Andrology*.

Lars Björndahl
Aleksander Giwercman
Herman Tournaye
Wolfgang Weidner

Contents

Contributors

Dimitrios A. Adamopoulos Department of Endocrinology, Diabetes, and Metabolism, Elena Venizelou Hospital, Athens, Greece

Luciano Adorini Bioxell, Milan, Italy

Massoud Afnan Assisted Conception Unit, Birmingham Women's Hospital, Birmingham, U.K.

Emre Akkus Professor in Urology-Andrology, Cerrahpasa School of Medicine, Istanbul University, Istanbul, Turkey

Peter Albers Department of Urology, Heinrich-Heine-University, Düsseldorf, Germany

Maria Alevizaki Endocrinology, Metabolism and Diabetes Unit, Evgenidion Hospital, and Department of Medical Therapeutics, Alexandra Hospital, Athens University School of Medicine, Athens, Greece

Davide Arcaniolo Department of Urology, University Federico II, Naples, Italy

Stefan Arver Centre for Andrology and Sexual Medicine, Department of Endocrinology, Metabolism and Diabetes, Karolinska University Hospital and Karolinska Institutet, Stockholm, Sweden

Dimitrios Baltogiannis Department of Urology, Ioannina University School of Medicine, Ioannina, Greece

Christopher L. R. Barratt Assisted Conception Unit and Reproductive & Developmental Biology Group, Division of Maternal and Child Health Sciences, Ninewells Hospital, University of Dundee, Dundee, Scotland, U.K.

Armin J. Becker Department of Urology, University Hospital Munich–Grosshadern, Ludwig-Maximilians-University, Munich, Germany

Mihály Berényi National Medical Center, Budapest, Hungary

Richard Berges PAN Klinik, Köln, Germany

Carlo Bettocchi Department of Urology, University of Bari, Bari, Italy

Lars Björndahl Centre for Andrology and Sexual Medicine, Clinic for Endocrinology, Department of Medicine, Huddinge Karolinska University Hospital and Karolinska Institutet, Stockholm, Sweden

Jens Peter Bonde Department of Environmental and Occupational Medicine, Copenhagen University Hospital, Bispebjerg Hospital, Copenhagen, Denmark

Nancy L. Brackett The Miami Project to Cure Paralysis, University of Miami Miller School of Medicine, Lois Pope Life Center, Miami, Florida, U.S.A.

Astrid E. P. Cantineau Isala Clinics Zwolle, Zwolle, The Netherlands

Ben J. Cohlen Isala Clinics Zwolle, Zwolle, The Netherlands

Elisabetta M. Colpi Biogenesi Reproductive Medicine Center, Istituti Clinici Zucchi, Monza, Italy

Giovanni M. Colpi Uro-Andrology and IVF Unit, Ospedale San Paolo – Polo Universitario, Milano, Italy

Giovanni Corona Endocrinology Unit, Ospedale Maggiore, Bologna, Italy

Thorsten Diemer Department of Urology, Pediatric Urology and Andrology, University of Giessen, Giessen, Germany

Fotios Dimitriadis Department of Urology, School of Medicine, Tottori University, Japan

Gert R. Dohle Erasmus Medical Centre, Rotterdam, The Netherlands

Jakob Eberhard Reproductive Medicine Centre, Skåne University Hospital Malmö, Lund University, Malmö, Sweden

Jens-Jørgen Elberg Department of Plastic Surgery, Rigshospitalet, University of Copenhagen, Copenhagen, Denmark

Nadja Engel Klinik Hirslanden, Zurich, Switzerland

Gianni Forti Endocrinology Unit, Department of Clinical Physiopathology, University of Florence, Florence, Italy

Mauro Gacci Department of Urology, University of Florence, Florence, Italy

Giulio Garaffa Institute of Urology, University College London, London, U.K.

Jemima Gaytant Bone Research Unit, Laboratory for Experimental Medicine and Endocrinology, Department of

Experimental Medicine, Katholieke Universiteit Leuven, Leuven, Belgium

Patrick de Geeter Department of Urology, Klinikum Kassel, Kassel, Germany

Dimitrios Giannakis Department of Urology, Ioannina University School of Medicine, Ioannina, Greece

Aleksander Giwercman Reproductive Medicine Centre, Skåne University Hospital Malmö, Lund University, Malmö, Sweden

Yvonne Lundberg Giwercman Molecular Genetic Reproductive Medicine, Department of Clinical Sciences, Lund University, Malmö, Sweden

Marc Goldstein Department of Urology and Cornell institute for Reproductive Medicine, Weill Medical College of Cornell University, and The Population Council at Rockefeller University, New York, New York, U.S.A.

Stavros Gratsias Department of Urology, Ioannina University School of Medicine, Ioannina

Levent Gurkan Department of Urology, Tulane University School of Medicine, New Orleans, Louisiana, U.S.A.

Uwe Hartmann Department of Urology, University Hospital Munich–Grosshadern, Ludwig-Maximilians-University, Munich, Germany

Ekkehard W. Hauck Department of Urology, Dr.-Otto-Gessler-Krankenhaus, Lindenberg, Germany, and Department of Urology and Pediatric Urology, University Hospital Giessen and Marburg GmbH, Justus-Liebig-University Giessen, Giessen, Germany

Wayne J. G. Hellstrom Department of Urology, Tulane University School of Medicine, New Orleans, Louisiana, U.S.A.

Ralf Henkel Department of Medical Biosciences, University of the Western Cape, Bellville, South Africa

Ilpo Huhtaniemi Department of Reproductive Biology, Imperial College London, Hammersmith Campus, London, U.K.

Ciro Imbimbo Department of Urology, University Federico II, Naples, Italy

Emmanuele A. Jannini School of Sexology, Course of Endocrinology and Medical Sexology, University of L'Aquila, L'Aquila, Italy

Hubert John Department of Urology, Kantonsspital Winterthur, Switzerland

Niels Jørgensen Department of Growth and Reproduction, Rigshospitalet, University of Copenhagen, Copenhagen, Denmark

Anders Juul Department of Growth and Reproduction, Rigshospitalet, University of Copenhagen, Copenhagen, Denmark

Axel Kamischke Centre for Reproductive Medicine and Andrology, University Clinic Münster, Münster, Germany

Vanessa J. Kay Assisted Conception Unit & Reproductive & Developmental Biology Group, Division of Maternal and Child Health Sciences, Ninewells Hospital, University of Dundee, Dundee, Scotland, U.K.

Howard H. Kim Department of Urology and Cornell Institute for Reproductive Medicine, Weill Medical College of Cornell University, and The Population Council at Rockefeller University, New York, New York, U.S.A.

Sabine Kliesch Department of Clinical Andrology, Centre for Reproductive Medicine and Andrology, University Clinic Münster, Münster, Germany

Zsolt Kopa National Medical Centre, Budapest, Hungary

Csilla Krausz Department of Clinical Physiopathology, Andrology Unit, University of Florence, Florence, Italy

Niels Kroman Department of Breast Surgery, Rigshospitalet, University of Copenhagen, Copenhagen, Denmark

Andrea Lenzi Department of Medical Pathophysiology, University of Rome "La Sapienza," Rome, Italy

Chi-Ying Li Institute of Urology, University College London, London, U.K.

Kersti Lundin Reproductive Medicine, Sahlgrenska University Hospital, Göteborg, Sweden

Charles M. Lynne Department of Urology, University of Miami Miller School of Medicine, Miami, Florida, U.S.A.

Maric Maggi Andrology Unit, Department of Clinical Physiopathology, University of Florence, Florence, Italy

Ahmed Mahmoud Section of Endocrinology/Andrology, Department of Internal Medicine, University Hospital Ghent, Ghent, Belgium

Roelof Menkveld Andrology Laboratory, Department of Obstetrics and Gynaecology, Tygerberg Academic Hospital and University of Stellenbosch, Tygerberg, South Africa

Vincenzo G. Mirone Urology Department, University Federico II, Naples, Italy

Giorgios Mitios Department of Endocrinology, Diabetes, and Metabolism, Elena Venizelou Hospital, Athens, Greece

Ikuo Miyagawa Department of Urology, Tottori University School of Medicine, Yonago, Japan

Francesco Montorsi Division of Urology, Istituto Scientifico San Raffaele, Milan, Italy

Table 3 Frequency Distribution of Male Infertility Diagnostic Categories in Two Periods of Time

1970s[a]		1980s[b]	
	%		%
Idiopathic infertility[c]	39.7	Idiopathic infertility	31.0
Varicocele	22.8	Varicocele	15.6
Infections	12.4	Endocrine hypogonadism	8.9
Seminal plasma abnormalities	6.3	Infections	8.0
Immunological factors	5.4	Maldescented testes	7.8
Congenital abn/ties	3.0	Sperm deposition problems	5.9
Sexual-ejaculatory problem	2.9	Immunological factors	4.5
Systemic diseases	2.5	Systemic diseases	3.1
Obstructive azoospermia	1.6	Obstructions	1.7
Endocrinopathies	1.2	Remainder (testicular tumors, cryo, etc.)	13.4
Various	2.2		

[a]Estimate from 3555 couples with a male factor infertility problem, extracted from Table 1 (1).
[b]Data from a reference reproductive medicine center, adapted from Table 5.2 (5).
[c]Oligo-terato-astheno-necro-zoo-spermia.

Table 4 Frequency Distribution of Male Infertility Diagnostic Classes Based on Recent Data (1996–2005)[a]

	% of each class	% of total no. of cases
1. *Single-cause class*[b]		
Idiopathic OTA syndrome	40.6	15.2
Varicocele	18.7	7.1
Epididymopathy	12.8	4.8
Environmental[c]	8.0	3.1
Genital infections	5.3	1.8
Acquired testicular damage	4.8	1.7
Congenital anomalies	3.4	1.3
Systemic causes	2.4	0.8
Endocrine dysfunction	1.6	0.6
Ejaculatory problems	1.5	0.5
Life-style	1.0	0.4
2. *Two-cause classes*[d]		
Combination of one other factor with		
Epididymopathy	31.3	9.8
Varicocele	26.5	8.5
Environmental	20.6	6.3
Remainder	21.6	6.7
3. *Three or more cause classes*[e]		
Combination of two or more factors with		
Epididymopathy	24.8	7.8
Varicocele	19.2	6.0
Environmental	19.0	6.0
Remainder	37.0	11.5

[a]Ref. 4.
[b]Single class, *n*: 289 (37.3%).
[c]Mainly occupational.
[d]Two-cause classes, *n*: 242 (31.3%).
[e]Three- or more-cause classes, *n*: 243 (31.4%).

context, the specific nature of the center (endocrinology, urology, etc.) might have been interfering with the representativeness of the population sample. Another important aspect was the time-related deviations in the relative incidence of etiological factors for compromised male reproductive capacity. These have been demonstrated in sets of data assembled in the 1970s or 1980s and observations made over the last decade. It appears that the main explanation for the differences observed was the updating of the investigative means available over the years passed.

Thus, in study from the 1970s (1), the highest incidence of male factor infertility was observed in subgroups of men with idiopathic dyspermia, varicocele, and accessory gland infections (39.7%, 22.8%, and 12.4%, respectively; Table 3). An intermediate, time-wise, distribution of diagnostic categories originated from a single reference center caring for a mid-European population showed similar findings, although the clinical material classified was not exclusively infertile (5). This picture has significantly changed as a result of an improved diagnostic approach applied in recent years. Thus, analysis of a set of data from a total of 774 dyspermic men investigated for couple infertility in an andrology clinic in the decade 1996 to 2005, using up-to-date investigative tools, showed marked differences from the early reports regarding both the number of categories listed and their relative frequency distribution (Table 4). It was of interest that despite applying sophisticated investigative means, the most frequently occurring diagnostic category was still that of idiopathic oligozoospermia [15.2% as compared to the 39.7% and 31.0% found in the earlier reports (1,5)]. Another interesting observation was the emergence of new categories listed as epididymopathy (12.8%), environmentally induced (8.0%), and life-style–related classes (including use/abuse of alcohol, tobacco, motorbike, etc., ~1.0%). Finally, of particular importance was the observation that single factor categories accounted for only 37.3% of the total study population, the remaining being combinations of 2 (31.3%) and 3 (31.4%) or more factor categories. This finding makes the relative distribution of diagnostic categories presented in the past not relevant today, because this classification was formulated on the assumption of a single factor etiology for each group. As it is noted, in the recent categorization, varicocele, as a part of the single-cause category, represents 18.7% of this subgroup, but only 7.1% of the whole sample (Table 4). However, its total incidence for all three subgroups was 21.6%. Moreover, two- or multi-cause factor classes were the commonest diagnostic categories (31.3% + 31.4% = 62.7%).

It is concluded that single-cause etiology of the problem is present only in approximately one-third of the cases, the great majority being bi- or multifactorial in origin, and this new distribution of causative factors is the result of improvement in the investigative tools employed. Moreover, a clearer picture of the distribution of causative factors is mandatory for decision making both for prevention policies and for therapeutic prognosis.

TRENDS IN MALE REPRODUCTIVE HEALTH

Conflicting data from epidemiological observations and large data bases have created a rather blurred picture of the prevailing trends in male reproductive capacity, with some extreme estimations ranging from those reporting no change or even improvement to some prophets of the doom, who have made catastrophic predictions. Some of the main constituents depicting male reproductive capacity trends include:

Sperm Parameter Changes

Since the 1992 meta-analysis demonstrating a significant decline of sperm parameters during the last 50 years (6), a number of reports from different parts of the world, mostly Europe and the United States, have either supported or refuted the findings of that study (7,8); this topic has been strongly debated in the early 1990s (9). To date, it is generally accepted that a deterioration of sperm parameters is a frequently observed phenomenon in certain populations, but there are also some notable exceptions. These differences should be properly analyzed on each particular case, and, if confirmed, it might be timely to consider a re-evaluation of normal sperm values as indeed was the case in the new WHO update (10) and introduction of new standards in specific populations on earth.

Trends in Male Factor Infertility

Up until the 1980s–1990s, overpopulation was a major global concern, particularly in high breeding countries in development. However, in recent years, this tide has been reversed and a marked drop in fertility rates has been observed, but most convincingly in the developed countries (11,12). This turn of events has not only been linked to the prevailing modern life-style but also to the environmental assault on men's reproductive health (13). In this context, it was of interest that a marked decline of total sperm number and seminal volume occurred over a two-decade period in reverse fashion, with an increase of some important environmental pollutants in a South-European Capital (14), and, most importantly, this change was concomitant with other reproductive health-compromising events occurring in both sexes (15). Moreover, a recent report on declining conception rates in a Northern European population related this finding with an overall compromise of the male reproductive health (16).

Direct information on the prevalence of male factor infertility is difficult to obtain from any source. In an early study, a prevalence of about 8% was reported as a couple's single male factor fertility problem (2,5). Another estimate of male factor infertility originated from the Society for Assisted Reproductive Technology, which listed in its Clinic Summary Report a male problem as the only factor in 17% of infertile couples, and a combination of male plus female factor in another 18% of ART trials performed for the year 2005 in the United States (17). Moreover, in a recent report, male factor problem was considered to be the cause in one-third of couple infertility cases, with an equal percentage attributed to a problem of both partners (18). However, the gravest piece of news came from the annual report of the U.S. Society on ART for the year 2003, which showed that an alarming 53% of the couples using in vitro fertilization (IVF) and intracytoplasmic sperm injection (ICSI) were admitted to these procedures because of male factor infertility (19).

Reproductive Organ Morbidities

During the last decade or so it became apparent, mostly through the pioneering work of Scandinavian workers, that poor semen quality is not a random observation but, indeed, a part of the consequences of a wider assault of the environment on male reproductive health (13,20). These pathologies were considered to be different morbidities developing on a common background and were manifested as separate problems including the following entities.

Compromised Testicular Function

Information regarding a declining trend in sperm parameters has been widely reported and published (6,8) and its impact on fertility rates has been well documented (11). This phenomenon, although not universal, has been considered as multifactorial in origin.

Increased Rate of Testicular Cancer

It appears that this malignancy, more common in young to middle adult ages, has been on the rise in the West during the second half of the 20th century and was a consistent finding in various Caucasian populations (21). It was thought that fetal gonads may be the target of various detrimental factors and, in this context, testicular cancer may not be but one of the deleterious consequences, the other one being sperm problems in adult age (13).

Congenital Anomalies of Male Genitalia

Cryptorchidism and hypospadias are two abnormalities for which an increasing incidence has been observed in recent decades in certain populations (22,23). These trends run concurrently with the rise of testicular cancer's incidence in the same populations, suggesting a common pathogenetic cause.

By and large, it appears that a rising tendency in reproductive organ morbidities occurred during the last few decades. In those compromising male fecundity conditions, one may add the recently described testicular dysgenesis syndrome (20).

IMPACT OF INFERTILITY ON SOCIETY

Health Care Services

As expected, any increase of infertility rate will have a direct impact on health care services in more than one aspects of the system. First line data on this area are scarce and most of the information available is derived from indirect sources. Even so, the magnitude of the problem is easily illustrated by the new infertility cases estimated to be about 2 million new couples per year, of which approximately 50% will be, directly or not, of male origin (2).

Of interest are the observations from an affluent North-European population in which the high demand for infertility treatment and particularly ICSI in a background of a high percentage of not natural conceptions (7%) and in association with a high demand for adoption amply illustrate not only the burden on health care services but also the social consequences of infertility (13). On the other hand, in a recent report from the United States, in-patient hospitalization for male infertility was low with an overall rate of 0.9/100,000 population, of which 55% were for varicocele management, whereas most of the out-patient visits came from the 24 to 34 years age group (24). However, this information is not truly representative, since, as was recently reported, men with the problem usually seek care outside the traditional reimbursement patterns so that the true prevalence of the infertility cannot be precisely established (24).

Expenditure Burden

The economy of male infertility treatment usually, if not always, submerges into the total cost of couple infertility treatment, and, therefore, it is very difficult to be accurately estimated. In an evaluation of the cost-effectiveness of treatment excluding varicocele ligation for male factor infertility, the diagnostic cost in the United Kingdom was estimated at £432 (in pre-2000 prices), being the highest among other causes of couple infertility (25). On the other hand, in a recent report from the United States, total expenses for male infertility treatment for the year 2000 were about US $17.0 million (24). Moreover, for 18- to -64-year-old males the average annual expenditure was US $3.515 per man treated for infertility, whereas 8% of employees with the problem missed some hours of work (19).

Cost-effectiveness studies regarding per os empiric treatments for oligozoospermia are not available, since such treatments are not universally accepted, although frequently used in various parts of the world. On the other hand, ARTs are also empiric interventions for cases of male infertility; however, a head-on comparison between the two modalities is lacking, although it may be instructive. Thus, using figures from specialized public and private clinics in Athens, the cost of empiric treatment [tamoxifen citrate and testosterone undecanoate (26)] in men with idiopathic oligozoospermia was estimated at €291 per six months or €851 per successful outcome (author's data). The corresponding figures for ICSI were multiple (public clinic: €1.863 per trial or €6.210 per successful outcome; private clinic: €4.460 per trial or €14.866 per pregnancy), as was the case for IVF trial in such cases (Fig. 1).

As it is obvious, marked deviations occur using different types of intervention in the cost of treating male factor infertility, and, therefore, it is important that their cost-effectiveness should be estimated and taken into account when considering therapeutic options.

Reproductive Medicine Practice

Not disputing the huge progress made in understanding the human reproduction process and the contribution in reproductive medicine since introduction of ART, one can not be but skeptical in witnessing the abuses of the approach as applied in everyday practice. To mention but a few of its shortcomings, one may cite concerns related to a deficit of supervision by the regulating authorities, a relative laxness of the referral policies, or the industry's driven exploitations.

To start with, regulatory bodies supervising the practice of ART have not been introduced, but only in North America and Europe. Moreover, there is a rather foggy state of affairs regarding referrals to ART centers by those who, traditionally, are the first to receive the anxious couple for consultation. It is imperative that those clinicians should have special training in order to evaluate, diagnose, and make a prognosis for the outcome of any therapeutic approach, before resorting to the services of an ART unit.

Finally, pharmaceutical and technology industries, for their own purposes, selectively promote research, fund scientific meetings, and support ART activities, sometimes to the exclusion of less promising research in male infertility.

Therefore, the public at large and in particular the medical profession should exercise a vigorous control over these activities, both for public money funding and for private spending.

AGING AND MALE INFERTILITY

In recent years, a drastic restructuring of age distribution frequencies of different populations has taken place which together with an overall delay in procreation planning, particularly in the West, has brought attention to a subgroup of men with advanced paternal age. In this context, a number of special aspects should be considered.

Sperm Parameters and Aging

Most of the information available comes from retrospective studies relating sperm parameters with advancing age. The consensus emerging from relevant observations is that sperm concentration and motility decline gradually with advancing age (27). This view is re-enforced by prospective studies in populations of healthy men from nonclinical (28) or clinical settings (29).

These changes appeared to be related not only to a testicular volume decrease (30) but also to a deterioration of testicular histology (27). Moreover, cytogenetic analysis studies have shown an increased frequency of numerical and structural sperm

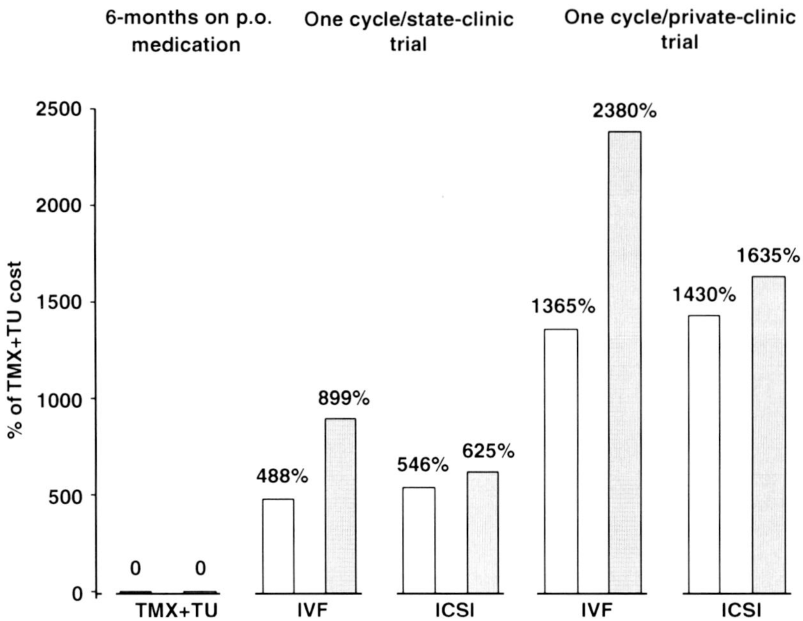

☐ Cost per treatment cycle irrespective of conception.

☐ Cost per treatment cycle for successful cases only, based on a pregnancy incidence of ~34% for TMX + TU (26), ~20% for IVF, and ~30% for ICSI (authors' data).

Vertical column: denotes increments above 100%.

Figure 1 Average cost per IVF or ICSI trial expressed as a percentage of medical treatment (considered as 0) with a combination of tamoxifen citrate-TMX (10 mg b.i.d.) and testosterone undecanoate-TU (40 mg t.i.d.) for six months in public or private clinics in Athens, in 2008.

chromosome abnormalities in aging men (59–74 years) as compared to a younger age group (23–29 years) of normal sperm donors (31).

By and large, it appears that sperm parameters show an age-related decline with concomitant testicular changes.

Fertility in Aging Men

Decline of sperm parameters with advancing age has an important bearing on fertility at the late stages of male reproductive life. This is particularly relevant since a rise of paternal age has been observed over the last few decades. Thus, population studies within the United States showed that the birth rate among fathers aged between 25 and 44 years has been increasing since 1970s (32). Moreover, although fathers aged <35 years accounted for 74% of the total number of live births, with only 25% coming from ages 35 to 54 years in 1993, a decade later these percentages changed to 60% and 40%, respectively (33). On the other hand, while a deterioration of the elements supporting fertility in aging men was to be expected, the ability to procreate is not excluded for a large proportion of these prospective fathers.

Age-Associated Risks for Pregnancy and Offspring

A number of sperm abnormalities associated with pregnancy's problematic outcome have been listed as contributing factors (Table 5) and appeared to deteriorate appreciably with advancing paternal age (34). As a result, the frequency of spontaneous abortions has been associated with advanced paternal age (35), independently of maternal age (31), and also with recurrent pregnancy loss (34).

With regard to the gene mutations involved, it appears that Y chromosome microdeletions, thrombophilia mutations, and HLA-G-polymorphisms are implicated. However, there is disagreement among the different studies. Thus, data from a large Scandinavian cohort showed no association between paternal age and birth defects (36). On the other hand, in a report from a Northern European population with increased reproductive health awareness and, possibly, problems, advanced paternal age was associated with an excess of specific offspring malformations (37). Finally, analysis of data from birth registrations in the United States (5,213,248 births) for the period 1999–2000 showed a slightly increased risk of birth defects (including heart

Table 5 Reproductive Problems Associated with Advanced Paternal Age

- Deterioration of sperm parameters (number, motility, volume)
- Decline in conception rates
- Increased chance for mutations aneuploidy
- Increased miscarriage rate
- Raised frequency of birth defects
- Increase in fetal demise
- Raised incidence of some 20 autosome dominant diseases in the offspring

Source: Adapted from Ref. 34.

malformations, musculoskeletal anomalies, Down's syndrome, etc.) in infants born to older fathers (38).

In conclusion, it appears that advanced paternal age is associated with a degree of sperm parameters' decline, subsequent decrease of fertility, and, perhaps, a small rise in the frequency of pregnancy risks and offspring problems.

COUNSELING THE INFERTILE MALE

Counseling men with a sperm problem has been hampered by the high proportion of cases with no definite diagnosis, categorized under the euphemism of "**idiopathic**" dyspermia or oligo-astheno-terato-zoospermia. This has turned the efforts for therapeutic interventions into a mess of different and often contradicting empiric treatments, aiming at activating or super-activating different components of the system. Moreover, most of these interventions did not satisfy the evidence-based criteria (39) and had completely ignored the female partner's role by not including pregnancy as the main outcome measure. In this context, Andrology has willingly deprived itself from one of the pillars of its activities this being helping men with reproductive problems and thus reducing its contribution to a narrower range of goals.

A precise diagnosis, when feasible, is the cornerstone of any attempt to council the male partner of a couple with infertility. Instrumental in this effort and in devising a proper therapeutic strategy is the consideration of the reproductive history of the couple. Moreover, in managing male infertility and since normalization or restoration of sperm is possible only on a few occasions, all efforts should be focused toward improving semen's quality, thus making the best possible use of the spermatozoa available.

Normalization or treatment of undisputedly recognized causal factors produce generally satisfactory results, depending on the individual diagnostic category. Thus, for example, normalizing an endocrine deviation is apparently the best prospect for this diagnostic category, whereas in other classes the prospects range from low to very low to nonexistent. On the other hand, in the largest category of all, the idiopathic oligozoospermia, empiric treatment, aiming at improving sperm parameters, has been proposed and tested, sometimes successfully.

The importance of simultaneous monitoring of the female partner with intervention, if need be, is a sine-qua non and cannot be stressed adequately. Obviously, when sperm improvement is substantial, there is no need but only for the normal partner's monitoring. However, very often sperm improvement may be partial so that, although natural conception has some reasonable chances to occur, downgrading of the requirements for ART application may be a legitimate task with all the economic, psychological, etc., advantages ensuing. Such an approach would reduce not only the treatment load for the female partner but also the pregnancy and offspring-related problems.

An important issue not adequately addressed so far is the overall future of dyspermic men not only in terms of genital organ morbidities but also regarding their gonadal hormone secretion in the years to come. It is therefore essential that these subjects are advised to keep-up their periodic visits to the clinic irrespective of their reproductive problem's outcome.

CLINICAL RECOMMENDATIONS

Based on the information presented, a number of clinical recommendations may be of help for the reader; these are as follows:

- Investigate the fertility potential of the male partner after pregnancy failure in efforts for more than a year, although this period should not necessarily be exhausted on certain occasions, and make use of the proper terminology in describing a problem.
- An effort to arrive to a precise diagnosis is of paramount importance and no investigative tools should not only be spared toward accurately establishing it for patients benefit, selection of therapeutic approach, prognosis, and therapeutic outcome but also for establishing a sound basis of reliable data for proper use in future.
- Investigate meticulously a possible impact on a man's reproductive health, particularly in relation to his individual, local or general, conditions of life.
- Make a proper estimation of the cost for any therapeutic intervention on evidence-based grounds so that the expense required is justified in terms of effectiveness both for the patient and the society at large.
- It is essential to council prospective fathers of advanced paternal age about the risks regarding pregnancy and the offspring at this period of their life.

REFERENCES

1. Comhaire FH, Lunenfeld B, Boukhzis R, et al.; World Health Organization. Towards more objectivity in diagnosis and management of male infertility. Int J Androl 1987; (suppl 7):1–53.
2. Rowe PJ, Comhaire FH, Hargreave TB, et al., eds. WHO Manual for the Standardized Investigation and Diagnosis of the Infertile Couple. Cambridge, U.K.: Cambridge University Press, 1993:1–7.
3. Rowe PJ, Comhaire FH, Hargreave TB, et al., eds. WHO manual for the standardized investigation, diagnosis and management of the infertile male. Cambridge, U.K.: Cambridge University Press, 2000:5–11.
4. Adamopoulos DA, Nicopoulou S, Michalakis C, et al. Incidence of dysspermia categories in a contemporary diagnostic setting [Abstract]. Andrologie 2006; 16:319–320.
5. Nieschlag E. Scope and goals of andrology. In: Nieschlag E, Behre HM, eds. Andrology: Male Reproductive Health and Dysfunction, 2nd ed. Berlin: Springer, 2000:1–8.
6. Carlsen E, Giwercman A, Keiding N, et al. Evidence for decreasing quality of semen during the past 50 years. Br Med J 1992; 305:609–613.

7. Bromwhich P, Cohen J, Stewart I, et al. Decline in sperm counts: an artifact of changed reference range of "normal"? Br Med J 1994; 309:19–22.
8. Swan SH, Elkin EP, Fenster L. The question of declining sperm density revisited: an analysis of 101 studies published 1934–1996. Environ Health Perspect 2000; 108:961–966.
9. Giwercman A. Declining semen quality and increasing incidence of abnormalities in male reproductive organs—fact or fiction? In: Edwards RG, Beard HK, eds. Modern Andrology. Oxford, U.K.: Oxford University Press, 1995:158–164.
10. Cooper GT, Noonan E, von Eckardstein S, et al. World Health Organization reference values for human semen characteristics. Hum Reprod Update 2009:1–15 doi: 10.1093/humupd/dmp048.
11. World Bank (2005) http://www.worldbank.org. Centers for Disease Control and Prevention. 2003 Assisted Reproductive Technology Report: Home. http://cdc.gov/ART/ART2005/index.htm.
12. Lutz W, O' Neill BC, Sherbov S. Demographics. Europe's population at a turning point. Science 2003; 299:1991–1992.
13. Skakkebaek NE, Jorgensen N, Main KM, et al. Is human fecundity declining? Int J Androl 2006; 29:2–11.
14. Adamopoulos DA, Pappa A, Nicopoulou S, et al. Seminal volume and total sperm number trends in men attending subfertility clinics in the Greater Athens Area during the period 1977–1993. Hum Reprod 1996; 11:1936–1941.
15. Adamopoulos DA, Koukkou E. Reproductive health problems in the Greater Athens Area. In: Nicolopoulou-Stamati P, Hens L, Howard CV, eds. Reproductive Health and the Environment. Dordrecht: Springer, 2007:337–352.
16. Jensen K, Sobotka T, Hansen MA, et al. Declining trends in conception rates in recent birth cohorts of native Danish women: a possible role of deteriorating male reproductive health. Int J Androl 2008; 31(2):81–92. http://www.ncbi.nlm.nih.gov/pmc/articles/PMC2440321/. doi: 10.111/ j.1365–2605.2007.00827.x
17. IVF success Rage Reports, 2006 Clinic Summary Report. www.sart.org.
18. Tielemans E, Burdof A, te Velde E, et al. Sources of bias in studies among infertility clients. Am J Epidemiol 2002; 156:86–89.
19. Centers for Disease Control and Prevention, 2003 ART Report: Home. www.cdc.gov.
20. Skakkebaek NE, Rajpert-DeMeyts E, Main KM. Testicular dysgenesis syndrome: an increasingly common developmental disorder with environmental aspects. Hum Reprod 2001; 16:972–978.
21. Moller H. Clues to the aetiology of testicular germ cell tumours from descriptive epidemiology. Eur Urol 1993; 23:8–15.
22. Boisen KA, Kaleva M, Main KM, et al. Difference in prevalence of congenital cryptorchidism in infants between two Nordic countries. Lancet 2004; 363:1264–1269.
23. Boisen KA, Chellakooty M, Schmidt I, et al. Hypospadias in a cohort of 1072 Danish newborn boys: prevalence and relationship to placental weight, anthropometrical measurements at birth and reproductive hormone levels at three months at age. J Clin Endocrinol Metab 2005; 90:4041–4046.
24. Meacham RB, Joyce GF, Wise M, et al. The urologic diseases in America Project, male infertility. J Urol 2007; 177:2058–2066.
25. Philips Z, Barraza-Lorens M, Posnett J. Evaluation of the relative cost-effectiveness of treatment for infertility in the UK. Hum Reprod 2000; 15:95–106.
26. Adamopoulos DA, Pappa A, Billa E, et al. Effectiveness of combined tamoxifen citrate and testosterone undecanoate treatment in men with idiopathic oligozoospermia. Fertil Steril 2003; 80:914–920.
27. Kühnert B, Nieschlag E. Reproductive functions of the ageing male. Hum Reprod Update 2004; 10:327–339.
28. Eskenazy B, Wyrobek AJ, Kidd SA, et al. The association of age and semen quality in healthy men. Hum Reprod 2003; 18:447–454.
29. Ng KK, Donat R, Chan L, et al. Sperm output of older men. Hum Reprod 2004; 19:1811–1815.
30. Mahmoud AM, Goemaere S, El-Garem Y, et al. Testicular volume in relation to hormonal indices of gonadal function in community-dwelling elderly men. J Clin Endocrinol Metab 2003; 88:179–184.
31. Kleinhaus K, Rerrin M, Friedlander Y, et al. Paternal age and spontaneous abortion. Obstet Gynecol 2006; 108:369–377.
32. Hamilton B, Martin J, Sutton P. Births: preliminary data for 2003. National Vital Statistics Report 2003; 53:9.
33. Bray I, Gunnell D, Smith GD. Advanced paternal age: how old is too old? J Epidemiol Community Health 2006; 60:851–853.
34. Puscheck EE, Jeyendran RS. The impact of male factor on recurrent pregnancy loss. Curr Opin Obstet Gynecol 2007; 19:222–228.
35. Slama R, Bonyer J, Windham G, et al. Influence of paternal age on the risk of spontaneous abortion. Am J Epidemiol 2005; 161:816–823.
36. Kazaura M, Lie RT, Skjaerven R. Paternal age and the risk of birth defects in Norway. Ann Epidemiol 2004; 14:566–570.
37. Zhu JL, Madsen KM, Vestergoard M, et al. Paternal age and congenital malformations. Hum Reprod 2005; 20:3173–3177.
38. Yung Q, Wen SW, Leader A, et al. Paternal age and birth defects: how strong is the association? Hum Reprod 2007; 22:696–701.
39. Tournaye H. Evidence-based management of male subfertility. Curr Opin Obset Gynecol 2006; 18:253–259.

2 Clinical investigation of the infertile male

Gert R. Dohle

Case: A couple has been visiting the urologist for primary infertility for two years. The husband is 32 years old and without urological complaints. There is no history of urogenital infection. He was operated for unilateral cryptorchidism at the age of seven. Sexual function is normal; ejaculations are antegrade. He uses no medication, does not smoke, and uses only limited alcoholic drinks. His partner is 30 years old, has no gynecological history, and has a menstrual cycle of 26–28 days.

Semen analysis shows a total count of 3.2 million spermatozoa (reference value >40 million) with 4% forward motility (reference value >40% A and B motile spermatozoa) and 1% normal forms (reference value >15% normal spermatozoa/strict criteria). Follicle stimulating hormone (FSH) is 12 IU/L (reference value 2–7), testosterone is 11 mmol/L (reference value 11–25).

Physical examination shows a small testis on the right side of 6 cm^3 and a 12 cm^3 testis on the left side, both without palpable abnormality. Further physical characteristics are normal; his body mass index is 28.

Scrotal ultrasound is performed and shows an inhomogeneous testis on the right side with a cluster of microcalcifications in the lower pole. The left testis appears normal and homogeneous. The epididymis has a normal appearance and diameter on both sides. A grade 1 varicocele is found on the left side (a scrotal venous diameter during Valsalva maneuver of 3.2 mm; no reflux).

The couple would like to be a candidate for assisted reproduction and have gathered information from the Internet about in vitro fertilization (IVF) and intracytoplasmic sperm injection (ICSI).

DEFINITION AND PROGNOSTIC FACTORS

According to the WHO definition, infertility is present if a sexually active couple is unable to conceive within one year (WHO, 1995) (1). About 15% of couples do not achieve pregnancy within one year: of these couples almost 50% will conceive spontaneously in the second year (2). Eventually, less than 5% will remain unwillingly childless.

The main factors influencing the prognosis in infertility are:

- Duration of infertility
- Primary or secondary infertility
- Results of semen analysis
- Age and fertility status of the female partner

At present, in many Western countries, women postpone their first pregnancy until they have finished their education and have started a professional career. However, the fertility of a woman aged 35 years is only 50% of the fertility potential of a woman aged 25 years. By the age of 38, this has reduced to only 25%, and over the age of 40 it is less than 5%. Female age is the most important single variable influencing outcome in assisted reproduction (3).

As a male fertility and urogenital expert, the urologist/andrologist should examine any male with fertility problems for urogenital abnormalities, so that a correct diagnosis is made and appropriate treatment can be given.

DIAGNOSIS

The diagnosis of male fertility must focus on a number of prevalent disorders (Table 1). Simultaneous assessment of the female partner is preferable, even if abnormalities are found in the male, because WHO data show that in one out of four couples who consult a physician with fertility problems, both male and female partners have abnormalities (1).

Reduced male fertility can be the result of congenital and acquired urogenital abnormalities, infections of the genital tract, increased scrotal temperature (varicocele), endocrine disturbances, genetic abnormalities, and immunological factors. No causal factor is found in 30% to 40% of cases (idiopathic male infertility) (4). These men present with no previous history associated with fertility problems and have normal findings on physical examination and endocrine laboratory testing. Semen analysis often reveals a decreased number of spermatozoa (oligozoospermia), decreased motility (asthenozoospermia), and many abnormal forms (teratozoospermia) on morphological examination. These abnormalities usually occur together and are described as the oligoasthenoteratozoospermia (OAT) syndrome.

Unexplained forms of male infertility may be caused by several factors, such as chronic stress, endocrine disruption due to environmental pollution, reactive oxygen species, and genetic abnormalities.

PHYSICAL EXAMINATION

Physical examination should focus on signs of hypogonadism (gynecomastia, increased body fat, abnormal hair distribution, small testes), congenital abnormalities of the reproductive tract (absence of the vas deferens, epididymis tail or the testes, prostatic cysts, absence or hypoplasia of the seminal vesicles, hypospadia and epispadia, phimosis), and acquired abnormalities (epididymal congestion, varicocele, signs of male accessory gland infection) (Table 2).

Table 1 Male Infertility-Associated Factors and Percentage of Distribution in 10,469 Patients (4)

Infertility-associated factor (male)	Percentage of patients affected ($n = 10{,}469$)
Idiopathic male infertility	31
Maldescended testes	7.8
Urogenital infection	8.0
Disturbances of semen deposition and sexual factors	5.9
General and systemic disease	3.1
Varicocele	15.6
Hypogonadism	8.9
Immunological factors	4.5
Obstructions	1.7
Other abnormalities	5.5

A varicocele can be found in 25% of subfertile men (1). The diagnosis should be made with the patient in a standing position in a warm examination room, with and without Valsalva maneuver. The following classification of varicocele (4) is useful in clinical practice:

- Subclinical: Not palpable or visible at rest or during Valsalva maneuver, but demonstrable by special tests (reflux found upon Doppler examination or during scrotal ultrasound)
- Grade 1: Palpable during Valsalva maneuver but not otherwise

Table 2 Typical Findings from the Physical Examination That May Be Present in a Male Patient with Reduced Fertility

General

- Obesity (body mass index, waist circumference)
- Signs of hypermasculinity (anabolic steroids)
- Abnormality or absence of hair distribution
- Gynecomastia (Tanner stage)
- Stature (normal, eunuchoid, undervirilization)
- Signs of pulmonary disease

Penis/urethra

- Penile and urethral abnormalities (phimosis, meatal stenosis, hypospadia, epispadia, urethral fibrosis/stricture)

Scrotum

- Absence or atrophy of the testes
- Cryptorchidism
- Abnormal testicular volume and/or consistency
- Varicocele

Rectal examination (if indicated)

- Swelling and/or pain of the prostate and the seminal vesicles (prostatitis/vesiculitis)
- Urethral discharge after rectal examination (MAGI)

Table 3 The Following Findings are Indicative of Obstructive Azoospermia

- At least one testis is >15 mL in volume (although a smaller testicular volume may be found in some patients with obstructive azoospermia and concomitant partial testicular failure)
- Enlarged and hardened epididymis
- Nodules in the epididymis or vas deferens
- Absence or partial atresia of the vas
- Signs of male accessory gland infection
- Prostatic abnormalities

- Grade 2: Palpable at rest, but not visible
- Grade 3: Visible and palpable at rest

Men with obstructive azoospermia normally present with normal size testes and normal FSH. On examination, enlargement of the epididymis may be found. Sometimes, the vas deferens appears absent due to congenital factors or previous inguinal or scrotal surgery (Table 3). Although obstructions in primary infertile men are often present at the epididymal level, other sites of obstruction are the ejaculatory ducts and the distal vas deferens, which are not palpable on physical examination. In 25% of men with obstruction, no spermatozoa are found in the epididymis during scrotal exploration, indicating an intratesticular obstruction (5).

SEMEN ANALYSIS

Further examination is indicated if semen analysis shows abnormalities. Because semen analysis still forms the basis of important decisions concerning appropriate treatment, standardization of the complete laboratory workup is highly desirable. Ejaculate analysis has been standardized by the WHO and propagated by continuing work and publications in the *WHO Laboratory Manual for Human Semen and Sperm-Cervical Mucus Interaction* (5th edition) (6).

If values are normal according to WHO criteria, one test should suffice. Only if the results are abnormal, semen analysis should be repeated once more. It is important to distinguish between oligozoospermia (<20 million spermatozoa/mL), asthenozoospermia (<50% motile spermatozoa), and teratozoospermia (<14% normal forms). These three pathologies often occur simultaneously (OAT syndrome). In extreme cases of the OAT syndrome (<1 million spermatozoa/mL), just as with azoospermia, there is an increased incidence of obstruction of the male genital tract and genetic abnormalities (see chapter 4).

HORMONAL INVESTIGATION

Endocrine malfunctions are more prevalent in infertile men than in the general population, but are still quite uncommon (1). Hormonal screening can be limited to determining FSH, luteinizing hormone (LH), and testosterone levels. In men diagnosed with azoospermia, it is important to distinguish between obstructive and nonobstructive causes. A criterion with reasonable predictive value for obstruction is a normal FSH with bilaterally a normal testicular volume. However, 29% of men with a normal FSH appear to have defective spermatogenesis (see chapter 22).

MICROBIOLOGICAL ASSESSMENT

Indications for microbiological assessment include abnormal urine samples, urinary tract infections, male accessory gland infections (MAGI), and sexually transmitted diseases (STDs) (7). The clinical implications of white blood cells detected in a semen sample are as yet undetermined. However, in combination with a small ejaculate volume, this may point to an obstruction (partial) of the ejaculatory ducts caused by an infection (chronic) of the prostate or seminal vesicles. Genital infections, especially epididymitis, may instigate the production of spermatotoxic free oxygen radicals that can impair semen parameters (8). Gonorrhea and Chlamydia trachomatis can also cause obstruction of the genital tract (see chapter 32).

GENETIC EVALUATION

A substantial number of male fertility disorders that used to be described as idiopathic male infertility will, in fact, have a genetic origin. By taking an extensive family history and carrying out a genetic analysis, a number of these disorders can be detected. This will not only yield a diagnosis, but also allow for appropriate genetic counseling. The latter may be very important with the advent of ICSI, because the fertility disorder and possibly the corresponding genetic defect may be transferred to the offspring.

Chromosomal abnormalities are more common in men with extreme OAT and with azoospermia. The most common sex chromosome abnormality is Klinefelter's syndrome (47,XXY) that affects around 10% of men diagnosed with azoospermia. Klinefelter's syndrome is characterized by gynecomastia and hypergonadotropic hypogonadism. Occasionally, a eunuchoid phenotype is found and sometimes psychological disorders. Both testicles are very small and they present with tubular sclerosis. In around 60% of all patients, testosterone levels decrease with age requiring androgen replacement (9).

In men presenting with extremely poor quality semen, chromosome translocations and deletions can be found, which may be hereditary and which may cause habitual abortion and congenital malformations in the offspring. In cases of azoospermia or severe OAT, deletions in the azoospermic factor (AZF) region of the Y chromosome can occur and testing is advised (10).

In men with congenital bilateral absence of the vas deferens (CBAVD), mutations of the cystic fibrosis transmembrane regulator (CFTR) gene can be found. Apart from causing cystic fibrosis (CF), this gene is also associated with CBAVD; 85% of all males diagnosed with CBAVD also test positive for one or two CFTR gene mutations. In cases where the partner is a carrier of a CFTR mutation, depending on the mutation involved, there is a 25% chance of having a child with CF or CBAVD. Genetic counseling is recommended in these cases (11) (see chapter 5).

ULTRASONOGRAPHY

Scrotal ultrasound can be helpful in finding signs of obstruction and of testicular dysgenesis, such as an inhomogeneous parenchyma and microcalcifications (12). Color Doppler flow studies can assist in detecting varicoceles and signs of inflammation.

Ultrasound of the scrotum is best performed with a linear high-resolution, high-frequency small parts transducer of 7.5–13 MHz (13). Most abnormalities can be visualized with gray-scale imaging, but adding color Doppler can be very helpful in case of inflammations and to detect a varicocele. A normal testis has a homogeneous parenchyma with a hyperechoic thin capsule, the tunica albuginea. The adult testis measures 35 to 50 mm in length (L), 25 to 35 mm in width (W), and 15 to 25 mm in height (H). The volume (V) of the testis is calculated by the formula $V = L \times W \times H \times 0.52$ (13). The epididymis can be visualized at the upper and posterior side of the testis. The caput epididymis has a maximum size of 10 to 12 mm and may show small cysts in 70% of cases. The body and the tail of the epididymis measure 5 to 7 mm and usually have a homogeneous aspect.

Frequent scrotal ultrasonography abnormalities found in infertile men are highlighted in Table 4.

Testicular tumors can be found in 0.5% to 1% of infertile males, and testicular microcalcifications are detected in around 5% of infertile males (14). Microcalcifications are defined as at least 20 calcifications per testis and are more often found in men with an inhomogeneous parenchyma, characteristic of testicular dysgenesis. Carcinoma in situ (CIS) is found in 20%

Table 4 Frequent Scrotal Ultrasonography Abnormalities Found in Infertile Men

Abnormalities of the testis
Small size
Inhomogeneous parenchyma (dysgenesis)
Testicular cysts
Microcalcifications (5%) (Fig. 1)
Dilatation of the rete testis (Fig. 2)
Intratesticular varicocele
Inflammation (orchitis) (Fig. 3)
Tumors (0.5–1%)
Hypoechoic lesions (Fig. 4)
Abnormalities of the epididymis
Dilatation (Fig. 5)
Epididymal cysts/spermatocele
Inflammation (epididymitis)
Other abnormalities
Varicocele (Fig. 6)
Absence of the vas deferens

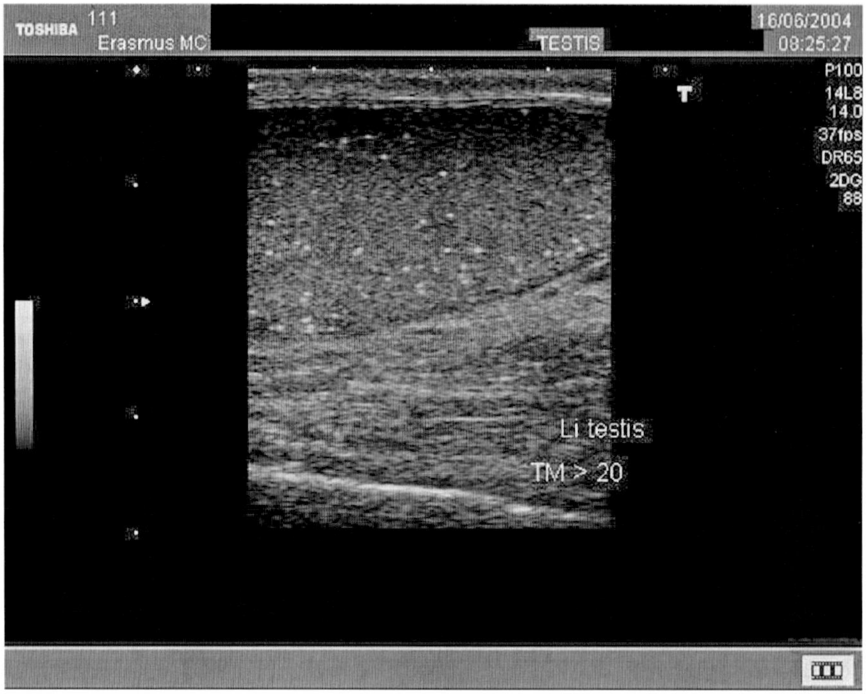

Figure 1 Testicular microcalcifications.

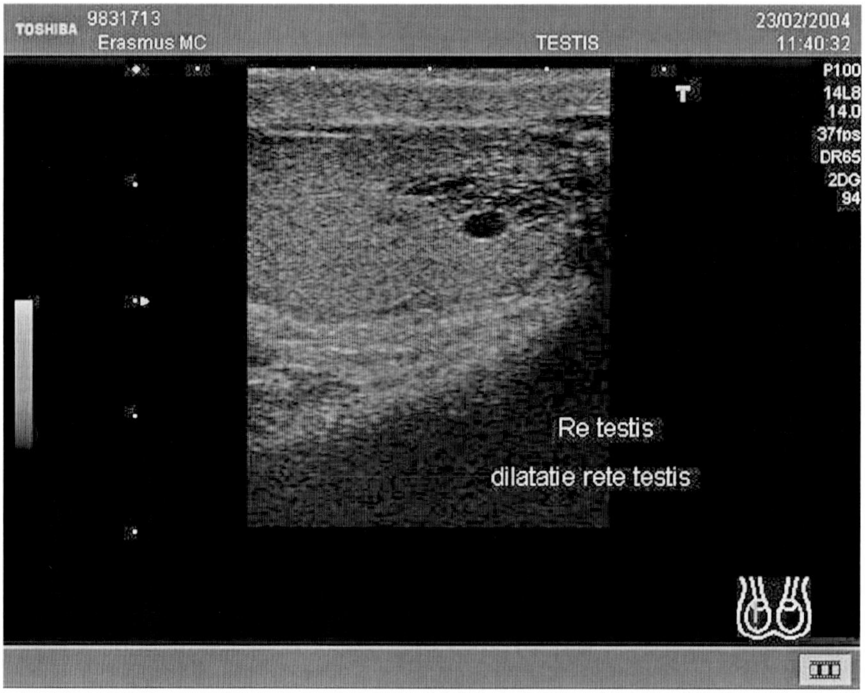

Figure 2 Dilatation of the rete testis.

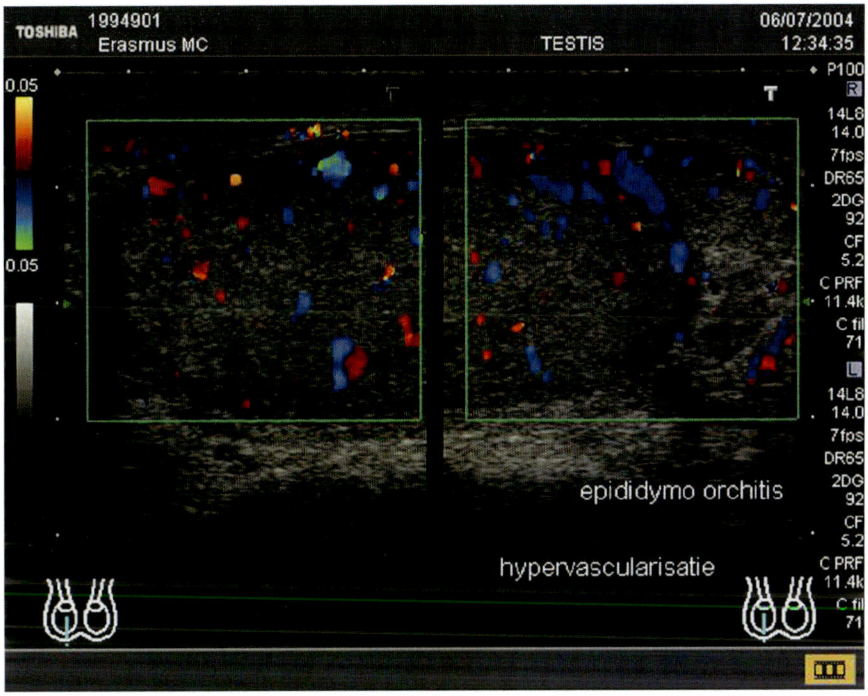

Figure 3 Epididymo-orchitis. There is an increased diameter of the epididymal caput and increased flow in the testis and epididymis.

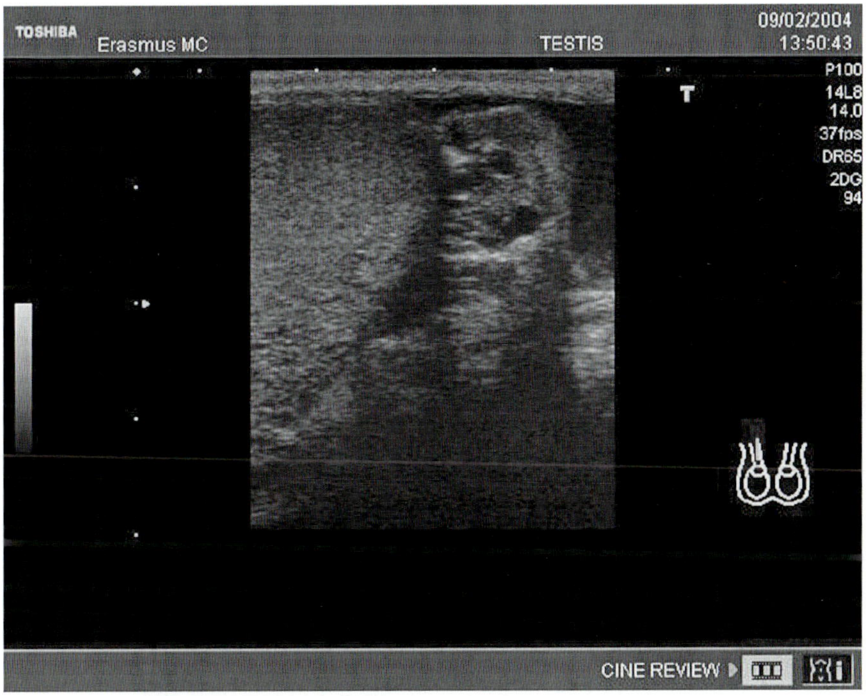

Figure 4 Cystic enlargement of the epididymal caput.

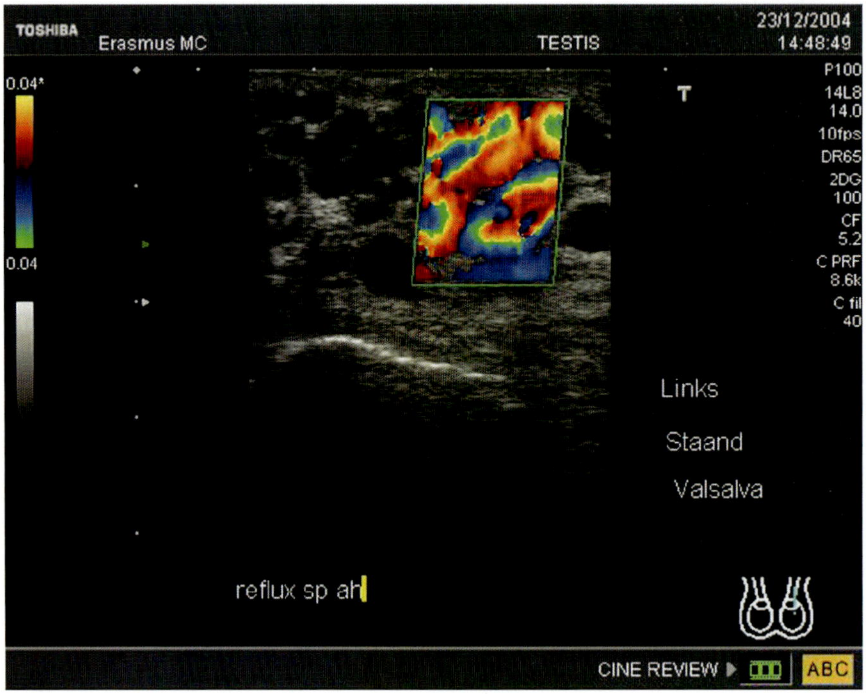

Figure 5 Varicocele/increased diameter of a scrotal vein.

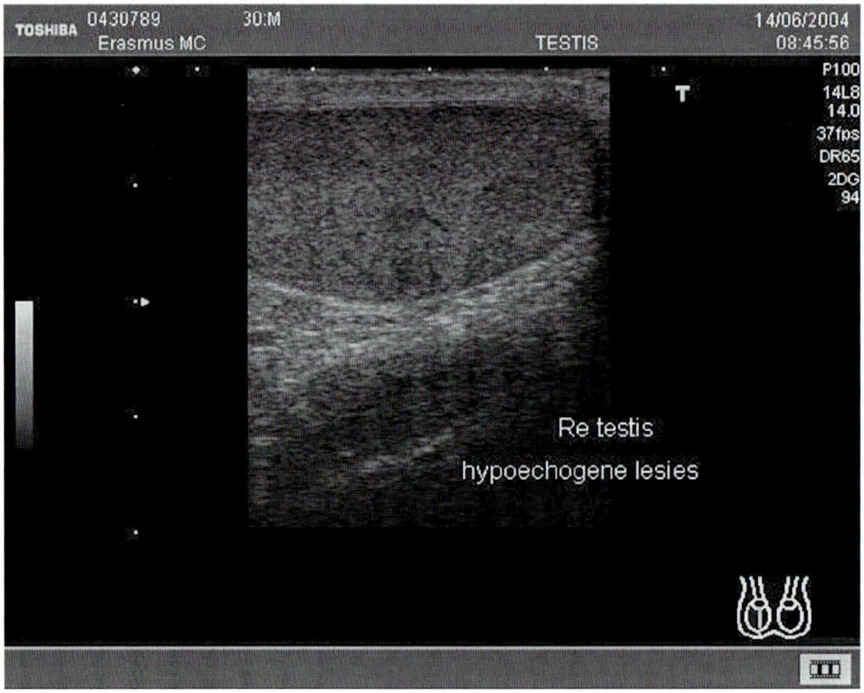

Figure 6 Hypoechoic lesion of the testis.

of such testis, especially if the microcalcifications are found bilaterally (15). CIS is found preferentially in men with a history of infertility, cryptorchidism, testicular tumor, and in atrophic testis (16).

Colour Doppler ultrasound of the scrotum can detect a varicocele in around 20% to 30% of infertile males (17). This part of the investigation should also be performed in a standing position. Accepted ultrasound criteria for the diagnosis of a varicocele is a venous diameter >3 mm with or without Valsalva maneuver, an increase of venous diameter during Valsalva maneuver, and venous blood flow reversal (reflux) for >2 seconds.

On the basis of the amount of reflux present, varicoceles can be graded as follows:

- Grade I, slight reflux (<2 seconds) during Valsalva
- Grade II, reflux (>2 seconds) during Valsalva, but no continuous reflux during the maneuver
- Grade III, reflux at rest during normal respiration or continuously during the entire Valsalva maneuver

Transrectal ultrasound (TRUS) of the prostate and the seminal vesicles is indicated in patients with a low seminal volume and in men with a history of male accessory gland infection. TRUS should be performed at high resolution and with high-frequency (7 MHz) biplane transducers. Seminal vesicle enlargement (anterior-posterior diameter 15 mm) and roundish, anechoic areas in the seminal vesicle are TRUS anomalies more often associated with ejaculatory duct obstruction, especially when semen volume is <1.5 cm^3. Other known anomalies in cases of obstructive azoospermia are Müllerian duct cysts or urogenital sinus/ejaculatory duct cysts and ejaculatory duct calcifications. TRUS may also be applied to aspirate seminal vesicle fluid in case of ejaculatory duct obstruction (18,19).

TESTICULAR BIOPSY

A diagnostic testicular biopsy is indicated in patients without evident factors (normal FSH and normal testicular volume) to differentiate between obstructive and nonobstructive azoospermia (NOA) (4). It is recommended to cryopreserve sperm if present in the biopsy for future ICSI.

Testicular biopsy is usually performed as part of a therapeutic process in patients with clinical evidence of NOA who decide to undergo ICSI. About 50% to 60% of men with NOA have some seminiferous tubules with spermatozoa that can be cryopreserved and used for ICSI. Many authors find a good

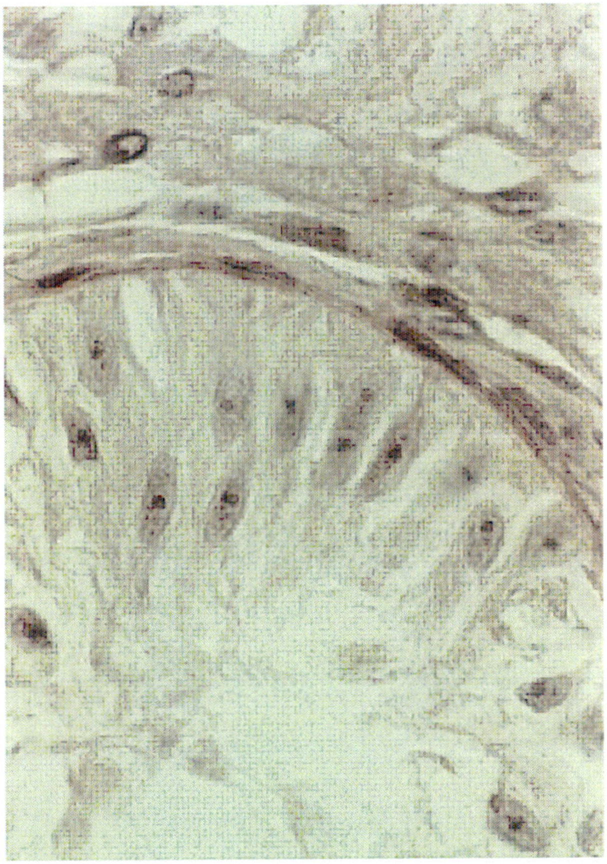

Figure 7 Sertoli cell only syndrome.

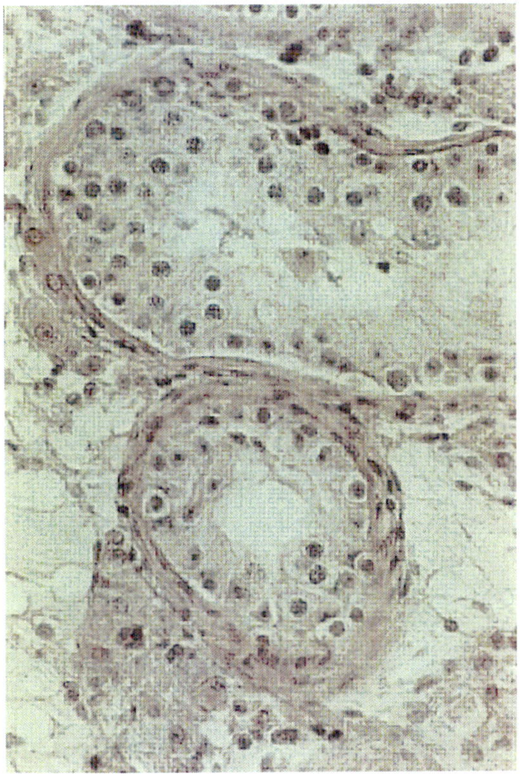

Figure 8 Maturation arrest.

correlation between diagnostic biopsy histology and the likelihood of finding mature spermatozoa during testicular sperm extraction (TESE) (20). Finally, a testicular biopsy is indicated for the diagnosis of CIS (21).

All too frequently in clinical practice, the value of testicular biopsy is diminished as a result of poor biopsy specimen handling and poor interpretation of samples by pathologists, not thoroughly familiar with the reproductive tract histology. A standardized approach of the fixation and staining procedure of the biopsy and the classification of the specimen is needed (22,23).

The four main pathological classifications are:

- Absence of seminiferous tubules (tubular sclerosis)
- Presence of Sertoli cells only (Sertoli cell-only syndrome) (Fig. 7)
- Maturation arrest—incomplete spermatogenesis, not beyond the spermatocyte stage (Fig. 8)
- Hypospermatogenesis—all cell types up to spermatozoa are present, but there is a distinct decline in the number of reproducing spermatogonia (Fig. 9)

Table 5 Scoring System for Testicular Biopsies (Johnsen Score) (24)

Score	Histological criteria
10	Full spermatogenesis (Fig. 10)
9	Slightly impaired spermatogenesis, many late spermatids, disorganized epithelium
8	Less than five spermatozoa per tubule, few late spermatids
7	No spermatozoa, no late spermatids, many early spermatids
6	No spermatozoa, no late spermatids, few early spermatids
5	No spermatozoa or spermatids, many spermatocytes
4	No spermatozoa or spermatids, few spermatocytes
3	Spermatogonia only
2	No germinal cells, Sertoli cells only
1	No seminiferous epithelium

A more quantitative histological grading is the Johnsen scoring system; in at least 100 seminiferous tubules the level of sperm maturation is determined (24). The total Johnsen score is determined by dividing the total score by the number of tubules (Table 5).

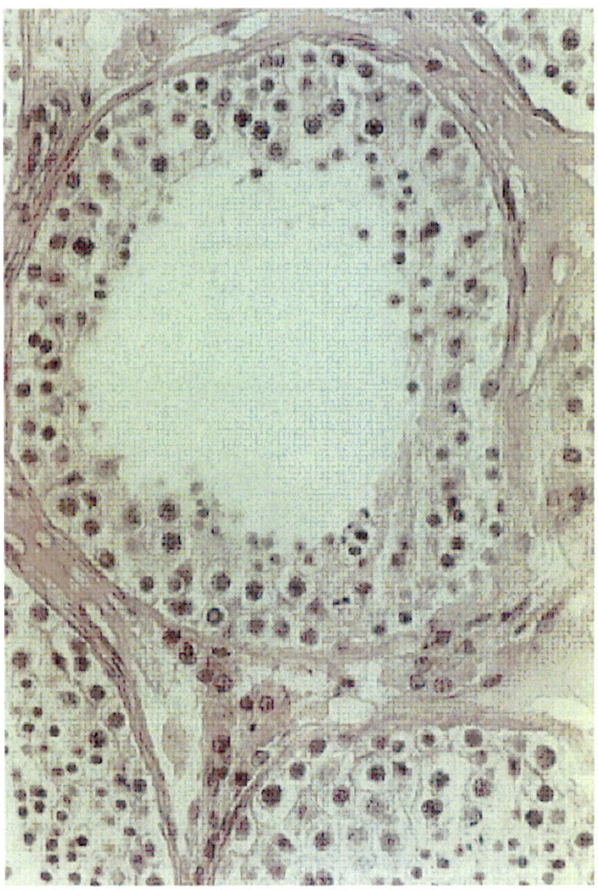

Figure 9 Hypospermatogenesis.

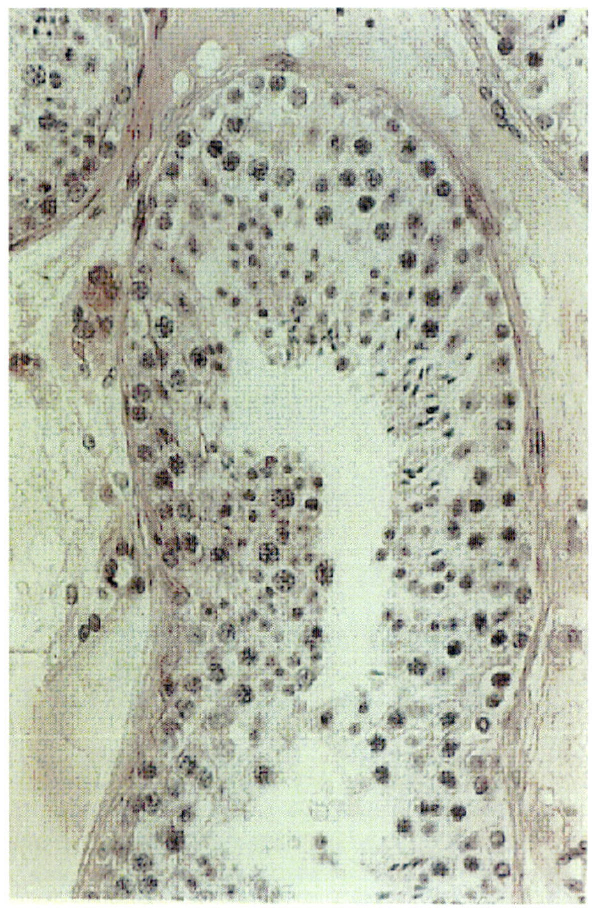

Figure 10 Normal spermatogenesis.

Testicular biopsy is important in the evaluation of men at risk of CIS or testicular cancer, such as those with idiopathic infertility, prior cryptorchidism, a history of testicular neoplasia, and in case of features on ultrasound suggestive for CIS, like an identified lesion or microcalcifications (25).

CASE DISCUSSION

On the basis of the fertility investigations, the male is diagnosed with primary infertility due to testicular insufficiency (small testis, high FSH). The findings on ultrasound in the atrophic right testis need further evaluation to exclude CIS; a testicular biopsy is indicated. The varicocele can be considered an infertility-associated factor. Although, there is a chance of a substantial sperm improvement of 40% to 50% after varicocele treatment, there is uncertainty in the literature if varicocele repair will also increase the chance of conception (26). Alternatively, the couple can be candidates for assisted reproduction such as IVF. Genetic evaluation is indicated before assisted reproduction is performed.

REFERENCES

1. World Health Organization. WHO Manual for the Standardised Investigation and Diagnosis of the Infertile Couple. Cambridge, UK: Cambridge University Press, 2000.
2. Te Velde ER, Eijkemans R, Habbema HD. Variation in couple fecundity and time to pregnancy, an essential concept in human reproduction. Lancet. 2000 Jun 3; 355(9219):1928–1929.
3. Rowe T. Fertility and a woman's age. J Reprod Med 2006:; 51(3):157–163.
4. Nieschlag E. Classification of andrological disorders. In: Nieschlag E, Behre HM, eds. Andrology: Male Reproductive Health and Dysfunction, 2nd ed. Berlin: Springer Verlag, 2000:83–87.
5. Dohle GR, Colpi GM, Hargreave TB, et al. The EAU Working Group on Male Infertility. EAU guidelines on male infertility. Eur Urol 2005; 48(5):703–711.
6. World Health Organization. WHO Laboratory Manual for the Examination of Human Semen and Sperm-Cervical Mucus Interaction. 5th edn. Cambridge: Cambridge University Press, 2010.
7. Weidner W, Krause W, Ludwig M. Relevance of male accessory gland infection for subsequent fertility with special focus on prostatitis. Hum Reprod Update 1999; 5(5):421–432.
8. Vicari E. Effectiveness and limits of antimicrobial treatments on seminal leucocyte concentration and related reactive oxygen species production in patients with male accessory gland infection. Hum Reprod 2000; 15(12):2536–2544.
9. Lanfranco F, Kamischke A, Zitzmann M, et al. Klinefelter's syndrome. Lancet 2004;364(9430):273–283.
10. Krausz C, Giachini C. Genetic risk factors in male infertility. Arch Androl 2007; 53(3):125–133.
11. Lipshultz LI, Lamb DJ. Risk of transmission of genetic diseases by assisted reproduction. Nat Clin Pract Urol 2007; 4(9):460–461.
12. Skakkebaek NE, Rajpert-De Meyts E, Main KM. Testicular dysgenesis syndrome: an increasingly common development disorder with environmental aspects. Hum Reprod 2001; 16:972–978.
13. Oyen RH. Scrotal ultrasound. Eur Radiol 2002; 12:19–34.
14. Pierik FH, Dohle GR, van Muiswinkel JM, et al. Is routine scrotal ultrasound advantageous in infertile men? J Urol 1999; 162(5):1618–1620.
15. De Gouveia Brazao CA, Pierik FH, Oosterhuis JW, et al. Bilateral testicular microlithiasis predicts the presence of the precursor of testicular germ cell tumors in subfertile men. J Urol 2004; 171:158–160.
16. Holm M, Hoei-Hansen CE, Rajpert-De Meyts E, et al. Increased risk of carcinoma in situ in patients with testicular germ cell cancer with ultrasonic microlithiasis in the contralateral testicle. J Urol 2003; 170:1163–1167.
17. Hoekstra T, Witt MA. The correlation of internal spermatic vein palpability with ultrasonographic diameter and reversal of venous flow. J Urol 1995; 153:82–84.
18. Jarow JP. Transrectal ultrasonography in the diagnosis and management of ejaculatory duct obstruction. J Androl 1996; 17:467–472.
19. Meacham RB, Hellerstein DK, Lipshultz LI. Evaluation and treatment of ejaculatory duct obstruction in the infertile male. Fertil Steril 1993; 59(2):393–397.
20. Tournaye H, Verheyen G, Nagy P, et al. Are there any predictive factors for successful testicular sperm recovery in azoospermic patients? Hum Reprod 1997; 12: 80–86.
21. Giwercman A, Bruun E, Frimodt-Moller C, et al. Prevalence of carcinoma in situ and other histopathological abnormalities in testes of men with a history of cryptorchidism. J Urol 1989; 142(4):998–1001.
22. McLachlan RI, Rajpert-De Meyts E, Hoei-Hansen CE, et al. Histological evaluation of the human testis–approaches to optimizing the clinical value of the assessment: mini review. Hum Reprod 2007; 22(1):2–16.
23. Cooperberg MR, Chi T, Jad A, Cha I, Turek PJ. Variability in testis biopsy interpretation: implications for male infertility care in the era of intracytoplasmic sperm injection. Fertil Steril 2005 84:672–677
24. Johnsen SG. Testicular biopsy score count – a method for registration of spermatogenesis in human testes: normal values and results in 335 hypogonadal males. Hormones 1970; 1(1):2–25.
25. Dieckmann KP, Pichlmeier U. Clinical epidemiology of testicular germ cell tumors. World J Urol 2004; 22:2–14.
26. Evers JL, Collins JA. Surgery or embolisation for varicocele in subfertile men. Cochrane Database Syst Rev 2004; (3):CD000479.

3 The female factor

Lynne Robinson and Masoud Afnan

INTRODUCTION

One in seven couples in the UK seek medical help for infertility, and of these, about half will require treatment with assisted conception. The increase in infertility rates in recent years is most likely because of a combination of factors including many women delaying the age at which they start trying for a family, declining sperm counts, and a rise in the incidence of sexually transmitted diseases such as chlamydia. The number of first-time mothers less than 25 years has halved over the last 20 years while it has trebled in those over 35 years. Approximately 30% of couples suffer from female factor infertility, the remainder being due to male factors or unexplained. However, of those that are unexplained, an increasing proportion is likely to be because of decreasing oocyte quality and ovarian reserve in older women. The current trend of increasing subfertility rates is also linked with obesity, leading to polycystic ovarian syndrome (PCOS) and hence anovulatory subfertility.

CASE HISTORY 1

A 36-year-old woman and a 40-year-old man attend the infertility clinic. They have been trying for three years for a baby. They both smoke and drink 20 units of alcohol per week. The semen analysis is normal. The woman has regular menstrual cycles and has been shown to ovulate. She is of normal weight. A hysterosalpingogram (HSG) has shown a normal uterine cavity and patent tubes. There is no significant medical history in either partner.

What advice would you give?
What investigations would you carry out?
What treatment options would you consider?
What are their chances of getting pregnant?

CASE HISTORY 2

A 40-year-old man and a 35-year-old woman wish to have children. The man had a vasectomy five years ago and is considering a vasectomy reversal. The woman had an HSG and was found to have bilateral cystic hydrosalpinges.

What is the best treatment option for this couple and what must be done before they are treated?

CASE HISTORY 3

A 40-year-old man and a 28-year-old woman want to have children. Semen analysis is normal. The woman has irregular menstrual cycles, a body mass index (BMI) of 32, and complains of hirsutism. Tubal patency testing is normal.

What is the likely diagnosis?
What investigations might be carried out?
Describe the treatment plan for this couple.
Are there any particular considerations that the couple should be aware of?

PRECONCEPTUAL ADVICE

At the subfertility clinic we have the perfect opportunity to ensure patients have up-to-date preconceptual advice. It is important to check rubella immunity because infection with the virus carries a high teratogenic risk, resulting in multiple congenital abnormalities or miscarriage (1). Cervical screening should be offered in line with the National Cervical Screening Programme guidance because any treatment necessary should be performed prior to pregnancy.

Periconceptual folic acid supplementation has been shown to reduce the incidence of neural tube defects in children (2). The recommendations are to take 400 μg of folic acid daily for at least 12 weeks preconceptually and for the first 12 weeks of pregnancy. For those who have previously had an infant with a neural tube defect, are diabetic, who suffer from celiac disease or sickle cell disease or thalassemia, or who are receiving antiepileptic medication, a higher dose of 5 mg per day is recommended.

Many complementary therapies are used by patients in the hope of increasing the chances of conceiving but these can be expensive and the effectiveness of these therapies have not been properly evaluated in clinical trials. Further research needs to be carried out before such therapies can be recommended (3).

As smoking has increased among women in recent years it is of increasing importance to counsel patients regarding it. There is a significant association between smoking and reduced fertility among female smokers (4) and passive smoking is associated with delayed conception (5). For those who achieve pregnancy there are increased risks of small for gestational age infants, stillbirth, and infant mortality (6,7). Smokers should be given advice and offered to be referred to a smoking cessation service.

The evidence for harm to the fetus during pregnancy and preconceptually with low levels of alcohol is inconsistent, although, it is known that high levels of alcohol intake can harm the unborn baby and in extreme cases cause fetal alcohol syndrome. It is recommended that women who are pregnant or trying to become pregnant restrict their alcohol intake to one to two units of alcohol once or twice per week and avoid binge drinking (8,9).

Women often worry about the effect caffeine may have on their fertility and on the fetus. However, there is no consistent evidence regarding a link between caffeine intake and infertility in women (3).

Obesity is fast becoming one of the biggest health problems in Western society, with 56% of women in the UK being either overweight or obese. BMI is the standard way we assess weight, and a BMI between 19 to 24.9 kg/m^2 is considered to be normal, although waist circumference as a marker of visceral fat mass is now thought to be a better predictor of insulin resistance. Obesity can have a profound effect on fertility. An increase in waist circumference (waist:hip ratio >0.85) and a BMI of >30 kg/m^2 has been shown to halve spontaneous conception rates in women who are ovulating (10). At least 40% of women with PCOS are obese and studies have shown that a modest reduction in weight can improve insulin resistance and restore ovulation (11). Obesity also increases the risk of spontaneous miscarriage and obese women do not respond well to drugs for ovulation induction. There are also increased risks with procedures such as laparoscopy and also technical difficulties with monitoring patients via ultrasound scan (USS). In pregnancy, there is an increased risk of hypertension, gestational diabetes, congenital anomalies, macrosomia, stillbirth, cesarean section, and perinatal death (10). It is therefore vital that patients are given dietary advice along with an exercise regimen and psychological support preconceptually. Weight-reducing drugs and bariatric surgery may be recommended. National guidelines for publicly funded treatment in the UK advise that women are not commenced on ovarian stimulation drugs until their BMI is <30 kg/m^2 (3).

FACTORS FOR INFERTILITY

Anovulation

Anovulation and oligo-ovulation are responsible for approximately 21% of female infertility (12). The World Health Organization (WHO) classifies this into three groups:

Group 1: Hypothalamic pituitary failure. This group accounts for 10% of ovulatory disorders and includes those with hypothalamic amenorrhea, anorexia nervosa, or exercise/weight loss–related amenorrhea. It also includes destruction of the anterior pituitary by a tumor (e.g., craniopharyngioma) or by infarction as in Sheehan's syndrome. Rare causes such as tuberculosis (TB) and irradiation also destroy the gland. Congenital conditions causing hypopituitarism include Kallmann's syndrome, Prader–Willi syndrome, and Laurence–Moon–Biedl syndrome. These patients have estrogen levels in the postmenopausal range, with normal-to-low follicle stimulating hormone (FSH) levels and normal prolactin (PRL) levels.

Those patients with hyperprolactinemia will also have low estrogen levels. Very high levels of prolactin may be caused by a prolactinoma. The symptoms from this may be oligomenorrhea, amenorrhea, galactorrhea, headaches, and visual field disturbances.

Group 2: This group includes patients with normal estrogen levels and normal FSH levels and accounts for 85% of ovulatory disorders. PCOS is included in this group and is thought to affect 6% to 7% of the general population (13). Approximately 80% of those with oligomenorrhea and 30% of those with amenorrhea have polycystic ovaries (14). Women with PCOS often suffer from weight gain, acne, hirsutism, and male pattern alopecia. The Rotterdam Criteria for the diagnosis of PCOS requires two out of the following three criteria (15,16):

1. Oligo-ovulation and/or anovulation
2. Clinical or biochemical evidence of hyperandrogenism
3. Ultrasound evidence of polycystic ovaries (at least 12 follicles 2–9 mm diameter or ovarian volume greater than 10 cm^3)

The biochemical abnormalities associated with the clinical picture include hypersecretion of luteinizing hormone (LH), hyperandrogenism, acyclic estrogen production, subnormal sex hormone binding globulin (SHBG) levels, and hyperinsulinemia. PCOS sufferers are at increased risk of developing type 2 diabetes and this risk is independent of obesity. It has also been suggested that these women may be at higher risk of cardiovascular disease although at present there is little direct evidence for this (13). Although women with PCOS have no increased risk of cervical or ovarian cancer, they are at risk of endometrial hyperplasia and cancer due to anovulation.

Group 3: The third group exhibits hypergonadotropic hypogonadism. These patients have elevated FSH and postmenopausal estrogen levels, including patients with premature ovarian failure and accounts for 4% to 5% of ovulatory disorders.

Age

Many women now choose to delay starting their families until their late thirties or beyond, and in the United States one in five women now have their first baby over the age of 35. While this may be more convenient with regard to developing a career, it may make conceiving more problematic. The probability of conceiving decreases by 3% to 5% every year after the age of 30 and the decline becomes more rapid after the age of 35. By the age of 40, 33% of couples are infertile.

The most important factor contributing to age-linked infertility is the aging ovum. At birth, each woman has about one million eggs but by menarche only about 400,000 eggs are available for fertilization. By the time menopause arrives, most women only have a few hundred eggs left in their ovaries. The quality of the eggs also declines with age, which also impacts on embryo quality and therefore decreases the success rate of in vitro fertilization (IVF). For those over 40, the success rate of IVF per cycle is only around 10% (17).

As women get older, their menstrual cycle often becomes more erratic and they become oligo-ovulatory or anovulatory. This obviously has an impact on conception, along with the endometrium becoming less receptive to implantation. Female age is a predictor of implantation as demonstrated by one study, which showed an intracytoplasmic sperm injection (ICSI) implantation rate of 25% in women with a mean age of 31 compared with 8.5% in a cohort of women aged 41 (18).

At the age of 20, a woman's risk of miscarriage is only 5% to 10%. By the age of 30 this increases to 20% and a 40- to 45-year old has a one in two risk of miscarrying. This is most likely due to chromosomal abnormalities in the embryo. The risk of trisomy 21 for a woman at the age of 40 is 1 in 100 compared with 1 in 1200 in her twenties.

If a woman is successful in conceiving later in life and the pregnancy is viable then there also are added risks during the pregnancy. Older mothers are more likely to develop pre-eclampsia and gestational diabetes. They are also more likely to have placental insufficiency, which leads to intrauterine growth retardation and are twice as likely to have a stillbirth. Other risks include premature delivery, placenta previa, and an increased chance of cesarean section.

Tubal Disease

Tubal disease is responsible for 20% to 25% of all cases of infertility. The most frequent cause of tubal damage is pelvic inflammatory disease (PID) and in approximately 70% of all cases of tubal infertility chlamydia is recognized as being the cause. There may be a history of pelvic pain, vaginal discharge, and dyspareunia but very often the infection is symptomless and only diagnosed on routine screening using urine testing or endocervical swabs. N. gonorrhea and tuberculosis are other rarer causes.

Pelvic endometriosis is another leading cause of tubal blockage. Endometriosis is seen in 10% to 15% of women undergoing diagnostic laparoscopy and 20% to 30% of subfertile women. A woman who has a mother or sister with endometriosis is six times more likely to develop endometriosis than a woman without this family history. The symptoms linked with the disease are pelvic pain, dysmenorrhea, deep dyspareunia, and occasionally dyschezia. Severe endometriosis (stage III–IV) is responsible for physical damage to the tubes; adhesion formation and endometriomas may also be present. However, even women with only stage I or II disease can suffer fertility problems, with an apparent halving of conception rates in spontaneous and artificial insemination treatment cycles (19).

Previous pelvic or abdominal surgery is another risk factor for tubal damage. This is particularly true if there has been previous peritonitis or a pelvic abscess. Another special group of patients with tubal blockage are those women previously sterilized. Success rates for reversal of sterilization (isthmo-isthmic anastomosis) can be as high as 80%.

Most tubal obstruction is due to distal tubal blockage and this is most likely due to PID. However, 10% to 15% of tubal obstruction is due to proximal tubal blockage (PTB) and the etiology of this may be very different. Salpingitis isthmica nodosa (SIN) can cause nodular occlusion, transluminal fibrosis may be present, or endometriotic nodules can cause obstruction. Mucus plugs or spasm of the tube may also be responsible for apparent obstruction (20). In fact, in 60% of resected proximal tubes no anatomical abnormality was detected (21). For this reason, selective tubal catheterization is recommended for the diagnosis and treatment for PTB.

Distal disease, especially hydrosalpinges is important to treat, either by salpingectomy or occlusion, prior to IVF or ICSI, as it halves the success rate of IVF (22), presumably due to the toxic effects of the fluid which communicate with the endometrial cavity.

Uterine Disease

Congenital uterine anomalies occur in between 1:200 to 1:600 women but many may go unnoticed. Uterine malformations from Müllerian duct defects are the most common of the female reproductive tract anomalies and most are related to polygenic and familial factors. The Müllerian ducts are bilateral structures that eventually fuse in their caudal portion to give rise to the uterus, cervix, and upper portion of the vagina. If fusion fails this can then give rise to various degrees of congenital abnormalities. These can range from a small partial septum in the uterus to a didelphic uterus where there are two completely separate horns and cervices present. In Rokitansky–Küster–Hauser (RKH) syndrome there is complete absence of the uterus, vagina, and cervix. This differs from testicular feminization because in RKH syndrome the karyotype is XX and that of testicular feminization is XY. Therefore patients with RKH have normal ovaries and those with testicular feminization have intra-abdominal testes, which require removal because of the high risk of testicular cancer. The teratogenic exposure to substances such as diethylstilbestrol (DES) in the past has also been linked with uterine abnormalities.

These abnormalities are generally symptomless until puberty, when outflow obstruction may present as amenorrhea with cyclical pain. This is usually due to the septum blocking menstrual flow causing a hematometra. However, most abnormalities will not be diagnosed until the woman presents with fertility problems, often recurrent miscarriage. A transvaginal ultrasound scan (TVUSS) may identify the congenital abnormality but an HSG or magnetic resonance imaging (MRI) is more accurate. As the renal system develops from the metanephric duct, renal anomalies can also occur and should be investigated in these patients.

Intrauterine adhesions or synechiae is an acquired uterine condition, also known as Asherman's Syndrome. Adhesions may only occur in a portion of the uterus, but in severe cases the anterior and posterior walls of the uterus may be stuck together. In 90% of cases the etiology is previous curettage causing damaged areas to stick together (23), especially in the presence of infection. However, rarely adhesions may be related to a previous cesarean section, polypectomy, or hysteroscopic resection of fibroid. Other rare causes are infections such as genital TB and schistosomiasis. Diagnosis is usually via hysteroscopy. Treatment of the condition is difficult and may involve hysteroscopic resection of the adhesions. However, adhesions can re-form, so estrogen can be used to encourage endometrial regeneration and a coil can be placed in the uterine cavity in the postoperative phase to help prevent apposition of the uterine walls (24).

Recurrent Miscarriage

Recurrent miscarriage is defined as the loss of three or more consecutive pregnancies and affects 1% of all women (25). Independent risk factors for this are age and the previous number of miscarriages. Other risk factors mentioned previously are PCOS and uterine anomalies. Genetic factors may be significant because in 3% to 5% of couples with recurrent miscarriage, at least one of the partners is a carrier of a balanced chromosomal anomaly (26).

Cervical incompetence is associated with painless cervical dilatation and mid-trimester miscarriages. Cone biopsies can increase the risk of this, but loop excisions are thought to pose much less of a risk unless they are repeated. With regard to infection, bacterial vaginosis (BV) is thought to increase the risk of second trimester miscarriages but a link with early miscarriages is unclear. A Cochrane review showed that screening and treating patients for BV may reduce preterm births and low birth weights (27).

Antiphospholipid syndrome (APS) is a condition diagnosed when antiphospholipid antibodies (aPL) are present and there has been an adverse pregnancy outcome or a vascular thrombosis. The most clinically important aPL are the lupus anticoagulant (LA) and the anticardiolipin antibodies (aCL). Approximately 15% of women with recurrent miscarriage are positive for either LA or aCL (28), and APS is now the most treatable cause of recurrent miscarriage. It seems likely that the APS affects trophoblast invasion and placentation, and also has an association with early onset pre-eclampsia and intrauterine growth restriction (IUGR) (29).

For a large proportion of couples with recurrent miscarriage, the cause will remain unexplained. These couples should not be treated empirically, but reassured that they have a 75% chance of having a successful pregnancy (30).

ASSESSING THE FEMALE

History Taking

Age

One of the most important aspects to take into consideration in history taking is age. As discussed previously, as a woman grows older so do her oocytes and their quality and quantity decline, making conceiving a more lengthy and difficult process. The average time to conception for women over 35 years is one to two years compared with 96% of couples who are under the age of 25 and who conceive within one year.

Menstrual History

Menstrual irregularity and any primary amenorrhea or secondary amenorrhea indicates anovulation and an increasingly short cycle may indicate a low ovarian reserve. A recent study found that the chance of delivery after IVF/ICSI was almost doubled for women with a cycle length >34 days compared with women with a menstrual cycle length <26 days (31). If amenorrhea is reported, pregnancy should be excluded and menopausal symptoms, weight loss or gain, and symptoms of hyperprolactinemia and hypothyroidism enquired about.

Sexual History

The frequency of sexual intercourse should be enquired about as well as the timing of intercourse around ovulation. However, the recommendations are now to have regular intercourse throughout the cycle rather than timed intercourse (3). An accurate smear history needs to be taken and any postcoital or intermenstrual bleeding identified. This may also indicate infection along with any symptoms such as pelvic pain, dyspareunia, and vaginal discharge.

Obstetric History

Previous pregnancies and their outcome need to be enquired about as well as any problems encountered during the pregnancies. It is important also to ask about pregnancies with a different partner. Any difficulties achieving a pregnancy or previous fertility treatments should be discussed (32).

Duration of Infertility

Duration of infertility is very relevant. It is clear from several studies that the duration of infertility is negatively correlated with the chance to conceive spontaneously (12,33) or by infertility treatment (32,34). *The chances of conceiving spontaneously remain high for three years and then decline by 25% per year and this has an impact on the treatment strategies (35).*

Contraception

Most contraceptives will allow for resumption of fertility immediately upon removal or withdrawal. These include intrauterine contraceptive devices (IUCD), the Mirena intrauterine system (IUS), Implanon, and the progesterone-only pill. Long acting injectable progestogens can delay the return of ovulation for a mean time of 5.3 months following the last injection but the delay may last 12 months or more. Although it is often thought women may suffer from post-pill amenorrhea after stopping the combined oral contraceptive pill (COCP), post-pill amenorrhea does not exist as a side effect of pills and warrants investigations as it can be due to any of the causes of secondary amenorrhea. IUDs (but not IUS) are associated with the risk of pelvic infection in 1% cases, which can lead to tubal disease and may reduce the chances of conception if severe. Complications usually occur within one month of insertion or removal of the IUCD.

Medical History

It is important to enquire about any previous medical disorders that may interfere with either fertility or pregnancy. Conditions such as heart disease or cancer may throw up an ethical dilemma regarding fertility treatment, considering the patient may have a high risk of maternal morbidity or mortality during a pregnancy. A careful drug history should be taken as some drugs will be teratogenic in pregnancy. Some medications may affect conception such as selective serotonin reuptake inhibitors (SSRIs) that cause hyperprolactinemia and nonsteroidal anti-inflammatory drugs (NSAIDs) can inhibit ovulation.

A family history should be taken because any familial condition may require genetic counseling prior to investigation and treatment, and preimplantation genetic diagnosis (PGD) may be required.

Examination of the Female Partner

One of the most important parts of assessing the female is calculation of the BMI and possibly the waist:hip ratio because being obese and underweight can both lead to anovulation. Any history of pelvic pain, dyspareunia, or suggestion of a pelvic mass should prompt a pelvic examination. Women with symptoms of hyperandrogenism should be examined for hirsutism and acne.

INVESTIGATIONS FOR THE FEMALE

Assessment of ovulation is done using a mid-luteal phase progesterone level. This should be timed seven days before the expected onset of the next menstrual cycle. In cases of amenorrhea or oligomenorrhea, FSH, LH, testosterone, SHBG, free androgen index, prolactin levels should be measured and thyroid function tests (TFTs) carried out (see Table 1). In women with a regular cycle, a day 3 FSH is useful to assess *ovarian reserve*. Anti-Müllerian hormone (AMH) is one of the best hormone markers to assess the quantitative aspect of ovarian reserve or dysfunction (36) and can be done at any time during the cycle, even while the woman is on the combined contraceptive pill. AMH levels correlate with the number of antral follicles. Women with lower AMH and antral follicle count (AFC) produce a significantly lower number of oocytes compared to women with higher levels.

Table 1 Evidence Levels for Investigations and Treatment Strategies

Key points	Evidence levels
Preconceptual advice	
Weight loss if BMI >30	1b
Stop smoking/decrease alcohol	2b
Check rubella, update smear	3
Folic acid supplement	1a
Ovulation assessment	
Regular cycles—check mid-luteal progesterone	2b
Irregular cycles—check prolactin, thyroid function, testosterone, LH, FSH	2b–3
Treatment of anovulation	
PCOS—anti-estrogens, gonadotropins, ovarian diathermy, IVF	1a
Hypothalamic/Pituitary failure—gonadotropins, pulsatile GnRH	1a–3
Ovarian failure—egg donation	2b–4
Tubal patency testing	
By HSG or HyCoSy, unless significant comorbidity, when a diagnostic laparoscopy and dye may be indicated	1b–2b
Treatment of tubal disease	
Proximal—selective salpingography, surgery, or IVF	1a–2b
Distal—surgery or IVF. If hydrosalpinges, should be treated prior to IVF	1a
Treatment of unexplained infertility/mild endometriosis	
Mild endometriosis can be treated with excision/ablation	1a
Unexplained infertility is treated with IUI or IVF	1a
Most significant prognostic determinants of pregnancy are female age and duration of infertility	3

Pelvic infection should be screened by using an endocervical swab or urine sample to test for chlamydia. Cervical screening should also be up to date. A pelvic USS should be arranged as it may reveal polycystic ovaries or uterine anomalies. An AFC can also be done as a measure of ovarian reserve.

For tubal patency the preferred investigation for those without risk factors is an HSG or hystero-contrast sonography (HyCoSy). Contrast medium is injected through the cervix into the uterine cavity and spill is seen along the fallopian tubes either radiologically or by ultrasonography. However, for women with an abnormal HSG, symptoms suggestive of endometriosis, or a past history of PID or pelvic surgery, a laparoscopy and hydrotubation offer more information; besides, treating mild-to-moderate endometriosis has also been shown to significantly increase the rate of spontaneous conception (see Table 1) (19, 37). Because laparoscopy requires a general anesthetic and carries a risk of visceral injury, it is not used as the first-line investigation. Selective salpingography may be used as a diagnostic and therapeutic measure in cases of proximal tubal occlusion also. Fertiloscopy can be considered a valid alternative to laparoscopy; it is a technique that combines transvaginal hydropelviscopy, dye-test, optional salpingoscopy, and hysteroscopy and can be performed on an outpatient basis under local anesthesia. It has the advantage of being minimally invasive and has some therapeutic role but as yet has not been widely used.

Hysteroscopy is not done routinely because the frequency of asymptomatic intrauterine lesions not seen on USS is low.

MANAGEMENT OF FEMALE INFERTILITY

Management of Anovulatory Infertility

There are several ways of achieving ovulation and the approach depends somewhat on the etiology. For women with hypogonadotropic hypogonadism, weight normalization may help. Otherwise they respond well to pulsatile administration of gonadotropin releasing hormone (GnRH) (see Table 1). For

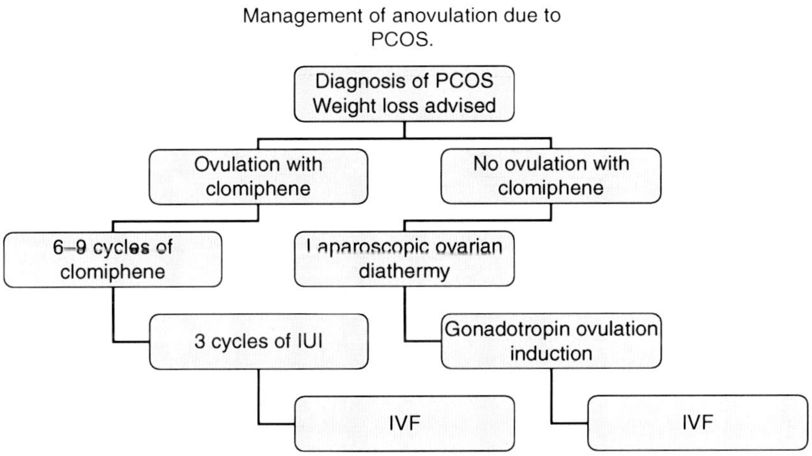

Figure 1 Management of anovulation due to PCOS.

women with hyperprolactinemia, medical treatment with dopamine agonists—such as bromocriptine, or more recently cabergoline or quinagolide, which have fewer side effects and are more effective—can help restore ovulation. For those women who are anovulatory because of a premature menopause (or even who are perimenopausal), ovulation induction would be unsuccessful; the most appropriate treatment would be the use of donor oocytes.

The vast majority of women with ovulatory problems will have PCOS (see Fig. 1).

In cases of obesity, weight loss should be advised in the first instance because even a 5% reduction in weight has been shown to improve reproductive outcome (see Table 1) (11), and obese women require more stimulation to ovulate (38). If they are of normal weight then anti-estrogens can be used in the form of clomiphene citrate or tamoxifen. They block estrogen receptors in the hypothalamus and therefore increase gonadotropins. Approximately 80% of women will ovulate on clomiphene and this can be used for up to 12 cycles. However, Clomiphene can also block estrogen receptors elsewhere possibly causing a thin endometrium and decreased cervical mucus. Treatment carries a 10% risk of multiple pregnancy (39), and a small increased risk of ovarian cancer (40). There is also a very small risk of ovarian hyperstimulation syndrome (OHSS) (41).

Metformin, an oral biguanide, is an insulin-sensitizing agent and has been used to increase ovulation rates. However, recent studies have shown it not to be as effective as clomiphene and it is now only recommended for those with glucose intolerance (42).

A potential alternative may be aromatase inhibitors such as letrozole. They inhibit estrogen synthesis, thereby causing an increase in GnRH pulsatility and consequently increased FSH secretion. This results in normal or enhanced follicular recruitment without risk of multiple ovulation and OHSS. Letrozole has a short half-life and is less likely to adversely affect the endometrium or cervical mucus.

For those who fail to ovulate with clomiphene, injectable human menopausal gonadotropin (hMG or FSH) can be used. This needs to be combined with follicular tracking for all cycles as it carries a higher risk (16%) of multiple births and a 1% risk of OHSS (41). Overall the cumulative singleton live birth rate for ovulation induction is 72% over 12 months (42).

For those who do ovulate with clomiphene but fail to achieve a pregnancy after six months of treatment, clomiphene-stimulated intrauterine insemination (IUI) should be offered (3).

A surgical method of inducing ovulation is ovarian drilling (see Table 1). This involves creating lesions on the surface of each ovary with diathermy and this in some unknown way, appears to trigger ovulation. It increases the pregnancy rate over 6 months, which is equivalent to three to six months of GnRH therapy (43) and has a lower risk of multiple pregnancy and OHSS. It tends to be reserved for clomiphene-resistant women as surgery carries risk of visceral injury and adhesion formation. In addition, there are increased surgical risks in obese women.

Management of Tubal Infertility

The various treatment options available for tubal infertility are tubal surgery, selective salpingography, or IVF.

For proximal tubal obstruction, selective salpingography may be useful. A catheter is placed in the cervix and a dye injected into the uterus and along the tubes, if there is no obstruction. If the tubes are blocked then a guidewire and catheter are used to effectively unblock them. This has been shown to be an effective technique for proximal blockage (44); it is noninvasive and can be done at the diagnostic stage.

Distal disease can be treated by surgery or IVF. Pregnancy rates after salpingostomy are generally low—5% (45,46), with a high risk of re-occlusion. In carefully selected patients, higher pregnancy rates can be achieved (see Table 1) (46). It is important therefore, before undertaking salpingostomy to make a careful evaluation of the hydrosalpinx to judge if it is unlikely to re-occlude or not.

Tubal surgery has become less commonplace since the advent of IVF and therefore there is less expertise in this area. There is no evidence of benefit or disadvantage of tubal surgery versus alternative treatments, so the patients' circumstances need to be taken into consideration (47). The cost of IVF may make surgery more attractive, and there is a decreased risk of multiple pregnancy as well as OHSS with tubal surgery. However, the risk of ectopic pregnancy is higher. With surgery there are risks of visceral damage and adhesion formation. If after 6 to 12 months of surgery a pregnancy does not occur then IVF is indicated.

IVF is the most commonly used treatment for tubal infertility. If hydrosalpinges are present, there is good evidence these should be removed or clipped as it is thought that the fluid from them may be toxic to embryo development and implantation (48).

Management of Unexplained Infertility

The main approaches to unexplained infertility are expectant management, ovulation induction with or without IUI and IVF. Approximately 60% of couples with unexplained infertility of less than three years' duration will fall pregnant in the next three years without any intervention. However, the woman's age needs to be taken into consideration when deciding on management.

With an average success rate of 33% (17) per cycle in women under the age of 35 (17), IVF is thought of as the most effective treatment for unexplained infertility, although there are few trials that compare it with other treatments (49). It also plays a diagnostic role that of providing information about fertilization and oocyte and embryo quality. The 25% multiple pregnancy rate is decreasing with the advent of elective single embryo transfer and the aim is to reduce the rate to 10% by 2011 (50,51,52).

IUI with ovarian stimulation is another option and is cheaper than IVF but less successful. There is evidence to show that stimulated IUI increases the chances of pregnancy when compared with gonadotropins and timed intercourse (53), and the conception rate is on average 11%. However, the risks of multiple pregnancy and ovarian stimulation need to be taken into account.

The usage of clomiphene for ovulation induction has been used in women with unexplained infertility because by producing more eggs, it is thought, the likelihood of pregnancy is greater. Similarly, unstimulated IUI has also been advocated (NICE guidance). A recent study indicated that there is little evidence of benefit over the background pregnancy rate (54).

The decision on management for the couple with unexplained infertility is dependent on the woman's age, duration of infertility, and the patient's wishes.

Management of Uterine Factor Infertility

The management of uterine problems is generally surgical. There is evidence that removing submucous fibroids which distort the uterine cavity increases the pregnancy rate (55). Submucous fibroids can be resected hysteroscopically but this carries a small risk of hemorrhage, perforation, and subsequent Asherman's syndrome. Myomectomy for significant subserous and intramural fibroids (>5 cm or which indent the uterine cavity) can be performed laparoscopically, but is more usually done by laparotomy. Depending on the size and number of fibroids, there is a small risk of hysterectomy. The resection of a uterine septum hysteroscopically can help decrease the risk of miscarriage. The main concern is the risk of postoperative adhesions interfering with fertility and the possibility of breaching the cavity, which may result in intrauterine adhesions.

Polyps can be dealt with hysteroscopically with relatively low morbidity. If uterine factors are thought to be preventing implantation, then they should be dealt with prior to other treatments.

Multifactorial Causes of Infertility

Where there are a combination of causes, IVF is the treatment of choice, as it is effective for tubal and ovulatory disorders.

FACTORS AFFECTING ART OUTCOME

When deciding the path of treatment to take with a couple, several factors need to be taken into consideration, which affect assisted reproductive techniques (ART) outcome.

Age

The age of the female patient is very important because success rates with IVF decrease from 28% per cycle in those who are younger than 35 years to 10% in those who are 40 years or older (17). However, if success rates between IVF patients using their own eggs and patients of the same age using donor eggs are compared, the age of the eggs used is the determining factor in achieving pregnancy. For example, a 40-year-old woman using the eggs of a 25-year-old donor has the same chance of conceiving as that of a 25-year-old woman using her own eggs.

Ovarian Reserve and Duration of Infertility

The next most important factor that affects IVF outcome is the number of eggs collected. This is determined by ovarian reserve and this can be evaluated by measuring the levels of FSH, AMH, or AFC throughout the cycle.

Studies have shown that couples with a long duration of infertility (three years or more) have a poorer outcome from IVF.

Obesity

Obesity, which is becoming increasingly common, has been shown to have a negative impact on the outcome of ART (56). It also requires higher levels of ovarian stimulation and if treatment is successful, can lead to a high-risk pregnancy. For this reason, some centers will not perform IVF on women with a BMI of more than 30 kg/m^2.

Hydrosalpinx

There is good evidence that the presence of a hydrosalpinx may impede implantation and should be removed or occluded prior to treatment (48).

CONCLUSION

As infertility rates have increased, so have the number of children born by ART. In the UK over 1% of all live births are through IVF or donor insemination and of the total number of IVF pregnancies, 24% are twins (17). As more couples require investigation and treatment with surgery or ART, we need to help them to optimize their chances of conceiving by reducing their weight and smoking. We also need to individualize management to suit each couple and keep in mind that for many couples the aging oocyte is the crucial factor and therefore expediting treatment is important.

ANSWERS TO CASE HISTORIES

Case 1

Pre-conception advice: Give general advice to stop smoking and to reduce alcohol intake. The woman should take 0.4 mg of folic acid daily and should be advised to have regular intercourse throughout the month.

As she has regular cycles, she almost certainly ovulates. A mid-luteal progesterone may be carried out, but is not considered essential. She should have her rubella immunity checked, and her tests of ovarian reserve (FSH, AMH, or AFC) should be carried out too. This will improve her chances of responding to ovulation induction with assisted conception.

Treatment options for unexplained infertility include expectant management, IUI in stimulated cycles, and IVF.

The chances of conceiving spontaneously at the age of 36 having had three years of infertility is low—about 1% per month. The chances with IUI are around 10% per cycle and with IVF 25% per cycle.

It is reasonable to offer three to six cycles of IUI and then proceed to IVF, or to go straight to IVF in view of the patient's age and her declining chances of conceiving as her age advances. Expectant management would have a very low chance of success, and treatment with clomiphene citrate would not increase the chance of conception.

CASE 2

As the male partner has had a vasectomy, IVF with ICSI following epididymal sperm aspiration would be the most efficient and effective way forward. Vasectomy reversal is less likely to be successful after five years have elapsed due to antisperm antibodies. Treatment of distal tubal disease has poor success rates and so IVF is usually the best way forward. However, prior to treatment, the woman should have the hydrosalpinges either removed, or occluded proximally, because it is known that hydrosalpinges reduce the chances of conceiving by half, and by removing the hydrosalpinges this condition can be reversed.

CASE 3

The likely diagnosis is anovulation due to PCOS.

Some of the investigations that would be helpful are FSH, LH, testosterone, pelvic scan. Other hormone investigations that can be carried out are TFTs and SHBG to determine the free androgen index. It is also important to screen overweight women with PCOS for diabetes.

The treatment plan would be to advise the woman to lose weight and to treat initially with anti-estrogens, and if she ovulates, to proceed to 6 to 12 cycles of treatment, then offer intrauterine insemination before progressing to IVF. If she does not ovulate with anti-estrogens, then laparoscopic ovarian diathermy, ovulation induction with gonadotropins, and IVF can be considered.

The couple should know that women with PCOS have a higher risk of miscarriage, especially if obese, and that they are at risk of multiple follicular ovulation, along with the risk of multiple pregnancy and OHSS.

REFERENCES

1. Miller CL, Miller E, Sequeira PJ, et al. Effect of selective vaccination on rubella susceptibility and infection in pregnancy. Br Med J (Clin Res Ed) 1985; 291(6506):1398–1401.
2. Lumley J, Watson L, Watson M, et al. Periconceptional supplementation with folate and/or multivitamins for preventing neural tube defects. Cochrane Database Syst Rev 2001; (3):CD001056.
3. National Institute for Clinical Excellence (NICE). Fertility Assessment and Treatment for People With Fertility Problems. London: RCOG Press, 2004.
4. Augood C, Duckitt K, Templeton AA. Smoking and female infertility: a systematic review and meta-analysis. Hum Reprod 1998; 13(6):1532–1539.
5. Hughes EG, Brennan BG. Does cigarette smoking impair natural or assisted fecundity? Fertil Steril 1996; 66(5):679–689.
6. Raymond EG, Cnattingius S, Kiely JL. Effects of maternal age, parity, and smoking on the risk of stillbirth. Br J Obstet Gynaecol 1994; 101(4):301–306.
7. Kleinman JC, Pierre MB Jr., Madans JH, et al. The effects of maternal smoking on fetal and infant mortality. Am J Epidemiol 1988; 127(2):274–282.
8. Royal College of Obstetricians and Gynaecologists. Alcohol Consumption and the Outcomes of Pregnancy. London: RCOG Press, 2006.
9. Department of Health. Sensible Drinking: The Report of an Inter-Departmental Working Group. 1995.
10. Balen AH, Anderson RA. Impact of obesity on female reproductive health: British Fertility Society, Policy and Practice Guidelines. Hum Fertil (Camb) 2007; 10(4):195–206.
11. Clark AM, Thornley B, Tomlinson L, et al. Weight loss in obese infertile women results in improvement in reproductive outcome for all forms of fertility treatment. Hum Reprod 1998; 13(6):1502–1505.

12. Hull MG, Glazener CM, Kelly NJ, et al. Population study of causes, treatment, and outcome of infertility. Br Med J (Clin Res Ed) 1985; 291(6510):1693–1697.
13. Azziz R, Woods KS, Reyna R, Key TJ, Knochenhauer ES, Yildiz BO. The prevalence and features of the polycystis ovarian syndrome in an unselected population. J Clin Endocrinol Metab 2004; 89(6):2745–2749.
14. Hull MG. Epidemiology of infertility and polycystic ovarian disease: endocrinological and demographic studies. Gynecol Endocrinol 1987; 1(3):235–245.
15. Rotterdam ESHRE/ASRM Sponsored PCOS consensus workshop. Revised 2003 consensus on diagnostic criteria and long-term health risks related to polycystic ovary syndrome (PCOS). Hum Reprod 2004; 19(1):41–47.
16. Rotterdam ESHRE/ASRM Sponsored PCOS consensus workshop. Revised 2003 consensus on diagnostic criteria and long-term health risks related to polycystic ovary syndrome. Fertil Steril 2004; 81(1):19–25.
17. HFEA Guide to Infertility 2006–2007: Fertility problems and treatment—facts and figures. Available at www.hfea.gov.uk/docs/facts_and_figures_03-04.pdf.
18. Devroey P, Godoy H, Smitz J, et al. Female age predicts embryonic implantation after ICSI: a case-controlled study. Hum Reprod 1996; 11(6):1324–1327.
19. Marcoux S, Maheux R, Berube S. Laparoscopic surgery in infertile women with minimal or mild endometriosis. Canadian Collaborative Group on Endometriosis. N Engl J Med 1997; 337(4):217–222.
20. Dunphy BC. Office falloposcopic assessment in proximal tubal occlusive disease. Fertil Steril 1994; 61(1):168–170.
21. Sulak PJ, Letterie GS, Coddington CC, et al. Histology of proximal tubal occlusion. Fertil Steril 1987; 48(3): 437–440.
22. Strandell A, Lindhard A, Waldenstrom U, et al. Hydrosalpinx and IVF outcome: cumulative results after salpingectomy in a randomized controlled trial. Hum Reprod 2001; 16(11):2403–2410.
23. Schenker JG, Margalioth EJ. Intrauterine adhesions: an updated appraisal. Fertil Steril 1982; 37(5):593–610.
24. Ventolini G, Zhang M, Gruber J. Hysteroscopy in the evaluation of patients with recurrent pregnancy loss: a cohort study in a primary care population. Surg Endosc 2004; 18(12):1782–1784.
25. Stirrat GM. Recurrent miscarriage. Lancet 1990; 336(8716): 673–675.
26. De BM, Dao TN. Cytogenetic studies in couples experiencing repeated pregnancy losses. Hum Reprod 1990; 5(5): 519–528.
27. Swadpanich U, Lumbiganon P, Prasertcharoensook W, et al. Antenatal lower genital tract infection screening and treatment programs for preventing preterm delivery. Cochrane Database Syst Rev 2008;(2):CD006178.
28. Rai RS, Regan L, Clifford K, et al. Antiphospholipid antibodies and beta 2-glycoprotein-I in 500 women with recurrent miscarriage: results of a comprehensive screening approach. Hum Reprod 1995; 10(8):2001–2005.
29. Wilson WA, Gharavi AE, Koike T, et al. International consensus statement on preliminary classification criteria for definite antiphospholipid syndrome: report of an international workshop. Arthritis Rheum 1999; 42(7):1309–1311.
30. Clifford K, Rai R, Regan L. Future pregnancy outcome in unexplained recurrent first trimester miscarriage. Hum Reprod 1997; 12(2):387–389.
31. Brodin T, Bergh T, Berglund L, et al. Menstrual cycle length is an age-independent marker of female fertility: Results from 6271 treatment cycles of in vitro fertilization. Fertil Steril 2007; 90(5):1656–1661.
32. Kupka MS, Dorn C, Richter O, et al. Impact of reproductive history on in vitro fertilization and intracytoplasmic sperm injection outcome: evidence from the German IVF Registry. Fertil Steril 2003; 80(3):508–516.
33. Evers JL. Female subfertility. Lancet 2002; 360(9327):151–159.
34. Templeton A, Morris JK, Parslow W. Factors that affect outcome of in-vitro fertilisation treatment. Lancet 1996; 348(9039):1402–1406.
35. Collins JA, Crosignani PG. Unexplained infertility: a review of diagnosis, prognosis, treatment efficacy and management. Int J Gynaecol Obstet 1992; 39(4):267–275.
36. Van RI, Broekmans FJ, Scheffer GJ, et al. Serum antimullerian hormone levels best reflect the reproductive decline with age in normal women with proven fertility: a longitudinal study. Fertil Steril 2005; 83(4):979–987.
37. Jacobson TZ, Barlow DH, Koninckx PR, et al. Laparoscopic surgery for subfertility associated with endometriosis. Cochrane Database Syst Rev 2002; (4):CD001398.
38. Balen AH, Platteau P, Andersen AN, et al. The influence of body weight on response to ovulation induction with gonadotrophins in 335 women with World Health Organization group II anovulatory infertility. BJOG 2006; 113(10):1195–1202.
39. Smitz J, Camus M, Devroey P, et al. Incidence of severe ovarian hyperstimulation syndrome after GnRH agonist/HMG superovulation for in-vitro fertilization. Hum Reprod 1990; 5(8):933–937.
40. Rossing MA, Daling JR, Weiss NS, et al. Ovarian tumors in a cohort of infertile women. N Engl J Med 1994; 331(12):771–776.
41. Venn A, Lumley J. Clomiphene citrate and pregnancy outcome. Aust N Z J Obstet Gynaecol 1994; 34(1):56–66.
42. Thessaloniki ESHRE/ASRM Sponsored PCOS consensus workshop. Consensus on infertility treatment related to polycystic ovary syndrome. Hum Reprod 2008; 23(3):462–477.
43. Farquhar C, Vandekerckhove P, Lilford R. Laparoscopic "drilling" by diathermy or laser for ovulation induction in anovulatory polycystic ovary syndrome. Cochrane Database Syst Rev 2001; (4):CD001122.

44. Papaioannou S, Afnan M, Girling AJ, et al. Diagnostic and therapeutic value of selective salpingography and tubal catheterization in an unselected infertile population. Fertil Steril 2003; 79(3):613–617.
45. Lilford RJ, Watson AJ. Has in vitro fertilization made salpingostomy obsolete? Br J Obstet Gynaecol 1990; 97(7):557–560.
46. Winston RM, Margara RA. Microsurgical salpingostomy is not an obsolete procedure. Br Obstet Gynaecol 1991; 98(7):637–642.
47. Ahmad G, Watson A, Vandekerckhove P, et al. Techniques for pelvic surgery in subfertility. Cochrane Database Syst Rev 2006; (2):CD000221.
48. Johnson NP, Mak W, Sowter MC. Surgical treatment for tubal disease in women due to undergo in vitro fertilisation. Cochrane Database Syst Rev 2004; (3):CD002125.
49. Pandian Z, Bhattacharya S, Vale L, et al. In vitro fertilisation for unexplained subfertility. Cochrane Database Syst Rev 2005; (2):CD003357.
50. Martikainen H, Tiitinen A, Tomas C, et al. One versus two embryo transfer after IVF and ICSI: a randomized study. Hum Reprod 2001; 16(9):1900–1903.
51. Gerris J, De ND, Mangelschots K, et al. Prevention of twin pregnancy after in-vitro fertilization or intracytoplasmic sperm injection based on strict embryo criteria: a prospective randomized clinical trial. Hum Reprod 1999; 14(10):2581–2587.
52. Cutting R, Morroll D, Roberts SA, Pickering S, Rutherford A; British Fertility Society and Association of Clinical Embryologists. Elective single embryo transfer: guidelines for practice. Hum Fertil (Camb) 2008; 11(3): 131–146.
53. Hughes EG. The effectiveness of ovulation induction and intrauterine insemination in the treatment of persistent infertility: a meta-analysis. Hum Reprod 1997; 12(9): 1865–1872.
54. Bhattacharya S, Harrild K, Mollison J, et al. Clomifene citrate or unstimulated intrauterine insemination compared with expectant management for unexplained infertility: pragmatic randomised controlled trial. BMJ 2008; 337: 716.
55. Pritts EA, Parker WH, Olive DL. Fibroids and Infertility: an updated systematic review of the evidence. Fertil Steril 2009; 91(4):1215–1223.
56. Lintsen AM, Pasker-de Jong PC, de Boer EJ, et al. Effects of subfertility cause, smoking and body weight on the success rate of IVF. Hum Reprod 2005; 20(7): 1867–1875.

4 Basic semen analysis and laboratory quality for clinicians

Lars Björndahl

CASE

A 32-year-old man consults because of infertility problems. His wife has been investigated by a gynecologist, and no causes for infertility have been discovered. The man was sent for semen analysis, and he is now worried because on the basis of the semen analysis the couple has now been categorized as "male factor" infertility, and he now wonders what is wrong and whether he can get some treatment. The laboratory report contains the following information:

Date	August 24	December 13	Unit	Reference limits
Sperm concentration	22.3	19.1	$\times 10^6$/mL	>20
Sperm motility				
% Motile	48.4	41.0	%	>40
% Rapid Progressive	30.3	32.5	%	>25
Sperm vitality	51.9	47.5	%	>75
Sperm morphology				
% Normal	8.5	11.1	%	>30

Clues for the proper interpretation of the data are given at the end of the chapter.

SEMEN ANALYSIS AND QUALITY ASPECTS

A basic understanding of the possibilities and limitations of semen analysis is important for correct interpretation of laboratory results from the semen laboratory. Today there are robust and reliable standardized laboratory methods available for all andrology laboratories (1,2) although several reports indicate very poor compliance with these basic recommendations (3–7). Therefore, it is essential for every clinician in the field of reproductive medicine to have sufficient insight into the laboratory methods to interpret results and to know when to call for improved laboratory standards. A list of possible indications for semen analysis is given in Table 1. The aim of this chapter is not to provide a full laboratory handbook (8) but to provide the clinician with guidelines on what to demand from the laboratory and how to interpret the results from semen analysis.

Uncertainty in Results

All laboratory results are more or less accurate. Repeated assessments of the same biological specimen will give a variety of results. If the method used for assessment is robust, the variation between repeated measurements will be relatively small, while the use of a less robust method will show a larger variation in results. Statistical analysis of repeated measurements is usually expressed as a measurement of the variation called the 95% confidence interval (95% CI). This interval represents, with a probability of 95%, the range within which the true value is calculated to be (i.e., there is a probability of only 5% that the true value is outside that interval).

Even if the technical quality of an analysis is good, results can vary a lot from one semen sample to another from the same individual as well as between different individuals. Variations between individuals can to a large extent be explained by general biological differences, and variations between different samples from the same man can often be explained by changes in the physiological conditions. These aspects will be discussed as *biological variation* (see section biological variation and pathological conditions).

There are a number of technical factors related to the laboratory investigation that can influence the numeric uncertainty of a result. Besides taking measures to minimize direct technical errors, it is the responsibility of the laboratory to ensure that the sample is collected and kept under standardized conditions until the start of the laboratory investigation.

Technical Variation

Especially important when particles (or cells) are counted is the total number of units (cells) assessed and also, for instance, how the semen volume used for dilution can be exactly determined, the precision in depth of a counting chamber, and the level of training of the laboratory staff. For the assessment of progressive sperm motility, the temperature of the specimen is very important. Some methods used for assessing sperm vitality can give wrong results due to osmotic effects that kill the sperm, and sperm morphology largely depends on which criteria are used for the evaluation as well as the quality of microscope optics.

Sample Collection, Transportation, and Keeping

It is essential that the patient be instructed to collect the entire ejaculate, and report especially if any of the early portions have not been collected, since the main part of motile sperm is normally expelled in the first ejaculation fractions. Furthermore, once collected the sample must be protected from cold shock (temperature drop to +15°C) since sperm motility may get severely reduced because of cold shock. Also, in the laboratory it is essential that the temperature be kept within a defined range. Otherwise, motility assessments will vary with the changes in temperature in the laboratory. The simplest way

Table 1 A List of Reasons for Performing Basic Semen Analysis with Comments on Aspects for the Referring Clinician to Consider

Man in a couple failing to achieve pregnancy after unprotected sexual intercourse for 6–12 mo	Men with severely decreased semen quality have a very low likelihood to contribute to a pregnancy. The best help for couples with a severe male factor is that the clinical andrology investigation be started as early as possible
Follow-up of treatment effect	Endocrine replacement therapy starting spermatogenesis—normalized sperm numbers and sperm functions Treatment of inflammatory disorders—normalized sperm motility Postvasectomy controls—detect any signs of remaining spermatozoa, failed surgery, or recanalization
Curiosity	A very sensitive subject—there could be very different reasons for the curiosity. It should always be clearly explained that results of semen analysis cannot guarantee fertility. It can often be wise to counsel the curious man that semen analysis can tell whether there are sufficient numbers of motile sperm, and that if that is the case the likelihood of being fertile is pretty good. • Adolescent boys may worry about "being normal," which could be expressed as a wish to know whether they are fertile or not. Since semen analysis cannot prove that completely, it is very important that the clinician gives the youth correct information and time to reflect. The clinician must also be prepared to take care of the patient for further counseling if semen analysis shows severe abnormalities. • An adolescent or young man who has suffered a case of severe mumps, especially if the testicles were swollen or painful, has a justified reason for semen analysis. • A chronologically more mature man with an undefined curiosity with regard to potential for fertility but without present or earlier partners should probably be referred for more extended counseling. • A man with history of genital infections may express interest for semen analysis for fear of having become infertile due to repeated infections. It is essential that the man is not referred until the man has been given a physical examination and undergone any antibiotic treatment due to the findings of the clinical examination. • A man asking for a semen analysis related to paternity issues should be informed that semen analysis is not very informative regarding paternity issues. For an earlier vasectomized man who suspects that he has caused a new pregnancy, semen analysis could be done without any further delay. In all other cases, referral to professional counseling should be considered. • A man who has been investigated for infertility in another center.

to keep a controlled temperature is to keep the samples in a +37°C incubator. At this temperature the liquefaction of the semen coagulum will be accomplished within 15 to 20 minutes in most samples but can take longer at lower temperatures. The recommendation is that semen analysis should start at 30 minutes after ejaculation, in order to reduce the variation in sperm parameters due to different duration of exposure of sperm to seminal plasma (1,2).

Correct Sample Volume

Assuming the density of human semen corresponds to 1.00 g/mL, the most accurate way to assess the semen sample volume is by weighing (9). Since weighing does not create losses of volume in sample container, tubes, and pipettes, this method is also preferable in the treatment situation when as little as possible of the sample should be wasted on diagnostic activities. The weighing method also means that the contact with different laboratory equipment is minimized, which is a great advantage for samples intended for treatment.

Numbers of Cells Assessed

When a semen sample is analyzed, random factors will influence which sperm are assessed and which are not. Presence or absence of sperm will depend not only on the actual sperm concentration but also on random factors influencing the distribution of sperm in the microscope field. Statistical calculations of the uncertainty of a result due to the total number of observations show that at low numbers the influence of random factors is very important. If only 100 sperm are counted, the 95% CI can be calculated to be approximately ±20% and when 400 sperm are counted, the 95% CI will be ±10% (Fig. 1) (2).

Correct Sampling Volume for Concentration Assessment

When an aliquot of semen is taken from the well-mixed semen sample in order to dilute sperm for determination of concentration, a positive displacement pipette with a piston in the tip of the pipette should be used (10) (Fig. 2). Air displacement pipettes are calibrated for watery solutions, that is, solutions with a viscosity far lower than that of semen—semen sampled

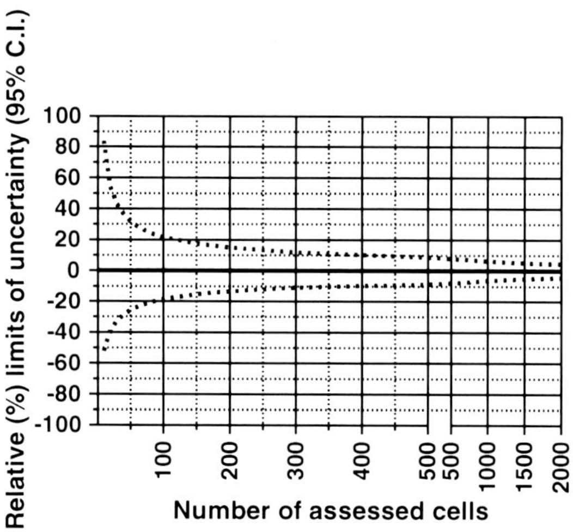

Figure 1 Variation in uncertainty of results for sperm counts due to different numbers of cells assessed.

with an air displacement pipette will always have a volume lower than the volume indicated by the pipette. How much lower the volume is depends on how high the viscosity is. In positive displacement pipettes, air bubbles will disclose any volume error due to filling problems in samples with very high viscosity. Furthermore, even in a macroscopically well-mixed semen sample, there may be "compartments" that are very heterogeneous with regard to the content of sperm. Thus, the recommended semen volume to dilute for sperm concentration assessment is 50 μL. If a smaller volume is used, there is an increased risk for random errors because the sampled aliquot may not be representative for the entire semen sample. To reduce this risk for sampling errors in small aliquots it is necessary to compare duplicate aliquots.

Depth of Counting Chamber

When the number of sperm is counted, the depth of the counting chamber is crucial for a correct result. Hemocytometers are in general 100 μm deep and the slight variations due to cover slip attachment are relatively small, whereas in chambers with a depth of only 10 to 20 μm and a cover slip that is not permanently mounted the variations in depth will be relatively more important. Furthermore, the concentrations obtained with disposable chambers with a fixed depth of 20 μm or less are consistently lower (11) due to the specific flow dynamics in such shallow chambers (12,13).

Semen Analysis as Postvasectomy Control

A general recommendation is to examine a first semen sample three months after surgery with frequent ejaculations after surgery to empty all spermatozoa remaining in any reservoirs (14). At least three completely sperm-free ejaculates at least a week apart and with intervening ejaculations are recommended before the surgery can be considered successful (15–17).

The laboratory should not perform a normal basic semen analysis but a focused investigation aimed at identifying any remaining spermatozoa. If initial overview of the neat sample ("wet preparation") under phase-contrast microscopy reveals motile or immotile spermatozoa in any of 10 to 20 fields (200× magnification), the patient should be contacted and given the information that there are still spermatozoa in the ejaculate. A new sample should be examined two to three weeks later after 5 to 10 unexamined ejaculations.

If no spermatozoa are detected in at least 20 fields of a wet preparation, the entire sample should be centrifuged and the supernatant should be saved for biochemical analyses (especially α-glucosidase as a marker for epididymal contribution to the ejaculate). The centrifugation pellet is carefully resuspended in a minute volume of seminal plasma and transferred to a microscopy slide and covered with a large cover slip (50 × 24 mm). The entire area is scanned under 200× phase-contrast microscope (400× if very dense layer of cells and debris in the pellet). If the entire centrifuge pellet is scanned without any spermatozoa identified, the likelihood of the presence of spermatozoa in the ejaculate is very low. However, it should be remembered that some spermatozoa may escape from the centrifugation pellet, as well as from the inspection under the microscope (18). If spermatozoa are identified, the number of immotile and motile spermatozoa should be given in the report.

If motile spermatozoa continue to appear in the ejaculate months after surgery and with high numbers of ejaculations,

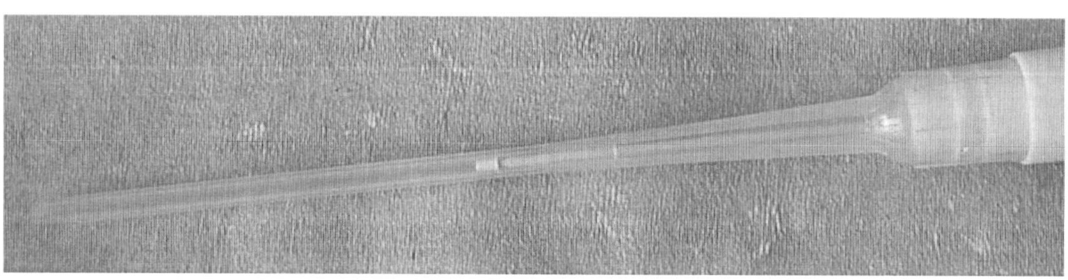

Figure 2 A positive-displacement pipette with a piston in the tip ensuring correct semen volume for sperm concentration assessment.

this could indicate a partially unsuccessful operation or signs of recanalization. Increasing numbers of motile spermatozoa under the same circumstances is indicative for recanalization.

Defined Temperature for Sperm Motility Assessment

Rapid progressive sperm motility is a property related to fertility success (19). Since the progressive motility decreases with lowering of the specimen temperature, it is necessary to standardize the temperature at which motility is assessed. Although maintaining the room temperature is less costly, it can vary between approximately 18°C and 25°C because of ambient temperature, climate, heating, and air conditioning. Therefore, the basic advice is to control the microscope stage at +37°C. Slides could easily be prewarmed in a +37°C incubator used to keep the samples at 37°C until assessments start.

Proper Microscope Equipment

Live, unstained sperm cannot be seen in ordinary light microscopes because of the very low contrast of these small cells. Therefore, phase-contrast microscopy (200–400×) is necessary to observe live sperm. On the other hand, smears of dried sperm that have been stained with, for example, Papanicolaou stain adapted for human sperm (2) are best assessed under bright field microscopy (1000× with oil immersion), since such optics have much higher resolution than phase-contrast optics. Still, there can be huge differences between observations taken with different microscopes due to differences in illumination (light source brightness and color temperature) as well as optic qualities (resolution, focal depth).

Sperm Vitality Assessment

The easiest way to see whether a sperm is alive is by observing it swim. The clinical situation when sperm vitality assessment should be done is when no—or very few—sperm are motile: to determine whether the immotile sperm are dead or alive. For this purpose, staining methods have been developed, based on the principle that live sperm do not take up the stain, while dead sperm with damaged cell membrane take up the stain. A problem with the methods recommended in the WHO manual (1) from 1999 is that the procedure actually kills a proportion of sperm (20). The recommendation is therefore to use a properly validated technique (2,20,21).

Another principle for detecting live sperm is the HOS test (hypo-osmotic swelling test) (22). Sperm are exposed to an environment with low osmolarity. Live sperm should be able to counteract the inflow of water to a certain degree, resulting in sperm with tails coiled within an expanded cell membrane. Dead sperm do not take up water so the tail will not coil within the membrane, and sperm with very poor function will not be able to adjust to water inflow and will therefore burst and die. The advantage of the method is that no harmful compounds (such as stains) are introduced, and identified live sperm can thus be used for treatment purposes.

Sperm Morphology Evaluation

There is a clear relationship between poor sperm morphology and poor fertility success (23). The main technical problem—and therefore also a problem for the interpretation and clinical use—with sperm morphology data is the lack of standardization of criteria. In the earlier history of semen analysis, sperm morphology criteria were based on observations of sperm in semen (24). Later studies of sperm with the capacity to move to the site of fertilization (i.e., passage through cervical mucus and binding to the zona pellucida) showed that such sperm are much more uniform in appearance. This is the base for the strict Tygerberg criteria (25), which are recommended by the WHO (1) and professional organizations such as the Nordic Association for Andrology (NAFA) and the European Society of Human Reproduction and Embryology Special Interest Group in Andrology (ESHRE-SIGA) (2). In general, the strict Tygerberg criteria have been used for several investigations indicating the usefulness of the assessment method, but the lack of external quality control systems makes it impossible to directly use data from one study for another clinic (26).

Basic to the detailed examination of sperm morphology is the need for proper techniques for smearing, fixation, staining, and mounting. The staining that gives the best overall results is the Papanicolaou staining specially adapted for human sperm (2).

Training for Semen Analysis

Reliable and comparable results from semen analysis depend not only on proper equipment and procedures (27,28) but also on the training of the laboratory staff, which is essential to obtain repeatable results (29,30). The ESHRE-SIGA has developed a standardized four-day course on basic semen analysis that has been given with great success in the local language in many different regions since 1994 (United Kingdom, Sweden, the Netherlands, Belgium, Denmark, Norway, Finland, Ukraine, South Africa, Spain, Greece, Portugal, and Canada). The principle of this course is to provide both a theoretical base and repeated practical training (31–34).

Quality Assurance

To control the technical variability and manual performance of assessments, it is essential that each andrology laboratory implements basic quality control procedures and complies with a comprehensive quality assurance system.

Robust Methods

Possible sources of errors must be minimized to reduce the variation between assessments taken at different times as well as between different individuals. Therefore, laboratory methods should be as simple as possible, with as few steps as possible.

Duplicate Assessments

A powerful tool to reduce the influence of random errors is the use of duplicate assessments if the results of the duplicate assessments are compared and the results accepted only if the two counts do not deviate too much from each other. The general recommendation is that sperm counts and sperm motility should always be done with duplicate assessments (1,2,35).

Internal Quality Control

The concept of internal quality control (IQC) comprises a number of different activities established to ensure that assessments are consistent over time and between different members of staff. One basic way to accomplish this is that a certain number of samples each month are assessed by all members of staff, and "archive" material is used for repeated assessments at different time points during the year. Another crucial point in IQC is that all members of staff are engaged in the interpretation of IQC results and take active part in discussions aiming at improving the results.

External Quality Assessment

Once the IQC is established to monitor the performance in the laboratory, it is of value to participate in an external quality assessment (EQA) program. In the EQA program, a number of laboratories receive QC material to evaluate. The results from the participating laboratories are put together so that each laboratory can see whether its results are consistent with the target values of the EQA program. Different programs exist but not all have target values determined by well-trained examiners. Instead there are often average values for all participating laboratories. This can cause problems, since the inclusion of less experienced laboratories in the program can influence the group average. In the nonprofit EQA scheme provided by the ESHRE-SIGA (36), the target values are based on the average results from several experienced staff members from five reference laboratories that use the same procedures and have trained in the same way and also trained together.

Biological Variation and Pathological Conditions

The total number of sperm in an ejaculate is determined by testicular production, transport through the male reproductive system, and recruitment at ejaculation. The testicular production among normal men is correlated to the total testicular volume, which, in turn, is related to the volume of the *tubuli seminiferi* and thereby to the number of spermatogonia. This is the reason why information about the testis volumes is of importance especially when semen analysis results with lower numbers of sperm are interpreted. In contrast to many other measurements of compounds and substances in the human body, sperm numbers in ejaculates do not show any sign of Gaussian distribution, at least not in men coming for infertility investigation (Fig. 3). It is very likely that the number of sperm in the ejaculate is determined by many, largely independent factors, including production, transport, and recruitment at ejaculation.

Obstructions in the male reproductive tract can completely hinder free transport from the testis to the urethra. Bilateral postinfectious scarring in the single canals from the epididymis to the urethra and of the ejaculatory ducts through the prostate can hinder the transport partially or completely (37). A genetic disorder closely related to the disease cystic fibrosis can cause congenital bilateral agenesis of vas deference (CBAVD) (38), which often is associated not only with azoospermia (absence of sperm in semen) but also with agenesis of other parts of the Wolffian duct system, including the seminal vesicles. Semen from men with this disorder thus often has a very low volume, no coagulum formation, and a low pH, since it is mainly prostatic secretion in the ejaculate and no seminal vesicular fluid and a total absence of sperm in the ejaculate.

A factor that has been given substantial attention regarding ejaculate production (volume, sperm number, sperm motility) is the time for sexual abstinence. Short abstinence time usually means lower total numbers, but quite often acceptable or good motility (39). Long abstinence time often leads to higher total numbers of sperm up to a certain limit. However, the effects of variation in abstinence time vary between individuals, where both large variations and lack of variation can be seen (40). Aspects influencing ejaculation that have been given less attention are the duration and quality of sexual stimulation preceding ejaculation. In addition, the duration of stimulation (41) and the use of visual stimulation (42) (video tapes) have been reported as factors influencing the quality of the ejaculate.

In contrast to the parameter total number of sperm, the parameter sperm concentration also includes the dilution of sperm by the accessory sex gland secretions (mainly seminal vesicular fluid and prostatic fluid). To evaluate sperm production and transport in the male reproductive tract, it is therefore not enough to evaluate the concentration without considering sperm volume and total sperm count. Abnormal secretory contributions from the prostate and seminal vesicles influence not only the final sperm concentration but also sperm functions negatively.

For sperm motility it is important that the composition of the seminal plasma does not create a hostile environment. Inflammatory reactions due to infections in the male reproductive tract are likely to also cause secretory changes in the prostate or seminal vesicles, which could lead to poor motility. Normally, sperm are expelled in the first ejaculate portions together with the zinc-rich prostatic secretion, while the later portions of the ejaculate contain mainly seminal vesicular fluid and much lesser sperm than in the first fractions. This normal sequence of ejaculation can be disturbed, probably because of inflammatory edema or postinfectious calcifications and cause decreased sperm motility, survival, and chromatin stability (43).

Presence of inflammatory cells in semen can be a sign of active infections. Methods to detect the presence of inflammatory cells include cytochemical assays (to show the presence of peroxidase positive leukocytes) and immunocytological tests (leukocyte surface antigen markers). Round cells in semen can be leukocytes but in the unstained wet preparation studied in

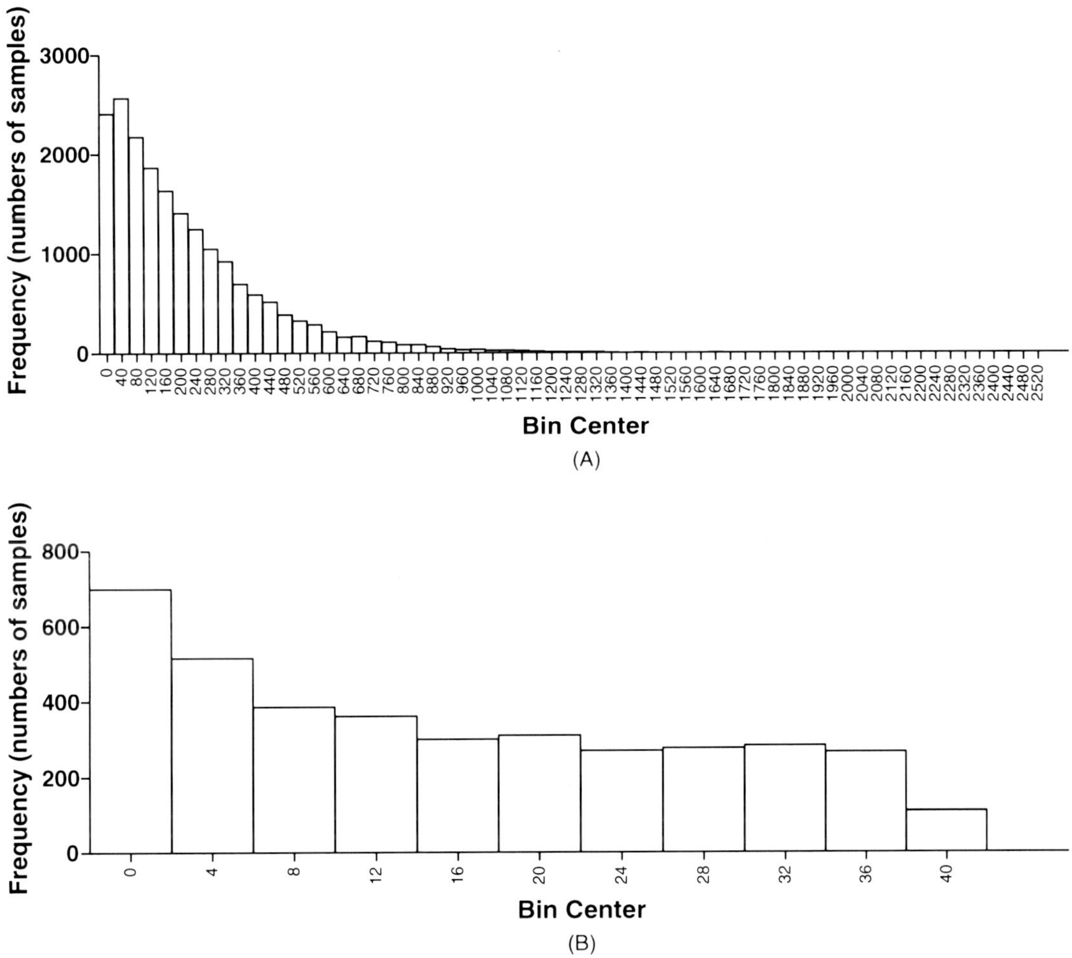

Figure 3 Frequency distributions of total sperm number in 19,356 complete semen samples collected after two to seven days of abstinence, investigated 1993–2007. (**A**) All samples; (**B**) samples up to 40 million/mL ($N = 3777$).

phase contrast microscopy it is not possible to distinguish leukocytes from round, immature germ cells. However, in the properly stained morphology smears differentiation between round cell types is less difficult.

Antisperm antibodies is a controversial field. In general, the haploid sperm need to be protected from the man's immune system. An inflammatory reaction in the male reproductive tract could allow the immigration of immuno competent cells into the reproductive tract, cells that could continue to produce antisperm antibodies even after the inflammation has subsided. Presence of antibodies of IgA-type has been found to hinder sperm passage through cervical mucus and therefore a substantial cause for infertility can now be cured with in vitro fertilization (IVF) (44). It has been speculated that antibodies of IgG-type binding to the postequatorial segment of the sperm head might interfere with sperm egg interaction, but this has not been consistently confirmed (45). Presently, there are two types of assays commercially available for detection of antisperm antibodies, but a problem is that the results of the tests do not always give similar results, indicating that the tests may not only reveal specific binding but could also be influenced by unspecific binding between sperm and beads. Thus, more knowledge is required in this field (46).

A testis under stress (e.g., systemic inflammatory reaction) or suffering from a genetic disorder is likely to produce fewer sperm and those produced are more likely to have an abnormal structure (35). A specific genetic disorder is characterized by round sperm heads without acrosomes—globozoospermia. Most cases with abnormal sperm morphology do however not show one singular abnormality—rather a panorama of different abnormalities. It has been shown that the presence of several categories of abnormalities (head, midpiece, tail, cytoplasmic residue) in each abnormal sperm is indicative of reduced fertilizing potential (47).

Table 2 A Flow Chart Suggesting a Systematic Approach to the Interpretation of Semen Analysis Results

Does the laboratory comply with internationally accepted and recommended standards?	See Table 3
Check that the sample is complete and according to standards	Complete collection by masturbation Abstinence time within limits
Check that analyses have been done according to standards	Time to investigation ideally 30 min (at least <60 min)
Are there signs of quantitatively normal sperm production?	Check: sperm number, sperm concentration, and semen volume If not OK—check motility and morphology, too. If these parameters are within acceptable limits, a slight decrease in sperm output is less likely to be significant. A general decrease in quality is likely to be more important. Differentiate between testicular and post testicular failure (see Table 4).
Sperm morphology—one qualitative aspect	Isolated moderate morphology decrease is not likely to be significant. If a significant proportion of the spermatozoa (arbitrarily set to >20%) have one specific defect, this is ascribed to a genetic defect.
Sperm motility—a basic functional property	Isolated motility decrease is most likely to be due to posttesticular (usually inflammatory or postinflammatory dysfunction): Check semen biochemistry, round cells, and leucocytes for signs of active inflammation. Consider investigation of split-ejaculate to explore disorder causing abnormal sequence of ejaculation. If rapid progressive spermatozoa are >25%, it is considered satisfactory. If not, it is still acceptable if the sum of slow and rapid progressive spermatozoa is >50%. Otherwise, the progressive motility is considered to be decreased. Note that these limits should only be applied to semen investigated at 37°C within 30 to 60 min after ejaculation. If all spermatozoa are immotile, it could either be due to severe inflammatory response (cytotoxic antisperm antibodies—test presence of antisperm antibodies) or in rare cases due to the genetic dyskinetic cilia syndrome—test sperm vitality.
Round cells—differentiation is not possible without further investigations	Immature germ cells from the testis—identified in stained morphology smears—usually more frequent in men with severe testicular problems. Inflammatory cells (leucocytes) that may be due to active inflammation; must be determined with specific methods (see below).
Inflammatory cells	Usually peroxidase positive granulocytes—determined with cytochemical or immunocytochemical staining methods. Peroxidase positive granulocytes are considered to be active inflammatory cells. Increased presence, especially together with other signs of negative effects of inflammatory activity, should lead to full clinical investigation of the man.
Antisperm antibodies	High proportion of spermatozoa with antisperm antibodies should be suspected for inflammatory reactions. Commercially available screening methods are dependent on motile sperm. Therefore, cytotoxic antisperm antibodies cannot be detected with these methods. Low proportions of sperm-binding antisperm antibodies are not considered significant and can be due to unspecific binding.
Semen biochemistry	Zinc (total amount and concentration) reflects the secretory contribution of the prostatic gland (usually ejaculated in the first fractions together with most of the spermatozoa). Fructose (total amount and concentration) reflects the secretory contribution of the seminal vesicles (normally ejaculated after prostatic fluid and most of the spermatozoa). α-Glucosidase (total amount and concentration) reflects the secretory function of the epididymal epithelium and can therefore be of help when evaluating the patency of the duct systems from the testicles.
Sequence of ejaculation—split ejaculate	Useful to explore whether spermatozoa and prostatic fluid are expelled in the first ejaculate fractions without significant addition of seminal vesicular fluid. Spermatozoa expelled mainly with seminal vesicular fluid have a shorter survival, exhibit worse motility, and have a less well-protected sperm chromatin. The latter could increase the vulnerability of the sperm DNA causing problems in the fertilized oocyte and early embryo.

Note that this template does not include consideration of the essential information obtained from interview, physical examination, and other laboratory investigations.

For the interpretation of sperm morphology it is important to know which criteria have been used. Earlier WHO manuals (48,49) described the morphology criteria very differently from the more recent editions (1,50). Furthermore, in the text in the fourth edition (1) there are discrepancies between different parts of the text with regard to definitions of normal and abnormal sperm morphology. A more consistent description can be found in the NAFA-ESHRE manual (2).

Interpretation of Semen Analysis Results

For the clinician to get the most out of a laboratory report with results from semen analysis it could be wise to follow a guideline, such as the one given in Table 2. A summary of common causes for some disorders seen in basic semen analysis is listed in Table 4.

Because of the lack of standardization and not uncommon use of poor techniques and less appropriate equipment by staff with suboptimal training, it is necessary for the clinician not to look at the laboratory report as such. The clinician should also be aware of how the laboratory providing the data has chosen to minimize errors and secure the quality of the service.

Besides these possible technical errors, it is not uncommon that laboratories uncritically adopt "reference ranges" from, for example, the WHO manual (1) but not necessarily concomitant with implementation of the techniques used to obtain the results on which the reference ranges are based. Furthermore, up to and including the fourth edition of the WHO manual, most of the reference limits, given as guidance, appear not to be based on real investigations of fertile men. The WHO manual gives information based on data from recent fathers and men in a general population. Still, the frequency distributions to be published reflect the methods and equipments used and cannot automatically be transferred to other laboratories. Ideally, common EQA should exist for laboratories to exchange and implement reference range data.

For the interpretation of data in comparison with reference limits, it is essential to keep in mind that a distribution of results from recent fathers still does not say very much about the probability that a specific man is subfertile. Results from the two populations—fertile and subfertile men—do overlap considerably. There is an important distinction between *correlation* between a semen parameter and, for example, *fertility success*, and the *predictive value* of the semen parameter. There are correlations between several semen parameters and fertility parameters, but the predictive value for a single parameter is poor. The predictive value of a test tells us whether the single test is useful to guide us in the individual case: a value on one side of the limit means with a certain probability that the man is likely to, for example, cause a pregnancy, whereas a result on the other side of the limit indicates the opposite outcome. It is likely that the use of terms such as teratozoospermia, asthenozoospermia, and oligozoospermia have contributed to the misunderstanding that semen parameters have a predictive value—not the least since these descriptive terms have been linked to specific numerical limits in the laboratory report. It is a severe misconception that "oligozoospermia" of 18 million sperm/mL is significantly different from "normozoospermia" of 22 million sperm/mL. The use of these terms also gives a false impression of semen analysis results as directly diagnostic.

Table 3 A Checklist to Determine Whether a Laboratory Complies with Standardized, Quality Controlled Methods for Semen Analysis

The laboratory uses standard operating procedures (SOPs) with validated methods	Minimum number of cells assessed (usually 400 or 2 × 200) As few dilution variants as possible Duplicate assessments with comparisons to detect random errors As few calculation steps as possible Wet preparations of sufficient depth for free sperm motility Papanicolaou staining adapted for spermatozoa for morphology assessment Sperm vitality staining that does not kill spermatozoa
The laboratory uses proper equipment	Phase contrast optics for unstained spermatozoa Bright field optics (1000–1250×) for stained smears Positive displacement pipettes for withdrawal of exact semen volume for sperm concentration assessment Glass hemocytometer (preferably with improved Neubauer ruling) for counting
All staff trained in a standardized way	Training based on internationally standardized methods, for example, the ESHRE Basic Semen Analysis Course (36) and plenty of in-house training
On-going internal quality control (IQC) as the basis for a continuous quality improvement program	Archives of test material (motility video clips, morphology and vitality slides) for IQC and in-house training Active program for follow-up of IQC results: investigation of causes of deviations, actions taken, and results of actions
Regular participation in an external quality assurance (EQA) program for the main methods	Program for follow-up of EQA results: investigation of causes of deviations, actions taken, and results of actions

Abbreviations: ESHRE: European Society of Human Reproduction and Embryology.

Table 4 A List of Common Causes for Disorders Observed in Basic Semen Analysis

Absence of spermatozoa—with open ducts	• Testicular failure (e.g., Sertoli cell–only syndrome • Endocrine failure (e.g., Kallman's syndrome)
Absence of spermatozoa—hindered passage from the testis	• Congenital bilateral agenesia of the vasa deferentia (CBAVD) • Bilateral postinflammatory atresia of ducts (postepididymitis; bacterial infections)
Decreased number of spermatozoa	• Disturbed production (testicular failure—genetics, failing endocrine stimulation; temporary reduction in testicular function) has been observed as a consequence of heat stress (daily hot baths, pizza bakers) and of severe inflammatory diseases (high fever influenza, general inflammatory conditions; reactions of pharmaceutical drugs, most known example salazopurine in severe inflammatory bowel disease)—usually combined with severe decrease in sperm morphology • Disturbed transport (malformations, unilateral or partial obstruction of duct system, partial retrograde ejaculation—neuropathy, sometimes due to diabetes)
Decreased motility	• Disturbed secretory function in the accessory sex glands, particularly the prostate (e.g., acute prostatitis), but also chronically decreased prostatic function after long-standing inflammations • Disturbed ejaculatory order (delayed emptying of prostatic glands, mixture of spermatozoa with seminal vesicular fluid) • Presence of moderately cytotoxic antisperm antibodies
Absence of motility	• Rare but distinct disorder (dyskinetic cilia syndrome). All sperm tails are stiff; patient often has a long history of chronic and iterated respiratory tract infections (sinusitis, bronchitis, could even be bronchiectasis on X-ray) and sometimes also situs inversus (the Kartagener syndrome) • Spermatozoa dead due to, for instance, cytotoxic antisperm antibodies
Hyperactivated motility in semen sample	• Increased presence of reactive oxygen species, ascribed to increased presence of leukocytes (inflammatory reaction) or extensive tobacco smoking
Presence of blood or red blood cells	• Could be due to active inflammation, but not directly linked to any known pathology. If repeatedly present, examination of a split ejaculate can give indications on the whereabouts of the source as guidance for further clinical investigations
Presence of white blood cells (leukocytes)	• May indicate active inflammation. Further clinical investigation must be done to determine whether, for instance, antibiotics should be given
Abnormal sperm morphology	• Low proportion of spermatozoa with morphology that is typical for spermatozoa that have passed through the cervical mucus and bind to the zona pellucida: decreased probability for pregnancy in vivo or in vitro • Increased average number of abnormalities on each abnormal spermatozoon is also indicative of decreased probability for pregnancy • All sperm with round heads—all lack acrosome and cannot fertilize an oocyte (globozoospermia). A genetic disorder • Increased appearance of amorphous and large sperm heads—may be due to physical stress (inflammatory disorders, see above; heat stress) • Acrosomal defects—besides globozoospermia—ascribed to testicular malfunction of unknown origin • Abnormal cytoplasmic residue is ascribed to disturbed epididymal function and could at least theoretically create problems by increasing the presence of reactive oxygen species because of excess cytoplasm and cell membrane

For a proper diagnosis of disorders in the male reproductive organs causing disturbances in the ejaculate, one cannot dispense with other information (51). A proper interview can tell whether the patient has had mumps after puberty, has a history of cryptorchism, has suffered from a severe infection the last half year, and has been exposed to toxic substances or other such circumstances. A physical examination will give information about secondary sexual characteristics and, for example, testis size, and blood samples for hormone analyses will tell about the function of the hypothalamic-pituitary-testis axis.

Clues to the Interpretation of the Case

It is expected that the reader has realized that the semen analysis report given at the beginning of this chapter is hard to interpret beyond the fact that there are quite many motile and progressively motile sperm.

There is a lack of information about time of abstinence and semen volume, why we actually do not know the total number of sperm. Considering a volume of 0.5 mL, the numbers are very low, but if the volume was 5 mL, the numbers are quite high. The reference limits have been "borrowed" from earlier editions of the WHO manual, and the morphology especially appears to be very poor. However, if strict criteria—as described in the fourth edition (1)—have been used, the results are quite good. In that specific edition of the WHO laboratory manual no reference limits were given for sperm morphology; it does occur that laboratories then use reference ranges from an earlier edition!

Sperm vitality results do not reach the "ideal" level of 75%, but on the other hand the motility is not so high. Vitality results are of interest mainly when there are few or no motile sperm to see whether the immotile sperm are dead or alive.

A strange, but too common, detail is that many results are given with one decimal place. If we consider the uncertainty due to the numbers of cells assessed (Fig. 1), there is at least a variation of ±10%, so the decimal place has no meaning!

KEYNOTES

To interpret semen analysis results, the informed clinician

- ... will ask not only for *sperm concentration*, and *proportions of motile*, *normal* , and *vital sperm*, but also for information about the
  - completeness of sample collection,
  - abstinence time,
  - time between sample collection and assessment, and
  - total semen volume and the total number of sperm in the ejaculate.
- ... *is aware of*
  - the number of sperm the laboratory bases their assessments on,
  - the temperature for motility analysis,
  - the staining procedures for morphology and the criteria used for assessment,
  - the vitality method used,
  - whether internal quality control is used,
  - whether the laboratory participates in an external quality assessment Program.

REFERENCES

1. World Health Organization. Department of Reproductive Health and Research. WHO Laboratory Manual for the Examination and Processing of Human Semen. Geneva: WHO, 2010.
2. Kvist U, Björndahl L, eds. Manual on Basic Semen Analysis. Oxford: Oxford University Press, 2002.
3. Jequier AM, Ukombe EB. Errors inherent in the performance of a routine semen analysis. Br J Urol 1983; 55:434–436.
4. Keel BA, Quinn P, Schmidt CF Jr, et al. Results of the American Association of Bioanalysts national proficiency testing programme in andrology. Hum Reprod (Oxford, England) 2000; 15:680–686.
5. Keel BA, Stembridge TW, Pineda G, et al. Lack of standardization in performance of the semen analysis among laboratories in the United States. Fertil Steril 2002; 78:603–608.
6. Keel BA. How reliable are results from the semen analysis? Fertil Steril 2004; 82:41–44.
7. Riddell D, Pacey A, Whittington K. Lack of compliance by UK andrology laboratories with World Health Organization recommendations for sperm morphology assessment. Hum Reprod (Oxford, England) 2005; 20:3441–3445.
8. Björndahl L, Barratt C, Mortimer D, et al. Practical Guide to Basic Semen Analysis. 1st ed. Cambridge: Cambridge University Press, 2009.
9. Eliasson R. Basic semen analysis. In: Matson P, ed. Current Topics in Andrology. Perth, Australia: Ladybrook Publishing, 2003:35–89.
10. Mortimer D, Shu MA, Tan R, et al. A technical note on diluting semen for the haemocytometric determination of sperm concentration. Hum Reprod (Oxford, England) 1989; 4:166–168.
11. Tomlinson M, Turner J, Powell G, et al. One-step disposable chambers for sperm concentration and motility assessment: how do they compare with the World Health Organization's recommended methods? Hum Reprod (Oxford, England) 2001; 16:121–124.
12. Douglas-Hamilton DH, Smith NG, Kuster CE, et al. Capillary-loaded particle fluid dynamics: effect on estimation of sperm concentration. J Androl 2005; 26:115–122.
13. Douglas-Hamilton DH, Smith NG, Kuster CE, et al. Particle distribution in low-volume capillary-loaded chambers. J Androl 2005; 26;107–114.
14. Hancock P, McLaughlin E. British Andrology Society guidelines for the assessment of post vasectomy semen samples (2002). J Clin Pathol 2002; 55:812–816.
15. Jouannet P, David G. Evolution of the properties of semen immediately following vasectomy. Fertil Steril 1978; 29:435–441.
16. Bedford JM, Zelikovsky G. Viability of spermatozoa in the human ejaculate after vasectomy. Fertil Steril 1979; 32:460–463.
17. Lewis EL, Brazil CK, Overstreet JW. Human sperm function in the ejaculate following vasectomy. Fertil Steril 1984; 42:895–898.
18. Cooper TG, Hellenkemper B, Jonckheere J, et al. Azoospermia: virtual reality or possible to quantify? J Androl 2006; 27:483–490.
19. Verheyen G, Tournaye H, Staessen C, et al. Controlled comparison of conventional in-vitro fertilization and intracytoplasmic sperm injection in patients with asthenozoospermia. Hum Reprod (Oxford, England) 1999; 14:2313–2319.
20. Björndahl L, Söderlund I, Johansson S, et al. Why the WHO recommendations for eosin-nigrosin staining techniques for human sperm vitality assessment must change. J Androl 2004; 25:671–678.
21. Björndahl L, Söderlund I, Kvist U. Evaluation of the one-step eosin-nigrosin staining technique for human sperm vitality assessment. Hum Reprod (Oxford, England) 2003; 18:813–816.

22. Wang FN, Suh BY. Revision of hypo-osmotic swelling (HOS) test with a proposition of classified grading system: its comparisons with four different types of human sperm separation technique. Arch Androl 2005; 51:317–326.
23. Menkveld R, Wong WY, Lombard CJ, et al. Semen parameters, including WHO and strict criteria morphology, in a fertile and subfertile population: an effort towards standardization of in-vivo thresholds. Hum Reprod (Oxford, England) 2001; 16:1165–1171.
24. MacLeod J, Gold RZ. The male factor in fertility and infertility. IV. Sperm morphology in fertile and infertile marriage. Fertil Steril 1951; 2:394–414.
25. Mortimer D, Menkveld R. Sperm morphology assessment—historical perspectives and current opinions. J Androl 2001; 22:192–205.
26. Ombelet W, Pollet H, Bosmans E, et al. Results of a questionnaire on sperm morphology assessment. Hum Reprod (Oxford, England) 1997; 12:1015–1020.
27. Auger J, Eustache F, Ducot B, et al. Intra- and inter-individual variability in human sperm concentration, motility and vitality assessment during a workshop involving ten laboratories. Hum Reprod (Oxford, England) 2000; 15:2360–2368.
28. Brazil C, Swan SH, Drobnis EZ, et al. Standardized methods for semen evaluation in a multicenter research study. J Androl 2004; 25:635–644.
29. Jorgensen N, Auger J, Giwercman A, et al. Semen analysis performed by different laboratory teams: an intervariation study. Int J Androl 1997; 20:201–208.
30. Brazil C, Swan SH, Tollner CR, et al. Quality control of laboratory methods for semen evaluation in a multicenter research study. J Androl 2004; 25:645–656.
31. Björndahl L, Kvist U. Basic semen analysis courses: experience in Scandinavia. In: Ombelet W, Bosmans E, Vandeput H, Vereecken A, Renier M, Hoomans E, eds. Modern ART in the 2000s—Andrology in the nineties. London, UK: The Parthenon Publishing Gorup, 1998:91–101.
32. Punjabi U, Spiessens C. Basic semen analysis courses: experience in Belgium. In: Ombelet W, Bosmans E, Vandeput H, Vereecken A, Renier M, Hoomans E, eds. Modern ART in the 2000s—Andrology in the nineties. London, UK: The Parthenon Publishing Group, 1998:107–113.
33. Vreeburg JTM. Basic semen analysis courses: experience in the Netherlands. In: Ombelet W, Bosmans E, Vandeput H, Vereecken A, Renier M, Hoomans E, eds. Modern ART in the 2000s. New York: The Parthenon Publishing Group, 1998:103–106.
34. Björndahl L, Barratt CL, Fraser LR, et al. ESHRE basic semen analysis courses 1995–1999: immediate beneficial effects of standardized training. Hum Reprod (Oxford, England) 2002; 17:1299–1305.
35. Jorgensen N, Andersen AG, Eustache F, et al. Regional differences in semen quality in Europe. Hum Reprod (Oxford, England) 2001; 16:1012–1019.
36. ESHRE SIGA External Quality Assessment Programme. http://www.eshre.eu/ESHRE/English/Specialty-Groups/SIG/Andrology/External-Quality-Control/page.aspx/104.
37. Dohle GR. Inflammatory-associated obstructions of the male reproductive tract. Andrologia 2003; 35:321–324.
38. Popli K, Stewart J. Infertility and its management in men with cystic fibrosis: review of literature and clinical practices in the UK. Hum Fertil (Cambridge, England) 2007; 10:217–221.
39. MacLeod J, Gold RZ. The male factor in fertility and infertility. V. Effect of continence on semen quality. Fertil Steril 1952; 3:297–315.
40. De Jonge C, LaFromboise M, Bosmans E, et al. Influence of the abstinence period on human sperm quality. Fertil Steril 2004; 82:57–65.
41. Pound N, Javed MH, Ruberto C, et al. Duration of sexual arousal predicts semen parameters for masturbatory ejaculates. Physiol Behav 2002; 76:685–689.
42. van Roijen JH, Slob AK, Gianotten WL, et al. Sexual arousal and the quality of semen produced by masturbation. Hum Reprod (Oxford, England) 1996; 11:147–151.
43. Björndahl L, Kvist U. Sequence of ejaculation affects the spermatozoon as a carrier and its message. Reprod Biomed online 2003; 7:440–448.
44. Hjort T. Do autoantibodies to sperm reduce fecundity? A mini-review in historical perspective. Am J Reprod Immunol 1998; 40:215–222.
45. Vujisic S, Lepej SZ, Jerkovic L, et al. Antisperm antibodies in semen, sera and follicular fluids of infertile patients: relation to reproductive outcome after in vitro fertilization. Am J Reprod Immunol 2005; 54:13–20.
46. Francavilla F, Santucci R, Barbonetti A, et al. Naturally-occurring antisperm antibodies in men: interference with fertility and clinical implications. An update. Front Biosci 2007; 12:2890–2911.
47. Jouannet P, Ducot B, Feneux D, et al. Male factors and the likelihood of pregnancy in infertile couples. I. Study of sperm characteristics. Int J Androl 1988; 11:379–394.
48. Belsey M, Eliasson R, Gallegos AJ, et al. Laboratory Manual for the Examination of Human Semen and Semen-Cervical Mucus Interaction. Singapore: Press Concern, 1980.
49. World Health Organization. WHO Laboratory Manual for the Examination of Human Semen and Sperm-cervical Mucus Interactions. 2nd ed. Cambridge, UK: Cambridge University Press, 1987.
50. World Health Organization. WHO Laboratory Manual for the Examination of Human Semen and Sperm-cervical Mucus Interactions. 3rd ed. Cambridge, UK: Cambridge University Press; 1992.
51. Jequier AM. The importance of diagnosis in the clinical management of infertility in the male. Reprod Biomed Online 2006; 13:331–335.

5 Genetic causes of male infertility and their impact on future generations

Csilla Krausz

INTRODUCTION

The etiology of impaired sperm production and function can be related to different factors acting at pretesticular, post-testicular, or directly at the testicular level (1). Genetic factors can be identified in each etiologic category and some of them are currently part of the diagnostic workup of selected groups of patients (Table 1). Males with impaired sperm production due to genetic anomalies may now benefit from the wide diffusion of assisted reproductive techniques (ART) and may generate their own biological children. This implies that mutations or karyotype anomalies associated with male infertility can be transmitted to the offspring. On the other hand even males with normal karyotype but impaired sperm production are at high risk to be carriers of numerical or structural chromosomal anomalies in their spermatozoa that, depending on the type of anomaly, may lead to fertilization failure, spontaneous abortion, or to offspring with genetic or epigenetic defects. This chapter will focus on genetic factors involved in male infertility and on the consequences of their transmission to future generations.

HERITABILITY OF CONGENITAL ENDOCRINE FORMS OF MALE INFERTILITY

Hypogonadotropic Hypogonadism

A fully efficient hypothalamic–pituitary–gonadal axis is requested for both endocrine and reproductive functions of the testis. Genetic factors causing deficit of gonadotropins (LH, FSH) may act at the hypothalamic or pituitary level and are responsible for the congenital forms of hypogonadotropic hypogonadism. The diagnosis of congenital hypogonadotropic hypogonadism is normally made before adulthood because in the majority of cases it is associated with delayed puberty. However, in some cases reduced spermatogenesis and mild hypoandrogenism may be the only symptoms and thus the diagnosis may be delayed till adulthood. A detailed clinical description of these forms is given in another chapter of this book.

A number of genes can be screened for mutations in **hypogonadotropic hypogonadism** with anosmia (Kallmann syndrome): ***KAL1*** encoding anosmin-1, ***KAL2*** encoding fibroblast growth factor receptor 1 (FGFR1), ***PROKR2*** encoding G protein-coupled prokineticin receptor-2, and ***PROK2*** encoding its ligand, prokineticin-2. On the other hand, *GnRH-R* and *GPR54/KiSS1* genes have been implicated in the etiology of normosmic hypogonadotropic hypogonadism as well as few mutations of the beta subunits of luteinizing hormone (LH) and follicle stimulating hormone (FSH) were described in patients with selective gonadotropin deficiency (see Ref. 2, 3, and 4).

Diagnostic Aspects and Inheritance

From a practical point of view the selection of genes to be screened in a given individual is based on the presence or absence of hyposmia/anosmia and on the type of inheritance patterns in the family. However, in sporadic cases and in normosmic idiopathic hypogonadotropic hypogonadism (IHH), because of the lack of a clear-cut genotype–phenotype correlation, each candidate gene should be tested in a sequential way. Because spermatogenesis can be relatively easily induced by hormonal treatment, genetic screening prior to therapy would be strongly suggested. The treatment with gonadotropins will allow natural conception in the large majority of cases (even with relatively low sperm count), hence the identification of the involved gene can provide a more accurate genetic counseling, i.e., a risk estimation for transmission to the offspring.

The inheritance of Kallmann syndrome can be X-linked (gene *KAL1*), therefore the affected father will transmit the mutation to his daughter who will have a 50% probability to generate a son with Kallmann syndrome, while all other listed genes are autosomal, and the transmission of the disease maybe autosomal dominant (*FGFR1*) or recessive. According to the Mendelian law of inheritance, the chance of generating an affected offspring will be 50% in the former condition, while the probability of disease occurrence in case of recessive inheritance pattern depends on the genetic background of the partner (high risk in case of a consanguinity).

It is difficult to predict the exact phenotype in the next generation, because phenotypic differences are found within carriers of the same mutation in the same family (5).

It is likely that environmental factors or epigenetic phenomena and/or modifier genes may influence the phenotype.

It is also interesting to note that in some cases of IHH, long-term testosterone treatment has lead to spontaneous reversibility of reproductive function (6). It is therefore plausible that in the future, the identification of mutations will have not only diagnostic but also prognostic value for treatment options and responsiveness.

Mutations and Polymorphisms in the Androgen Receptor

The androgen receptor (*AR*) gene is located on the long arm of the X chromosome (Xq11-q12). Mutations in the *AR* gene may result in mild-to-complete androgen insensitivity (7). The phenotypic features of complete androgen insensitivity

Table 1 Diagnostic Genetic Testing in Male Infertility

Gene or region	Indication for testing
Pretesticular	
KAL1	Kallmann syndrome
KAL2 (*FGFR1*)	Kallmann syndrome or normosmic IHH
PROK2/*PROK2R*	Kallmann syndrome or normosmic IHH
GnRHR	IHH (normosmic)
KiSS1/*GPR54*	IHH (normosmic)
FSH	Isolated FSH deficiency
LH	Isolated LH deficiency
Post-testicular	
CFTR	Congenital Absence of Vas Deferens (mono/bilateral) Idiopathic epididymal obstruction
Testicular	
Chromosomal Anomalies (structural or numerical)	Azoospermia or sperm concentration <10 million/mL
Y chromosome microdeletions	Azoospermia or sperm concentration <5 million/mL
AR	Hypoandrogenized infertile male
gr/gr[a]	Oligozoospermia

[a]The diagnostic value of "gr/gr" deletions varies depending on the ethnic background; they are considered "risk factors" in certain populations. IHH: Idiopathic Hypogonadotropic Hypogonadism.

syndrome are female external genitalia and absence of pubic hair (Morris syndrome). In partial androgen insensitivity syndrome (8), several different phenotypes are evident, ranging from predominantly female phenotype (female external genitalia, pubic hair with or without clitoromegaly, and partial-to-completely fused labia) through ambiguous genitalia to predominantly male phenotype with micropenis, perineal hypospadias, and cryptorchidism. The latter phenotype is also termed as Reifenstein syndrome. In the above-mentioned severe forms of androgen resistance there is no risk of transmission because affected men cannot generate their own biological children.

Patients with mild androgen insensitivity syndrome (MAIS) (9) have male infertility as their primary or even sole symptoms.

Only a few mutations have been reported in infertile men (10,11) and most of them were found in the first exon (coding for the transactivation domain of the protein) with predicted reduction of transactivation potential of the mutant protein.

Also a polymorphism in exon 1 of the *AR* gene, called **(CAG)n repeats** (encoding for a polyglutamine stretch) has been extensively studied for its relationship with male infertility. Because in vitro experiments demonstrated that the length of the polyglutamine tract, while remaining within the polymorphic range, is inversely correlated with the transactivation activity of the receptor (12), it was proposed that high (CAG)n repeats may lead to impaired sperm production. Although some studies reported an association between longer polyglutamine stretch and oligozoospermia, the large majority of studies failed to find such a relationship (13–15).

Diagnostic Aspects and Genetic Counseling in MAIS

A standard indication for *AR* mutation should be based on the phenotype (hypoandrogenization) and high Androgen Sensitivity Index (ASI). However, in case of MAIS there has been no correlation between the type of *AR* mutation and the subtype of infertility (azoospermia, oligozoospermia, or oligoteratozoospermia) and not all carriers had high ASI. Apart from the difficulty to preselect patients for the analysis, the need for routine testing in infertile subjects without high ASI is further questioned by reports in which none or very few mutations were detected in large series of idiopathic infertile men (16,17). Similarly, given the lack of a cutoff value for (CAG)n repeat number with clear association with impaired sperm production, the screening for this polymorphism is not performed as a routine genetic analysis in idiopathic infertile men. Also, in *AR* mutation screening, this polymorphism can be analyzed in selected cases in which mild androgen insensitivity is suspected.

In case a functionally relevant mutation responsible for impaired sperm production is detected in the *AR* gene, the mutation can be transmitted through ART from the affected father to his daughter, who will transmit MAIS to her male descendent with a 50% probability. Concerning the (CAG)n repeat polymorphism, because of the well-known phenomenon of microsatellite instability, (CAG)n too are prone to further expansion which may exceed the polymorphic range (8–39). Consequently, the transmission of a long polyglutamine stretch near the upper limits of the polymorphic range to the female offspring, represents a potential risk for Kennedy syndrome (lethal spinobulbar atrophy) in her male descendents if the expansion will be >40 repeats. The probability to transmit the paternal X chromosome is 50% but still the exact risk estimation for Kennedy syndrome is difficult because both expansion and contraction phenomenon may occur during meiosis and their entity is unpredictable.

POST-TESTICULAR FORMS OF MALE INFERTILITY DUE TO *CFTR* MUTATION

The autosomal *CFTR* (*cystic fibrosis transmembrane conductance regulator*) gene (7q31.2) (18,19) is highly mutated with more than 1500 mutations and variants described in the gene bank. Depending on the severity of the reduction of functionally normal CFTR protein, the phenotype can be cystic fibrosis (CF) (generally due to the presence of two "severe" mutations) or "mild forms" of CF (combination of less severe mutations with a consequent reduction of functional CFTR protein below 50% but above 10%); congenital agenesis of vas deferens (CAVD) is considered a "mild form" of CF (20,21). The most widely diffused mutation both in CF and CAVD is the severe delta F508 mutation (about 70% of the total CF mutations in patients). The role of intron-8 variants (IVS8–5T, IVS8–7T, IVS8–9T) in the phenotypic expression of mutations is now well established. The three variants include different numbers of thymidines within the acceptor splice site of intron 8, i.e,. 5, 7, and 9, respectively. The length of the T tract affects the splicing efficiency of exon 9 and thus the percent of normal CFTR mRNA. The 5T tract is less efficient and allows about 8% to 10% of CFTR mRNA to be completed with exon 9. The lack of exon 9 leads to a nonfunctional Cl channel and thus the combination of 5T with other mutations (severe or mild) may cause the development of CF or CAVD, respectively. There is a five- to sixfold increase in the frequency of the 5T variant among CAVD chromosomes (21).

Genetic Testing and Counseling

Currently the *CFTR* mutation screening should be limited to obstructive defects which can be correlated to the reduction of functional CFTR protein, i.e., CAVD and idiopathic epydidymal obstruction. Given that the frequency of a particular CF mutation is variable between different geographic areas and shows important ethnic differences, the routine mutation screening is based on a panel of mutations (normally 30) which are the most common for a given population. Because the 5T-tract variant is now considered a mild *CFTR* mutation rather than a polymorphism, it should be analyzed in each CAVD patient.

Patients affected by CAVD may have sperm in their ejaculate (monolateral absence of vas deferens) or be azoospermic (congenital bilateral absence of vas deferens; CBAVD). All patients with CF have CBAVD. Thanks to the possibility to combine testis biospy (22) with intracytoplasmic sperm injection (ICSI), both CF or CBAVD patients may now generate their own biologial children therefore they can transmit their *CFTR* mutations to their descendents. Because the carrier frequency of *CFTR* mutations in persons with Northern European descent is high (1:25), the screening for CF gene mutations in the female partners of men with CAVD without congenital kidney anomalies or with CF should be performed before assisted reproduction. If mutations are detected in both partners (possibly performing a whole gene screening), the risk of an offspring with CF (or mild forms of CF such as CAVD, depending on the type and combination of mutations) is very high so preimplantation genetic diagnosis (PGD) should be advised to the couple. However, in most cases it remains difficult to make precise risk estimates due to the different degree of penetrance of the same genotype between different individuals (23).

GENETIC FACTORS ACTING AT THE TESTICULAR LEVEL

Genetic anomalies related to primitive testicular failure can be detected in leukocytes or directly in spermatozoa. Among the firsts, karyotype evaluation and Y chromosome microdeletion screening have become routine genetic tests for men with severe spermatogenic failure. Among the seconds, sperm DNA integrity testing and sperm aneuploidy analysis by fluorescence in situ hybridization (FISH) should be advised only for distinct pathologies.

Chromosomal Abnormalities

Karyotype abnormalities occur in about 0.4% of the general population and can affect the number or the structure of chromosomes. The majority of chromosome abnormalities are generated during meiosis. Severely impaired sperm production is associated with a significantly higher frequency of both numerical and structural chromosomopathies (24).

The more severe is the testicular phenotype, the higher is the frequency of chromosomal abnormalities. Patients with spermatozoa <10 million/mL show already a 10 times higher incidence (4%) of mainly autosomal structural abnormalities in respect to the general population. Among severe oligozoospermic men (with spermatozoa <5 million/mL), the frequency increases to 7%, whereas in nonobstructive azoospermic men it reaches the highest value, 15%. Klinefelter syndrome (47,XXY) represents the most common karyotype abnormality in severe male factor infertility, followed by Y chromosome terminal deletions (Yq-) and structural autosomal abnormalities.

Sperm Chromosome Abnormalities

The human sperm–hamster oocyte fusion system is used to analyze in detail sperm chromosomes (sperm karyotyping). Using this method it has been clearly demonstrated in normal controls that structural abnormalities are more common (average of 6–7%) than numerical chromosome abnormalities (1–2%) in spermatozoa (25). However, despite the fact that this technique is used to study each individual chromosome, its elevated cost and time consumption, the difficulty of performing the assay, the necessity of providing hamster oocytes, lead to the rapid diffusion of a faster and easier (although still rather expensive) method such as the sperm–FISH analysis with chromosome-specific DNA probes. This method does not assess structural anomalies and is currently limited to five to nine probes per sample, which can make interpretation of the results difficult (26). After using this method it became clear that even subjects with normal chromosomal constitution in their lymphocytes, but affected by infertility, have an increased risk for sperm autosomal and sex chromosomal abnormalities (varying from 2–10 times higher than controls). Specific infertile phenotypes are at even higher risk than others such as round-head only syndrome, macrocephaly, or a high percentage of multiflagellated sperm (25).

Klinefelter Syndrome

Klinefelter syndrome is the most common sex chromosome abnormality in humans with an incidence of 1 in 600 live births and 1 in 300 spontaneous abortion (27). It is also the most frequent chromosomal anomaly in azoospermic men (14%). About 80% of patients bear a 47,XXY karyotype, whereas the other 20% are represented either by 47,XXY/46,XY mosaics or higher grade sex chromosomal aneuploidy or structurally abnormal X chromosome (28).

The clinical description of this syndrome is provided in other chapters of this book.

Genetic Counseling

Although the large majority of subjects affected by Klinefelter syndrome are azoospermic, they may generate their own genetic children by undergoing TESE/ICSI, because they have an average of 30% to 50% of testicular sperm recovery rate (28–32). Moreover, spermatozoa can be even found in the ejaculate of mainly mosaic patients or in nonmosaic but young patients (28), indicating the potential importance of an early diagnosis. Although men in their early twenties may not desire immediate conception, a preventive sperm cryopreservation of ejaculated spermatozoa should be a correct way to preserve their fertility. Based on sperm–FISH studies showing an increased frequency of sex chromosomal abnormalities and increased incidence of autosomal aneuploidies (disomy for chromosomes 13, 18, and 21), concerns have been raised about the chromosomal normality of the embryos generated through ICSI (see Ref. 33 and references therein). To date, 49 healthy children have been born using ICSI without PGD and the conception of one 47,XXY fetus has been reported (see Ref. 34, 35, and references therein). However, a study based on ICSI combined with PGD on 113 embryos shows that there is a significant fall in the rate of normal embryos for couples with Klinefelter syndrome, in respect to controls (54% vs. 77.2%). Due to the significant increase of sex chromosomal and autosomal abnormalities in the embryos of Klinefelter patients, ICSI along with PGD should be strongly advised (34).

Autosomal Abnormalities

The most frequently found autosomal karyotype abnormalities are Robertsonian translocations, reciprocal translocations, paracentric inversions, and marker chromosomes. Robertsonian translocation consists of the fusion of two acrocentric chromosomes and the most frequent combinations are t(13;14) and t(14;21). This abnormality is rarely observed in azoospermic men (0.2%) but is often found in oligozoospermic patients (about nine times higher in infertile men than in newborns). However, since Robertsonian translocations have been found also in normospermic fertile males in the same pedigree (36), the contribution of this chromosomal defect to disturbed spermatogenesis remains to be clarified. Reciprocal translocations are defined as an exchange of chromosome material between arms of two nonhomologous chromosomes; usually the exchange is conservative without loss of genetic material. The frequency of balanced reciprocal translocations is estimated to be 5 to 10 times higher in infertile men than in the general population. Pericentric inversions result from two breaks within a single chromosome followed by a 180° rotation of the chromatin between these breaks. These rearrangements are 13 times higher in infertile men and probably interfere with meiosis, leading to a reduced rate of postmeiotic sperm development.

Genetic Counseling

The importance of the detection of these structural chromosomal anomalies is related to the increased risk of aneuploidy or unbalanced chromosomal complements in the fetus. Translocations and inversions may affect the sperm genome by altering both the dosage of genes by the production of spermatozoa with an unbalanced translocation, or by affecting meiotic segregation negatively and inducing generalized aneuploidy (37,38). The percentage of unbalanced spermatozoa varies according to the translocation and a normal cutoff level for a good prognosis with PGD would be approximately 65% unbalanced spermatozoa (39,40). Sperm–FISH analysis and/or PGD should be performed to give a more accurate risk estimation of affected offspring. In case of Robertsonian translocations, a special risk is represented by uniparental disomies that are generated through a mechanism called "trisomy rescue" (repairing of trisomy) during the first division of the zygote. For chromosome 14 (the most frequently involved chromosome) and 15, both paternal and maternal uniparental disomies are pathological and give rise to severe disease such as Angelman syndrome or Prader–Willi syndrome despite an apparently normal or balanced karyotype.

Other Chromosomal Abnormalities

47,XYY Male

The frequency of males with this karyotype is 1:750. Carriers of this abnormality show a great diversity in the degree of spermatogenic impairment, ranging from severe oligozoospermia to apparent normality (41). Distortion of sex vesicle formation is probably the major cause of disturbed spermatogenesis in these men (42).

XX-male

This is a disorder of sex determination and occurs in about 1:20,000 newborns. In about 80% of cases, XX maleness can be explained by the translocation of the SRY gene (encoding the testis-determining factor) (43) to the X chromosome. The cause of SRY-negative XX maleness remains to be elucidated (44,45).

The phenotypic features of the syndrome are gynecomastia, female hair pattern, and small testes with azoospermia. Genital malformations such as hypospadias are rare. In SRY-negative patients, ambiguous genitalia is a frequent finding (46).

Aneuploidies of autosomes

Most numerical aneuploidies of autosomes are lethal. Patients affected by Down's syndrome may be either fertile or infertile (47).

The Y Chromosome–Linked Infertility

The long arm of the human Y chromosome (Yq) hosts a number of genes involved in spermatogenesis and several types of

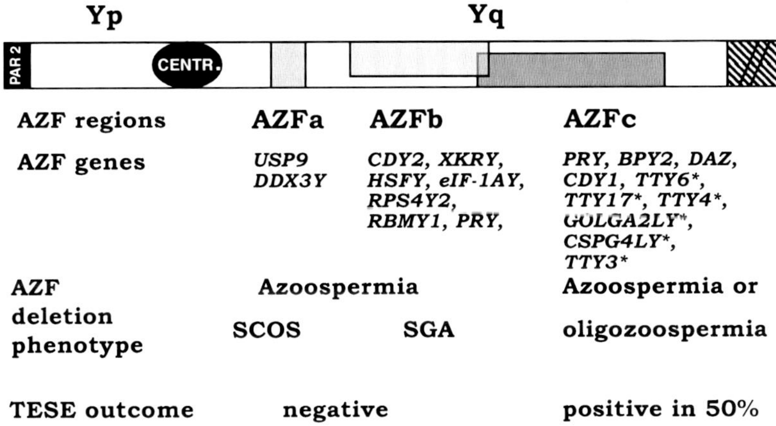

Figure 1 Schematic representation of the Y chromosome and genotype–phenotype correlation. Genes of the three AZoospermia Factor (AZF) regions are listed. Transcription unit families are indicated with asterisk (*). Deletions of these regions result in spermatogenic failure. AZFb deletions (two subtypes) overlap with the AZFc region. Yq: long arm of the Y chromosome; Yp: short arm of the Y chromosome; PAR: pseudoautosomal region; SCOS: Sertoli Cell-Only Syndrome; SGA: SpermatoGenic Arrest; TESE: Testicular Sperm Extraction.

recurrent Yq deletions are firmly associated with spermatogenic failure (Fig. 1) (see Ref. 48, 49, 50, and references therein). However, such observations do not allow attribution of spermatogenic function to any particular Y chromosome–encoded protein, because each of these deletions removes multiple genes. Despite the efforts of many laboratories only four cases of confirmed isolated Yq gene mutation have been reported to date, and all are related to the AZFa region (51–54).

The rarity of single azoospermia factor (AZF) gene mutations or deletions is in sharp contrast with the relatively high frequency of AZF deletions (classically divided into three regions, AZFa, AZFb, and AZFc) (55) which represent the most frequent molecular genetic cause of azoospermia and severe oligozoospermia (spermatozoa <5 million/mL) (see Ref. 56 and references therein). A likely explanation is that the peculiar structure and the sequence organization of the Y chromosome make prone this chromosome to the loss of large regions such as the AZF regions (50).

The clinical significance of Yq deletions have been debated for a long time mainly because of the large variability in deletion frequencies reported by different authors and because Yq deletions have also been reported in "fertile" men. After more than 10 years of clinical research, it can be now concluded that: (*i*)Y deletions were not found in normospermic men and thus have a clear-cut cause–effect relationship with spermatogenic failure (49); (*ii*) the highest frequency is found in azoospermic men (8–12%) followed by oligospermic men (3–7%); (*iii*) deletions are extremely rare with a sperm concentration of spermatozoa >5 million/mL (approximately 0.7%); (*iv*) the most frequently deleted region is AZFc (approximately 65–70%), followed by deletions of the AZFb and AZFb+c or AZFa+b+c regions (25–30%), whereas deletions of the AZFa region are extremely rare (5%); (*v*) the complete removal of the AZFa and AZFb regions are associated with severe testicular phenotype, Sertoli cell-only syndrome and spermatogenic arrest, respectively. The complete removal of the AZFc region causes a variable phenotype, which may range from azoospermia to oligozoospermia.

The specificity and the above-reported genotype–phenotype correlation confers to Y deletion analysis a diagnostic and a prognostic value for testicular sperm retrieval (56).

Genetic Counseling

Those Y deletions that are compatible with the presence of spermatozoa in the testis or in the ejaculate, are obligatory transmitted to the male offspring, therefore genetic counseling is mandatory. The extent of spermatogenic failure of the son may vary substantially, however, given the strict cause–effect relationship between AZF deletions and impaired spermatogenesis, normal spermatogenesis cannot be expected.

We and others have reported that a significant proportion of spermatozoa from men with Y microdeletion are nullisomic for sex chromosomes (57,58).

This result indicates a potential risk for the offspring to develop 45,X0 Turner's syndrome and other phenotypic anomalies associated with sex chromosome mosaicism, including ambiguous genitalia. The screening for Y chromosome microdeletions in patients bearing a mosaic 46,XY/45,X0 karyotype with sexual ambiguity and/or Turner stigmata, has shown a relatively high incidence of AZFc deletions (33%) (59). Additional data (60,61) support that Yq microdeletions could be associated with an overall Y chromosomal instability leading to the formation of 45,X0 cell lines.

Despite this theoretical risk, the 36 babies (18 male and 18 female) born from fathers affected by Yq microdeletions are phenotypically normal (see Ref. 56, 62, and references therein). This could be due to the reduced implantation rate and a likely higher risk of spontaneous abortions of embryos bearing a 45,X0 karyotype. However, only PGD together with the abortion rate would provide a more accurate estimation about the real risks of 46,XY/45,X0 mosaicism and Turner's syndrome.

PGD can be offered to the couple both for sex selection and for avoiding the transfer of 45,X0 embryos. The first indication may raise some ethical concerns because infertility may not be considered a disease, whereas the second remains a theoretical indication in the absence of any direct evidence.

The gr/gr Deletions of the AZFc Region

It is now widely accepted that complete deletions of the AZFc region (b2/b4 deletion) is the most common known genetic cause of spermatogenic failure. Recently, new types of AZFc deletions, called "partial deletions," have been reported (63) that remove approximately half of the AZFc gene content, including two *DAZ* copies and one *CDY1* copy. Among them, gr/gr partial deletion is considered a genetic risk factor for spermatogenic impairment by a number of research groups, including ours (64–66), while "b2/b3" and "b1/b3" deletions seem to not to have significant effects on male fertility with the exception of one study in the Han Chinese population (see Refs. 66, 67, and references therein).

Genetic Counseling

Given that fathers bearing gr/gr deletion will obligatory transmit this genetic variant (together with their Y background) to the male offspring, it is likely that their sons will have a similar spermatogenic disturbance in the future. gr/gr deletions are more likely to cause oligozoospermia than azoospermia, and the calculated OR in our central Italian population (1043 subjects tested) is OR = 7.9 (95% CI 1.8−33.8) (65). Thus, gr/gr deletion screening should be introduced among genetic diagnostic tests in those ethnic groups in which it resulted as a significant risk factor, especially prior to ART (64,65).

Gene Mutations and Polymorphisms

A number of autosomal and X-linked spermatogenesis candidate genes have been identified (mainly based on animal models) and they represent the most obvious target for mutation analysis in men with spermatogenic failure. The screening for mutations in genes with predicted specific spermatogenic function did not allow the identification of clinically relevant mutations. An overview on this topic is given in a recent review by Nuti and Krausz (68). The paucity of gene mutations in male infertility is surprising if we consider that the expected number of genes involved in spermatogenesis has been calculated to be over 1000 (69). Whether this is due to the real rarity of gene mutations or due to the inappropriateness of the currently used approaches, remains to be established.

Polymorphisms are genetic variants with a frequency of $>1\%$ in the general population. They can be divided into structural polymorphisms of the genome (deletions, duplications, gene copy number variants), single nucleotide polymorphisms and microsatellites (70). Polymorphisms should be considered as risk factors rather than direct etiological causes for spermatogenic disturbances or male infertility. It is likely that they lead to testicular dysfunction only in association with a specific genetic background or with environmental factors (71). Similarly, in many other fields of medicine, the search for genetic risk factors in male infertility reached to rather disappointing results. Published studies are all based on case–control association studies and are focusing on distinct genes, or rarely on a group of functionally related genes. In many cases, only sporadic data are available, or when more studies are published on the same polymorphism, results are often contradictory. Inadequate sample size, pathogenetic heterogeneity of infertility, inappropriate control subjects, and ethnic–geographic differences (probably related also to environmental factors) may be responsible for discrepancies among case–control studies (67). With the exception of the gr/gr deletions and the MTHFR 677C>T polymorphism, no other polymorphisms have clinical relevance (72).

EPIGENETIC ASPECTS OF MALE INFERTILITY

Epigenetic genomic control encompasses all of the mechanisms by which regulation of genes can be attained without any additional alterations on part of the DNA sequence. Epigenetic reprogramming of germ cells is responsible for the phenomenon of imprinting. This process regulates the mode of inheritance of some genes in a monoallelic fashion by transcriptionally silencing one of the homologue genes, dependent on its parental origin. DNA methylation is an epigenetic regulator of gene expression and acts as an important molecular mark underlying the parental specific expression of genes subject to genomic imprinting. DNA methylation is the most widely studied epigenetic modification. A number of genes regulated by imprinting contain differential methylation regions inherited from the gametes (73,74). Imprint resetting involves erasure of imprints in the primordial germ cells and the acquisition of new sex-specific imprints. To date only few studies have focused on the analysis of imprinting abnormalities in spermatozoa. Two studies focusing on single imprinted domain gave contradictory results, one reporting abnormal imprinting of H19 in oligozoospermic patients (75), whereas the other found appropriate genomic imprinting in infertile men (76). A recent study examined 7 imprinted genes in 97 infertile men and found both abnormal paternal and maternal methylation imprint (14.4% and 20.6%, respectively), mainly in patients with moderate or severe oligozoospermia. Although the outcome of ART with sperm shown to have methylation errors was generally poor, one child with normal appearance was conceived by ICSI from men bearing spermatozoa with abnormal paternal and maternal imprints (77).

The importance of nonequivalence of the parental genomes and their different developmental roles is clearly shown both in animal models and in humans in relationship with uniparental disomies for individual chromosomes or chromosomal regions. Uniparental disomies (discussed under section autosomal abnormalities) lead to a broad range of phenotypic abnormalities. Disorders related to epigenetic dysregulation can be roughly divided into three clinical categories: defects in growth and development, neurology disorders, and hormonal and metabolic disorders.

New insights into the epigenetic contributions of sperm chromatin to embryo development have been recently provided by Carrell and co-workers (78) showing that epigenetic marking in sperm is extensive, and correlated with developmental regulators. Since some studies have suggested that there is an increased incidence of rare imprinting disorders in babies conceived by ART (79–83), and clearly men affected by spermatogenetic impairment have a higher risk for both being carriers of chromosomal anomalies and of sperm methylation errors, there is an urgent need for further research in this field (see Ref. 84 and references therein).

CONCLUSIONS

Infertility in both men and women is closely associated with genetic risks. Both constitutional and sperm chromosomal abnormalities (aneuploidies or structural chromosomal abnormalities) are more frequent in men with impaired sperm production than in normospermic subjects. These abnormalities have a profound effect on the outcome of ART, on abortion rate, and on the rate of congenital malformations. It is well known that ICSI babies have a higher risk of *de novo* sex chromosomal aberrations and paternally inherited structural abnormalities (85). Given the higher rate of sperm chromosomal anomalies in infertile men, they are at higher risk to transmit chromosomal anomalies to the offspring and thus to generate children with mental and physical disabilities or infertility. In the diagnostic setting of the infertile male it is now very important that couples be adequately counseled about their increased risks.

In specific cases, such as impaired sperm production related to Y chromosome microdeletions, infertility will be obligatory transmitted to the male offspring. In case of autosomal gene mutations such as *CFTR* mutation much care must be taken for the screening of the partner in order to provide an accurate estimate for the risk of CF.

Although a large proportion of men with idiopathic infertility are likely to be carriers of genetic anomalies, the screening for mutations in genes with predicted specific spermatogenic function did not allow the identification of clinically relevant mutations or risk factors. Up to now candidate spermatogenesis genes have been identified mainly through model organisms, expression studies, linkage analysis, or cytogenetic findings (see Ref. 86). Recently, transcriptomics and proteomics approaches started to be applied also in this field and opened a new perspective to the understanding of male infertility (87–89). Similarly, a substantial advancement is expected with the use of array-based SNP typing (90) and analysis of large cohorts of patients and controls, which already have lead to the identification of genetic risk factors for various other complex diseases (91).

REFERENCES

1. Forti G, Krausz C. Clinical review 100: Evaluation and treatment of the infertile couple. J Clin Endocrinol Metab 1998; 83(12):4177–4188.
2. Huhtaniemi I, Alevizaki M. Mutations along the hypothalamic-pituitary-gonadal axis affecting male reproduction. Reprod Biomed Online 2007; 15(6):622–632.
3. Layman LC. Hypogonadotropic hypogonadism. Endocrinol Metab Clin North Am 2007; 36(2):283–296.
4. Trarbach EB, Silveira LG, Latronico AC. Genetic insights into human isolated gonadotropin deficiency. Pituitary 2007; 10(4):381–391.
5. Beranova M, Oliveira LM, Bedecarrats GY, et al. Prevalence, phenotypic spectrum, and modes of inheritance of gonadotropin-releasing hormone receptor mutations in idiopathic hypogonadotropic hypogonadism. J Clin Endocrinol Metab 2001; 86(4):1580–1588.
6. Pitteloud N, Acierno JS Jr., Meysing AU, et al. Reversible Kallmann syndrome, delayed puberty, and isolated anosmia occurring in a single family with a mutation in the fibroblast growth factor receptor 1 gene. J Clin Endocrinol Metab 2005; 90(3):1317–1322.
7. Quigley CA, De Bellis A, Marschke KB, et al. Androgen receptor defects: historical, clinical, and molecular perspectives. Endocr Rev 1995; 16(3):271–321.
8. Pais VM, Vasudevan P. Infertility in an XX male. J Urol 1977; 118(4):690–691.
9. Higuchi RI, Arienti KL, Lopez FJ, et al. Novel series of potent, nonsteroidal, selective androgen receptor modulators based on 7H-[1,4]oxazino[3,2-g]quinolin-7-ones. J Med Chem 2007; 50(10):2486–2496.
10. Gottlieb B, Beitel LK, Wu JH, et al. The androgen receptor gene mutations database (ARDB): 2004 update. Hum Mutat 2004; 23(6):527–533.
11. Ferlin A, Vinanzi C, Garolla A, et al. Male infertility and androgen receptor gene mutations: clinical features and identification of seven novel mutations. Clin Endocrinol (Oxf) 2006; 65(5):606–610.
12. Tut TG, Ghadessy FJ, Trifiro MA, et al. Long polyglutamine tracts in the androgen receptor are associated with reduced trans-activation, impaired sperm production, and male infertility. J Clin Endocrinol Metab 1997; 82(11):3777–3782.
13. Dowsing AT, Yong EL, Clark M, et al. Linkage between male infertility and trinucleotide repeat expansion in the androgen-receptor gene. Lancet 1999; 354(9179):640–643.
14. Rajpert-De Meyts E, Leffers H, Petersen JH, et al. CAG repeat length in androgen-receptor gene and reproductive variables in fertile and infertile men. Lancet 2002; 359(9300):44–46.
15. Asatiani K, von Eckardstein S, Simoni M, et al. CAG repeat length in the androgen receptor gene affects the risk of male infertility. Int J Androl 2003; 26(5):255–261.
16. Rajender S, Singh L, Thangaraj K. Phenotypic heterogeneity of mutations in androgen receptor gene. Asian J Androl 2007; 9(2):147–179.
17. Singh R, Shastry PK, Rasalkar AA, et al. A novel androgen receptor mutation resulting in complete androgen insensitivity syndrome and bilateral Leydig cell hyperplasia. J Androl 2006; 27(4):510–516.
18. Riordan JR, Rommens JM, Kerem B, et al. Identification of the cystic fibrosis gene: cloning and characterization of complementary DNA. Science 1989; 245(4922):1066–1073.

19. Kerem B, Rommens JM, Buchanan JA, et al. Identification of the cystic fibrosis gene: genetic analysis. Science 1989; 245(4922):1073–1080.
20. Dumur V, Gervais R, Rigot JM, et al. Abnormal distribution of CF delta F508 allele in azoospermic men with congenital aplasia of epididymis and vas deferens. Lancet 1990; 336(8713):512.
21. Patrizio P, Leonard DG. Mutations of the cystic fibrosis gene and congenital absence of the vas deferens. Results Probl Cell Differ 2000; 28:175–186.
22. Ottesen AM, Garn ID, Aksglaede L, et al. A simple screening method for detection of Klinefelter syndrome and other X-chromosome aneuploidies based on copy number of the androgen receptor gene. Mol Hum Reprod 2007; 13(10):745–750.
23. Cuppens H, Cassiman JJ. CFTR mutations and polymorphisms in male infertility. Int J Androl 2004; 27(5):251–256.
24. Vincent MC, Daudin M, De MP, et al. Cytogenetic investigations of infertile men with low sperm counts: a 25-year experience. J Androl 2002; 23(1):18–22; discussion 44–45.
25. Martin RH. Meiotic errors in human oogenesis and spermatogenesis. Reprod Biomed Online 2008; 16(4):523–531.
26. Carrell DT, Emery BR. Use of automated imaging and analysis technology for the detection of aneuploidy in human sperm. Fertil Steril 2007; 90(2):434–437.
27. Nielsen J, Wohlert M. Chromosome abnormalities found among 34,910 newborn children: results from a 13-year incidence study in Arhus, Denmark. Hum Genet 1991; 87(1):81–83.
28. Kamischke A, Baumgardt A, Horst J, et al. Clinical and diagnostic features of patients with suspected Klinefelter syndrome. J Androl 2003; 24(1):41–48.
29. Tournaye H, Liu J, Nagy PZ, et al. Correlation between testicular histology and outcome after intracytoplasmic sperm injection using testicular spermatozoa. Hum Reprod 1996; 11(1):127–132.
30. Westlander G, Ekerhovd E, Bergh C. Low levels of serum inhibin B do not exclude successful sperm recovery in men with nonmosaic Klinefelter syndrome. Fertil Steril 2003; 79(suppl 3):1680–1682.
31. Westlander G, Ekerhovd E, Granberg S, et al. Testicular ultrasonography and extended chromosome analysis in men with nonmosaic Klinefelter syndrome: a prospective study of possible predictive factors for successful sperm recovery. Fertil Steril 2001; 75(6):1102–1105.
32. Rucker GB, Mielnik A, King P, et al. Preoperative screening for genetic abnormalities in men with nonobstructive azoospermia before testicular sperm extraction. J Urol 1998; 160(6, pt 1):2068–2071.
33. Martin RH. Clinical relevance of sperm aneuploidy. In: Carrell DT, ed. The Genetics of Male Infertility. Totowa, NJ: Humana Press, 2007; 129–144.
34. Staessen C, Tournaye H, Van Assche E, et al. PGD in 47,XXY Klinefelter's syndrome patients. Hum Reprod Update 2003; 9(4):319–330.
35. Lanfranco F, Kamischke A, Zitzmann M, et al. Klinefelter's syndrome. Lancet 2004; 364(9430):273–283.
36. Chandley AC, Edmond P, Christie S, et al. Cytogenetics and infertility in man. I. Karyotype and seminal analysis: results of a five-year survey of men attending a subfertility clinic. Ann Hum Genet 1975; 39(2):231–254.
37. Carrell DT. Contributions of spermatozoa to embryogenesis: assays to evaluate their genetic and epigenetic fitness. Reprod Biomed Online 2008; 16(4):474–484.
38. Gianaroli L, Magli MC, Ferraretti AP, et al. Possible interchromosomal effect in embryos generated by gametes from translocation carriers. Hum Reprod 2002; 17(12):3201–3207.
39. Escudero T, Lee M, Carrel D, et al. Analysis of chromosome abnormalities in sperm and embryos from two 45,XY,t(13;14)(q10;q10) carriers. Prenat Diagn 2000; 20(7):599–602.
40. Munne S. Analysis of chromosome segregation during preimplantation genetic diagnosis in both male and female translocation heterozygotes. Cytogenet Genome Res 2005; 111(3–4):305–309.
41. Skakkebaek NE, Zeuthen E, Nielsen J, et al. Abnormal spermatogenesis in XYY males: a report on 4 cases ascertained through a population study. Fertil Steril 1973; 24(5):390–395.
42. Berthelsen JG, Skakkebaek N, Perboll O. Electron microscopic demonstration of the extra Y chromosome in spermatocytes from human XYY males. In: Byskov AG, Peters H, eds. Development and Function of Reproductive Organs. Amsterdam: The Nertherlands: Excerpta Medica, 1981:328–337.
43. Sinclair AH, Berta P, Palmer MS, et al. A gene from the human sex-determining region encodes a protein with homology to a conserved DNA-binding motif. Nature 1990; 346(6281):240–244.
44. McElreavey K, Barbaux S, Ion A, et al. The genetic basis of murine and human sex determination: a review. Heredity 1995; 75 (Pt 6):599–611.
45. Lalli E, Ohe K, Latorre E, et al. Sexy splicing: regulatory interplays governing sex determination from Drosophila to mammals. J Cell Sci 2003; 116(pt 3):441–445.
46. Abbas NE, Toublanc JE, Boucekkine C, et al. A possible common origin of "Y-negative" human XX males and XX true hermaphrodites. Hum Genet 1990; 84(4):356–360.
47. Zuhlke C, Thies U, Braulke I, et al. Down syndrome and male fertility: PCR-derived fingerprinting, serological and andrological investigations. Clin Genet 1994; 46(4):324–326.
48. McElreavey K, Krausz C. Sex Chromosome Genetics '99. Male infertility and the Y chromosome. Am J Hum Genet 1999; 64(4):928–933.

49. Krausz C, Forti G, McElreavey K. The Y chromosome and male fertility and infertility. Int J Androl 2003; 26(2):70–75.
50. Skaletsky H, Kuroda-Kawaguchi T, Minx PJ, et al. The male-specific region of the human Y chromosome is a mosaic of discrete sequence classes. Nature 2003; 423(6942):825–837.
51. Brown GM, Furlong RA, Sargent CA, et al. Characterisation of the coding sequence and fine mapping of the human DFFRY gene and comparative expression analysis and mapping to the Sxrb interval of the mouse Y chromosome of the Dffry gene. Hum Mol Genet 1998; 7(1):97–107.
52. Sun C, Skaletsky H, Birren B, et al. An azoospermic man with a de novo point mutation in the Y-chromosomal gene USP9Y. Nat Genet 1999; 23(4):429–432.
53. Krausz C, Degl'Innocenti S, Nuti F, et al. Natural transmission of USP9Y gene mutations: a new perspective on the role of AZFa genes in fertility. Hum Mol Genet 2006; 15(18):2673–2681.
54. Tyler-Smith C, Krausz C. The will-o-the-wisp of genetics–hunting for the azoospermia factor gene. N Engl J Med 2009; 360(9):925–927.
55. Vogt PH, Edelmann A, Kirsch S, et al. Human Y chromosome azoospermia factors (AZF) mapped to different subregions in Yq11. Hum Mol Genet 1996; 5(7):933–943.
56. Krausz C, Degl'Innocenti S. Y chromosome and male infertility: update, 2006. Front Biosci 2006; 11:3049–3061.
57. Siffroi JP, Le Bourhis C, Krausz C, et al. Sex chromosome mosaicism in males carrying Y chromosome long arm deletions. Hum Reprod 2000; 15(12):2559–2562.
58. Jaruzelska J, Korcz A, Wojda A, et al. Mosaicism for 45,X cell line may accentuate the severity of spermatogenic defects in men with AZFc deletion. J Med Genet 2001; 38(11):798–802.
59. Patsalis PC, Sismani C, Quintana-Murci L, et al. Effects of transmission of Y chromosome AZFc deletions. Lancet 2002; 360(9341):1222–1224.
60. Patsalis PC, Skordis N, Sismani C, et al. Identification of high frequency of Y chromosome deletions in patients with sex chromosome mosaicism and correlation with the clinical phenotype and Y-chromosome instability. Am J Med Genet A 2005; 135(2):145–149.
61. Le Bourhis C, Siffroi JP, McElreavey K, et al. Y chromosome microdeletions and germinal mosaicism in infertile males. Mol Hum Reprod 2000; 6(8):688–693.
62. Simoni M, Bakker E, Krausz C. EAA/EMQN best practice guidelines for molecular diagnosis of Y-chromosomal microdeletions. State of the art 2004. Int J Androl 2004; 27(4):240–249.
63. Repping S, Skaletsky H, Brown L, et al. Polymorphism for a 1.6-Mb deletion of the human Y chromosome persists through balance between recurrent mutation and haploid selection. Nat Genet 2003; 35(3):247–251.
64. Giachini C, Guarducci E, Longepied G, et al. The gr/gr deletion(s): a new genetic test in male infertility? J Med Genet 2005; 42(6):497–502.
65. Giachini C, Laface I, Guarducci E, et al. Partial AZFc deletions and duplications: clinical correlates in the Italian population. Hum Genet 2008; 124(4)399–410.
66. Visser L, Westerveld GH, Korver CM, et al. Y chromosome gr/gr deletions are a risk factor for low semen quality. Hum Reprod 2009; 24(10):2667–2673.
67. Krausz C, Giachini C. Genetic risk factors in male infertility. Arch Androl 2007; 53(3):125–133.
68. Nuti F, Krausz C. Gene polymorphisms/mutations relevant to abnormal spermatogenesis. Reprod Biomed Online 2008; 16(4):504–513.
69. Venables JP, Cooke HJ. Lessons from knockout and transgenic mice for infertility in men. J Endocrinol Invest 2000; 23(9):584–591.
70. Krausz C. Polymorphisms and male infertility. In: Carrell DT, ed. The Genetics of Male Infertility. Totowa, NJ: Humana press, 2007:275–289.
71. Guarducci E, Nuti F, Becherini L, et al. Estrogen receptor alpha promoter polymorphism: stronger estrogen action is coupled with lower sperm count. Hum Reprod 2006; 21(4):994–1001.
72. Tuttelmann F, Rajpert-De Meyts E, Nieschlag E, et al. Gene polymorphisms and male infertility–a meta-analysis and literature review. Reprod Biomed Online 2007; 15(6):643–658.
73. Gosden R, Trasler J, Lucifero D, et al. Rare congenital disorders, imprinted genes, and assisted reproductive technology. Lancet 2003; 361(9373):1975–1977.
74. Lucifero D, Chaillet JR, Trasler JM. Potential significance of genomic imprinting defects for reproduction and assisted reproductive technology. Hum Reprod Update 2004; 10(1):3–18.
75. Marques CJ, Carvalho F, Sousa M, et al. Genomic imprinting in disruptive spermatogenesis. Lancet 2004; 363(9422):1700–1702.
76. Hartmann S, Bergmann M, Bohle RM, et al. Genetic imprinting during impaired spermatogenesis. Mol Hum Reprod 2006; 12(6):407–411.
77. Kobayashi H, Sato A, Otsu E, et al. Aberrant DNA methylation of imprinted loci in sperm from oligospermic patients. Hum Mol Genet 2007; 16(21):2542–2551.
78. Hammoud SS, Nix DA, Zhang H, et al. Distinctive chromatin in human sperm packages genes for embryo development. Nature 2009; 460(7254):473–478.
79. Cox GF, Burger J, Lip V, et al. Intracytoplasmic sperm injection may increase the risk of imprinting defects. Am J Hum Genet 2002; 71(1):162–164.
80. DeBaun MR, Niemitz EL, Feinberg AP. Association of in vitro fertilization with Beckwith-Wiedemann syndrome and epigenetic alterations of LIT1 and H19. Am J Hum Genet 2003; 72(1):156–160.
81. Maher ER, Brueton LA, Bowdin SC, et al. Beckwith-Wiedemann syndrome and assisted reproduction technology (ART). J Med Genet 2003; 40(1):62–64.

82. Nikolettos N, Asimakopoulos B, Papastefanou IS. Intracytoplasmic sperm injection–an assisted reproduction technique that should make us cautious about imprinting deregulation. J Soc Gynecol Investig 2006; 13(5):317–328.
83. Orstavik KH, Eiklid K, Van der Hagen CB, et al. Another case of imprinting defect in a girl with Angelman syndrome who was conceived by intracytoplasmic semen injection. Am J Hum Genet 2003; 72(1):218–219.
84. Carrell DT, Hammoud SS. The human sperm epigenome and its potential role in embryonic development. Mol Hum Reprod 2010; 16(1):37–47.
85. Van Steirteghem A, Bonduelle M, Devroey P, et al. Follow-up of children born after ICSI. Hum Reprod Update 2002; 8(2):111–116.
86. Matzuk MM, Lamb DJ. Genetic dissection of mammalian fertility pathways. Nat Cell Biol 2002; 4(suppl):s41–s49.
87. Ostermeier GC, Dix DJ, Miller D, et al. Spermatozoal RNA profiles of normal fertile men. Lancet 2002; 360(9335):772–777.
88. Martinez-Heredia J, Estanyol JM, Ballesca JL, et al. Proteomic identification of human sperm proteins. Proteomics 2006; 6(15):4356–4369.
89. Platts AE, Dix DJ, Chemes HE, et al. Success and failure in human spermatogenesis as revealed by teratozoospermic RNAs. Hum Mol Genet 2007; 16(7):763–773.
90. Aston KI, Carrell DT. Genome-wide study of single-nucleotide polymorphisms associated with azoospermia and severe oligozoospermia. J Androl 2009; 30(6):711–725.
91. Ropers HH. New perspectives for the elucidation of genetic disorders. Am J Hum Genet 2007; 81(2):199–207.

6 Conventional Treatment of the male in infertile couples

Herman Tournaye and Aleksander Giwercman

INTRODUCTION

Infertility is a problem of the couple, not only from a psychosocial but also from a functional point of view. It means that in each case the situation of an infertile couple should be evaluated in an integrated manner. Even when the investigation of the male partner has disclosed some minor to moderate impairment of the semen quality, it does not mean that improvement of semen parameters is the only way of helping the couple to achieve spontaneous pregnancy. When specific, that is nonempirical treatments have failed or were not indicated, optimalization of the female partner is the first-line approach to improve a couple's fecundity. Even when the female factor was found to be normal, an attempt should be made to increase the wife's fecundity.

The goal of the therapeutic attempts towards the male can be one of following:

1. To help the couple to achieve a spontaneous pregnancy.
2. To use a less invasive method of assisted reproduction like conventional intrauterine insemination (IUI) or in-vitro fertilization (IVF) instead of intracytoplasmatic sperm injection (ICSI).
3. To improve the success rate from either method of assisted reproduction.

Because of the variability of semen parameters in men (chapter 5) and the phenomenon of "regression towards the mean," studies evaluating treatment of male subfertility must include placebo (1) and should have pregnancy as their main outcome measure. Unfortunately very few randomized controlled trials with pregnancy as the main outcome measure do exist in the field of male subfertility. The Cochrane library currently includes nine reviews on male infertility and the majority of these trials have not been updated for a long time because of the lack of new evidence. Clinical practice is thus subject to authority-based guidelines.

In the last decade most progress has been made in understanding and treating the azoospermic male. For the oligozoospermic subfertile male efficient specific treatments are still scarce and as a result there has been an increase in the application of assisted reproduction (ART) to "treat" male subfertility.

Good medical practice implies that once the causative factor for a condition has been diagnosed, an efficient, safe and specific treatment has to be applied. Unfortunately in 40% of men presenting with a "male factor" the causative factor remains unknown and in another 50%, no specific treatment with a proven efficiency is currently available (2).

In the following we will go through different modalities of treating the male partner of infertile couples and put them in the context of the different types of goals to be achieved (see item 1–3 above) and their levels of evidence.

TREATMENTS WITH A PROVEN BENEFIT

Apart from preventive treatments such as cryobanking semen before gonadotoxic therapy (chapter 16), treatments for anejaculation and retrograde ejaculation (chapter 14) and surgical treatments for reversing obstructive azoospermia (chapter 12), only hormonal treatments for inducing spermatogenesis in men with hypogonadothrophic hypogonadism have a proven efficiency (3,4-level of evidence 3). The goal of this therapy, which is successful in 80% to 90% of cases, is to give the couples a possibility of achieving pregnancy without use of ART. However, it should be kept in mind that even among the couples in whom hypogonadotropic hypogonadism is diagnosed in the male partner, there may be accompanying disturbances in the female reproductive function and/or dysfunction of testes or accessory sex glands, making the use of ART necessary although a sufficient gonadotropin stimulation has been given.

TREATMENTS FOR WHICH NO CLEAR EVIDENCE HAS BEEN PROVIDED

Several treatment modalities have been suggested as efficient in making a couple capable to achieve pregnancy without use of ART. For decades, empirical treatments have yet been very popular. Thanks to meta-analyses, however, there is now a growing consensus that most of these treatments have no proven benefit for treating male subfertility.

The use of once popular drugs such as androgens, antiestrogens, gonadotrophins, bromocriptine, kinine-enhancers and corticoids is not recommended. Table 1 summarizes the current consensus. Although more clinical evidence is needed, the administration of tamoxifen alone or in combination with androgens appears promising (5-level of evidence 1b). Some randomized controlled trials (RCTs) have indicated both α-blockers and mast-cell blockers as empirical treatments to alleviate unexplained male subfertility, but clinical evidence remains poor because of limitations in the design of these RCTs.

Varicocele is diagnosed in a quarter of subfertile men but the role of varicocele correction in improving an adult man's fecundity is still under debate (6,7-level of evidence 1a).

Male accessory gland infection (MAGI) is another frequently encountered condition during the work-up of infertile men. According to the WHO, MAGI is present when more than 10^6 white blood cells per ml semen are observed (8-level of

Table 1 Summary of the Current Consensus on the Treatment of Unexplained Male Subfertility[a]

Studies with pregnancy as an outcome measure	
HMG / FSH	No benefit
Androgens	No benefit
Antiestrogens	No benefit in general, but need for more research in subgroups
Dopamine agonists	No benefit
Glucocorticoids	No benefit
Kalikrein	No benefit
Aromatase inhibitors	No benefit, based on only one RCT
Mast cell blocker	Potential benefit but needs further evaluation
Antioxidants	Potential benefit but needs further evaluation
Studies with sperm parameters as an outcome measure	
GnRH	No benefit
Growth hormone	No benefit

[a]Based on the Cochrane Library data, the NICE guidelines and the EAU guidelines on male infertility.

evidence 4). A small randomized-controlled trial evaluated the effect of treatment on the fecundity associated with this condition, but failed to show any difference between antibiotherapy and placebo (9-level of evidence 2a).

Some recent studies have indicated that sperm DNA strand breaks may have an impact on the fertility potential of the couple. Using Sperm Chromatin Structure Assay (SCSA) it was shown that a DNA Fragmentation Index (DFI) more than 30% excludes more or less the possibility of achieving pregnancy *in vivo* spontaneously or by use of IUI (10–12-level of evidence 3). Since some cases of high DFI may be due to increased levels of reactive oxygen species (ROS) attempts with use of antioxidant drugs have been made. However, so far the results of available reports are rather contradictory (13). In contrast to spontaneous conception and IUI, there is currently no evidence of any adverse impact of DNA fragmentation in *in vitro fertilization* (14-level of evidence 1a).

ASSISTED REPRODUCTION FOR MALE SUBFERTILITY

When specific, that is nonempirical treatments have failed or were not indicated, optimization of the female partner is the first-line approach to improve a couple's fecundity. Even when the female factor was found to be normal, an attempt should be made to increase the wife's fecundity. This may be achieved by timed intercourse combined with mild ovarian stimulation. This treatment must be monitored by ovarian ultrasonography in order to avoid multiple pregnancies.

When optimization of the female partner failed, techniques of assisted reproduction come in because they may be more beneficial to compensate for the reproductive failure of the male partner (15). The common rationale behind these techniques is to bring the spermatozoa closer in the oocyte's vicinity trying to enhance fertilization. Although assisted reproductive techniques have become fairly successful, they have not made clinical work-up or specific treatment of the male partner pointless. Any correction of a specific dysfunction in the male should be completed since this may avoid the use of assisted reproductive techniques or may enhance their outcome. Assisted-reproductive techniques cannot be viewed as a primary treatment option but rather as a complimentary treatment. The objective in assisted reproductive techniques is to bring more functional spermatozoa closer to the oocyte. Assisted reproductive techniques are thus not a cure in se.

The most popular techniques of assisted reproduction for the treatment of male subfertility and infertility are intrauterine insemination (IUI) (chapter 8) and in-vitro fertilization and embryo transfer (IVF-ET) (chapter 10). In the latter technique fertilization can be obtained after bringing oocyte and motile spermatozoa together in the insemination medium, that is "conventional" IVF, or by microinjecting one single spermatozoon directly into the oocyte's cytoplasm, a technique referred to as intracytoplasmic sperm injection or ICSI.

REFERENCES

1. Baker HW, Kovacs GT. Spontaneous improvement in semen quality: Regression towards the mean. Int J Androl 1985; 8:421–426.
2. Baker HW. Requirements for controlled therapeutic trials in male infertility. Clin Reprod Fertil 1986; 4:13–25.
3. Büchter D, Behre HM, Kliesch S, et al. Pulsatile GnRH or human chorionic gonadotropin/human menopausal gonadotropin as effective treatment for men with hypogonadotropic hypogonadism: A review of 42 cases. Eur J Endocrinol 1998; 139(3):298–303.
4. Christiansen P, Skakkebaek NE. Pulsatile gonadotropin-releasing hormone treatment of men with idiopathic hypogonadotropic hypogonadism. Horm Res 2002; 57 (1–2):32–36.
5. Adamopoulos DA, Pappa A, Billa E, et al. Effectiveness of combined tamoxifen citrate and testosterone undecanoate treatment in men with idiopathic oligozoospermia. Fertil Steril 2003; 80:914–920.
6. Evers JL, Collins JA. Assessment of efficacy of varicocele repair for male subfertility: A systematic review. Lancet 2003; 361:1849–1852.
7. Kamischke A, Nieschlag E. Varicocele treatment in the light of evidence-based andrology. Hum Reprod Update 2001; 7:65–69.
8. Rowe P, Comhaire F, Hargreave T, et al; World Health Organisation (WHO). WHO Manual for the standardized

investigation, diagnosis and management of the infertile male. Cambridge, UK: Cambridge University Press, 2000.

9. Comhaire FH, Rowe PJ, Farley TM. The effect of doxycycline in infertile couples with male accessory gland infection: A double blind prospective study. Int J Androl 1986; 9:91–98.
10. Bungum M, Humaidan P, Axmon A, et al. Sperm DNA integrity assessment in prediction of assisted reproduction technology outcome. Hum Reprod 2007; 22:174–179.
11. Evenson DP, Jost LK, Marshall D, et al. Utility of the sperm chromatin structure assay as a diagnostic and prognostic tool in the human fertility clinic. Hum Reprod 1999; 14:1039–1049.
12. Spanò M, Bonde JP, Hjøllund HI, et al. Sperm chromatin damage impairs human fertility. The Danish First Pregnancy Planner Study Team. Fertil Steril 2000; 73: 43–50.
13. Tremellen K. Oxidative stress and male infertility–a clinical perspective. Hum Reprod Update 2008; 14:243–258.
14. Collins JA, Barnhart KT, Schlegel PN. Do sperm DNA integrity tests predict pregnancy with in vitro fertilization? Fertil Steril 2008; 89:823–831.
15. O'Donovan PA, Vandekerckhove P, Lilford RJ, et al. Treatment of male infertility: Is it effective? Review and meta-analyses of published randomized trials. Hum Reprod 1993; 8:1209–1222.

7 Nonsurgical methods for sperm retrieval in patients with anejaculation and retrograde ejaculation

Axel Kamischke

INTRODUCTION

This chapter focuses on the diagnosis and nonsurgical treatment of infertile male patients with anejaculation (AE) and retrograde ejaculation (RE). Relevant studies were identified as outlined in our previous publications (1,2). Regarding general diagnostic and therapeutic aspects of male infertility and hypogonadism, reference is made to other chapters of the EAU/ESAU Clinical Andrology Course Guidelines and to established andrology textbooks (3).

The methodological quality of the studies analyzing patients with AE or RE being treated for fertility disturbances remains mostly unsatisfactory (1,2,4). Despite various treatment modalities only six randomized controlled clinical trials could be identified while the remaining evidence is based on case reports and mostly small observational studies. Furthermore, a considerable publication bias in the papers is apparent, as pregnancy rates per patient with some treatments are unexpectedly high compared to other fields of male infertility. Therefore caution is advised when comparing the results of different types of drugs and electrostimulation procedures. Nonetheless, under consideration of the methodological quality of the studies some general recommendations can be drawn. Whenever possible, the levels of evidence and the nature of recommendations are rated according to the levels of evidence published by the U.S. Department of Health and Human Services, Public Health Service, Agency for Health care Policy and Research (5).

PHYSIOLOGY OF EJACULATION

For physiological ejaculation afferent stimuli via the pudendal nerve travel from the glans penis to the brain. Efferent response of the sympathetic nerves from sympathetic motor neurons emerging in segments T12–L3, passes through the inferior mesenteric ganglion and produces emission of semen from the ampulla of the vas deferens into the posterior urethra (6). Following the initial emission of semen into the posterior urethra, sympathetic contraction of the posterior urethra and closure of the bladder neck, together with parasympathetically (originating from S2 to S4) induced contraction of the bulbocavernosus and ischiocavernosus muscles and pelvic-floor activity leads to antegrade ejaculation through the urethral meatus (7).

Failures of the initial emission of semen from the ampulla of the vas deferens into the posterior urethra by stimulation of the sympathetic nerves leads to AE. Failures of the sympathetic contraction of the posterior urethra and closure of the bladder neck or parasympathetically induced contraction of the bulbocavernosus and ischiocavernosus muscles lead to RE.

DIAGNOSIS OF ANEJACULATION AND RETROGRADE EJACULATION

Compared to other reasons for ejaculatory dysfunction AE and RE are rare causes of infertility. Valid international guidelines and flow-charts for the evaluation of the infertile men are generally not existent. However, the Male Infertility Best Practice Policy Committee of the American Urological Association and the Practice Committee of the American Society for Reproductive Medicine and the European Society of Human Reproduction & Embryology Capri Workshop Group provide some guidance (8–10).

In the absence of an antegrade ejaculation suspicion of AE or RE can often (Table 1) be made by the medical history. According to the American consensus in order to diagnose possible RE and to exclude AE, the physician should perform a postejaculatory urinalysis for any man whose ejaculate volume is less than 1.0 mL, and who has not been diagnosed with hypogonadism or Congenital Bilateral Absence of the Vas Deferens (CBAVD). It is also important to assure that improper or incomplete collection, or a very short abstinence period (less than 1 day) is not the cause of the low-volume ejaculate (10).

Diagnosis of Retrograde Ejaculation

Definition: Retrograde ejaculation is substantial propulsion of seminal fluid from the posterior urethra into the bladder. Retrograde ejaculation can appear as complete retrograde ejaculation (no antegrade fraction) or incomplete retrograde ejaculation (only minimal antegrade emission).

Retrograde ejaculation (RE) accounts for around 0.3 % of male infertility (11) and is the most common cause for ejaculatory dysfunction in the absence of antegrade ejaculation. Retrograde ejaculation is mainly caused by injury to the lumbar sympathetic nerves or by surgery that damages the neck of the bladder (Table 1). Transurethral prostatectomy or transurethral incision for BPH most commonly leads to RE in ≈ 75% of patients (11). However, as BPH is mainly a disease of the ageing male, the most common reason for RE in patients consulting for infertility is retroperitoneal lymph node dissection (RLND) that

Table 1 Aetiology of Retrograde Ejaculation and Anejaculation and Reported Frequency in Patients Treated for Infertility (1)

			RE (%)	AE (%)
Anatomic (myotonic)	Acquired	Prostatectomy (transurethral/open)	8.5	
		Bladder neck surgery/Bladder neck fibrosis	10.2	
	Congenital	Abnormal location of the ejaculatory duct orifice into the urethra	0.3	
		Bladder neck incompetence	1.5	
		Urethral stricture	2.3	
		Epispadias extrophy	0.9	
		Posterior urethral valves	2.6	
Neurogenic	Acquired	Retroperitoneal lymph node dissection	29.2	6.1
		Sympathectomy		
		Trauma/retroperitoneal surgery	2.1	0.2
		Spinal cord injury	1.8	86.9
	Acquired	Diabetes mellitus	13.5	0.8
		Multiple sclerosis		0.1
Toxic		Alcohol, morphine, cocaine		
Drugs		α-Receptor blockers, antihypertensiva, antipsychotics, antidepressants	0.3	
Idiopathic (psychogenic)			6.4	7.1

accounts for 42% of patients treated for infertility (1). However, modified unilateral RLND, as performed today, reduces the initial loss of antegrade ejaculation to 10% to 15% (12). Common additional reasons include idiopathic and pharmacological causes (α-blockers) and neurological diseases. Especially diabetic polyneuropathy can also cause RE although less often than it leads to erectile dysfunction (7). When, apart from organic reasons, no cause can be identified for ejaculatory dysfunction it is classified as idiopathic or psychogenic (13,14) ejaculatory dysfunction.

Recommendation: Level 3 Grade B

Diagnostic evidence of RE includes absent or intermittent emission of ejaculate, orgasm without ejaculation and ability to empty the bladder during erection. Retrograde ejaculation must be differentiated from several other diseases (Fig. 1). Diagnostically, reproductive hormone analysis, scrotal and transrectal sonography and microscopic investigations of the postcoital or postmasturbatory urine are most important. The postejaculatory urinalysis is performed by centrifuging the specimen for 10 minutes at a minimum of 300 g, and microscopically inspecting the pellet at 400× magnification (9). Diagnosis is suggestive by the presence of any sperm in a postejaculatory urine analysis of a patient without apparent antegrade ejaculation. In addition, in patients with RE, which are azoospermic due to other disturbances, a postmasturbatory detection of fructose may indicate RE (Fig. 1). Significant numbers of sperm must be found in the urine of patients with low ejaculate volume oligozoospermia in order to suggest the diagnosis of additional RE. Expert consensus on the definition of significant numbers of sperm in the urine does not exist (1,9).

Diagnosis of Anejaculation

Definition: Anejaculation is defined as the total failure of seminal emission into the posterior urethra.

Although erections after spinal cord injury (SCI) were reported in 63% of 2461 patients, ejaculations were reported in only 14% of these patients and only 1.8% were able to achieve a pregnancy with their spouse (15). As the average age at injury is below 30 years spinal cord injury is the most common diagnosis in patients with AE and accounts for 87% of the cases reported (Table 1). To less extent compared to RE also patients with RLND and idiopathic disturbances attribute to the patients consulting for infertility.

Recommendation: Level 3 Grade B

Diagnostic clues to AE are the complete absence of an antegrade ejaculation combined with a nonviscous, fructose-negative and sperm-negative postorgasmic urinanalysis (16). AE has to be differentiated from several other diseases (Fig. 1). Diagnostically scrotal and transrectal sonography and microscopic investigations of the postcoital or postmasturbatory urine are most important (9). Diagnosis is confirmed when despite regular

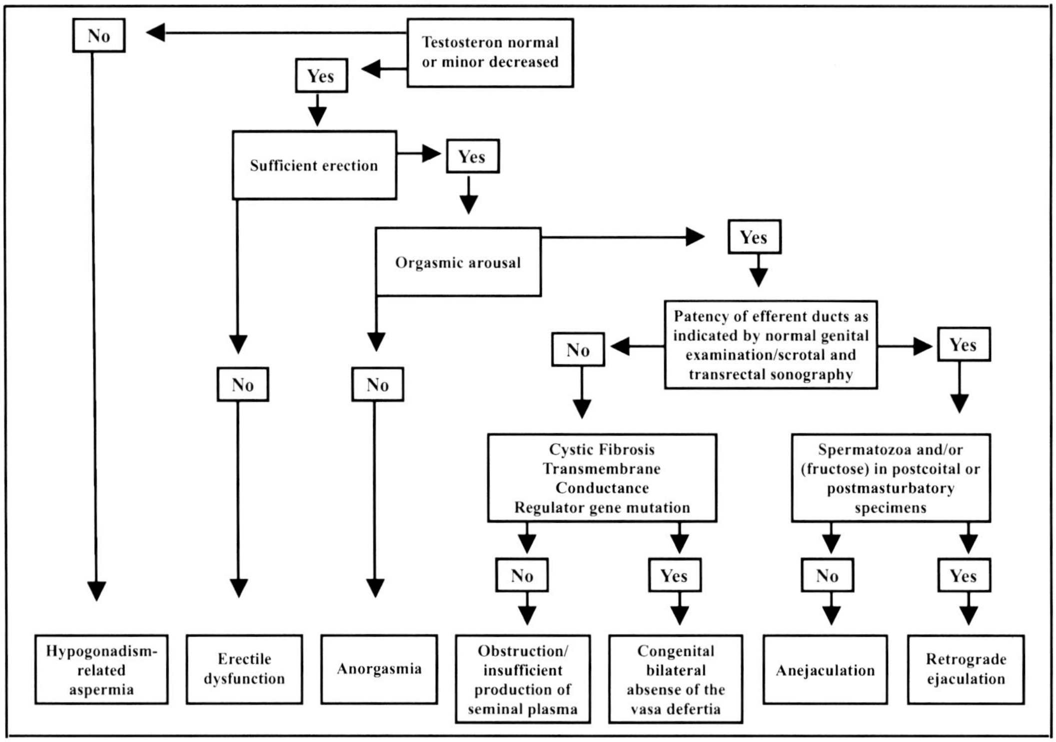

Figure 1 Flow-chart for diagnosis of anejaculation and retrograde ejaculation in patients without apparent normal antegrade ejaculation (< 1 mL) despite normal abstinence time (> 2 days) and proper and complete ejaculate collection.

erection and orgasmic sexual contact no antegrade or RE can be detected in the urine after ejaculation (1).

NONSURGICAL TREATMENT OF ANEJACULATION AND RETROGRADE EJACULATION

For treatment of AE and RE depending on the origin and degree of the disorder medical treatment, electrovibration stimulation (EVS), electroejaculation (EE) and operative procedures have been used successfully since decades. Concern has been raised regarding a higher miscarriage rate in patients with RE and AE. However, analyzing all studies which present pregnancy outcome in their data, the miscarriage rates were 14% for auto-IUI/IUI, 23% for IVF/GIFT and 12% for ICSI in men with AEs or REs (update from 2). This is comparable to the general population in which the total rate of pregnancy loss after implantation, including clinically recognized spontaneous abortions, was 31% (17).

Nonsurgical Treatment of Retrograde Ejaculation

Compared to our previous systematic review (2) no further studies have been published dealing with medical treatment for reversal of RE. For detailed analysis of single studies (e.g., success rates, ejaculate parameters) therefore reference is made to our previous systematic reviews (1,2).

Methods used for retrieval of sperms in patients with RE involve medical treatment with alpha agonistic, anticholinergic or antihistaminic drugs, sperm recovery from urine, EVS and operation with the Abraham's or Young-Dees technique, and testicular sperm extraction (TESE). As in other infertile patients most patients with RE wish to conceive offspring naturally. However, apart from occasionally reports of patients who voided postcoitally into the vagina of their spouse and patients who had been operated with the Abraham's or Young-Dees technique, spontaneous pregnancies were only reported in patients with medical treatment of RE. In addition, compared to the other methods medical treatment of RE is the less invasive method and should therefore be considered the first choice for patients with RE.

Drugs used for medical treatment of RE include alpha agonistic or anticholinergic and antihistaminic drugs which either increase the sympathetic or decrease the parasympathetic tone of the bladder (Table 2). Drugs frequently used in the 264 patients reported in the literature are 25 to 75 mg/day p.o. imipramine (Tofranil®, Pryleugan®) given 3 to 14 days prior to desired ejaculation, 5 to 40 mg iv milodrin (Gutron®) given 30 minutes to 2.5 hours prior to desired ejaculation, 50 to 100 mg/day p.o. ephedrine given two hours to four weeks prior to desired ejaculation, 50 mg/day p.o. chlorpheniramine + phenylpropanalamine (Ornade®) given one hour to 10 days prior

Table 2 If Possible Ejaculate Volume, Sperm Concentration, Sperm Motility Are Given as Mean Numbers of Patients With Retrograde Ejaculation, Success Rate, Numbers of Cycles and Spontaneous Pregnancies Are Given as Total Numbers.

Drug	No. of patients	No. of successful patients	Ejaculate volume (mL)	Sperm concentration (Mill/mL)	Sperm motility (%)	No. of patients desiring pregnancy	No. of cycles	No. of pregnancies
Imipramine	121	78	2.1	68.4	25	76 (7)	Unclear (unclear)	30 (4)
Midodrin	40	21	4		39	4	Unclear	0
Ephedrine	30	6	Unclear	Unclear	Unclear			
Chlorpheniramine+ phenylpropanalamine	14	11	0.05–5	1–160	20	7 (4)	20 (unclear)	1 (>2)
Brompheniramine+ phenylephrine	10	3	0.77	239.3	53	None	——	——
Pseudoephedrine	10	3	Unclear	50.9	40	None	——	——
Brompheniramine	8	3	2	50	60	2	Unclear	0
Brompheniramine + phenylephrine+ phenylprpopylamine	7	4	0.3	Unclear	Unclear	Unclear	Unclear	1
Synephrine	6	3	1.12	68.8	30	6	Unclear	0
Ephedrine+imipramine	5	0	——	——	——	None	——	——
Amezinium (18)	3	3	Unclear	28.7	36.7	3	18	2
Dextroamphetamine	1	1	Unclear	2	11.5	None	——	——
Ephedrine+chlorpheniramine	1	1	Unclear	2.5	11	None	——	——
Phenylpropanalamine	1	1	Unclear	2.75	1.5	None	——	——
Unclear	11	0	——	——		None	——	——
Medical treatment total	264	133	2.0	69.6	29	95 (11)		32 (>6)

Numbers of patients, numbers of cycles and assisted pregnancies are given as total numbers in brackets. For detailed references refer to Ref. (2).

to desired ejaculation and brompheniramine (Diametane®) given 12 hours to 14 days prior to desired ejaculation. Frequent side effects at the given doses are various degrees of dizziness, sleep disturbances, weakness, restlessness, dry mouth, nausea or sweating.

Recommendation: Level 3 Grade C

The underlying diagnosis has no significant influence on the overall 50% success rate of the various medical treatments (2). However, in the 264 patients reported in the literature there are considerable differences in the success rates between idiopathic RE (78%), urethral stricture (67%), RLND (53%) and SCI (50%) compared to bladder neck insufficiency (20%) and Diabetes Mellitus (31%). Due to the low value of the existing evidence combined with the various treatments applied, it remains to be elucidated whether these differences have any clinical relevance.

Recommendation: Level 3 Grade B

Neither from systematic review nor from statements of single authors there is evidence nor rational provided regarding which from the thirteen treatments, various dosages or durations of treatment to be chosen. Compared to ephedrine, imipramine and chlorpheniramine + phenylpropanalamine showed significantly higher reversal rates, while the differences between the other treatments were not significant (2). Imipramine was the drug most used (46% of all patients reported for reversal of RE) and accounts for 80% of the treatments where pregnancy was desired (Table 1). As imipramine also accounts for 94% of the spontaneous pregnancies achieved and has a success rate (65%) above the combined mean success rate of all treatments (50%) 25 to 75 mg/day p.o. imipramine should be applied first in patients with RE.

Recommendation: Level 3 Grade C

The second choice for reversal of RE appear to be the commercially distributed combination of 50 mg/day p.o. chlorpheniramine + phenypropanalamine (Ornade), and 5 to 40 mg iv milodrin. Although experience with chlorpheniramine + phenypropanalamine is limited (n = 14 patients) in comparison to imipramine, the success rate of 79% favors the use as a second choice. Alternatively 5 to 40 mg iv milodrin appear to be a favorable second choice as it is the second most used drug (n = 40 patients) for reversal of RE and shows a success rate slightly above the mean (Table 2). In contrast, ephedrine, although widely used, appears to be a poor choice because of the relatively low reversal rate (19). However, whether these

Table 3 Numbers of Patients, Pregnancies and Cycles are Given as Total Numbers, Pregnancy Rate Per Cycle Is Given as Percentages. IVF and GIFT were Evaluated Together.

Intervention	Patients desiring pregnancy (No)	Artificial method	Cycles (No)	Pregnancies (No)	Pregnancy rate per cycle (%)
Alkalizing	2	Auto-IUI	7	2	28.6
Alkalizing	44	IUI	232	47	20.3
Alkalizing	4	IVF	7	4	57.1
Alkalizing	2	ICSI	2	2	100
Alkalizing/medium instillation	18	IUI	113	11	9.7
Medium instillation	1	Auto-IUI	16	1	6.2
Medium instillation	12	IUI	At least 59	12	20.3
Medium instillation	6	IVF	Unclear	3	Unclear
Fluid intake/medium instillation	3	IUI	12	2	16.7
None	11	IUI	72	9	12.5

Source: From Ref. 1.

statements are justified has to be proven in comparative controlled clinical studies.

Recommendation: Level 3 Grade B

If medical treatment of RE fails, the next choice is sperm recovery from urine to retrieve sperm for artificial procedures in men with RE. Urine is known to have a detrimental effect on sperm quality and may decrease sperm motility by at least half within five minutes of mixing with urine (21). Therefore most studies aiming for retrieval of the retrograde ejaculates from the bladder induce alkalization of the urine pH with $NaHCO_3$ (dose 1.2–16 g) given orally for a duration of a few hours up to three days prior to ejaculation to adjust pH between 7 and 8 prior to masturbation. However, in addition to the detrimental effect of urine pH, there is evidence that osmolarity rather than pH decreases sperm motility (20,21) In order to reduce osmolaric stress to sperm some studies either install buffered media into the bladder prior to ejaculation or try to manipulate the osmolarity of the urine via the fluid intake of the patient in addition to pH adjusting. However, the pregnancy rates per IUI cycle (Table 3) between alkalization of urine, instillation of medium, alkalization of urine plus instillation of medium and no intervention prior to RE were not different ($p = 0.2$; power $= 0.5$), which argues at least against invasive medium instillation.

Recommendation: Level 3 Grade B

Most studies published in the eighties and nineties have performed intrauterine inseminations (IUI) with sperm recovered from urine despite sometimes markedly reduced semen parameters (1). However, as ICSI has been shown to be superior to other ART in other cases of severe male infertility, it should be considered as first choice if only sperm of poor quality could be retrieved. As in case of ICSI the detrimental effect of the urine on quality of sperm motility is of secondary interest, the importance of alkalization of urine and medium instillation is even more reduced compared to IUI. However, so far no benefit of ICSI compared to IUI or IVF could be observed (probably due to the low number of patients treated with ICSI) this consideration should be confirmed in controlled clinical trials. In the absence of such studies, the choice whether to perform IUI, IVF or ICSI should be made on the basis of the sperm quality. If no viable sperm can be retrieved in the urine TESE should be considered as a last resort as in other cases of male infertility.

Case Story

Medical History:

A 32-year-old man consulted our clinic with primary infertility since two years. The patient had a known Insulin dependent Diabetes Mellitus since 20 years. Due to his Diabetes Mellitus, he has compensated renal malfunction with arterial hypertension and diabetic retinopathy. His 29 year old, healthy wife had normal ovulatory cycles. Due to his illnesses, he received daily medications with Insulin and a renin-angiotensin inhibitor. In a former examination outside he was not able to provide an ejaculate due to a "dry ejaculation". After sexual intercourse he reported to have more foamic urine. Occasionally he reported to have an erectile dysfunction, which can be successfully treated with a PDE 5 inhibitor.

Physical Examination:

General physical examination as well as the examination of the penis were normal. Testicular volume was 12 mL on the left side and 16 mL on the right side with firm consistency. Evaluation of the Plexus Pampiniformis revealed a Varicocele I on the left side. Both epididymis appeared enlarged in the caput with normal Deferent Ducts on both sides. In the scrotal sonography, both testes showed a homogenous structure with normal echogenicity and confirmed the alterations in the epididymis and the Varicocele I. Transrectal ultrasonography of the prostate gland and the seminal vesicles showed no abnormalities.

Hormones:
LH: 3.5 (normal range 1.7–8.7 U/L), FSH: 8.1 (normal range 1–7 U/L), Testosterone 11.6 (normal range > 10 nmol/L), free testosterone 228 (normal range > 200 pmol/L); Östradiol 32 (normal range < 43 ng/mL), SHBG 34 (normal range 14.5 – 48.4 nmol/L)

Semen Analysis:
The patient was not able to provide an ejaculate after masturbation. However, postmastubatory urine analysis revealed after centrifugation (15 min at 3000 g) sperms in the pellet.

Diagnoses:
Complete RE, Varicocele I, Diabetes Mellitus, compensated renal malfunction, arterial hypertension, and diabetic retinopathy.

Process:
After informing the patients about the possible side effects of imipramine (Tofranil) treatment was started with daily oral doses increasing from 25 mg in the evening for four days to 50 mg in the evening for three days. In addition the patient was asked to take a urine alkalizing substance per os (*4.8 g* potassium-sodium-hydrogen citrate three times a day) on day 7 and on the morning of the planned ejaculation. On day 8 of the patient was asked to provide an ejaculate again. Semen analysis showed reduced volume (1.2 mL) with 7 million sperms/mL and reduced progressive motility (20%) and morphology (2% normal morphology using strict criteria). The postmasturbatory urine sample after centrifugation still revealed spermatozoa in the urine. Due to the partial success of the medical treatment, the couple tried to conceive naturally under clomiphene stimulation of the wife for five months. However, as no pregnancy occurred and as an antegrade fraction could not achieved always despite dose escalation the couple was scheduled for an ICSI cycle. However, on the day of oocyte aspiration the patient was able to provide an antegrade fraction [ejaculate volume (0.9 mL) with 10.1 million sperms/mL, progressive motility (15%), normal morphology (4%)] and ICSI was done with fresh spermatozoa. Out of thirteen, six oocytes showed pronuclei formation and two embryos were transferred, leading to a singleton pregnancy and birth of a boy. The remaining fertilized oocytes with pronuclei formation were cryopreservated for potential later use.

Recommendation: Level 4 Grade C

Other occasional approaches include electrovibration stimulation (EVS), electroejaculation (EE), vas deferens aspiration, and ejaculation in a standing position with full bladder, tamponade of the bladder neck during masturbation with the balloon of a Foley catheter and postcoital voiding into the vagina. However, as long as no bigger or even controlled clinical trials showing any major benefit of such procedures they should not be used outside from clinical studies.

Nonsurgical Treatment of Anejaculation

As in patients with RE, medical treatment offers AE patients the only chance to conceive naturally. Medical treatment of AE has to be divided according to the underlying causes. In patients not suffering from SCI, nearly exclusively the alpha agonists (ephedrine (30–100 mg/day p.o.), imipramine (20–00 mg/day p.o), milodrin (15 mg/day p.o. or 10–30 mg intravenous) and pseudoephedrine (30–240 mg/day p.o.) have been used while in patients with AE due to SCI, only the parasympathomimetics physostigmine and neostigmine were used (1,2,22).

Recommendation: Level 3 Grade B

For patients suffering from AE but not SCI the underlying diagnosis has no significant influence on the overall disappointing 20% success rate of the various medical treatments (2). Frequent side affects at the given doses of the alpha agonistic drugs were comparable to the treatment of RE with alpha agonistic drugs. The drug most used for reversal of AE was imipramine (38% of the patients). In contrast to the situation in RE patients, however, imipramine is a poor choice for treating AE, as it is significant inferior to milodrin (Fig. 2). Furthermore, the overall reversal rate (antegrade plus retrograde) of 5–30 mg iv milodrin (61%) mainly in patients with RLND is significantly better than with pseudoephidrine and ephedrine while all other treatments were not significantly different (2). Although the overall reversal rate is better, the proportion of patients with antegrade ejaculation after milodrin treatment remains low (18%). In addition, in the few studies where semen parameters are reported especially sperm motility shows impairments and consequently only two spontaneous pregnancies in partners of patients with AE after alpha agonistic drug therapy have been reported (23,24). Therefore medical treatment of AE not due to SCI cannot be recommended generally as treatment of first choice and warrants further investigation.

Recommendation: Level 3 Grade B

For the treatment of patients with AE due to SCI, only the parasympathomimetics physostigmine and neostigmine were used (Fig. 2). Both were equally effective with respect to the general success rate (1,22). However, only earlier studies mainly in the seventies used intrathecal neostigmine administration. Because of severe side effects (including the death of one patient), and as physostigmine can traverse the blood-brain barrier and can be administered subcutaneously, neostigmine was abandoned and has to be considered obsolete. However, at the given doses (1–2 mg s.c.) physostigmine also has the potential for severe autonomic dysreflexia in men with lesions above T6 (22), which include nausea, vomiting, abdominal cramps, diarrhea as well as orthostatic hypotension for one hour after ejaculation. Pretreatment with 20–40 mg N-butylhyocine bromide, an inhibitor of the peripheral parasympathetic system, or metoclopramide or atropine 10 to 30 minutes before medication with the parasympathetic drugs decreases its peripheral adverse events while permitting the central action of physostigmine and

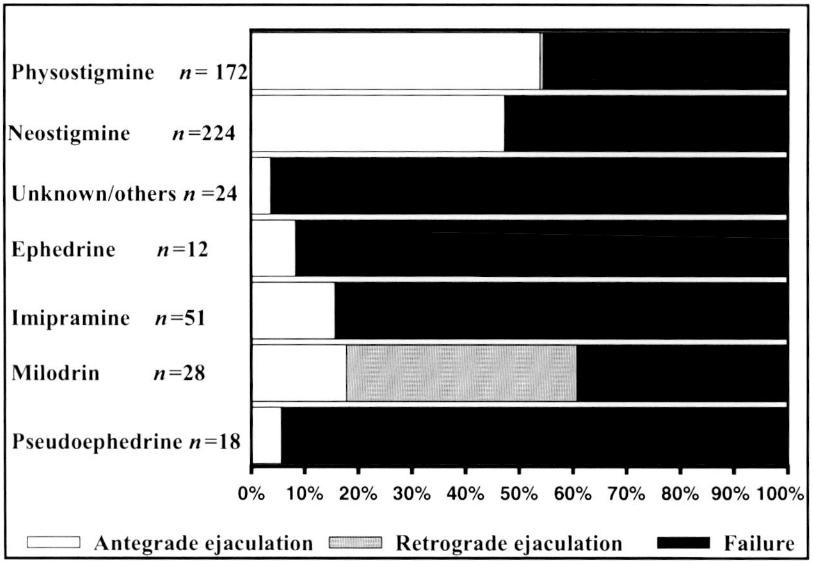

Figure 2 Reversal rates for drugs used for treatment of anejaculation. Shown is the percentage of patients achieving antegrade ejaculation (*white bar*) retrograde ejaculation (*grey bar*) and unchanged anejaculation (*Failure/black bar*). For detailed analysis we refer to our systematic reviews (1,2).

should therefore be recommended (25). Nevertheless with one exception (26) physostigmine has only been applied in a clinical setting. Only a few studies reported semen parameters and as in patients with AE due to other reasons semen parameters of anejaculatory patients with SCI especially of sperm motility are far from normal. From patients receiving parasympathetic drugs six spontaneous pregnancies and nine pregnancies by auto-IUI were reported (26). In addition, from 20 patients seven pregnancies could be induced by artificial IUI (for details see 1). Because of the potential side effects which require a clinical setting, medical treatment of AE in SCI patients cannot be recommended generally as treatment of first choice and warrants further investigation.

The quality of semen obtained by assisted ejaculation by EVS or EE especially from men with chronic SCI is nearly almost always poor. It is characterized particular by poor sperm motility. This pattern of semen abnormality has been attributed to many factors (21,27). However, the major etiology of poor sperm quality remains largely unknown (28). Recent evidence implies that the seminal plasma of spinal cord injured men is deleterious to sperm and that a primary cause of poor sperm quality in SCI men is disordered storage of sperm with stagnation of sperm in the seminal vesicles. (29,30)

Recommendation: Level 1b Grade A

Two small randomized controlled clinical trials (31,32) and a case control study (27) suggested that SCI men should undergo repeated ejaculations to improve sperm quality prior to assisted reproduction procedures. However, the majority of studies could not show this effect (6,30,33–36). As the literature remains inconclusively and under consideration of the small sample size of the randomized controlled clinical studies and the potential side effects of the procedures for the time being repeated procedures seems not justified for improving the sperm quality as long as larger studies prove the concept.

Recommendation: Level 1a Grade B

Although no spontaneous pregnancies could be achieved, EVS together with auto-IUI (EVS: 140 patients, 66 pregnancies vs. EE: 18 patients, 5 pregnancies) offers the couple more than EE the possibility of achieving a pregnancy in the privacy of their home (1). In our analysis of semen parameters in SCI patients evaluated in our previous systemic review (2) and new included studies here sperm motility and sperm concentration were significantly better in patients after EVS compared to EE stimulation. Furthermore evidence from controlled clinical trials indicates that sperm obtained with vibratory stimulation had better quality, side effects were generally lower and EVS has the marked advantage of better patient acceptance compared to EE (22,37,38). However here too, SCI patients with lesions above T6 should be treated with caution to prevent autonomic dysreflexia, for which pretreatment with nifedipine or prazosin and careful monitoring should be performed.

EVS stimulation initiates reflex spinal cord activity causing ejaculation. The patient is seated upright in a chair or is placed in a supine position. To induce ejaculation the vibrating disc is applied against the frenulum for periods of 2.5 to 3 minutes or until antegrade ejaculation occurs. In the literature various vibrators ranging from 60 to 120 HZ, with peak-to-peak amplitude of excursion ranged from 1.5 to 4.5 mm have been applied. However, controlled clinical trials indicated that high amplitude is superior ($\geq$ 2.5 mm) to low amplitude (39,40). Therefore actual commercially available vibrators (FertiCare®, Careclinic®, Relax®) use a frequency of 100 HZ and peak amplitude of excursion of greater than 2.5. Every cycle should be followed by a rest period of twominutes and should be terminated when no further ejaculate can be obtained or when a maximum of approximately six stimulation cycles is completed. In general, the duration of stimulation lies between 10 seconds and 18 minutes. In a recent study antegrade or RE was achieved in 102 out of 185 SCI men (64.6%) with 7.5 to 30 mg p.o. Milodrine, which failed to respond to EVS in a first attempt indicating that PVS on midodrine may be considered second line treatment for AE after PVS and before EE (41). In general, PVS is a well-tolerated procedure with very few potential complications (42). Criteria for discontinuation of the procedure were blood pressure exceeding 200 mm Hg systolic or 130 mm Hg diastolic or reported headache and signs of autonomic dysreflexia. For prevention of autonomic dysreflexia in SCI patients nifedipine or prazosin should be given in all patients with lesions above T6. Most studies additionally perform pre- and post-vibration catheterization of the bladder with instillation of a buffer medium into the bladder for better sperm recovery in case of RE.

For detailed analysis of studies evaluating EVS for sperm retrieval and pregnancy rates we refer to our previous systematic review (1). However added new publications (30,32,35,36,41,43) are here appropriate.

Recommendation: Level 2b Grade B

With rare exceptions EVS has only been applied to anejaculatory men with SCI or idiopathic AE and was equally effective in inducing either antegrade or RE in both groups (SCI 1612 patients 59% success; Idiopathic AE 79 patients 70% success). However, men with idiopathic AE have been reported only with antegrade ejaculation while men with SCI could have both or only a retrograde fraction. Important prognostic factors for overall success of EVS therapy in SCI patients includes in patients with SCI the high of the spinal lesions. (≥ T11). Patients with lesions including T11 and above (424 patients/286 responders) had a significantly higher response to EVS than patients with lesions below T11 (127 patients/55 responders). Other factors seem to have no major prognostic relevance for EVS (39). If one restricts analysis of EVS success only to SCI patients with an intact ejaculatory reflex arc (above T10) using modern vibration output to induce ejaculation success rate can be approximately 80% of all SCI patients (39).

Most studies have performed inseminations with the sperm obtained by EVS. Altogether 184 patients have achieved 74 (50%) pregnancies in an unknown number of auto-IUI cycles. In addition with IUI (64 patients, > 90 cycles, 47 pregnancies), IVF (31 patients, 50 cycles, 19 pregnancies) and ICSI pregnancies (1 reported) have been achieved (1). However, in light of the advantage of IVF/ICSI over IUI in other fields of infertility, ICSI should be considered as first choice, if only sperm of poor quality could be seen (44).

Case Story

Medical History:

A 38-year-old man consulted our clinic with secondary infertility since one year. Together with his 35 year old, healthy wife who had normal ovulatory cycles, the couple had together a healthy 5-year-old girl. The patient was diagnosed to have a testicular cancer (nonseminoma clinical stage IIB) three years ago. He received a left sided orchidectomy together with three cycles of BEP first-line chemotherapy and subsequent surgery for residual masses by nerve sparing RLND. No cryopreser vation of semen was done. Libido and erectile function were normal. However, since the RLND he reported to have a "dry ejaculation".

Hormones:

LH: 6.7 (normal range 1.7–8.7 U/L), FSH: 16.1 (normal range 1–7 U/L), Testosterone 10.4 (normal range > 10 nmol/L), free testosterone 249 (normal range > 200 pmol/L:); Östradiol 18 (normal range < 43 ng/mL), SHBG 23 (normal range 14.5 – 48.4 nmol/L)

Semen Analysis:

The patient was not able to provide an ejaculate after masturbation. Postmastubatory urine analysis revealed after centrifugation (15 min at 3000 g) no spermatozoa in the pellet. Furthermore no fructose could be detected in the postmastubatory urine.

Diagnoses:

Anejaculation, history of testicular cancer with consecutive chemotherapy and RLND.

Process:

Initially a treatment cycle with milodrin (Gutron 25 mg iv 30 min prior to masturbation) was done. However, postmastubatory urine analysis revealed no spermatozoa after centrifugation and no antegrade ejaculation was achieved. After the failure of medical treatment prostatic massage and subsequent vibratory stimulation with the FertiCare device were tried without achievement of an antegrade or retrograde fraction. Under consideration of the advanced age of the wife, the marked increased FSH values after unilateral orchidectomy and chemotherapy a diagnostic and therapeutic testicular biopsy was performed. Testicular histology showed mixed atrophy with elongated spermatids in a few tubules. ICSI was performed after hormonal stimulation therapy of the wife with the cryopreserved testicular tissue from the testicular biopsy. Pronuclei formation was observed in one-third oocytes after injection of testicular spermatids. However, embryo transfer did not resulted in a pregnancy and the couple refused to undergo further treatment cycles.

Recommendation: Level 2b Grade B

As EE has a higher success rate in inducing ejaculation it can be used when EVS is not successful and twelve studies could retrieve sperm with EE after EVS failure (1). The patient is positioned in the right lateral decubitus position on a table, thighs and knees slightly flexed. Blood pressure is measured continuously until the procedure is completed. Digital rectal examination and rectoscopy is performed prior to the procedure to confirm that there are no preexisting rectal lesions and after the procedure to exclude injury to the rectum. As EE leads in many individuals to a substantial portion of RE most studies, like in EVS, perform a pre- and post-catheterization of the bladder with instillation of a buffer medium into the bladder. Starting the stimulation a modern commercially available, solid bar, rectal stimulator (e.g., Seager Model 14 Electroejaculator, Dalzell Medical System, USA) is stabilized against the anterior wall at the area of the prostate gland and the seminal vesicles. The overall ejaculatory response rate of EE with solid bars was significant superior compared to previous used finger cot electrodes, which should not be used anymore (1). Electrical current should be delivered in a progressively increasing wave like pattern with voltage progressively increasing in 1 to 2 V increments until ejaculation occurs, which normally requires one to seven minutes and between 15 and 35 stimulations (42). The voltage and current that have been reported to successfully produce ejaculation range from 5 to 25 V and 100 to 600 mA, respectively (45). It is usually recommended that a low level of electrical baseline (100 mA) be maintained between voltage peaks and during ejaculation (42). However, the sustained nature of the response to EE suggests that electrical stimulation should be stopped completely during ejaculation to allow more relaxation of the external sphincter (43,46). In interrupted trials therefore the current was delivered for five seconds and then turned off for five seconds. Each time the current was turned back on it was increased by 2 V until antegrade ejaculation occurred or until the physician or patient stopped the procedure. (43,46). During the EE procedure the pendulous and bulbar urethra is continuously milked to collect the ejaculate. Forceful contraction of the external sphincter followed by contraction of the internal sphincter always precedes ejaculation during EE. Antegrade ejaculate is not produced in a projectile fashion, but rather as an intermittent release of semen during the course of the procedure (42).

Side effects of EE include rectal mucosa injury and transitory erythema, thermal-electrical injury to the rectum. As in SCI patients treated with EVS, SCI patients with lesions above T6 require careful monitoring of signs of autonomic dysreflexia.

Table 4 All EE Stimulation Studies Presented in this Table Were Done with Solid Bar Electrodes.

Source of data extraction	No. of patients	No. of success antegrade	No. of success retrograde	No. of success total
SCI	**777**	**224**	**88**	**642**
(1)	604	211	80	488
(46)	1	1	Unclear	1
(31)	34	Unclear	Unclear	32
(33)	84	Unclear	Unclear	84
(48)	2	2	2	2
(49)	27	10	6	11
(35)	17	Unclear	Unclear	17
(30)	2	Unclear	Unclear	2
(43)	6	Unclear	Unclear	6
Idiopathic	**108**	**12**	**10**	**106**
(1)	41	4	2	39
(48)	8	8	8	8
(48)	59	Unclear	Unclear	59
RLND				
(1)	**85**	**45**	**16**	**83**
Diabetes mellitus				
(1)	**13**	**1**	**1**	**12**
Multiple sclerosis				
(1)	**3**	**Unclear**	**Unclear**	**3**
Others Myelitis, Retroperitoneal-OP or trauma				
(1)	**3**	**1**	**Unclear**	**3**

Numbers of patients, success rates (if provided) are given as total numbers. Detailed references are only given to studies published after our previous publication (1) to which we refer for detailed analysis of the summarized data provided here.

Table 5 Numbers of Patients, Number of Cycles (if Provided) and Pregnancies Are Given as Total Numbers.

	Treatment	Source of data extraction	Patients desiring pregnancy (No)	Cycles (No)	Fertilization rate (%)	Pregnancies (No)	Pregnancy rate per cycle (%)
SCI							
	Auto-IUI	(1)	**18**	**Unclear**	**n.a.**	**5**	**Unclear**
	IUI		**148**	**267**	**n.a**	**42**	**< 10**
		(1)	123	207	n.a.	35	< 10
		(33)	15	33	n.a.	5	15
		(49)	9	25	n.a.	1	4
		(51)	1	2	n.a.	1	50
	IVF		**65**	**115**	**49**	**28**	**24**
		(1)	62	112	49	27	24
		(49)	3	3	Unclear	1	33
	ICSI		**68**	**119**	**63**	**40**	**34**
		(1)	6	8	63	4	67
		(47)	1	1	63	1	100
		(31)	32	32	64	9	28
		(33)	20	68	Unclear	18	27
		(49)	2	2	Unclear	1	50
		(51)	7	8	Unclear	7	88
RLND	IUI	(1)	**47**	**170**	**n.a.**	**14**	**8**
	IVF	(1)	**21**	**24**	**41**	**12**	**50**
	ICSI	(1)	**5**	**8**	**47**	**4**	**50**
Idiopathic	IUI	(1)	**18**	**59**	**n.a.**	**4**	**7**
	IVF	(1)	**4**	**8**	**55**	**4**	**50**
	ICSI		**39**	**61**	**45**	**10**	**16**
		(1)	14	22	25	3	14
		(19)	17	29	55	3	10
	(cryopreserved ejaculate)	(19)	8	10	57	4	40
Others	IUI		**73**	**219**	**n.a.**	**21**	**10**
		(1)	66	198	n.a.	21	11
		(50)	7	21	n.a.	0	0
	IVF	(1)	**17**	**31**	**54**	**14**	**45**
	ICSI		**39**	**52**	**67**	**25**	**48**
		(1)	32	38	72	19	50
		(50)	7	14	60	6	43

Fertilization and pregnancy rates were only calculated for studies were all needed data are available. Detailed references are only given to studies published after our previous publication (1) to which we refer for detailed analysis of the summarized data provided here.
Abbreviations: n.a., not applicable.

Pretreatment with 10 to 30 mg nifedipine reduces the side effects of autonomic dysreflexia. Electroejaculation can cause significant discomfort in men with incomplete injuries and pinprick sensations in the sacral or L4 or L5 dermatome and unpredictable intolerance in those with intact sensation in the L1 to L3 dermatome. All men except those with spinal cord injuries require general anesthesia for EE. Criteria for discontinuation of the procedure are signs of autonomic dysreflexia or if rectal temperature reaches 40°C.

Success rates, ejaculate parameters and pregnancy rates are evaluated according to the criteria as outlined in our previous systematic review (1). New publications regarding the success of EE on ejaculate parameters (30,31,33,34,43,47–49) and pregnancies (19,31,33,35,49–51) were added where appropriate and are presented in Tables 4 and 5.

Recommendation: Level 3 Grade B

The underlying diagnosis of AE has no significant influence on the overall success rate of EE and no differences could be detected between the total response rates to EE between anejaculatory patients due to SCI, idiopathic AE, diabetes mellitus or RLND (Table 4). However, a strong systematic error could be expected in Table 4 as in experienced hands 80% to 100% of men after EE have at least a RE (42). Analyzing all available studies, which reported antegrade semen parameters, mean ejaculate volume between SCI patients (n = 215, 1.81 mL) and patients with idiopathic AE (n = 12, 2.30 mL) was not different. As expected by the underlying disease and its potential treatment mean sperm concentration in patients with RLND (n = 17, 26.6 million/mL) was significantly lower compared to SCI patients (n = 342, 104.7 million/mL) and patients with idiopathic AE (n = 92, 105.4 million/mL). In contrast mean total sperm motility was significantly higher in patients with RLND (n = 35, 29%) compared to SCI patients (n = 350, 17%) and patients with idiopathic AE (n = 101, 14 %). Other factors seem to have no major influence on success prognosis. In the studies where the level of the lesion is presented, no significant difference between patients with lesions including T11 and above (603 patients/457 overall responders) and patients with lesions below T11 (116 patients/72 overall responders) could be detected.

Recommendation: Level 3 Grade C

Still today, most published studies have performed inseminations with the sperm obtained with EE (Table 5). Comparing IUI, IVF and ICSI success per cycle no differences between patients with SCI, RLND and idiopathic anejaculatory patients could be observed. As expected in all different subgroups of patients ICSI showed significant higher pregnancy rates per cycle compared to IUI. Compared to IVF ICSI failed to show its advantage in the subgroup analysis. However, in patients with SCI oocyte fertilization rate was significantly higher in ICSI compared to IVF. As ICSI has shown its advantage over IUI and IVF also in other fields of infertility, ICSI should be considered as first choice, especially with the poor sperm quality often seen after EE. In addition, ICSI requires less sperm quality to be used for ART as all other methods. In a case control study the fertilization and pregnancy rates with cryopreserved sperm from EE were as good as those of freshly obtained sperm (19). As cryopreserving of sperms further reduces the poor quality of electroejaculated sperm in most cases only ICSI should be able to further reduce the number of electrostimulations needed for retrieval of sperms.

Recommendation: Level 3 Grade B

In recent years prostatic massage seems to offer an interesting alternative to the established methods. Although the overall reversal rates remains lower than with vibratory stimulation and electroejaculation (1) the simplicity of the method, the low rate of side effects and low costs makes an attempt with prostatic massage for reversal of AE attractive. For sperm retrieval by prostatic massage the patient is placed in knee–chest position. After rectal examination the prostatic massage was performed from lateral to mid-line by firm rolling motion massage of the prostate. The other prostatic lobe was palpated and the procedure repeated several times. The hypotonic anal sphincter facilitated the massage. During the massage the patient hold a sterile wide container to collect the drops from the glans penis (52,53). So far no side effects or discomfort of the procedure were reported. However, due to the low numbers it can not be excluded that prostatic massage might also induce autonomic dysreflexia requiring medical pretreatment and a clinical setting in SCI patients with lesions above T6. In addition to our previous evaluation (1) one study (35) can be added. In total 74 patients (44 SCI, 18 idiopathic AE, 9 RLND, 2 Diabetes Mellitus) have been treated. Antegrade ejaculation was achieved in 57% of non-SCI patients and 32% of men with SCI. Semen parameters showed severe impairments of motility (mean ejaculate volume 1.5 mL; mean sperm concentration 66.0 million/mL; mean total motility 7%). In 10 patients undergoing successful prostatic massage, 15 IVF cycles were performed without any clinical pregnancies. However, in the 13 patients in whom a total of 27 ICSI cycles were performed, 10 clinical pregnancies (pregnancy rate per cycle 66%) resulted in 14 live births. Whether prostatic massage offers an alternative to vibratory stimulation and EE remains to be further elucidated in more patients before it can be generally recommended outside clinical studies.

Other occasional reports on successful approaches include psychological therapy in patients with idiopathic AE and microsurgical vas deferens aspiration and an alloplastic spermatocele formation according to Wagenknecht. However, as in other cases of severe male infertility, testicular sperm extraction (TESE) in combination with ICSI provides a good alternative for sperm retrieval in anejaculatory men and is performed as first line treatment in many centres (2,54).

REFERENCES

1. Kamischke A, Nieschlag E. Treatment of retrograde ejaculation and anejaculation. Hum Reprod Update 1999; 5(5):448–474.
2. Kamischke A, Nieschlag E. Update on medical treatment of ejaculatory disorders. Int J Androl 2002; 25(6):333–344.
3. Nieschlag E, Behre HM. Andrology: Male Reproductive Health and Dysfunction, 2nd ed. Heidelberg: Springer, 2000.
4. Beckerman H, Becher J, Lankhorst GJ. The effectiveness of vibratory stimulation in anejaculatory men with spinal cord injury. Review article. Paraplegia 1993; 31(11):689–699.
5. US Department of Health and Human Services. Public Health Service. Agency for Health Care Policy and Research. 1992.
6. Das S, Dodd S, Soni BM, et al. Does repeated electro-ejaculation improve sperm quality in spinal cord injured men? Spinal Cord 2006; 44(12):753–756.
7. Hershlag A, Schiff SF, DeCherney AH. Retrograde ejaculation. Hum Reprod 1991; 6(2):255–258.
8. ESHRE Capri Workshop Group. Male infertility update. Hum Reprod 1998; 13(7):2025–2032.
9. The Male Infertility Best Practice Policy Committee of the American Urological Association and, the Practice Committee of the American Society for Reproductive Medicine.

Report on optimal evaluation of the infertile male. Fertil Steril 2006; 86(5 suppl):S202–S209.
10. The Male Infertility Best Practice Policy Committee of the American Urological Association and, the Practice Committee of the American Society for Reproductive Medicine. Report on evaluation of the azoospermic male. Fertil Steril 2006; 86(5 Suppl):S210–S215.
11. Yavetz H, Yogev L, Hauser R, et al. Retrograde ejaculation. Hum Reprod 1994; 9(3):381–386.
12. Donohue JP, Thornhill JA, Foster RS, et al. Retroperitoneal lymphadenectomy for clinical stage A testis cancer (1965 to 1989): Modifications of technique and impact on ejaculation. J Urol 1993; 149(2):237–243.
13. Chung PH, Palermo G, Schlegel PN, et al. The use of intracytoplasmic sperm injection with electroejaculates from anejaculatory men. Hum Reprod 1998; 13(7):1854–1858.
14. Köhn FM, Schill WB. The alpha-sympathomimetic midodrin as a tool for diagnosis and treatment of sperm transport disturbances. Andrologia 1994; 26(5):283–287.
15. Otani T, Kondo A, Takita T. A paraplegic fathering a child after an intrathecal injection of neostigmine: Case report. Paraplegia 1986; 24(1):32–37.
16. Murphy JB, Lipshultz LI. Abnormalities of ejaculation. Urol Clin North Am 1987; 14(3):583–596.
17. Wilcox AJ, Weinberg CR, O'Connor JF, et al. Incidence of early loss of pregnancy. N Engl J Med 1988; 319(4):189–194.
18. Ichiyanagi O, Sasagawa I, Suzuki Y, et al. Successful treatment of retrograde ejaculation with amezinium. Arch Androl 2003; 49(3):215–217.
19. Hovav Y, Almagor M, Yaffe H. Comparison of semen quality obtained by electroejaculation and spontaneous ejaculation in men suffering from ejaculation disorder. Hum Reprod 2002; 17(12): 3170–3172.
20. Crich JP, Jequier AM. Infertility in men with retrograde ejaculation: The action of urine on sperm motility, and a simple method for achieving antegrade ejaculation. Fertil Steril 1978; 30(5):572–576.
21. Linsenmeyer TA, Perkash I. Infertility in men with spinal cord injury. Arch Phys Med Rehabil 1991; 72(10):747–754.
22. Brackett NL. Semen retrieval by penile vibratory stimulation in men with spinal cord injury. Hum Reprod Update 1999; 5(3):216–222.
23. Goldwasser B, Madgar I, Jonas P, et al. Imipramine for the treatment of sterility in patients following retroperitoneal lymph node dissection. Andrologia 1983; 15 Spec No:588–591.
24. Schill WB. Pregnancy after brompheniramine treatment of a diabetic with incomplete emission failure. Arch Androl 1990; 25(1):101–104.
25. Jesionowska H, Hemmings R. Good-quality semen recovered from a paraplegic man with physostigmine salicylate treatment. A case report. J Reprod Med 1991; 36(3):167–169.
26. Chapelle PA, Roby-Brami A, Yakovleff A, et al. Neurological correlations of ejaculation and testicular size in men with a complete spinal cord section. J Neurol Neurosurg Psychiatry 1988; 51(2): 197–202.
27. Mallidis C, Lim TC, Hill ST, et al. Necrospermia and chronic spinal cord injury. Fertil Steril 2000; 74(2):221–227.
28. Ohl DA, Sonksen J, Wedemeyer G, et al. Canine model of infertility after spinal cord injury: Time course of acute changes in semen quality and spermatogenesis. J Urol 2001; 166(3):1181–1184.
29. Brackett NL, Lynne CM, Aballa TC, et al. Sperm motility from the vas deferens of spinal cord injured men is higher than from the ejaculate. J Urol 2000; 164(3 Pt 1):712–715.
30. Ohl DA, Menge AC, Jarow JP. Seminal vesicle aspiration in spinal cord injured men: Insight into poor sperm quality. J Urol 1999; 162(6):2048–2051.
31. Giulini S, Pesce F, Madgar I, et al. Influence of multiple transrectal electroejaculations on semen parameters and intracytoplasmic sperm injection outcome. Fertil Steril 2004; 82(1):200–204.
32. Hamid R, Patki P, Bywater H, et al. Effects of repeated ejaculations on semen characteristics following spinal cord injury. Spinal Cord 2006; 44(6):369–373.
33. Heruti RJ, Katz H, Menashe Y, et al. Treatment of male infertility due to spinal cord injury using rectal probe electroejaculation: The Israeli experience. Spinal Cord 2001; 39(3):168–175.
34. Hovav Y, Sibirsky O, Pollack RN, et al. Comparison between the first and the second electroejaculate qualities obtained from neurologically intact men suffering from anejaculation. Hum Reprod 2005; 20(9):2620–2622.
35. Momen MN, Fahmy I, Amer M, et al. Semen parameters in men with spinal cord injury: Changes and aetiology. Asian J Androl 2007; 9(5):684–689.
36. Sonksen J, Ohl DA, Giwercman A, et al. Effect of repeated ejaculation on semen quality in spinal cord injured men. J Urol 1999; 161(4):1163–1165.
37. Brackett NL, Padron OF, Lynne CM. Semen quality of spinal cord injured men is better when obtained by vibratory stimulation versus electroejaculation. J Urol 1997; 157(1):151–157.
38. Ohl DA, Sonksen J, Menge AC, et al. Electroejaculation versus vibratory stimulation in spinal cord injured men: Sperm quality and patient preference. J Urol 1997; 157(6):2147–2149.
39. Sonksen J, Biering-Sorensen F, Kristensen JK. Ejaculation induced by penile vibratory stimulation in men with spinal cord injuries. The importance of the vibratory amplitude. Paraplegia 1994; 32(10):651–660.
40. Brackett NL, Ferrell SM, Aballa TC, et al. (1998). An analysis of 653 trials of penile vibratory stimulation in men with spinal cord injury. J Urol 1998; 159:1931–1934.

41. Soler JM, Previnaire JG, Plante P, et al. Midodrine improves ejaculation in spinal cord injured men. J Urol 2007; 178(5):2082–2086.
42. Sonksen J, Ohl DA. Penile vibratory stimulation and electroejaculation in the treatment of ejaculatory dysfunction. Int J Androl 2002; 25(6):324–332.
43. Sonksen J, Ohl DA, Wedemeyer G. Sphincteric events during penile vibratory ejaculation and electroejaculation in men with spinal cord injuries. J Urol 2001; 165(2):426–429.
44. Dahlberg A, Ruutu M, Hovatta O. Pregnancy results from a vibrator application, electroejaculation, and a vas aspiration programme in spinal-cord injured men. Hum Reprod 1995; 10(9):2305–2307.
45. Ohl DA, Bennett CJ, McCabe M, et al. Predictors of success in electroejaculation of spinal cord injured men. J Urol 1989; 142(6):1483–1486.
46. Brackett NL, Ead DN, Aballa TC, et al. Semen retrieval in men with spinal cord injury is improved by interrupting current delivery during electroejaculation. J Urol 2002; 167(1):201–203.
47. Chen SU, Shieh JY, Wang YH, et al. Successful pregnancy achieved by intracytoplasmic sperm injection using cryopreserved electroejaculate sperm in a couple both with spinal cord injury: A case report. Arch Phys Med Rehabil 2005; 86(9):1884–1886.
48. Hovav Y, Sibirsky O, Davarashvili A, et al. Electroejaculation with a foley catheter in the bladder. J Androl 2004; 25(6):960–962.
49. Kolettis PN, Lambert MC, Hammond KR, et al. Fertility outcomes after electroejaculation in men with spinal cord injury. Fertil Steril 2002; 78(2):429–431.
50. Schatte EC, Orejuela FJ, Lipshultz LI, et al. Treatment of infertility due to anejaculation in the male with electroejaculation and intracytoplasmic sperm injection. J Urol 2000; 163(6):1717–1720.
51. Shieh JY, Chen SU, Wang YH, et al. A protocol of electroejaculation and systematic assisted reproductive technology achieved high efficiency and efficacy for pregnancy for anejaculatory men with spinal cord injury. Arch Phys Med Rehabil 2003; 84(4):535–540.
52. Fahmy I, Kamal A, Metwali M, et al. Vigorous prostatic massage: A simple method to retrieve spermatozoa for intracytoplasmic sperm injection in psychogenic anejaculation: case report. Hum Reprod 1999; 14(8):2050–2053.
53. Marina S, Marina F, Alcolea R, et al. Triplet pregnancy achieved through intracytoplasmic sperm injection with spermatozoa obtained by prostatic massage of a paraplegic patient: Case report. Hum Reprod 1999; 14(6):1546–1548.
54. Löchner-Ernst D, Mandalka B, Kramer G, et al. Conservative and surgical semen retrieval in patients with spinal cord injury. Spinal Cord 1997; 35(7):463–468.

8 Sperm preparation for ART and IUI

Kersti Lundin

KEY POINTS

- Sperm preparation is performed to select and isolate a population of highly motile, functional spermatozoa with low levels of anomalies.
- Swim-up and density gradient centrifugation methods are the most widely used sperm preparation techniques at present.
- Currently existing data does not show any significant differences in fertilization and pregnancy rates when comparing these methods.

Preparation of the ejaculated sperm before use for insemination fulfils several purposes, where isolation and selection of spermatozoa may be considered the most important. An optimal preparation method should separate the motile spermatozoa from dead sperm and debris as well as from the seminal plasma itself that contains substances that inhibit capacitation, thereby reducing the sperms capacity to fertilize the oocyte. The ejaculate may also be contaminated by for example bacteria, virus and/or leukocytes, which should be removed by the preparation process (1–4).

ART treatments today have shifted from being primarily focused on female subfertility factors to also include severe male factors, such as low numbers of sperm, low motility and/or poor sperm morphology. This requires refined methods of sperm preparation in order to obtain a final result consisting of a concentrated and clean sperm sample also from a poor quality ejaculate or a testicular biopsy with low numbers of sperm, much debris and other cells. Correspondingly, methods have moved from a sole washing step to more advanced methods where high-quality spermatozoa are being concentrated.

Throughout the years a large number of sperm preparation techniques have been invented, published, tried, and often discarded. It seems clear that clinical ART laboratories require methods that are not only effective and rapid but also easy to use and inexpensive, and therefore more complicated methods do not seem to become adopted. Thus, the consistently most common ways to prepare sperm for ART are still to use a swim-up method or discontinuous density gradient centrifugation (1,5–14).

SEPARATION FROM SEMINAL PLASMA

Prolonged exposure of spermatozoa to other cells present in the ejaculate such as leukocytes and dead spermatozoa can result in impaired sperm motility and sperm DNA fragmentation (15–19). It is therefore of importance to isolate the spermatozoa from the seminal plasma as soon as possible, preferably within an hour after ejaculation. However, before the preparation is started, the ejaculate should be allowed to liquefy at room temperature for 20 to 30 minutes.

In the beginning of assisted reproduction the practice of collecting a split ejaculate was sometimes used. This method, where the patient is asked to collect his sperm sample split into two or three pots, is based on the physiological concept that the spermatozoa are not normally present in the last portion of the ejaculate. By separating the sperm-rich first portion of the ejaculate from the following portions the sperm will be less subjected to negative factors from the seminal plasma and it has been discussed (20) that this could improve fertilization and pregnancy rates. However, the split method is more awkward for the patient, especially in a stressed situation, and there are no studies showing improved ART results when split ejaculates are used. The method is therefore very rarely practiced in the clinical situation today.

SPERM PREPARATION METHODS

Direct Washing

In the early days of IVF, sperm were prepared by a simple washing method, where the ejaculate is diluted with cell culture medium and then centrifuged (21). Later, this direct washing method was mostly combined with a swim-up from the centrifugation pellet. However, although most of the seminal plasma will be removed with this direct centrifugation method by repeated washing, both live and dead spermatozoa, and in addition debris and other cells such as epithelial cells and leukocytes will be concentrated together in the pellet. This has been shown to induce the production of reactive oxygen species, known to cause membrane and nuclear damage to the spermatozoa and impair their fertilizing capacity (1,16–17,22). Thus, the method of direct washing of the ejaculate should be avoided. However, it may be acceptable when only occasional spermatozoa are found in the ejaculate or in a biopsy from the testicle. In these cases it may be necessary to concentrate the sample by direct washing before starting the sperm selection.

Density Gradient Separation

Centrifugation of the ejaculate through a series of gradients of different viscosity enriches highly motile spermatozoa by utilizing the density difference between live spermatozoa and dead sperm, other cells and debris in the ejaculate. The motility of the spermatozoa will increase the selection capacity of this method.

Typically, discontinuous gradients of silane coated particles are used. Originally, the method was developed with Percoll, but due to high endotoxin levels this product was withdrawn from clinical use in 1996. New silica products such as PureSperm®, IxaPrep or Isolate or iohexol molecules (Nycodenz®) products have been found to be equivalent to Percoll in aspects of sperm yield, motility and normal sperm morphology (11,23–25).

The gradients can be purchased ready-to-use, or bought as a 100% stock solution to be diluted with the sperm preparation medium normally used in the clinic. The gradients should be layered on the same day they are to be used, since this will conserve more distinct boundaries between the layers. Most common is the use of two layers (45/90% or 40/80%), but an increased number of layers can be used. A comparison of two-layer versus four-layer PureSperm gradients showed that four-layer gradient yielded a higher proportion of motile spermatozoa and slightly higher rates of spermatozoa with normal morphology (11). However, it is more time-consuming and more expensive to increase the number of layers, and it has not been shown to improve fertilization rates.

Example of How to Perform a Density Gradient Separation (see also Fig. 1)

Load 1 mL (if more than two layers are used) or 2 mL (if two layers are used) of each gradient in a 15 mL centrifugation tube, with the most diluted gradient on top. For commercial media—which is recommended to use—specified instructions for use will be included upon purchase. Each gradient has to be carefully loaded onto the previous, in order not to mix the boundary surfaces. Above the gradients 1 to 2 mL ejaculate is loaded. Centrifugate the gradients at 300 rpm for 20 to 30 minutes (the longer time if a higher number of layers are used). The seminal plasma will stay on top, some debris, dead sperm and other cells end up in between the layers, while the pellet will contain mainly motile spermatozoa. If the ejaculate is very contaminated by cells and debris the amount of ejaculate loaded on top should be decreased, otherwise the debris may pass through the gradients down to the pellet. After centrifugation, the seminal plasma together with the top gradient layer is pipetted off and discarded. Then collect the pellet from the bottom of the tube with a clean Pasteur pipette and transfer to a new 15 mL centrifugation tube. Wash the pellet twice by adding approximately 5 mL medium, centrifugate, resuspend, repeat and finally dilute to the preferred concentration before use for IUI, IVF or ICSI.

Swim-up

The so called swim-up technique utilizes the spermatozoa's own swimming ability. Swim-up generally results in a lower total yield of sperm than gradient centrifugation but with a higher proportion of motile spermatozoa (11,26–27). During the preparation there may be a risk for contamination of the swim up medium with compounds from the seminal plasma (28), especially if the seminal plasma has a high viscosity. In addition to being a technique for isolation of motile spermatozoa, the yield and motility after a standardized swim-up procedure can be used as a functional test to discriminate between whether to perform conventional IVF or ICSI. When a yield of less than one million motile sperm are obtained from a good quality ejaculate after a standardized swim-up procedure, this may be regarded as an indication for performing ICSI (29,30).

Example of How to Perform a Swim-up (see also Fig. 2)

Load 1 mL of ejaculate in the bottom of a 15 mL centrifugation tube, and carefully add 1.5 mL medium on top. It is important to use exact volumes if the swim-up is to be used as a functional test. The procedure can also be performed by underloading when the medium is first loaded in the tube, and thereafter the ejaculate is added underneath the medium. This will usually result in less mixing of the surface between the ejaculate and the medium.

Incubate the tube (37°C) for 30 to 60 minutes at an 45° angle. This increases the surface area between the ejaculate and the medium, facilitating sperm transfer from seminal plasma to medium. After incubation, use a sterile Pasteur pipette to collect 1 mL of the supernatant and transfer into a clean tube.

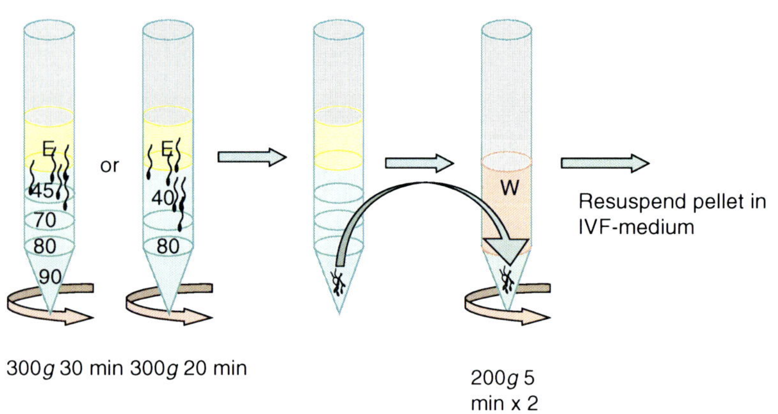

Figure 1 Gradient separation. Examples of gradient centrifugation are here shown using four or two gradients of different viscosity. E = ejaculate; 45, 70, 80, 90 = viscous gradients; W = washing medium. See text for explanation.

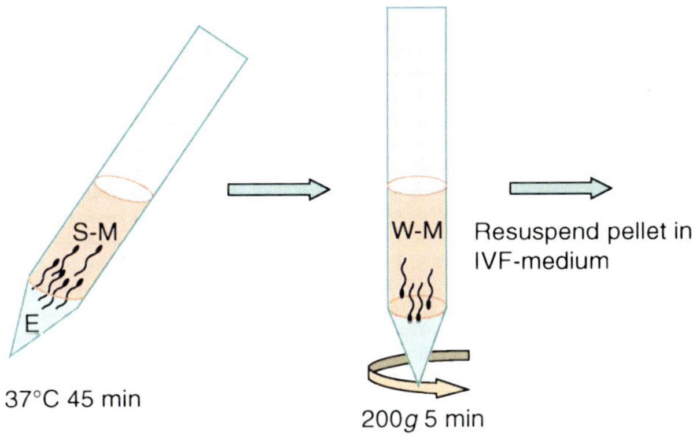

Figure 2 Swim-out. Example of how to perform a swim-up. E = ejaculate, S-M = swim-up medium, W-M = washing medium. See text for explanation.

Be careful not to include any of the underlying seminal plasma. Wash and concentrate the supernatant by adding approximately 5 mL medium and centrifuge at 300 g for five minutes. Often, two tubes are loaded for swim-up, and the supernatant from them pooled and washed.

Performing swim-up is not optimal for sperm samples with a low sperm concentration (< 1 million). In these cases it is possible to do so called mini-swim-ups, when several tubes with a low volume of ejaculate (0.1–0.5 mL) and a correspondingly low volume of medium (0.5–1.0 mL) in each are used. This will increase the total area between the ejaculate and the medium phases, allowing more sperm in total to swim up into the medium. For ejaculates with a high presence of other cells and debris it is usually more optimal to perform a density gradient centrifugation.

Side Migration "Swim-out"

When an extremely low number of spermatozoa are present in the ejaculate or in a biopsy from the testicle or the epididymis, regular swim-up or gradient separation techniques will usually not produce good results, since there is a high loss of spermatozoa when using these methods. Instead, a kind of horizontal swim-up ("swim-out") or side migration procedure can be used (31) (Fig. 3), where a few μL of ejaculate or washed sperm sample is placed either into a large medium droplet (100–200 μL) connected with a number of smaller droplets, or directly into one or several small (10–20 μL) medium droplets. The spermatozoa will swim out to the droplet edges, where they can be picked up directly with the ICSI needle. The side migration technique produces a considerably cleaner sample than a simple washing/centrifugation procedure, and will thus facilitate the ICSI procedure. It was also shown in a small study (31), that for oligospermic samples, this technique compared with direct wash/swim-up and gradient centrifugation resulted in highest rates of motile spermatozoa and normal morphology spermatozoa, as well as sperm with normal chromatin condensation (evidence level 3).

Other Sperm Preparation Techniques

A large number of different techniques for enhancing sperm quality and capacity for fertilization have been proposed. The glass wool filtration (GWF) technique has in several reports been shown to result in a high yield of spermatozoa with equal or

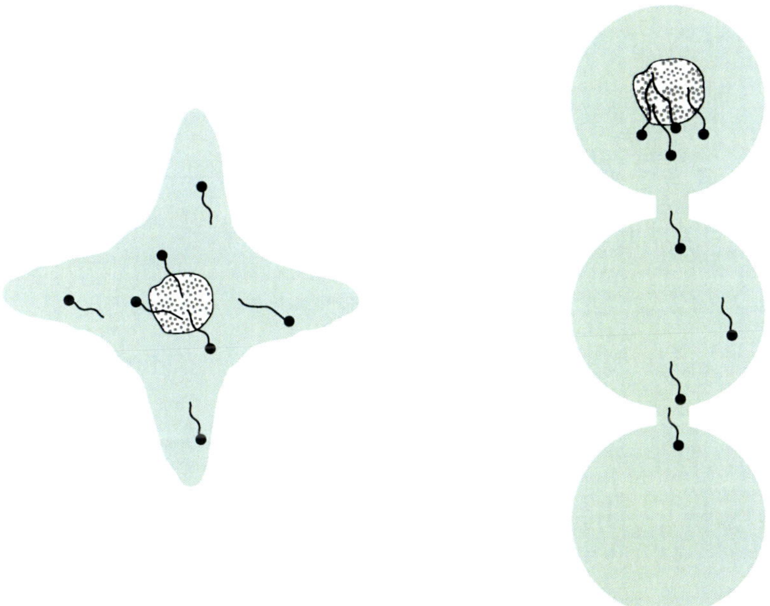

Figure 3 When the ejaculate contains very few sperm, the "swim-out" or side migration method can be used. Two examples of the method is shown here. A single droplet of medium (15–20 μL) is put into a Petri dish, and a pipette is used to draw out a number of elongations. The sperm sample (2–3 μL ejaculate or washed sperm) is added into the middle. The spermatozoa will swim away from the seminal plasma and out to the "arms" of the droplet where they can be picked up with a microinjection pipette. To the right another variant is shown. Here three droplets are made, with narrow channels drawn between them. The sperm sample is added to the first droplet and the sperm can be picked up after swimming into the second or third droplet.

improved morphology and nuclear integrity compared to swim-up and gradient separation (12–15,32–35) (evidence level 2a). Despite this and the early introduction of GWF, the method is not commonly used in the clinical setting. A recently published study presented a molecular based GWF technique, where the traditional GWF was combined with annexin V binding (36).

Another novel method, electrophoretic separation (37), has been suggested as a rapid method to isolate spermatozoa of high quality with low rates of DNA damage. It has been shown to be comparable to discontinuous gradient centrifugation regarding yield, motility, and DNA fragmentation. There were also no significant differences found regarding fertilization, pregnancy and implantation rates (38) (evidence level 2b).

Magnetic activated cell separation (MACS) in combination with density gradient separation has shown to enrich the fraction of nonapoptotic spermatozoa (evidence level 2b) and result in comparable rates of fertilization, embryo development and implantation (39–41) compared with only gradient separation (evidence level 3).

A method where Petri dishes coated with hyaluronic acid (HA) are used to bind single mature spermatozoa to be used for ICSI (42) has been developed. The sperm HA receptors play a role in sperm-zona and sperm-oolemmal binding. The method is thus based on the principle that HA-bound sperm would be similar to those that bind to the zona pellucida, and thereby hypothesised to have a high fertilization potential. The method was shown to increase the proportion of haploid spermatozoa with normal morphology compared with the native semen population (42,43) (evidence level 2b). However, there are no results published of comparisons with other sperm selection methods regarding outcome after preparation, or regarding IVF success parameters such as fertilization, embryo development, pregnancy or implantation rates. In addition, this method can only be used in combination with ICSI.

Many other methods for optimal isolation of sperm have been proposed, for example the dual-chamber capillary dish (44), the microchamber (45), nuclepore membranes (46), and swim-up in media containing for example hyaluronidase (47) or dextran (17). However, the majority of these techniques are either more complicated, more expensive, and/or result in a very low yield of spermatozoa compared to current methods, and have so far not gained widespread clinical use.

SPERM PREPARATION MEDIUM

Usually a swim-up or a gradient separation with subsequent washing are performed in a HEPES buffered medium supplemented with albumin. Sperm preparation medium can also be supplemented with antibiotics and/or antioxidants. The final dilution before IVF/ICSI should be made in a medium optimized for fertilization, without HEPES buffer.

A number of different motility enhancers have been investigated, in particular pentoxifylline (PF), a phosphodiesterase inhibitor. This substance has been used in order to increase fertilization rates, especially in patients with asthenozoospermia (13,48). Although several studies have shown pentoxyfylline to increase sperm motility in poor quality sperm samples (48–50) (evidence level 2b), other studies have shown no effect on motility on normospermic samples and/or fertilization rates (50,51) (evidence level 2a). Most existing studies are small and retrospective, and no large conclusive studies have been performed. Pentoxyfylline has also been used to initiate motility in immotile fresh and frozen-thawed testicular sperm, thus discriminating between live and dead spermatozoa for ICSI in these samples (52–54) (evidence level 3).

WHICH METHOD TO CHOOSE?

So which method of preparation is the best choice for an ART laboratory? In a research setting, more advanced and elaborate methods are sometimes used. However, for a routine ART laboratory the sperm preparation should be fast, easy to perform, efficient and preferably inexpensive, which excludes many of the developed methods. Most clinics stick to one method and use it for all samples and situations, although perhaps the ideal would be to choose method according to the quality of the ejaculate and treatment method that is to be used (Table 1) (55). For intrauterine insemination a higher volume and a higher

Table 1 Comparison Between the Most Common Techniques for Sperm Preparation

	Advantage	Evidence level	Disadvantage
Direct wash	No loss of sperm cells		Contamination by other cells and debris
	Easy to perform		Negative influence by seminal plasma
Swim-up	Highest rates of motile sperm	2a	Possible contamination by seminal plasma
	Gives a clean sample		
	Easy to perform		
Gradient centrifugation	Highest total sperm yield	2a	Possible contamination of gradient substance
	Highest rate of normal morphology	2a	
	High rates of nuclearly normal sperm	2a	
	Easy to perform		
Side migration	Gives a clean sample with motile sperm when very few sperm are available		Only for ICSI
			Not applicable for good quality ejaculates
	Easy to perform		

concentration of spermatozoa is desirable. A standard procedure usually requires that 3 to 5 million motile sperm to be used for insemination are obtained after preparation (56–58). Thus, the density gradient centrifugation method can be recommended for IUI, since it will produce a high total sperm count compared with other methods.

The impact of sperm morphology in ART has been much discussed. It seems clear that sperm morphology correlates at least to a certain extent with fertilization capacity in conventional IVF although there are conflicting reports (30,59–61) (evidence level 2b). Many ART laboratories are now abandoning the analysis of strict sperm morphology, due to that it is time-consuming and difficult to obtain consistency in results.

Different preparation methods will affect the ratio of normal forms, which might be considered when preparing sperm for conventional IVF. It can be concluded from several studies that gradient separation results in a higher rate of normal forms than swim-up (12,62–63) (evidence level 2a). It is important to note though, that in some of these studies the semen was washed by centrifugation before swim-up, which may have caused damage to the spermatozoa as previously discussed. It can also be concluded that swim-up results in a higher proportion of motile spermatozoa than density gradient separation with either Percoll or PureSperm (11,26,27,64) (evidence level 2a).

A number of studies have shown correlations between abnormal sperm DNA integrity and fertilization rates, pregnancy rates and/or early spontaneous abortions (65–69) (evidence level 2a). Both gradient separation and glass wool filtration have shown to be superior to swim-up for selection of sperm with normal nuclear DNA (12,70,71) (evidence level 3).

When performing conventional IVF, the prepared sperm and oocytes are incubated together, either in an open volume in a Petri dish, or in microdroplets under oil. In general, a couple of hundred thousand spermatozoa are required for conventional IVF (depending on how many oocytes that are being inseminated). Thus, sperm preparation for conventional IVF can usually be performed equally well by swim-up or by gradient separation, whichever is considered most convenient for the laboratory. Ejaculates of very high viscosity and/or with a very high presence of other cells and debris might be of advantage to prepare by gradient centrifugation. During a swim-up procedure, cells and debris can stick to the sperm, which may contaminate the supernatant. When handling ejaculates of a very high viscosity the ejaculate can be mixed with medium (1:1) before preparation to facilitate the isolation of the spermatozoa.

Intracytoplasmic sperm injection requires only a low number of--preferably motile—spermatozoa. It facilitates the immobilization and aspiration into the microinjection needle if the sample contains a high proportion of motile sperm as is possible. This implies that swim-up may be preferential to gradient centrifugation. Another advantage with swim-up compared with gradient separation is that only "pure" medium is used throughout the whole preparation. When using the viscous gradients, in some poor quality sperm samples residues of the gradients may cause stickiness during the ICSI procedure. For samples with extreme low sperm concentration a side migration technique can be more optimal.

When ICSI is used as treatment method, fertilization and pregnancy rates are less influenced by sperm factors such as concentration, morphology, motility and chromatin decondensation (66,72–76). Thus, the sperm preparation method does not need to be aimed at sperm selection to the same extent as when IUI or conventional IVF is used.

SPERM PREPARATION AND ART RESULTS

In a meta-analysis, five randomised control trials (RCTs) where different sperm preparation techniques (gradient, direct wash and swim-up) were compared regarding pregnancy rates after IUI (262 couples) were included (75). No difference in pregnancy rates was found (evidence level 1a) and it was concluded that at present, no specific technique could be recommended, but that larger RCTs are needed.

For conventional IVF, no significant differences were found when comparing swim-up and gradient separation regarding fertilization rates, proportion of good quality embryos or pregnancy rates (11–12) (evidence level 2a). In the study by Söderlund and Lundin (11), the swim-up procedure was recommended for the reasons that a higher proportion of motile spermatozoa is obtained, and that no other substances than the ordinary culture media are used in the preparation process.

In conclusion, although both of the two most utilized techniques for semen preparation are efficient for selecting a sperm population of high quality, the highest proportion of morphologically normal spermatozoa and the lowest contamination of bacteria are seen after semen processed using density centrifugation. In contrast, when swim-up is performed, the highest proportion of motile sperm are obtained. No conclusive differences in the fertilization, implantation and pregnancy rates between the different preparation methods have been shown, and it should thus be choice of the laboratory to decide when to use which method. The more novel methods such as electrophoretic or magnetic separation and hyaluronic acid binding need more evaluation before introduction into the clinical setting.

REFERENCES

1. Bolton VN, Braude PR. Preparation of human spermatozoa for in vitro fertilization by isopycnic centrifugation on self-generating density gradients. Arch Androl 1984; 13:167–176.
2. Merino G, Carranza-Lira S, Murrieta S, et al. Bacterial infection and semen characteristics in infertile men. Arch Androl 1995; 35:43–47.
3. Cottell E, Lennon B, McMorrow J, et al. Processing of semen in an antibiotic-rich culture medium to minimize microbial presence during in vitro fertilization. Fertil Steril 1997; 67:98–103.

4. Nicholson CM, Abramsson L, Holm SE, et al. Bacterial contamination and sperm recovery after semen preparation by density gradient centrifugation using silane-coated silica particles at different g forces. Hum Reprod 2000; 15:662–666.
5. Lopata A, Patullo MJ, Chang A, et al. A method for collecting motile spermatozoa from human semen. Fertil Steril 1976; 27:677–684.
6. Pertoft H, Laurent TC, Laas T. Density gradients prepared from collodial silica particles coated by polyvinylpyrrolidone (Percoll). Anal Biochem 1978; 88:271–277.
7. Gorus FK, Pipeleers DG. A rapid method for the fractionation of human spermatozoa according to their progressive motility. Fertil. Steril 1981; 35:662–665.
8. Mahadevan M, Baker J. Assessment and preparation of semen for in vitro fertilisation. In: Wood C, Trounson A, eds. Clinical in Vitro Fertilisation. Berlin: Springer-Verlag, 1984: 83–97.
9. Makler A, Murillo O, Huszar G, et al. Improved techniques for collecting motile spermatozoa from human semen. I. A self-migratory method. Int J Androl 1984; 7:61–70.
10. World Health Organization (WHO) Laboratory Manual for the Examination of Human Semen and Sperm–Cervical Mucus Interaction, 4th ed. Cambridge: Cambridge University Press, 1999.
11. Söderlund B, Lundin K. The use of silane-coated silica particles for density gradient centrifugation in in-vitro fertilization. Hum Reprod 2000; 15:857–860.
12. Hammadeh ME, Kühnen A, Amer AS, et al. Comparison of sperm preparation methods: Effect on chromatin and morphology recovery rates and their consequences on the clinical outcome after in vitro fertilization embryo transfer. Int J Androl 2001; 24:360–368.
13. Henkel RR, Schill WB. Sperm preparation for ART. Reprod Biol Endocrinol 2003; 108.
14. Paasch U, Grunewald S, Glander HJ. Sperm selection in assisted reproductive techniques. Soc Reprod Fertil Suppl 2007; 65:515–525.
15. Aitken RJ, Clarkson JS. Significance of reactive oxygen species and antioxidants in defining the efficacy of sperm preparation techniques. J Androl 1988; 9:367–376.
16. Mortimer D. Sperm preparation techniques and iatrogenic failures of in-vitro fertilization. Hum Reprod 1991; 6:173–176.
17. Alvarez JG, Lasso JL, Blasco L, et al. Centrifugation of human spermatozoa induces sublethal damage; separation of human spermatozoa from seminal plasma by a dextran swim-up procedure without centrifugation extends their motile lifetime. Hum Reprod 1993; 8:1087–1092.
18. Parinaud J, Le Lannou D, Vieitez G, et al. Enhancement of motility by treating spermatozoa with an antioxidant solution (Sperm-Fit) following ejaculation. Hum Reprod 1997; 12:2434–2436.
19. Twigg J, Fulton N, Gomez E. et al. Analysis of the impact of intracellular reactive oxygen species generation on the structural and functional integrity of human spermatozoa: Lipid peroxidation, DNA fragmentation and effectiveness of antioxidants. Hum Reprod 1998; 13:1429–1436.
20. Björndahl L, Kvist U. Sequence of ejaculation. Reprod Biomed Online 2003; 7:440–448.
21. Tarlatzis BC, Laufer N, Murillo O, et al. Semen evaluation following preparation for in vitro fertilization of human oocytes. Arch Androl 1986; 17:215–222.
22. Marchetti C, Obert G, Deffosez A, et al. Study of mitochondrial membrane potential, reactive oxygen species, DNA fragmentation and cell viability by flow cytometry in human sperm. Hum Reprod 2002; 17:1257–1265.
23. Serafini P, Blank W, Tran C, et al. Enhanced penetration of zona-free hamster ova by sperm prepared by Nycodenz and Percoll gradient centrifugation. Fertil Steril 1990; 53:551–555.
24. Claassens OE, Menkveld R, Harrison KL. Evaluation of three substitutes for Percoll in sperm isolation by density gradient centrifugation. Hum Reprod 1998; 13:3139–3143.
25. Chen MJ, Bongso A. Comparative evaluation of two density gradient preparations for sperm separation for medically assisted conception. Hum Reprod 1999; 14:759–764.
26. Englert Y, Van den Bergh M, Rodesch C, et al. Comparative auto-controlled study between swim-up and Percoll preparation of fresh semen samples for in-vitro fertilization. Hum Reprod 1992; 7:399–402.
27. Ng FLH, Liu DY, Baker HWG. Comparison of Percoll, mini-Percoll and swim-up methods for sperm preparation from abnormal semen samples. Hum Reprod 1992; 7:261–266.
28. Björndahl L, Mohammadieh M, Pourian M, et al. Contamination by seminal plasma factors during sperm selection. J Androl 2005; 26:170–173.
29. Westlander G, Levkov L. Spermaanalys och preparation. In: Hreinsson J, Hamberger L, Hardarson TH, eds. Infertilitet. Studentlitteratur 2005:61–75.
30. Söderlund B, Lundin K. Choosing fertilization method by analyzing sperm morphology or by performing swim-up preparation. Acta Obstet Gynecol Scand 2006; 85:306–311.
31. Hinting A, Lunardhi H. Better sperm selection for intracytoplasmic sperm injection with the side migration technique. Andrologia 2001; 33:343–346.
32. Paulson JD, Polakoski K, Leto S. Further characterization of glasswool column filtration of human serum. Fertil Steril 1979; 32:125–126.
33. Jeyendran RS, Perez-Pelaez M, Crabo BG. Concentration of viable spermatozoa for artificial insemination. Fertil Steril 1986; 45:132–134.
34. Johnson DE, Confino E, Jeyendran RS. Glass wool column filtration versus mini-Percoll gradient for processing poor quality semen samples. Fertil Steril 1996; 66:459–462.
35. Nani JM, Jeyendran RS. Sperm processing: Glass wool column filtration. Arch Androl 2001; 47:15–21.

36. Grunewald S, Miska W, Miska G, et al. Molecular glass wool filtration as a new tool for sperm preparation. Hum Reprod 2007; 22:1405–1412.
37. Ainsworth C, Nixon B, Aitken RJ. Development of a novel electrophoretic system for the isolation of human spermatozoa. Hum Reprod 2005; 20:2261–2267.
38. Fleming SD, Ilad RS, Griffin AM, et al. 2008; 23:2646–2651.
39. Said TM, Agarwal A, Grunewald S, et al. Evaluation of sperm recovery following annexin V magnetic-activated cell sorting separation. Reprod Biomed Online 2006; 13:336–339.
40. Grunewald S, Paasch U, Glander HJ. Enrichment of non-apoptotic human spermatozoa after cryopreservation by immunomagnetic cell sorting. Cell Tissue Bank 2001; 2:127–133.
41. Dirican EK, Ozgün OD, Akarsu S, et al. Clinical outcome of magnetic activated cell sorting of non-apoptotic spermatozoa before density gradient centrifugation for assisted reproduction. J Assist Reprod Genet. 2008; 25:375–381.
42. Huszar G, Jakab A, Sakkas D, et al. Fertility testing and ICSI sperm selection by hyaluronic acid binding: Clinical and genetic aspects. Reprod Biomed Online 2007; 14:650–663.
43. Jakab A, Sakkas D, Delpiano E, et al. Intracytoplasmic sperm injection: A novel selection method for sperm with normal frequency of chromosomal aneuploidies. Fertil Steril 2005; 84:1665–673.
44. Sills ES, Wittkowski KM, Tucker MJ, et al. Comparison of centrifugation- and noncentrifugation-based techniques for recovery of motile human sperm in assisted reproduction. Arch Androl 2002; 48:141–5.
45. Lih CH, Obasaju M, McCaffrey C, et al. Development of a microchamber which spontaneously selects high-quality sperm for use in in vitro fertilization or micromanipulation. J Assist Reprod Genet 1996; 13:657–662.
46. Chijioke PC, Crocker PR, Gilliam M, et al. Importance of filter structure for the trans-membrane migration studies of sperm motility. Hum Reprod 1988; 3:241–244.
47. Wikland M, Wik O, Steen Y, et al. A self-migration method for preparation of sperm for in-vitro fertilization. Hum Reprod 1987; 2:191–195.
48. Yovich JL. Pentoxifylline: Actions and applications in assisted reproduction. Hum Reprod 1993; 8:1786–1791.
49. Tarlatzis BC, Kolibianakis EM, Bontis J, et al. Effect of pentoxifylline on human sperm motility and fertilizing capacity. Arch Androl 1995; 34:33–42.
50. Dimitriadou F, Rizos D, Mantzavinos T, et al. The effect of pentoxifylline on sperm motility, oocyte fertilization, embryo quality, and pregnancy outcome in an in vitro fertilization program. Fertil Steril 1995; 63:880–886.
51. Tournaye H, Janssens R, Verheyen G, et al. An indiscriminate use of pentoxifylline does not improve in-vitro fertilization in poor fertilizers. Hum Reprod 1994; 9:1289–1292.
52. Terriou P, Hans E, Giorgetti C, et al. Pentoxifylline initiates motility in spontaneously immotile epididymal and testicular spermatozoa and allows normal fertilization, pregnancy, and birth after intracytoplasmic sperm injection. J Assist Reprod Genet 2000; 17:194–199.
53. Kovacic B, Vlaisavljevic V, Reljic M. Clinical use of pentoxifylline for activation of immotile testicular sperm before ICSI in patients with azoospermia. J Androl 2006; 27: 45–52.
54. Griveau JF, Lobel B, Laurent MC, et al. Interest of pentoxifylline in ICSI with frozen-thawed testicular spermatozoa from patients with non-obstructive azoospermia. Reprod Biomed Online 2006; 12:14–18.
55. Leonetti T, Causio F, Cagnazzo G. Techniques of sperm selection and in vitro fertilization results. Acta Eur Fertil 1995; 26:31–34.
56. Khalil MR, Rasmussen PE, Erb K, et al. Homologous intrauterine insemination. An evaluation of prognostic factors based on a review of 2473 cycles. Acta Obstet Gynecol Scand 2001; 80:74–81.
57. Strandell A, Bergh C, Söderlund B, et al. Fallopian tube sperm perfusion: The impact of sperm count and morphology on pregnancy rates. Acta Obstet Gynecol Scand 2003; 82:1023–1029.
58. Wainer R, Albert M, Dorion A, et al. Influence of the number of motile spermatozoa inseminated and of their morphology on the success of intrauterine insemination. Hum Reprod 2004; 19:2060–2065.
59. Lundin K, Söderlund B, Hamberger L. The relationship between sperm morphology and rates of fertilization, pregnancy and spontaneous abortion in an in-vitro fertilization/intracytoplasmic sperm injection programme. Hum Reprod 1997; 12:2676–2681.
60. Høst E, Ernst E, Lindenberg S, et al. Morphology of spermatozoa used in IVF and ICSI from oligozoospermic men. Reprod Biomed Online 2001; 3:212–215.
61. Keegan BR, Barton S, Sanchez X, et al. Isolated teratozoospermia does not affect in vitro fertilization outcome and is not an indication for intracytoplasmic sperm injection. Fertil Steril 2007; 88:1583–1588.
62. Prakash P, Leykin L, Chen Z, et al. Preparation by differential gradient centrifugation is better than swim-up in selecting sperm with normal morphology (Strict Criteria). Fertil Steril 1998; 69:722–726.
63. Vanderzwalmen P, Bertin-Segal G, Geerts L. et al. Sperm morphology and IVF pregnancy rate: Comparison between Percoll gradient centrifugation and swim-up procedures. Hum Reprod 1991; 6:581–588.
64. Le Lannou D, Blanchard Y. Nuclear maturity and morphology of human spermatozoa selected by Percoll density gradient centrifugation or swim-up procedure. J Reprod Fertil 1988; 84:551–556.
65. Tomlinson MJ, Moffatt O, Manicardi GC, et al. Interrelationships between seminal parameters and sperm nuclear

DNA damage before and after density gradient centrifugation: Implications for assisted conception. Hum Reprod 2001; 16:2160–2165.
66. Bungum M, Humaidan P, Axmon A, et al. Sperm DNA integrity assessment in prediction of assisted reproduction technology outcome. Hum Reprod 2007; 22:174–179.
67. Evenson DP, Jost LK, Marshall D, et al. Utility of the sperm chromatin structure assay as a diagnostic and prognostic tool in the human fertility clinic. Hum Reprod 1999; 14:1039–1049.
68. Larson KL, DeJonge CJ, Barnes AM, et al. Sperm chromatin structure assay parameters as predictors of failed pregnancy following assisted reproductive techniques. Hum Reprod 2000; 15:1717–1722.
69. Virro MR, Larson-Cook KL, Evenson DP. Sperm chromatin structure assay (SCSA) parameters are related to fertilization, blastocyst development, and ongoing pregnancy in in vitro fertilization and intracytoplasmic sperm injection cycles. Fertil Steril 2004; 81:1289–1295.
70. Larson KL, Brannian JD, Timm BK, et al. Density gradient centrifugation and glass wool filtration of semen remove spermatozoa with damaged chromatin structure. Hum Reprod 1999; 14:2015–2019.
71. Sakkas D, Manicardi GC, Tomlinson M, et al. The use of two density gradient centrifugation techniques and the swim-up method to separate spermatozoa with chromatin and nuclear DNA anomalies. Hum Reprod 2000; 15:1112–1116.
72. Svalander P, Jakobsson AH, Forsberg AS, et al. The outcome of intracytoplasmic sperm injection is unrelated to 'strict criteria' sperm morphology. Hum Reprod 1996; 11:1019–1022.
73. Katsoff B, Check ML, Summers-Chase D, et al. Absence of sperm with rapid motility is not detrimental to IVF outcome measures when ICSI is used. Arch Androl 2005; 51:413–417.
74. Check JH, Bollendorf A, Wilson C, et al. A retrospective comparison of pregnancy outcome following conventional oocyte insemination vs intracytoplasmic sperm injection for isolated abnormalities in sperm morphology using strict criteria. J Androl 2007; 28:607–612.
75. Boomsma CM, Heineman MJ, Cohlen BJ, et al. Semen preparation techniques for intrauterine insemination. Cochrane Database Syst Rev 2007; 17:CD004507.
76. van Weert JM, Repping S, van der Steeg JW, et al. A prediction model for ongoing pregnancy after in vitro fertilization in couples with male subfertility. J Reprod Med 2008; 53:250–256.

9 Intrauterine insemination for male subfertility

Astrid E. P. Cantineau and Ben J. Cohlen

INTRODUCTION

Once idiopathic male subfertility has been diagnosed as a contributor to the subfertility of a couple therapeutic options should be discussed. One option is to abstain from treatment when the chance of spontaneous conception is considered moderate or good (1,2). When on the other hand sperm counts are extremely low immediate treatment might be offered with intracytoplasmatic sperm injection (ICSI) (chapter 10). For couples with male subfertility, reasonable sperm counts and moderate to poor prognosis of spontaneous conception intrauterine insemination (IUI) is a favorable treatment option.

The rationale for performing IUI in case of a male factor is clear: one tries to increase the number of motile sperm with a high proportion of normal forms at the site of fertilization. But does this strategy work? In other words, is IUI for male subfertility effective in increasing pregnancy and live birth rates? And should we combine IUI with mild ovarian hyperstimulation (MOH) in these couples to further improve treatment outcome? How should we prepare the semen and when and how often should it be inseminated? Can we predict success before hand?

We will try to answer these important clinical questions using the best available evidence. But how should we interpret this existing evidence?

LEVEL OF EVIDENCE

The highest level of evidence (level 1A) is described as a systematic review of high-quality randomised controlled trials (NICE Guidelines) (3). These trials should be truly randomized by centralized randomization scheme or on-site computer system with adequate concealment of allocation (e.g., third party or sealed opaque envelopes). Ideally, a power analysis should be performed to detect relevant differences and intention to treat analysis should be applied. This should be done following the guidelines of performing and presenting randomized controlled trials (for instance the CONSORT-checklist). However, one should realize that the quality of a systematic review depends on the quality of the study with the lowest methodological quality included. The levels of evidence are defined in table 1.

Since evidence based medicine gained its popularity large prospective multicenter international studies have been started and published with a perspicuous style. This will eventually lead to medical interventions based on convincing evidence. Regretfully many medical interventions are still based upon older evidence from small randomized trials. Many of these trials have been published before the foundation of the Cochrane Collaboration and its guidelines for performing and publishing randomized trials. Thus, results were often presented as pregnancy rates per completed cycle only, instead of live birth rates per couple. Many trials had a crossover design and intention to treat analysis was often not performed. However, evidence based on older studies, which do not always comply with the newer methodological requirements might be the best available current evidence, and should be used, but considered critically.

Confounding factors should always be taken into account when data is interpreted. Therefore, validation of evidence in your own population can be worthwhile.

EFFECTIVENESS OF IUI FOR MALE SUBFERTILITY

To (dis)prove the efficacy of IUI in couples with male subfertility IUI should be compared with (unrestricted) intercourse in a large randomized controlled trial (RCT) (4). This trial should present its results as live birth rates per couple after a maximum period of time or maximum number of treatment cycles. Regretfully, such a large RCT does not exist until now, but smaller randomized trials performing the comparison mentioned have been published and appraised in a systematic Cochrane review (5,6).

When in 2000 the first version of the Cochrane review was published 13 RCTs could be included that compared IUI with (timed) intercourse either in natural or in stimulated cycles (6). A statistically significant difference was found favoring IUI in natural and stimulated cycles (OR 3.1 with 95% CI 1.5–6.3 and OR 2.1 with 95% CI 1.3–3.5 respectively).

In 2007, this review has been updated applying more strict inclusion criteria such as including RCTs that presented results as live birth rates or pregnancy rates per couple only (5). Precross-over data were included and intention to treat analysis was performed. Because of these strict inclusion criteria one RCT remained that compared IUI with intercourse in natural cycles including 21 couples! Because of the lack of power a significant difference in pregnancy rates per couple was no longer found (OR 5.3, 95% CIs 0.42–66) (level IB) (Fig. 1). Comparing IUI with intercourse in stimulated cycles the results of three RCTs could be combined with a total of 202 couples. Again no significant difference in pregnancy rates per couple was found (OR 1.7, 95% CIs 0.83–3.4) (level IA) (Fig. 1).

What can we conclude? First of all, that there is still a need for large multicenter RCTs, with enough power to detect small but clinically relevant differences in live birth rates per couple, comparing the efficacy of IUI with intercourse in couples with a male factor. Secondly, a beneficial effect is to be expected when IUI is applied in couples with a moderate semen defect, despite

Table 1 Levels of Evidence

IA	A systematic review of high-quality randomized controlled trials
IB	At least one randomized controlled trial
2A	At least one well-designed controlled study without randomization
2B	At least one other type of well-designed quasi-experimental study
3	Well-designed nonexperimental descriptive studies
4	Expert committee

the fact that this conclusion is supported by 'older' evidence only and that 'modern' trials are lacking.

EFFECTIVENESS OF MILD OVARIAN HYPERSTIMULATION/IUI FOR MALE SUBFERTILITY

Mild ovarian hyperstimulation is applied to increase the number of available oocytes and thus to increase the probability of conception. Furthermore, MOH might correct subtle cycle disorders. On the other hand, MOH increases the probability of achieving a multiple pregnancy, an outcome that is regarded as unfavorable (7).

Both the first version of the Cochrane review and the updated version conclude that there is no place for MOH in an IUI program when a male factor is present (4,5) (level IA). These results, expressed as pregnancy rate per couple, are based on four RCTs with a total of 409 couples (OR 1.5 with 95% CI 0.91–2.4) (Fig. 2).

In couples with unexplained subfertility MOH has been proven effective to increase live birth rates (OR 2.1 with 95% CI 1.3–2.5) (8) (level IA). The distinction between normal sperm parameters in couples with unexplained subfertility and mild male factor is of course not a straight line. It seems logical therefore, to assume a positive effect of MOH in couples with a mild factor subfertility (resembling unexplained subfertility). In the literature a mild semen factor has been defined as an average total motile sperm count of two separate semen analyses of more than 10 million (9).

When MOH is applied gonadotropins are clearly superior to clomiphene citrate (10) (level IA). Combining the results expressed as pregnancy rates per couple of seven randomized trials in a meta-analysis shows a significant difference in favor of gonadotropins (OR 1.8 with 95% CI 1.2–2.7) (Fig. 3).

Prevention of multiple pregnancies is an important issue in modern infertility treatment. In the Netherlands, a nation wide study revealed a multiple pregnancy rate per pregnancy of approximately 9% after IUI in stimulated cycles when the Dutch guideline was used (level 3). This guideline advises the use of a mild low dose step-up stimulation protocol starting with 50 to 75 IU gonadotropin per day, close ultrasound monitoring, counting all follicles > 10 mm and strict cancellation criteria (11).

Intrauterine insemination in cycles with MOH is cost-effective only when the number of multiple pregnancies is kept to a minimum and there is an acceptable pregnancy rate per couple.

SEMEN PREPARATION

Several types of semen preparation techniques have been described as follows:

(a) A simple wash and centrifuge
(b) Swim-up
(c) Gradient technique

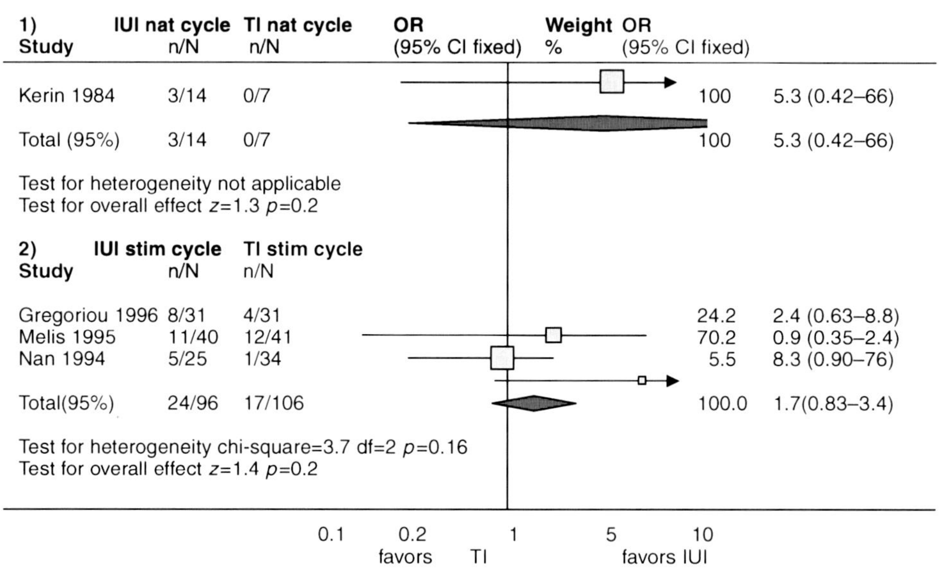

Figure 1 IUI versus timed intercourse (TI) in natural cycles (1) and stimulated cycles (2). Outcome: pregnancy rate per couple.

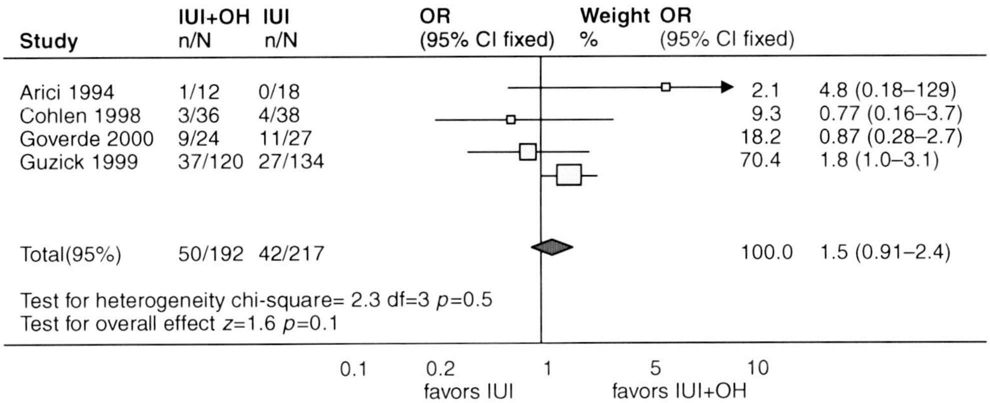

Figure 2 IUI in stimulated cycles versus IUI in natural cycles for male subfertility. Outcome: pregnancy rate per couple.

Regretfully, these different types of preparation techniques have been poorly standardized. Furthermore, the methodological quality of most published trials on this subject is low. Recently Boomsma and co-workers updated their Cochrane review on the subject of semen preparation techniques for IUI (level IA) (12). Of the 32 studies found that investigated semen preparation techniques in relation to outcome after IUI, five could be included only. The authors concluded that there is insufficient data to recommend any of the three semen preparation techniques over another. From clinical practice (level 4), it is known that gradient techniques yield the highest recovery rates. It might therefore be advised to apply this technique in case of a male factor where motile sperm are scarce.

TIMING OF INTRAUTERINE INSEMINATION

Optimal timing of IUI depends on various factors such as the method of timing and the time-interval between ovulation and insemination. Luteinizing hormone (LH) detection in urine or blood, ultrasound combined with human chorionic gonadotropin (hCG) injection, basal body temperature charts (BBTC), GnRH agonist injection or a combination of these methods can be used for inducing or detection of ovulation and to time the insemination. A few randomized studies (13,14) compared hCG injection with urinary LH detection reporting no significant difference in pregnancy rates (level IB). However, the dropout rate with LH detection was high due to failure to detect an LH surge (31% vs. 11%), which is disappointing for women undergoing this treatment. Regarding other methods of timing randomised controlled studies are lacking for couples suffering from male subfertility.

Regarding the optimal time-interval between ovulation and IUI it is known that approximately 38 hours after hCG administration the largest follicle ruptures (15). This suggests that the optimal timing for insemination would be around 38 hours after hCG administration. Randomized controlled studies comparing different time-intervals (24 hours vs. 36 hours after hCG and

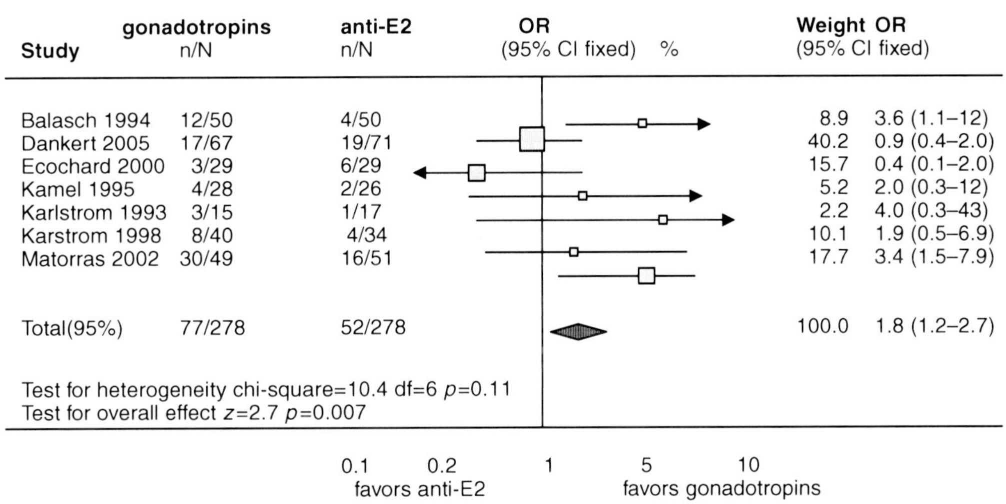

Figure 3 Antioestrogens versus gonadotropins combined with Intrauterine insemination. Outcome: pregnancy rate per couple.

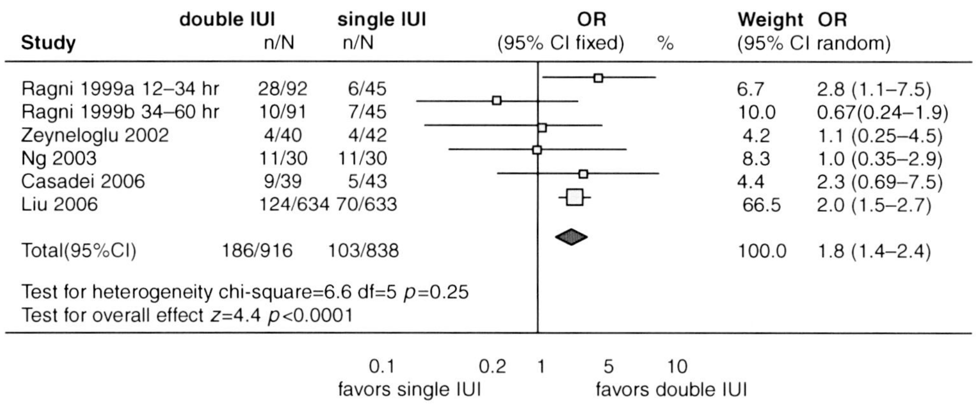

Figure 4 One IUI versus double IUI in stimulated cycles. Outcome: pregnancy rate per couple.

32–34 hours vs. 38–40 hours after hCG) reported no significant difference in pregnancy rates (16,17) (level IB). A large retrospective trial (18) reported the highest number of live births 24–42 hours after a positive urinary LH test (11.7% vs. 5.6% when insemination took place 18–23 hours after a positive urinary LH test) (level 3). Thus, it can be hypothesised that an optimal window of several hours seems to exist in which IUI can be performed. How large this window is and when it begins and ends needs to be investigated further in future randomized trials.

ONE OR TWO INSEMINATIONS

In cases of male subfertility the spermatozoa probably survive for a shorter time period in the female genital tract, compared with normal sperm (9). Increasing the number of inseminations per cycle from one to two might increase the probability of conception.

A systematic review of the existing literature (19) comparing single with double IUI revealed a statistically significant higher pregnancy rate per couple when double insemination was performed (level IA) (Fig. 4). This was based on six trials of which one trial (20) comprised 60% of the included couples. This study reported pregnancy rates as high as obtained with in vitro fertilization (IVF). Furthermore, this positive effect of double insemination was seen in the subgroup suffering from male subfertility (WHO criteria) only and not for the group suffering from unexplained subfertility. The studies that reported a significant effect of double IUI stated a mean of three dominant follicles compared to a mean of 1.7 dominant follicles in studies which did not report a significant difference between single or double IUI, which might imply that double IUI results in higher pregnancy rates when more dominant follicles are available, since these follicles will release their ova at different time-intervals (range of 34–46 hours) (15).

Another review (21) reported significant higher pregnancy rates with double IUI compared to single IUI when clomiphene citrate (CC) was used for ovarian hyperstimulation (level IA). This effect was not observed in gonadotropins stimulated cycles in the same review. A good explanation is lacking.

One can conclude that double insemination might be effective only when more dominant follicles are available which rupture at different time intervals after hCG. A second consecutive IUI adds significantly to the costs and psychological burden, but if the number needed to treat with double IUI is low it might be cost-effective. Up till now there is insufficient data to advise double IUI on a large scale.

There is also insufficient evidence from large prospective trials to advice how many cycles IUI treatment should be continued. General practice is to apply this treatment option three to six consecutive cycles (Level 4).

PREDICTION OF SUCCESS

Different prediction models have been developed to predict the probability of spontaneous conception for subfertile couples using various criteria such as age of the woman, duration of subfertility, primary or secondary subfertility, postcoital testing and sperm-parameters (22–24). These models are used in daily practice for decision making to start treatment or to advise expectant management and seem to be successful in distinguishing between couples with good and poor prognosis (25). In couples with unexplained subfertility and an intermediate prognosis IUI does not seem to improve the probability of conception (26) (level IB). A prediction model for outcome of IUI in couples with subfertility of various origins have been developed (25). Regretfully this model has a relatively poor discriminative capacity and allows distinction between couples with a poor and good prognosis only.

In couples with a male factor it seems logic to assume that the number of motile sperm that is inseminated is related to the probability of conception. A meta-analysis of a diagnostic test that investigated this relation found that the postwash total motile count was able to predict failure (when less than 0.8 to 5 million motile sperm were inseminated) but not to predict success (26). The large difference between various centers was obvious and it is therefore advised to detect a postwash motile count cut-off level for each center individually. In a second retrospective cohort study of this group, the authors concluded that adding antisperm antibodies and postwash total motile count in a predictive model might increase the accuracy of selecting couples for IUI, and by excluding couples with a poor prognosis treatment outcome might be improved (27).

CONCLUSION

A beneficial effect is to be expected when IUI is applied in couples with a mild to moderate semen defect. In cases of severe male factor subfertility (total motile sperm count after semen preparation below 1 million), ICSI should probably be the treatment of choice because at least 0.8 to 5 million motile spermatozoa should be obtained after semen preparation to make IUI worthwhile. There is insufficient data to recommend any of the three types of semen preparation techniques.

Additional MOH is advised for mild male subfertility only (total motile sperm count of more than 10 million per ejaculate) otherwise IUI in natural cycle should be performed. Only when the number of multiple pregnancies are kept to a minimum this treatment will be cost-effective.

The optimal time-interval for IUI is not known, but it can be hypothesised that an optimal window of several hours seems to exist in which IUI can be performed. Double insemination might only be effective when more dominant follicles are available which rupture at different time intervals after hCG. A second consecutive IUI adds significantly to the costs and psychological burden, but if the number needed to treat with double IUI is low it might be cost-effective. Up till now there is insufficient data to advise double IUI on a large scale.

Whether or not a couple will benefit from IUI depends on various prognostic factors. Optimal cut-off levels for these confounding factors are hard to give in general and it is therefore advised that each individual center should collect their own data to calculate their own optimal cut-off levels using ROC curves.

Although newer techniques like IVF-ET or ICSI give higher pregnancy rates per cycle, IUI might result in comparable cumulative pregnancy rates. Compared with these newer techniques IUI still remains a cost-effective treatment option (28). However, the road to take is longer for the couple, which they have to be willing to take.

REFERENCES

1. van der Steeg JW, Steures P, Eijkemans MJ, et al. Pregnancy is predictable: A large-scale prospective external validation of the prediction of spontaneous pregnancy in subfertile couples. Hum Reprod 2007; 22(2):536–542.
2. Steures P, van der Steeg JW, Hompes PG, et al. Intrauterine insemination with controlled ovarian hyperstimulation versus expectant management for couples with unexplained subfertility and an intermediate prognosis: A randomised clinical trial. Lancet 2006; 368(9531):216–221.
3. National Collaborating Centre for Women's and Children's Health. Fertility: Assessment and Treatment for People With Fertility Problems. London: National Institute for Clinical Excellence, 2004.
4. Cohlen BJ. Should We Continue Performing Intrauterine Inseminations in the Year 2004? Gynecol Obstet Invest 2004; 59(1):3–13.
5. Bensdorp AJ, Cohlen BJ, Heineman MJ, et al. Intra-uterine insemination for male subfertility. Cochrane Database Syst Rev 2007; (4):CD000360.
6. Cohlen BJ, Vandekerckhove P, te Velde ER, et al. Timed intercourse versus intra-uterine insemination with or without ovarian hyperstimulation for subfertility in men. Cochrane Database Syst Rev 2000; (2):CD000360.
7. Fauser BJCM, Devroey P, Macklon NS. Multiple birth resulting from ovarian stimulation for subfertility treatment. Lancet 2005; 365(9459):5000.
8. Verhulst SM, Cohlen BJ, Hughes E, et al. Intra-uterine insemination for unexplained subfertility. Cochrane Database Syst Rev 2006(4):CD001838.
9. Cohlen BJ, te Velde ER, van Kooij RJ, et al. Controlled ovarian hyperstimulation and intrauterine insemination for treating male subfertility: A controlled study. Hum Reprod 1998; 13(6):1553–1558.
10. Cantineau AE, Cohlen BJ, Heineman MJ. Ovarian stimulation protocols (anti-oestrogens, gonadotrophins with and without GnRH agonists/antagonists) for intrauterine insemination (IUI) in women with subfertility. Cochrane Database Syst Rev 2007; (2):CD005356.
11. Cohlen BJ, van Dop P. Prevention of multiple pregnancies after non-in vitro fertilization treatment. In: Gerris J, Olivennes F, de Sutter P, eds. Assisted Reproductive Technologies. Quality and Safety. London, England: The Parthenon Publishing Group London, 2004:39–48.
12. Boomsma CM, Heineman MJ, Cohlen BJ, et al. Semen preparation techniques for intrauterine insemination. Cochrane Database Syst Rev 2007; (4):CD004507.
13. Lewis V, Queenan J Jr, Hoeger K, et al. Clomiphene citrate monitoring for intrauterine insemination timing: A randomized trial. Fertil Steril 2006; 85(2):401–406.
14. Zreik TG, Garcia-Velasco JA, Habboosh MS, et al. Prospective, randomized, crossover study to evaluate the benefit of human chorionic gonadotropin-timed versus urinary luteinizing hormone-timed intrauterine inseminations in clomiphene citrate-stimulated treatment cycles. Fertil Steril 1999; 71(6):1070–1074.
15. Andersen AG, Als-Nielsen B, Hornnes PJ, et al. Time interval from human chorionic gonadotrophin (HCG) injection to follicular rupture. Hum Reprod 1995; 10(12):3202–3205.
16. Claman P, Wilkie V, Collins D. Timing intrauterine insemination either 33 or 39 hours after administration of human chorionic gonadotropin yields the same pregnancy rates as after superovulation therapy. Fertil Steril 2004; 82(1): 13–16.

17. Wang YC, Chang YC, Chen IC, et al. Comparison of timing of IUI in ovarian stimulated cycles. Arch Androl 2006; 52(5):371–374.
18. Khattab AF, Mustafa FA, Taylor PJ. The use of urine LH detection kits to time intrauterine insemination with donor sperm. Hum Reprod 2005; 20(9):2542–2545.
19. Cantineau AE, Heineman MJ, Cohlen BJ. Single versus double intrauterine insemination (IUI) in stimulated cycles for subfertile couples. Cochrane Database Syst Rev 2003; (1):CD003854.
20. Liu W, Gong F, Luo K, et al. Comparing the pregnancy rates of one versus two intrauterine inseminations (IUIs) in male factor and idiopathic infertility. J Assist Reprod Genet 2006; 23(2):75–79.
21. Osuna C, Matorras R, Pijoan JI, et al. One versus two inseminations per cycle in intrauterine insemination with sperm from patients' husbands: A systematic review of the literature. Fertil Steril 2004; 82(1):17–24.
22. Eimers JM, te Velde ER, Gerritse R, et al. The prediction of the chance to conceive in subfertile couples. Fertil Steril 1994; 61(1):44–52.
23. Hunault CC, Eijkemans MJ, te Velde ER, et al. Validation of a model predicting spontaneous pregnancy among subfertile untreated couples. Fertil Steril 2002; 78(3):500–506.
24. Snick HK, Snick TS, Evers JL, et al. The spontaneous pregnancy prognosis in untreated subfertile couples: The Walcheren primary care study. Hum Reprod 1997; 12(7):1582–1588.
25. Steures P, van der Steeg JW, Mol BW, et al. Prediction of an ongoing pregnancy after intrauterine insemination. Fertil Steril 2004; 82(1):45–51.
26. van Weert JM, Repping S, Van Voorhis BJ, et al. Performance of the postwash total motile sperm count as a predictor of pregnancy at the time of intrauterine insemination: A meta-analysis. Fertil Steril 2004; 82(3):612–620.
27. van Weert JM, Repping S, van der Steeg JW, et al. IUI in male subfertility: Are we able to select the proper patients? Reprod Biomed Online 2005; 11(5):624–631.
28. Goverde AJ, McDonnell J, Vermeiden JP, et al. Intrauterine insemination or in-vitro fertilisation in idiopathic subfertility and male subfertility: A randomised trial and cost-effectiveness analysis. Lancet 2000; 355(9197):13–18.

10 IVF and ICSI for treating male infertility

Herman Tournaye

INTRODUCTION

A couple's fecundity is the result of an interaction between both partners. For infertile men who suffer from azoospermia, a "male factor" is a certain cause for the couple's, however, in case of oligozoospermia, the couple's inability to have children may be influenced by a "female factor" as well. Given the trend of postponing pregnancy to a later age, female age has become the most important prognostic factor for a couple's fecundity. The consequence of this interaction is that it is difficult to evaluate treatments that try to alleviate the "male factor". On top of this, semen parameters show huge intraindividual variations over time. Because of the phenomenon of "regression towards the mean", studies evaluating treatment of male subfertility must include placebo (1) and must have pregnancy as the main outcome measure. Yet, very few randomized controlled trials with pregnancy as outcome measure have been published in our field. The Cochrane library includes only nine reviews on male subfertility or infertility, including one on IVF and ICSI, and most have not been updated because of the lack of new evidence (2).

CASE 1

A 45-year old man visits the andrology clinic. For two years he is trying to have a child. He has been referred because his sperm count is 10 million spermatozoa per mL (he produced 3 mL of semen). Progressive motility is 20% and morphology according to strict criteria is 7%.

According to the referring doctor, he has never been ill, neither has he got any surgery. His wife has no gynecological problems. His physical examination is normal including normal virilization and andrological examination. A scrotal ultrasound has been performed and was normal. However, further history-taking reveals he has two children from a previous marriage which are now aged 10 and 12. Further enquiry on his current partner reveals that his current wife has no children and is aged 40 years.

This case clearly shows how relative a "male factor" can be: if this man would have got remarried with a 30-years old wife he would probably not sitting in front of you! This is not a male problem: this is a female problem!

Although our knowledge of the etiology of male subfertility has expanded over the last decade, little progress has been made in treating the subfertile male. Good medical practice implies that once the causative factor for a condition or inability has been identified, an efficient, safe and specific treatment should be applied that remedies this factor in order to alleviate the condition or inability. Unfortunately for the treatment of male subfertility, the causative factor remains unknown in 40% of men presenting with a "male factor" (3) and in another 50%, no specific treatment with a proven efficiency is available (3). Any critical review of conventional treatments of male subfertility—and unexplained male subfertility especially—will conclude that few subfertile men can benefit from an evidence-based treatment (4–6) (level of evidence: A). Efficient specific, that is nonempirical, treatments are thus scarce and as a result there has been an exponential increase in the practice of assisted reproductive techniques (ART) to remedy male subfertility.

WHEN TO OPT FOR ASSISTED REPRODUCTIVE TECHNIQUES?

Being also empirical *in se*, the aim of IVF and ICSI is to bring the spermatozoon closer to the oocyte in an attempt to enhance fertilization. This is also what intra-uterine insemination (IUI) aims for.

While these techniques should not be viewed as primary treatment options, they are indicated when no specific treatment with a proven benefit is available and optimalization of the female factor has failed or is not indicated.

According to meta-analysis (7), IUI is an efficient technique to increase fecundity in couples with male subfertility: compared to timed intercourse, three times more couples will achieve pregnancy thanks to IUI (level of evidence: A).

Unfortunately, the total motile sperm count after semen preparation cannot predict whether a couple undergoing IUI will conceive; it is more likely to predict whether a couple will not conceive (8) (level of evidence: A). How many cycles of IUI are needed is difficult to answer because of the complete lack of prospective studies that take into account the female age factor. Based on the currently available retrospective life-table studies, at least three IUI cycles and maximum IUI six cycles can be proposed depending on the age (level of evidence: D).

CASE 2

A 31-year-old man is referred by his GP for ICSI because he and his wife are now trying for 18 months to get pregnant. His sperm count is 10 million spermatozoa per mL and the semen volume 3 mL. Progressive motility is 20% and morphology according to strict criteria is 7%.

History-taking and physical examination, including andrological examination does not reveal any abnormality or dysfunction. His wife, 30 years old, has no detectable gynecological problems.

Since his semen was only checked once, you refer him to an andrology laboratory, which is included in a quality control program for semen analysis and ask for a standard semen analysis and a sperm preparation test. Because of their age and the result of the sperm preparation test you propose them to have IUI in a natural cycle with LH-timing. His wife conceives after the third cycle of insemination. She has a singleton pregnancy.

If no pregnancy is obtained, the next step would be IVF or ICSI. There is currently no solid evidence regarding cut-off values before or after sperm preparation for accepting a couple with male subfertility for IVF treatment with anticipated success rates comparable to non-male indications. Results after semen preparation of 0.2 (9), 0.5 (10) to 2 million (11) motile spermatozoa have been proposed for accepting couples for conventional IVF treatment (level of evidence: D).

Only two prospective studies have compared IUI with IVF for male subfertility (12,13). Neither of the two studies showed any difference in pregnancy rates between IUI and IVF in moderate male subfertility (level of evidence: A). In addition, the study by Goverde et al. concluded that IUI is more cost-effective than IVF even in case of male subfertility (13). The main criticism that can be leveled at this, otherwise valuable study, is that the pregnancy rates after IUI were higher than generally expected, while those after IVF were much lower.

SHOULD I OPT FOR IVF OR ICSI?

Making a Choice Between IVF and ICSI

Defining when to opt for either IVF or ICSI is an important issue because it has not only a repercussion on the success rate the treatment, but may have an important psychological impact on the couple too. Complete fertilization failure is an unwanted event because apart from financial implications, it has an important negative psychological impact on the couple. The prevalence of fertilization failure in conventional in-vitro fertilization is reported to occur for non-male indications in 5% to 15% of cycles, when IVF is performed for male indications, the complete fertilization failure rate can be as high as 50% (14–17) (level of evidence: C). The causes of complete fertilization failure after IVF are related to either oocytes factors or sperm factors (especially in male indications) or laboratory factors, that is poor injection technique. A review on the role of sperm morphology on fertilization in-vitro reported an overall fertilization failure and failure to perform an embryotransfer in 24% of patients when the husband had a sperm morphology less than 5% according to strict criteria (18) (level of evidence: C). Furthermore, complete fertilization failure after IVF has been reported to be repetitive in 30% to 50% of cycles. In contrast, after ICSI, complete fertilization failure occurs in less then 3% of started cycles (19,20) (level of evidence: C) and can be present in subsequent cycles in up to 25%. Although ICSI has been proposed as the most robust technique for achieving fertilization in an IVF program, the aim of any method of assisted reproduction should always be to use the simplest and least expensive procedure with the greatest long-term chance of healthy children (21). But even apart from these considerations, the question remains whether ICSI is the method of choice for all IVF indications. The Cochrane Library of Systematic Reviews includes one meta-analysis on IVF versus ICSI (2). The last update of 2003 dealing with non-male indications only comprised 10 randomized control trials (RCTs) all, except for one (22) (level of evidence: A), had a sibling oocyte set-up design. In this set-up, oocytes obtained after ovum pick up are randomly assigned to either conventional IVF or ICSI. Because the nine RCTs on sibling oocytes do not allow any valid conclusion towards implantation and pregnancy rates, the Cochrane review only selects the study by Bhattacharya (22) as best evidence. This study is a large multicentre RCT powered to detect a 10% difference in implantation rate. It comprises 206 conventional IVF cycles versus 209 ICSI cycles. Although there was no difference in complete fertilization failure between IVF and ICSI (5% vs. 2% respectively), the fertilization rate per oocyte was significantly higher after IVF then after ICSI (58% vs. 47% respectively). Furthermore, the implantation rate per embryo after IVF was also higher then after ICSI (30% vs. 22%, $p = 0.03$). The lower implantation rate after ICSI may be attributed to the denuding step in ICSI, which may alter the implantation potential of the eventual embryo. Given the results of this adequately powered multicentre study, there is obviously no benefit in performing ICSI for non-male indications. The choice between IVF and ICSI for these indications is thus easy.

Making a Choice Between IVF and ICSI in Male Indications

Although clinical evidence is lacking for many typical ICSI indications, there are strict male indications for ICSI: use of surgically retrieved sperm, use of spermatozoa with flagellar dyskinesia (immotile cilia syndromes), use of round-headed spermatozoa (globozoospermia). The prevalence of relevant titers of antisperm antibodies may also be an indication for performing ICSI (23–25) (level of evidence: D). The same goes for cryopreserved sperm from cancer patients. Again, no prospective comparative studies are available in the literature, however, based on retrospective case series it may be assumed that for most of these patients, given the poor quality of sperm cryopreserved, the postthaw sperm damage and the limited numbers of spermatozoa frozen, ICSI is the method of choice when assisted reproduction is indicated (26) (level of evidence: C).

But what about oligoasthenoteratozoospermia? In the past functional assays were proposed as a screening method by which to select patients for conventional IVF. However these methods are expensive, show an important interobserver variability and cannot predict fertilization failure (27).

Most studies will propose certain cut-off values in sperm parameters in order to opt for either IVF or ICSI. The cut-off values used for conventional IVF are mostly experience-based and extrapolated from small, older studies not always using the same laboratory standards as of today. Apart from the motile count after sperm preparation, motile count in the native semen sample as well as morphology according to Tygerberg criteria has been used for accepting couples for conventional IVF treatment. *Kastrop et al.* proposed a motile count of at least one million spermatozoa in the native semen sample (28) (level of evidence: D). When the motile progressive count after sperm preparation is taken as a criterion, numbers vary from 1 million (29,30) to 0.5 million progressive motile spermatozoa (31) or even 0.2 million motile progressive spermatozoa! (32) (all studies with a D level of evidence). When morphology is taken as a criterion, in general 5% normal morphology is the cut-off value below which a low fertilization after conventional IVF is anticipated (33,34) (level of evidence: C). Exceptionally, a combination of morphology and motile count is used: Plachot et al. proposed 0.5 million normal motile progressive count in the ejaculate for accepting couples for conventional IVF (35) (level of evidence: D). Nowadays, strategies for defining the limits between IVF and ICSI are either based on these experience-based preset cut-off values or are based on the assumption that ICSI is the more robust insemination technique. Then, a split IVF-ICSI set up is also proposed as a strategy.

But even when the preset cut-off values for conventional IVF are met, as in "border-line male infertility", the choice between conventional IVF and ICSI may be difficult. A meta-analysis, dealing only with borderline oligoasthenoteratozoospermia, concluded that the fertilization and fertilization failure rate after IVF can be highly depended on the insemination protocol used for conventional IVF (10). Although corrective measures have been proposed many years ago (36) still today, many IVF programs use suboptimal insemination concentrations for couples with borderline oligoasthenoteratozoospermia. In one RCT (10) fertilization rate after conventional IVF was 37.5% per oocyte versus 64.2% after ICSI when an insemination concentration of 0.2 million progressively motile spermatozoa per mL were used for conventional IVF. However, after correcting the insemination concentration to the 0.8 million progressively motile spermatozoa per mL, the fertilization rate after IVF was 59.7% versus 67.6% (difference not significant). With the suboptimal insemination concentration complete failure of fertilization occurred in 25.7% of cycles while with the optimized protocol total fertilization failure only occurred in 5.26% of cycles (level of evidence: A). The results of the above-mentioned meta-analysis corroborate these findings: RCTs with a suboptimal insemination concentration report a significant higher fertilization rate per oocyte after ICSI than after conventional IVF. However, subanalysis of the three RCTs in which a high insemination concentration was used shows no significant benefit of ICSI over IVF (level of evidence: A). Although the current evidence is limited, the result of this meta-analysis calls for caution when promoting ICSI for borderline oligoasthenoteratozoospermia.

CASE 3

A couple is now trying for 24 months to get pregnant. The wife is 33 years old and has no detectable gynecological problems according to her gynecologist.

Her husband's semen, however, revealed moderate oligoasthenoteratozoospermia. He had a full investigation by an andrologist but no cause for this finding was found.

They had four cycles of intrauterine insemination. At each cycle follicular development was normal and insemination was properly timed with more than five million rapid progressively motile sperm being inseminated each time.

They want ICSI, because they read on the internet that this is a very successful technique for their case. You propose them conventional IVF with increased numbers of sperm for in-vitro insemination. They are not happy with your proposal.

Seven months later they show up again. They had one ICSI cycle with another doctor. Seven eggs were retrieved of which five looked mature and were subsequently injected with a single sperm. Two eggs were damaged during the ICSI procedure and only one embryo developed from the two normally fertilized eggs. However, this embryo showed a lot of fragmentation and therefore no transfer took place.

Now they want IVF.

Is a Split IVF-ICSI Set Up the Way to Go?

Performing a split IVF-ICSI strategy in a clinical setting as performed in the RCTs mentioned above, has been proposed as the method of choice when attempting a first IVF cycle in couples with borderline male infertility because it may avoid unnecessary fertilization failure. Eventually embryos transferred are derived both from conventional IVF and ICSI, and therefore this approach is not allowed in all countries. But even then, it is far from clear whether this approach is indeed the first choice. One study concluded that "this strategy enabled... to avoid 32.8% of complete fertilization failures after IVF" (35) (level of evidence: C). However, in another study with a similar set-up, the complete fertilization failure after conventional IVF was only 7.1% (37) (level of evidence: C). Strikingly, the main methodological difference between both studies was that in the former study an insemination concentration of only 0.06 million motile spermatozoa was used. Another study also failed to show any benefit of a split set up in patients with moderate oligoasthenotera-tozoospermia (38) (level of evidence: C). Yet, a recent RCT showed that a split IVF-ICSI could avoid fertilization failure in one out of four cycles where conventional IVF was applied for borderline male infertility and where even a high insemination concentration was applied (39) (level of evidence: A).

From the above it may be concluded that we need better methods to define the limits between IVF and ICSI and that the outcome of the two methods are closely related to the methodology used in the IVF laboratory. Preferentially, each IVF program should try to define its own limits based on a prediction of fertilization failure after conventional IVF in its own setting. Rhemrev et al. published a perfect example of this approach (40). In their study, first they constructed a multiple regression model based on a set of 2366 couples undergoing IVF with a complete fertilization failure rate of 25% as being acceptable. Then, they validated their model on a subsequent set of 917 other couples. They used a high insemination concentration of one million motile spermatozoa per mL. They showed that apart from the postpreparation motile count, the number of follicles is an important predictor for complete fertilization failures. For example, if a pick up is scheduled in a couple in which the wife shows less then 5 follicles, at least 1.11 million motile spermatozoa are to be obtained after sperm preparation for accepting the couple for conventional IVF with an anticipated risk for complete fertilization failure of 25%. On the other hand, when more than 15 follicles are present, the postpreparation motile count can be as low as 0.35 million before the risk for complete fertilization failure after conventional IVF exceeds 25%. They also calculated, based on the number of follicles, probabilities of a total fertilization failure according to the postwash total progressive motile count. For example, when the number of follicles in their model is between 10 and 15, the probability of a complete fertilization failure is 23% when the postwash total progressive motile count was one million. But the probability drops to 14% when this count is three million. The approach as proposed by Rhemrev seems to be very rational and hopefully more studies will be performed with center-specific adaptations proving that it is a valuable strategy. Depending on the local situation towards reimbursement and costs of IVF versus ICSI, a predefined and acceptable total fertilization failure rate can be introduced in the predictive model. When complete fertilization failure is totally unacceptable, a split IVF-ICSI set up can be proposed although clinical evidence for the superiority of this approach is currently lacking.

CHILDREN AFTER IVF OR ICSI

CASE 4

A couple conceived a son after ICSI in your clinic some three years ago. Now they have read in the local newspaper that children born after IVF treatment 'face higher health risks'. They are very confused and contact you to have more explanations.

Assisted reproductive technologies have been under debate since the introduction of ICSI in the early 1990s especially since one study conducted in Australia found that babies conceived after IVF or ICSI, were more than twice as likely as naturally conceived infants to have major birth defects (9% vs. 4.2%), mainly problems with the heart and urinary or genital tracts (41) (level of evidence: B).

Large follow up studies as published by Bonduelle et al. in 2002 have shown a significantly higher incidence of chromosomal abnormalities (3.0%) as compared to the general population (42) (level of evidence: B). All couples referred for ICSI must therefore have chromosomal analysis whenever extreme oligo-astheno-terato-zoospermia (OAT) is present. After ICSI more urogenital malformations such as undescended testis and hypospadias were observed when compared to the general population (43,44) (level of evidence: B). It is important to mention that well-designed studies showed that not the technique per se, but rather the risk profile of the candidate-patients themselves is involved in the increased prevalence of congenital malformations (45) (level of evidence: B). Also psychomotor and mental development were subject to further study but at present up to the age of 10 years old, children conceived after either ICSI or IVF do not show any delay compared to children obtained after natural conception (46,47) (level of evidence: B).

Reports were published in genetics journals concluding that children with Beckwith–Wiedemann syndrome, a syndrome affecting one in 15,000 newborns, were four to six times more likely to have been conceived through IVF or ICSI than not and that IVF was associated with a five- to seven-fold increased risk of a rare form of eye cancer known as retinoblastoma (48,49) (level of evidence: C). Another report linked ICSI with Angelman syndrome, yet another rare condition (50) (level of evidence: C). At present the precise risks of these imprinting diseases and childhood cancer after IVF and ICSI remain unclear and further long-term follow-up are needed. Yet these abnormalities are uncommon even if the risk is increased.

CASE 4, Continued

The couple can be told that in spite of information given by layman press, evidence from larger well-designed studies demonstrates that ICSI has so far appeared to be a safe procedure, allowing couples with severe male factor infertility and low fertilization rate, a chance to conceive. The slight increase in risk for either congenital malformations or karyotype anomalies are assumed to be associated to the risk profile of the candidate-parents rather than to the reproductive techniques themselves.

Yet because this evidence is built on few well-designed studies, this couple should be encouraged to participate in long-term children follow-up programs.

REFERENCES

1. Baker HW, Kovacs GT. Spontaneous improvement in semen quality: Regression towards the mean. Int J Androl 1985; 8:421–426.
2. van Rumste MM, Evers JL, Farquhar CM. ICSI versus conventional techniques for oocyte insemination during IVF in patients with non-male factor subfertility: A Cochrane review. Hum Reprod 2004; 19:223–227.
3. Baker HW. Requirements for controlled therapeutic trials in male infertility. Clin Reprod Fertil 1986; 4:13–25.
4. Kamischke A, Nieschlag E. Analysis of medical treatment of male infertility. Hum Reprod 1999; 14(suppl 1):1–23.
5. O'Donovan PA, Vandekerckhove P, Lilford RJ, et al. Treatment of male infertility: Is it effective? Review and meta-analyses of published randomized trials. Hum Reprod 1993; 8:1209–1222.
6. Tournaye H. Evidence-based management of male subfertility. Curr Opin Obstet Gynecol 2006; 18(3):253–259.
7. Cohlen BJ. Should we continue performing intrauterine inseminations in the year 2004? Gynecol Obstet Invest 2005; 59:3–13.
8. van Weert JM, Repping S, Van Voorhis BJ, et al. Performance of the postwash total motile sperm count as a predictor

of pregnancy at the time of intrauterine insemination: A meta-analysis. Fertil Steril 2004; 82:612–620.

9. Payne D, Matthews CD. Intracytoplasmic sperm injection-clinical results from the reproductive medicine unit, Adelaide. Reprod Fertil Dev 1995; 7:219–227.
10. Tournaye H, Verheyen G, Albano C, et al. Intracytoplasmic sperm injection versus in vitro fertilization: A randomized controlled trial and a meta-analysis of the literature. Fertil Steril 2002; 78:1030–1037.
11. Baker HW. Clinical management of male infertility. In: De Groot L, Jamieson JL, eds. Endocrinology. Philadelphia, PA: Elsevier Saunders, 2006:3199–3225.
12. Crosignani PG, Walters DE. Clinical pregnancy and male subfertility; the ESHRE multicentre trial on the treatment of male subfertility. European Society of Human Reproduction and Embryology. Hum Reprod 1994; 9:1112–1118.
13. Goverde AJ, McDonnell J, Vermeiden JP, et al. Intrauterine insemination or in-vitro fertilisation in idiopathic subfertility and male subfertility: A randomised trial and cost-effectiveness analysis. Lancet 2000; 355: 13–18.
14. Molloy D, Harrison K, Breen T, et al. The predictive value of idiopathic failure to fertilize on the first in vitro fertilization attempt. Fertil Steril 1991; 56:285–289.
15. Ben-Shlomo I, Bider D, Dor J, et al. Failure to fertilize in vitro in couples with male factor infertility: What next? Fertil Steril 1992; 58:187–189.
16. Lipitz S, Rabinovici J, Goldenberg M, et al. Complete failure of fertilization in couples with mechanical infertility: Implications for subsequent in vitro fertilization cycles. Fertil Steril 1994; 61:863–866.
17. Coates TE, Check JH, Choe J, et al. An evaluation of couples with failure of fertilization in vitro. Hum Reprod 1992; 7:978–981.
18. Coetzee K, Kruger TF, Lombard CJ. Predictive value of normal sperm morphology: A structured literature review. Hum Reprod Update 1998; 4:73–82.
19. Liu J, Nagy Z, Joris H, et al. Analysis of 76 total fertilization failure cycles out of 2732 intracytoplasmic sperm injection cycles. Hum Reprod 1995; 10:2630–2636.
20. Flaherty SP, Payne D, Matthews CD. Fertilization failures and abnormal fertilization after intracytoplasmic sperm injection. Hum Reprod 1998; 13(suppl 1):155–164.
21. Tucker M, Wiker S, Massey J. Rational approach to assisted fertilization. Hum Reprod 1993; 8:1778.
22. Bhattacharya S, Hamilton MP, Shaaban M, et al. Conventional in-vitro fertilization versus intracytoplasmic sperm injection for the treatment of non-male factor infertility: A randomised controlled trial. Lancet 2001; 357:2075–2079.
23. Nagy ZP, Verheyen G, Liu J, et al. Results of 55 intracytoplasmic sperm injection cycles in the treatment of male-immunological infertility. Hum Reprod 1995;10:1775–1780.
24. Lahteenmaki A, Reima I, Hovatta O. Treatment of severe male immunological infertility by intracytoplasmic sperminjection. Hum Reprod 1995; 10(11):2824–2828.
25. Vazquez-Levin MH, Notrica JA, Polak de Fried E. Male immunologic infertility: Sperm performance on in vitro fertilization. Fertil Steril 1997; 68:675–681.
26. Kelleher S, Wishart SM, Liu PY, et al. Long-term outcomes of elective human sperm cryostorage. Hum Reprod 2001; 16:2632 2639.
27. Mahutte NG, Arici A. Failed fertilization failure: Is it predictable? Curr Opin Obstet Gynecol 2003; 15:211–218.
28. Kastrop PM, Weima SM, Van Kooij RJ, et al. Comparison between intracytoplasmic sperm injection and in-vitro fertilization (IVF) with high insemination concentration after total fertilization failure in a previous IVF attempt. Hum Reprod 1999; 4:65–69.
29. Fisch B, Kaplan-Kraicer R, Amit S, et al. The relationship between sperm parameters and fertilizing capacity in vitro: A predictive role for swim up migration. J In Vitro Fert Embryo Transf 1990; 7: 38–43.
30. Söderlund B, Lundin K. Choosing fertilization method by analyzing sperm morphology or by performing swim-up preparation. Acta Obstet Gynecol 2006; 85:306–311.
31. Verheyen G, Tournaye H, Staessen C, et al. Controlled comparison of conventional in-vitro fertilization and intracytoplasmic sperm injection in patients with asthenozoospermia. Hum Reprod 1999; 14:2313–2319.
32. Payne D, Flaherty SP, Jeffrey R, et al. Successful treatment of severe male factor infertility in 100 consecutive cycles using intracytoplasmic sperm injection. Hum Reprod 1994; 9:2051–2057.
33. Kruger TF, Acosta AA, Simmons KF, et al. Predictive value of abnormal sperm morphology in in vitro fertilization. Fertil Steril 1988; 49:112–117.
34. Grow DR, Oehninger S, Seltman HJ, et al. Sperm morphology as diagnosed by strict criteria: Probing the impact of teratozoospermia on fertilization rate and pregnancy outcome in a large in vitro fertilization population. Fertil Steril 1994; 62:559–567.
35. Plachot M, Belaisch-Allart J, Mayenga JM, et al. Outcome of conventional IVF and ICSI on sibling oocytes in mild male factor infertility. Hum Reprod 2002; 17:362–369.
36. Oehninger S, Acosta AA, Morshedi M, et al. Corrective measures and pregnancy outcome in in vitro fertilization in patients with severe sperm morphology abnormalities. Fertil Steril 1988; 50:283–287.
37. Elizur SE, Levron J, Seidman DS, et al. Conventional in vitro fertilization versus intracytoplasmic sperm injection for sibling oocytes in couples with mild oligoteratoasthenozoospermia and couples with normal sperm. Fertil Steril 2004; 82:241–243.
38. Hershlag A, Paine T, Kvapil G, et al. In vitro fertilization-intracytoplasmic sperm injection split: An insemination

method to prevent fertilization failure. Fertil Steril 2002; 77:229–232.

39. Van der Westerlaken L, Naaktgeboren N, Verburg H, et al. Conventional in vitro fertilization versus intracytoplasmic sperm injection in patients with borderline semen: A randomized study using sibling oocytes. Fertil Steril 2006; 85:395–400.
40. Rhemrev JP, Lens JW, McDonnell J, et al. The postwash total progressively motile sperm cell count is a reliable predictor of total fertilization failure during in vitro fertilization treatment. Fertil Steril 2001; 76:884–891.
41. Hansen M, Kurinczuk JJ, Bower C, et al. The risk of major birth defects after intracytoplasmic sperm injection and in vitro fertilization. N Engl J Med 2002; 346:725–730.
42. Bonduelle M, Liebaers I, Deketelaere V, et al. Neonatal data on a cohort of 2889 infants born after ICSI (1991–1999) and of 2995 infants born after IVF (1983–1999). Hum Reprod 2002; 17:671–694.
43. Bonduelle M, Wennerholm UB, Loft A, et al. A multi-centre cohort study of the physical health of 5-year-old children conceived after intracytoplasmic sperm injection, in vitro fertilization and natural conception. Hum Reprod 2005; 20:413–419.
44. Ludwig AK, Katalinic A, Thyen U, et al. Physical health at 5.5 years of age of term-born singletons after intracytoplasmic sperm injection: Results of a prospective, controlled, single-blinded study. Fertil Steril 2009; 91:115–124.
45. Ludwig M, Katalinic A. Malformation rate in fetuses and children conceived after ICSI: results of a prospective cohort study. Reprod Biomed Online 2002; 5:171–178.
46. Leunens L, Celestin-Westreich S, Bonduelle M, et al. Follow-up of cognitive and motor development of 10-year-old singleton children born after ICSI compared with spontaneously conceived children. Hum Reprod 2008; 23:105–111.
47. Ludwig A, Katalinic A, Thyen U, et al. Neuromotor development and mental health at 5.5 years of age of singletons born at term after intracytoplasmatic sperm injection ICSI: Results of a prospective controlled single-blinded study in Germany. Fertil Steril 2009; 91:125–132.
48. Chang AS, Moley KH, Wangler M, et al. Association between Beckwith-Wiedemann syndrome and assisted reproductive technology: A case series of 19 patients. Fertil Steril 2005; 83:349–354.
49. Moll AC, Imhof SM, Schouten-van Meeteren AY, et al. In-vitro fertilisation and retinoblastoma. Lancet 2003; 361:1392.
50. Cox GF, Bürger J, Lip V, et al. Intracytoplasmic sperm injection may increase the risk of imprinting defects. Am J Hum Genet 2002; 71:162–164.

11 Surgery for male infertility: surgical treatment of obstructive azoospermia

Laurent Vaucher and Peter N. Schlegel

SURGERY FOR MALE INFERTILITY: OBSTRUCTIVE AZOOSPERMIA

When an urologist is presented with an azoospermic semen sample, specific questions arise, such as: Should any diagnostic tests be run on the sample? Is an obstruction in the ductal system the cause of the lack of sperm? and What are the therapeutic options that can be offered to the patient? In this chapter, each of these questions will be discussed to provide the urologist with the tools necessary to deal with these issues.

The most clinically useful classification for azoospermia is nonobstructive versus obstructive etiologies. Obstruction accounts for 40% of azoospermia cases (1). Obstructive disorders may be congenital or acquired and can result from a blockage at any point along the outflow tract of the sperm, from the testis to the urethra. Severe genitourinary infections or iatrogenic injuries during scrotal and inguinal procedures are common causes of obstructive azoospermia. Some of these disorders such as congenital bilateral absence of vas deferens (CBAVD) can only be dealt with using assisted reproduction. However, other causes such as ejaculatory duct obstruction and vasal obstruction can be surgically treated. Men with obstructive azoospermia can father a child either by surgical correction of the obstruction, which may lead to pregnancy after intercourse without the need of assisted reproductive technology, or by retrieval of sperm from male reproductive system for use with in vitro fertilization (IVF) and intracytoplasmic sperm injection (ICSI). The advantages and drawbacks of these options should be discussed with consideration of the couple's history and desired outcome.

EJACULATORY DUCT OBSTRUCTION

Ejaculatory duct obstruction is reported to be a cause of azoospermia in up to 5% of patients (2). Although rare, this obstruction is a surgically correctable cause of male infertility. Various symptoms, signs, transrectal ultrasound (TRUS), and cystoscopic findings have been associated with ejaculatory duct obstruction, but none of these is pathognomonic for this disorder. Moreover, the clinical picture may be complicated when obstruction is unilateral, partial, or functional (3).

Anatomy

The ejaculatory ducts are formed by the confluence of the vasa deferentia and the ducts of the seminal vesicle. They pass 1 to 2 cm caudal and anteriorly through the prostate gland, converging as they approach their separate openings on the verumontanum (4). The existence of a sphincter located distal to the ductus has been described, but its role in functional or partial obstruction remains unclear (5). The prostatic utricle lies between the two ejaculatory ducts. It is a blind glandular grouping that is not connected to the main prostatic ducts, but has access to the superior aspect of the verumontanum through an independent orifice. Its exact embryogenesis is still a matter of controversy (6,7). Kato et al. (8) suggest that the cystic lesions arise at a later stage of embryogenesis, and that their development is probably due to a narrowing (cystic dilatation of the prostatic utricle) or an obstruction (prostatic utricular cyst) of the communication through the urethra. Some authors differentiate midline cysts into utricular cysts and Müllerian duct cysts (9). Utricular cysts are of endodermal origin, usually smaller than Müllerian duct cysts, and communicate with prostatic urethra. Müllerian duct cysts are of mesodermal origin and do not communicate with prostatic urethra. However, these distinctions, if any, are irrelevant to the management of these conditions. Midline cysts are thought to cause obstruction by extrinsic compression of the ejaculatory duct. Wolffian cysts or ejaculatory duct cysts, produce para median or lateral intraprostatic cysts and have connection with either vas deferens or seminal vesicles. They are often associated with abnormalities of the urogenital tract derived from the Wolffian duct and are rarely found in clinical practice (10).

ETIOLOGIES OF OBSTRUCTION

Ejaculatory duct obstruction can be classified as congenital or acquired. Congenital causes include atresia or stenosis of the ejaculatory ducts, and utricular or Wolffian cysts. Acquired causes include trauma, inflammation, infection, and iatrogenic etiologies. They are listed in Table 1.

Symptoms

As previously mentioned, there are no pathognomonic symptoms for ejaculatory duct obstruction. Patients may complain of nonprojectile ejaculation and decreased ejaculatory volume, a decreased sensation of orgasm, pain on or after ejaculation, hematospermia, or perineal or testicular pain. Many of these patients have no symptoms (11). In patients with partial obstruction, these symptoms may be mild or absent.

Signs

The clinical examination of patients with suspected obstruction of the vas is usually normal. The testes are normal in size and

Table 1 Etiologies of Ejaculatory Duct Obstruction

Congenital
Agenesia
Stenosis
Prostatic utricular cyst
Müllerian cyst
Wolffian cyst
Acquired
Trauma or iatrogenic lesion
Endoscopic resection
Excision of seminal cysts
Rectal surgery in childhood
Infection
Genital infection
Urinary infection
Prostatic abcess
Prolonged catheterization
Tuberculosis
Post-infectious calculus
Neoplasia
Idiopathic

consistency. There are palpable vasa and normal secondary sexual characteristics. Occasionally, there can be prostatic or epididymal tenderness, a palpable prostatic cystic lesion, or palpable seminal vesicle (12). In most cases even larger prostatic cysts are not palpable, but sometimes may be appreciated as a soft area in the midline of the prostate. Ejaculatory disorders, by excluding spermatozoa in urine after ejaculation as well as presence of vas deferens by clinical palpation, should of course be ruled out before suggesting this diagnosis. Because the hypothalamic–pituitary axis is intact, the serum follicle stimulating hormone (FSH) level is usually normal. Complete bilateral ejaculatory duct obstruction results in lack of secretions from seminal vesicles in the ejaculate. Typical semen analysis findings show low volume (less than 1.5 mg), oligospermia or azoospermia, low pH, and absent or very low fructose concentration. These clinical features may be modified if the obstruction is partial or unilateral. Motility is usually also decreased (13). The absence of fructose, consistently low volume ejaculate, or acidic semen (pH < 7.4) should lead one to consider the possibility of ejaculatory duct obstruction or CBAVD (14). Nevertheless, fructose may be present, reflecting a partial obstruction in most cases. In partial obstruction, semen analysis may approach normal values (15). Ejaculatory volume, however, is consistently decreased. Any male with infertility characterized by decreased ejaculate volume, impaired sperm count and/or motility, as well as normal findings on physical examination and normal hormonal profile should have ejaculatory duct obstruction considered.

Intraoperative vasography after vasopuncture was the standard diagnostic method for ejaculatory duct obstruction for several decades. The risk of iatrogenic strictures and vasal obstructions required finding a less invasive method. TRUS is a convenient and noninvasive method to examine these patients (16), which allows demonstration of the anatomical relationship between the prostate, seminal vesicles, and ejaculatory ducts (Fig. 1). It should be performed with a high frequency (7 MHz) biplane transducer. Theoretically, obstruction of the ejaculatory ducts should be associated with dilation of the seminal vesicle. Previous authors have suggested that a transaxial seminal width >1.5 cm is the cutoff value for dilation (17,18). However, Jarow (19) observed a weak correlation between seminal vesicle width and ejaculatory volume, and showed that there is significant overlap of the seminal vesicle area between fertile and infertile men. Nevertheless, a low ejaculate volume (< 1 mL) associated with seminal vesicle enlargement is highly suggestive of ejaculatory duct obstruction.

TRUS findings in suspected ejaculatory duct obstruction include anechoic areas within the seminal vesicle, midline cysts, ejaculatory duct dilation, seminal vesicle size asymmetry, and hyperechoic areas suggestive of calcifications. Hyperechoic findings near the ejaculatory ducts are found in normal men. These lesions can be associated with prior inflammation of the prostate or can be corpora amylacea (18). However, calcifications within the ejaculatory ducts may reflect calculi causing obstruction (20). TRUS-guided seminal vesicle aspiration and vesiculography may be helpful in the diagnosis of ejaculatory duct obstruction. This technique, although not widely used, allows an accurate visualization of the ducts, without the risks of standard vasography. Under TRUS guidance, a 22-gauge needle is inserted, and after localization is confirmed by seminal fluid aspiration, radiographic contrast medium is injected. Moreover, as sperms are normally found at very low levels within the seminal vesicles, >1 to 2 sperms per high power field (HPF) in the seminal vesicle fluid diagnose a ductal obstruction (21).

Although MRI has already been described as an imaging modality, its use is not recommended on the basis of lack of evidence-based studies.

In the absence of clear sonographic alterations of the distal seminal tract or in cases in which the level of obstruction cannot be evaluated clearly (12), as is often the case in partial obstructions, vaso-vesiculography and a diagnostic seminal tract washout has been suggested by some authors as a diagnostic and therapeutic maneuver (3).

Treatment

Originally described by Farley and Barnes in 1973 (22), transurethral resection of ejaculatory ducts (TURED) has become a standard treatment for ejaculatory duct obstruction. A variety of transurethral procedures were used, including Collings knife incision, loop resection lateral to the verumontanum, or loop resection of the verumontanum itself. TURED is performed using pure cutting current without coagulation (23), to avoid stricturing of the newly opened ejaculatory duct

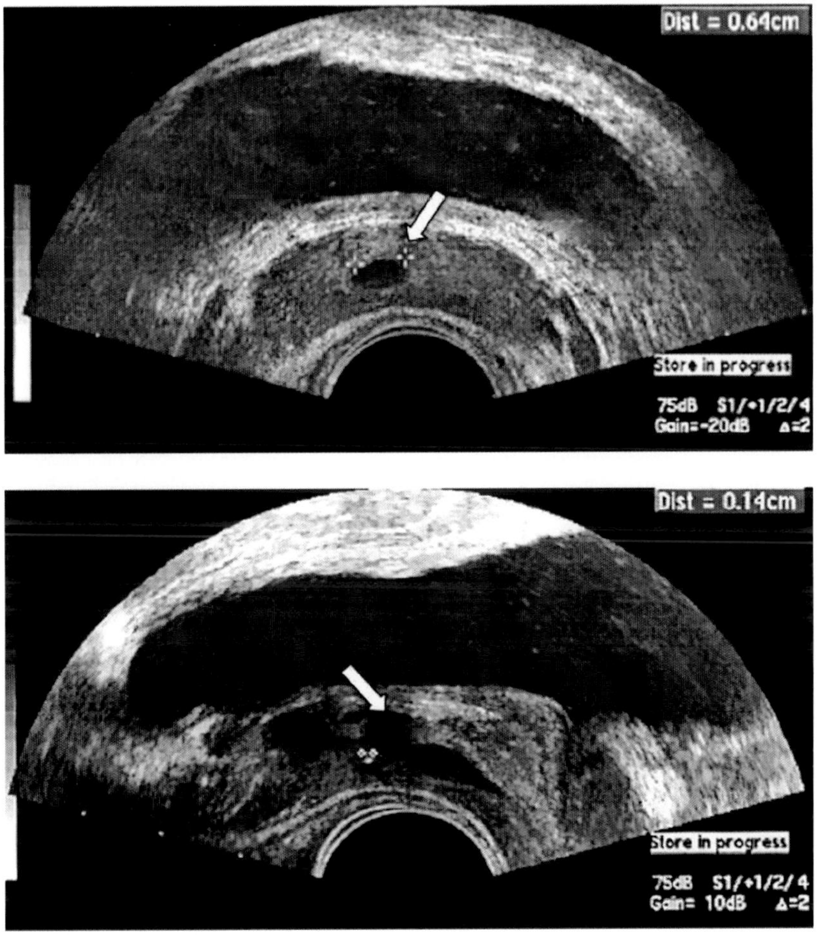

Figure 1 Transrectal Ultrasound (TRUS): coronal and sagittal sections. Note the dilated seminal vesicles (*white arrow*).

(Fig. 2). The resection technique may vary, from incising or unroofing the midline cyst in cases of obstruction due to a midline intraprostatic cyst (to relieve extrinsic compression on the ducts), to deep resection along the course of the ejaculatory ducts in case of long post-inflammatory obstruction. Because the anatomy of the ejaculatory duct running parallel to the urethra likely helps to prevent urinary reflux to the vasa, extensive resection of the ejaculatory ducts should only be undertaken with caution. Preoperative or intraoperative TRUS can make this procedure safer and more effective, allowing precise localization of the cyst and distance measurement from the bladder neck (16). Transurethral resection can also be facilitated by placing a gloved finger in the rectum to squeeze the seminal vesicles and allowing efflux of seminal fluid (and dye), as well as localizing the proximity of the resection loop to the rectum. The ducts are considered opened when the distal portion is visualized (24). Another older but reliable technique involves localization of the stenotic levels by intraoperative microsurgical hemivasotomy and vasography. The vasotomy is made at the time of the resection. During vasography, the fluid from the testicular end of the vas is examined for spermatozoa, in order to exclude an additional epididymal blockage. Using vasal injection of a dye during resection also allows intraoperative confirmation of patency. This approach limits the rash caused by stenotic complications when microsurgical closure of the vasotomy is performed (25). This procedure should be done by urologists with microsurgical experience. Semen analysis should be obtained one month following resection.

The outcome on fertility varies between the different available studies. Schroeder-Printzen et al. (26) demonstrate an improvement in sperm concentration, ejaculate volume, and fructose content for 8 out of 16 patients. Two patients fathered a child after the procedure. The low 25% pregnancy rate for patent cases is confirmed by Weintraub et al. (14), with two pregnancies achieved in eight patients. In a retrospective study, Meacham et al. (12) showed a 50% increase in sperm density and motility, and a postoperative pregnancy rate of 29% after TURED. Most interestingly, the success of TURED can vary according

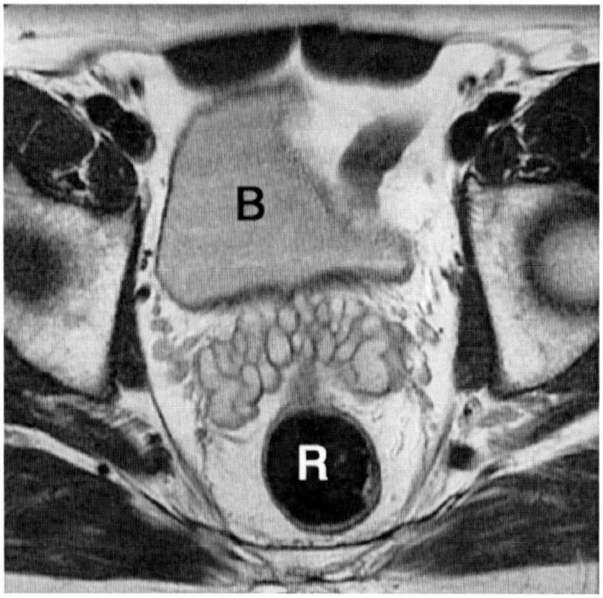

Figure 2 (A) Endoscopic view of intraprostatic cyst. (B) Unroofing the midline cyst (C) Using vasal injection of a dye during resection allows also intraoperative confirmation of patency. (D) Relationship of cyst and bladder neck.

to the etiology of obstruction as demonstrated by Netto et al. (24). Men with partial obstruction due to congenital abnormalities did significantly better after transurethral resection (100% improvement in semen volume and motility) than those with inflammatory or traumatic conditions (37.5%). Other investigators confirm the better outcome in the case of central cystic lesions, although some of the increase in ejaculate may occur because of urinary contamination (27).

Johnson et al. (11) demonstrated that men with symptomatic duct obstruction have subjective and objective relief in symptoms and signs after TURED, including the resolution of painful ejaculation or improvement in ejaculate volume. They advocated that the symptoms of ejaculatory duct obstruction can also have a major impact on sexual satisfaction, and should hence be taken into consideration.

Complications of TURED include rectal injuries, external sphincter injuries, bladder neck injury with resulting retrograde ejaculation, and the possibility of urine reflux into the ejaculatory ducts. This latter complication may cause poor sperm motility, acid semen pH, and epididymitis (28). One study also showed a 4% rate of secondary postoperative azoospermia after return of sperm to the ejaculate (2). In that same study, complications were reported by 20% of patients, including prolonged catheterization for gross hematuria, urinary tract infection, post-void dribbling, and premature ejaculation. Excessive postoperative fibrosis may also result in reocclusion of ejaculatory ducts. In this case, a repeated TURED could be necessary (12).

Given the potential complications, alternative treatments for ejaculatory duct obstruction were proposed. Jarow and Zagoria (29) published a report on the use of antegrade balloon dilation of an obstructed ejaculatory duct. The antegrade approach was suggested because the catheterization of the ejaculatory duct orifice was difficult to perform via a transurethral approach. An alternative approach was for limited resection of the verumontanum followed by retrograde balloon dilation of the ejaculatory ducts with a 4-mm vascular balloon dilation system as proposed by Schlegel (30). The durability of this approach is less clear, but is applicable for extraprostatic obstruction, which cannot be treated with TURED. The alternatives to TURED are MESA, TESE, proximal vas deferens aspiration, seminal vesicle aspiration, and direct ultrasonically guided cyst aspiration. Spermatozoa retrieved by any of the mentioned surgical techniques should always be cryopreserved and can be used for assisted reproduction.

Summary

Ejaculatory duct obstruction is a rare but curable cause of male infertility. Although there are no pathognomonic findings in ejaculatory duct obstruction, this diagnosis should be suspected in any infertile man with normal testis and hormonal profile, but with a decreased ejaculatory volume, an impaired sperm count and/or motility, and low fructose concentration, or acidic semen pH. Dilated seminal vesicles or midline prostatic cyst on TRUS is also highly suggestive of the diagnosis. In selected cases, TURED has resulted in marked improvement in semen parameters, and pregnancies have been reported. Improvement in semen parameters can be expected in 50–100% of patients (24), depending on the extent of obstruction. Pregnancy typically occurred without assisted reproduction in only 25% to 30% of cases. Sperm retrieval with assisted reproduction is an alternate approach.

EPIDIDYMAL AND VASAL OBSTRUCTION

Etiologies

Epididymal obstruction is a common cause of obstructive azoospermia in men with a normal ejaculate volume and FSH value below 7.6 mIU/mL (31). Its etiology may be congenital (CBAVD, idiopathic epididymal obstruction) or acquired. The acquired causes of epididymal blockage include traumatic injury of the epididymis (typically iatrogenic, e.g., posthydrocelectomy or orchidopexy) and infectious or inflammatory damage (32). The obstruction may also be secondary to chronic vasal obstruction (post vasectomy), associated with back pressure–induced rupture of the epididymal tubule. Many cases are idiopathic. Surgery for epididymal cyst is also a reported cause of obstruction (33). Silent chronic infection by Chlamydia trachomatis, although a common etiology of epididymitis, is an uncommon cause of male reproductive tract obstruction (34), unlike what is seen for women.

Obstruction of the vas may be proximal or distal. Vasectomy for sterilization is the most common cause of proximal

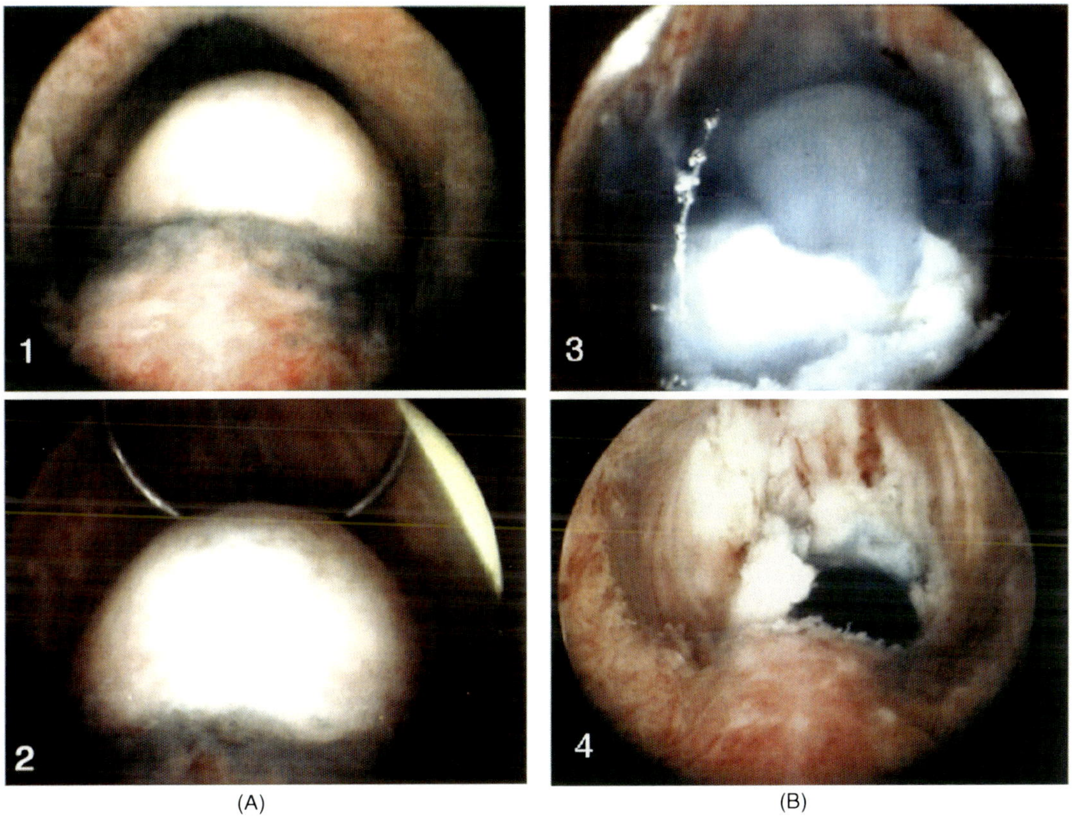

Figure 2b

acquired obstruction. Vasectomy remains one of the most popular methods for contraception; between 500,000 and one million men undergo this procedure each year in North America (35). There are many hypothesis-seeking studies on the possible effect of vasectomy (33,36,37). However, there are no definitive studies suggesting an adverse effect of vasectomy on a patient's health or spermatogenesis. Despite preoperative counseling, 2% to 6% of vasectomized men will undergo vasectomy reversal (38). Proximal obstructive vasal lesions can also occur after hydrocelectomy.

Distal obstructions are usually traumatic or iatrogenic. Orchidopexy and herniorrhaphy during childhood or hernia repairs in adults (39) are frequently described etiologies (40).

Treatment

Vasovasostomy

There is general agreement that results of vasovasostomy are better after microsurgical than after macrosurgical anastomosis (41). Microsurgical vasovasostomy was described by Owen and popularized by Silber in 1976 (42). Multiple modifications were introduced, all based on the surgical principles of a tension-free, watertight anastomosis with mucosa-to-mucosa apposition (43) (Fig. 2b). The intervention can be performed under local, regional, or general anesthesia, depending on preferences of the surgeon and patient. After a scrotal incision, the two ends of the vas are excised and the patency of the distal end is tested with injection of saline solution. The fluid obtained from the proximal or testicular end is observed, and from its gross and microscopic appearance as well as the surgeon's experience, a decision to perform vasovasostomy or vasoepididymostomy is made. A grade from 1 to 5 can be applied to the vasal fluid. The grading scale, based on gross appearance and microscopic findings, is described in Table 2. If the sperm quality is graded from 1 to 4, vasovasostomy can be performed. The Practice Committee of the American Society for Reproductive Medicine advocated to perform a vasovasostomy if sperm was identified in the vas fluid or if the fluid was copious, crystal clear, and watery, or perform a vasoepididymostomy otherwise (44). Vasoepididymostomy requires substantial clinical skills and can cause measurable scarring in the epididymis, so only surgeons experienced in vasoepididymostomy should perform this procedure. Note that the gross aspect of the fluid is important mainly for grade 4 and 5, and clear, because watery fluid carries a better prognosis of return of sperm to the semen than thick and creamy fluid. A one-layer or two-layer microsurgical

Table 2 Vasal Fluid Grading, and Surgical Recommendation Based on Gross Appearance of Vasal Fluid and Microscopic Findings

Grade	Microscopic findings	Vasal fluid appearance	Surgical procedure recommended
1	Mainly normal motile sperm	Copious, cloudy, water soluble	Vasovasostomy
2	Mainly normal non motile sperm	Copious, cloudy, water soluble	Vasovasostomy
3	Mainly sperm head	Copious, cloudy, water soluble	Vasovasostomy
4	Only sperm head	Copious, cloudy, water insoluble	Vasovasostomy
5	No sperm	Copious, crystal clear, watery	Vasovasostomy
5	No sperm	Copious, thick white toothpaste-like, water insoluble	Vasoepididymostomy
5	No sperm	Scant white thin fluid	Vasoepididymostomy

If the vas fluid has a thick, creamy consistency it should be diluted with normal saline to allow observation of sperm that otherwise may be overlooked because they are packed together tightly, and obscured by debris in the viscous fluid.

technique for vasovasostomy seems to carry similar results (41). Cryopreservation of the sperm harvested intraoperatively should be discussed with patients with consideration to the costs of IVF/ICSI. There are relatively few complications after vasovasostomy, the most common of which are postoperative hematomas and infections.

Iatrogenic injuries causing distal lesions may be associated with longer vasal defects, impaired blood supply, and longer obstructive intervals, frequently resulting in secondary epididymal obstruction and testicular atrophy (40). In selected cases, the vas of the contralateral atrophic testis can be used for a crossover vasovasostomy or vasoepididymostomy.

Vasoepididymostomy

Microsurgical vasoepididymostomy can be performed using an end-to-end, an end-to-side (45), or an intussusception end-to-side method (46). The first step of each method involves identifying the level of epididymal obstruction, starting from cauda to caput epididymis. For end-to-end anastomosis the epididymis is cut and the dominant effluxing tubule is examined. When fluid is found, it is aspirated and observed in the operating room (33). The mucosa is then approximated to the opened edges of the epididymal tubule with 10-0 nylon or polypropylene, and the vas muscular layer is approximated to the epididymal tunic with 9-0 suture. This approach is limited because of profuse bleeding from the cut end of the epididymis and the difficulty in identifying a single effluxing tubule.

For end-to-side anastomosis, and for the most recent intussusception end-to-side method (46,47) (Fig. 3), the tunic of the epididymis is incised with a microblade, and the fascia overlying the epididymal tubule is dissected carefully. Double-armed 10-0 nylon sutures are placed longitudinally within the chosen tubule. The tubulotomy is performed between the suture needles, and the epididymal fluid is examined. The four needles are placed 1 mm into the vas lumen and out through the muscularis on the cut edge, which allows invagination of the epididymal tubule into the vas lumen. The anastomosis is completed with at least three to four 9-0 nylon sutures through the muscularis of the vas and epididymal tunic. In a retrospective study of four different techniques of microsurgical vasoepididymostomy, the intussusception technique showed comparable results to the traditional end-to-end and end-to-side, but late failures seemed to be less common (48).

Better postoperative fertility rates are achieved with caudal anastomosis, presumably because spermatozoa that pass

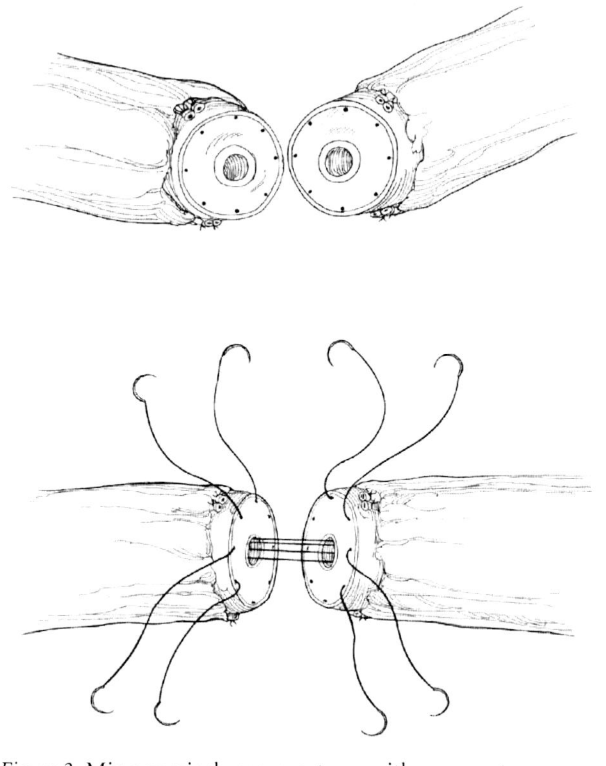

Figure 3 Microsurgical vasovasostomy with mucosa-to-mucosa apposition.

through at least part of the epididymis to mature show better mobility and have greater functional capacity as well.

Semen analyses are performed three months after the intervention and repeated at that frequency until sperm parameters are normal or a pregnancy occurs. Because the possibility of late failure exists, periodic semen testing is recommended in couples desiring pregnancy. Cryopreservation should be considered when motile sperm return to the ejaculate. For bilateral vasovasostomy, the overall patency rate is 87% and the pregnancy rate is 53%, and for bilateral vasoepididymostomy, overall patency rate is 50% and pregnancy rate is 29% (41). These values are highly influenced by several features, such as preoperative factors (prior fertility, medical, and surgical history subsequent to vasectomy, obstruction interval, partner's age and fertility status, prior reversal failure) and intraoperative factors (presence of sperm granuloma, length of the vas from the testis to the level of obstruction, quality of sperm and vasal fluid, unilateral or bilateral procedure performed). The more important features for subsequent patency and pregnancy rate will be discussed later.

Obstructive Interval

The postoperative rate of return of sperm to the ejaculate and the pregnancy rate decrease according to the duration of time since vasectomy. The Vasovasostomy Study Group reported rate of return of sperm to the semen and of pregnancy at, respectively, 97% and 76% if the interval is less than 3 years, 88% and 53% if 3 to 8 years, 79% and 44% if 9 to 14 years, and 71% and 30% if 15 years or longer.

Partner Factor

Of all pre- and perioperative factors, age of the wife has the most significant impact on pregnancy rate (49). The pregnancy rate for vasectomy reversal is good regardless of female age, as long as the female partner is 39 years or younger. Pregnancy rates for couples with the female partner aged 35 to 39 are reported to be 54%, and drop to 14% for female partners aged 40 years or older. Although advancing male age is associated with declining fertility, the magnitude of this change is far smaller than the effect of female age (50). The outcome of vasectomy reversal in men with the same partner seems to be better than for men with a new partner (51). Kim et al. (52) debated that this difference is probably due to the previously proven female partner fecundity.

Sperm Granuloma

A grossly identifiable sperm granuloma occurs in 15% to 40% of men after a vasectomy. This immune reaction to leaking sperm at the cut end of the vas was thought to have a positive effect on vasovasostomy outcome. The granuloma is thought to benefit the reconstruction by allowing sperm leakage to be reabsorbed within the microcanaliculi of the sperm granuloma, preventing secondary pressure buildup and damage to the epididymis. The Vasovasostomy Study Group showed that patency and pregnancy rates are not significantly different whether or

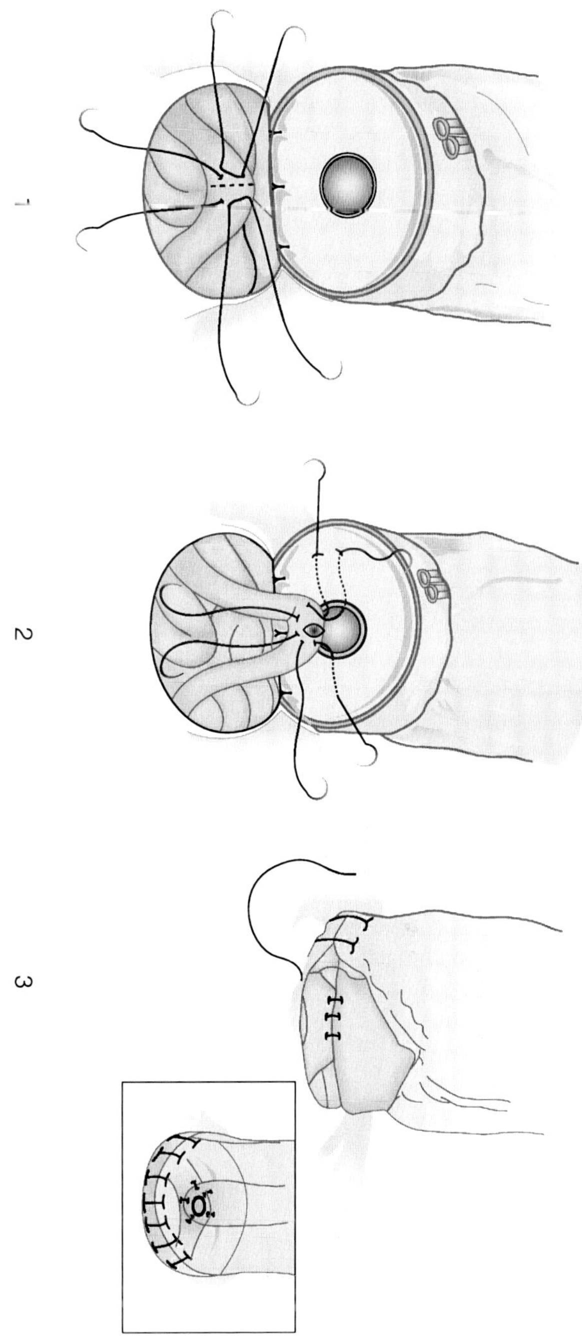

Figure 4 Microsurgical vasoepididymostomy. (A) 10-0 nylon double-armed sutures are placed longitudinally or transversally to the chosen tubule. (B) The tubulotomy is performed between the retracted sutures, and the epididymal fluid is examined. (C) The anastomosis is completed with 9-0 nylon sutures through the muscularis of the vas and epididymal tunic.

not a histologically confirmed granuloma is present; this may be a reflection of the nearly universal development of microscopic (but not macroscopic) granulomas.

Antisperm Antibodies

High titer antibodies that bind to specific sperm antigens are a potential cause of infertility in humans (53). Although vasectomy is an important risk factor for the development of antisperm antibodies, preoperative antisperm antibody levels do not preclude the success of vasectomy reversal and do not need to be tested. The antisperm antibodies associated with vasectomy reversal seem to disappear if a vasectomy is technically reversed successfully and spermatozoa do not have to be reabsorbed at high levels.

Prior-Reversal Failure

The return of sperm to the ejaculate occurs significantly late for vasoepididymostomy (1 year or longer) than for vasovasostomy (6 months) (54). Absence of sperm in ejaculate more than six months after vasovasostomy is usually due to unrecognized epididymal obstruction, and late failure following initial patency suggests a compromised anastomosis. Though the patency and pregnancy rates are lower than in successful first-time procedures, a repeat attempt remains a good option for men who have failed vasovasostomy or epididymostomy. When performing reoperative vasovasostomy, the surgeon should bypass the entire scarred portion of the vas and dissect a sufficient length of the vas to avoid anastomotic tension. On a total of 222 repeated procedures, the Vasovasostomy Study Group reported 75% patency and 43% pregnancy, which was confirmed by other reports (55). Because stenosis rates are greater following reoperation, intraoperative and postoperative sperm cryopreservation is recommended.

The first pregnancies via ICSI were reported in 1992 by Palermo et al. (56). From that time, the most controversial issue for vasectomy-associated infertility is whether to perform vasectomy reversal or sperm retrieval with ICSI. Randomized controlled clinical trials to determine the optimal treatment have not been undertaken, nor are they considered feasible. Cost-effectiveness studies are one way to analyze the benefit of an intervention and compare the value of vasectomy reversal to assisted reproduction. These studies suggest that vasectomy reversal is the preferred initial approach, unless female factors require IVF to be performed.

In one of the first cost-effectiveness studies, Pavlovich and Schlegel (57) clearly showed that vasoepididymostomy is as successful and more cost-effective than microsurgical epididymal sperm aspiration (MESA) and ICSI. Vasectomy reversal also does not expose the woman to the complications of IVF treatment or to the increased risk of multiple pregnancies (58), while treating a male factor problem. Nevertheless, information such as the number of desired children, economic situation of the couple, and presence of female factor requiring IVF/ICSI should be taken into account when counseling couples regarding the more appropriate treatment.

CONCLUSION

Since the development of microsurgical reconstructive techniques, the surgical treatment of obstructive azoospermia has dramatically improved. The results of reconstructive microsurgery depend on the cause and location of the obstruction as well as on the expertise of the surgeon. In the case of vasectomy-induced infertility, the treatment of choice is often vasectomy reversal. Nevertheless, parameters including obstruction interval, partner's age and reproductive status, as well as specific goals and desire of the individual couple must be considered before initiating therapy.

TAKE-HOME MESSAGE

The possibility of ejaculatory duct obstruction should not be overlooked in the differential diagnosis of obstructive azoospermia, as it can be successfully treated with transurethral resection of ejaculatory ducts.

Microsurgical reconstruction of the vas and/or epididymis is a valid therapeutic alternative for obstructive azoospermia in selected cases (grade B).

Prior to performing microsurgery in the male, the female partner should be evaluated to determine if female infertility factors are present.

Vasectomy reversal is more successful and cost-effective than MESA and ICSI (Grade B)

REFERENCES

1. ASRM Practice Committee. Report on evaluation of the azoospermic male. Fertil Steril 2004; 82(suppl 1):S131–S136.
2. Turek PJ, Magana JO, Lipshultz LI. Semen parameters before and after transurethral surgery for ejaculatory duct obstruction. J Urol 1996; 155:1291–1293.
3. Colpi GM, Negri L, Nappi RE, et al. Is transrectal ultrasonography a reliable diagnostic approach in ejaculatory duct sub-obstruction? Hum Reprod 1997; 12:2186–2191.
4. Pryor JP, Hendry WF. Ejaculatory duct obstruction in subfertile males: analysis of 87 patients. Fertil Steril 1991; 56:725–730.
5. Hellerstein DK, Meacham RB, Lipshultz LI. Transrectal ultrasound and partial ejaculatory duct obstruction in male infertility. Urology 1992; 39:449–452.
6. Mayersak JS. Urogenital sinus-ejaculatory duct cyst: a case report with a proposed clinical classification and review of the literature. J Urol 1989; 142:1330–1332.
7. Elder JS, Mostwin JL. Cyst of the ejaculatory duct/urogenital sinus. J Urol 1984; 132:768–771.
8. Kato H, Hayama M, Furuya S, et al. Anatomical and histological studies of so-called Mullerian duct cyst. Int J Urol 2005; 12:465–468.

9. Kirkali Z, Yigitbasi O, Diren B, et al. Cysts of the prostate, seminal vesicles and diverticulum of the ejaculatory ducts. Eur Urol 1991; 20:77–80.
10. Surya BV, Washecka R, Glasser J, et al. Cysts of the seminal vesicles: diagnosis and management. Br J Urol 1988; 62:491–493.
11. Johnson CW, Bingham JB, Goluboff ET, et al. Transurethral resection of the ejaculatory ducts for treating ejaculatory symptoms. BJU Int 2005; 95:117–119.
12. Meacham RB, Hellerstein DK, Lipshultz LI. Evaluation and treatment of ejaculatory duct obstruction in the infertile male. Fertil Steril 1993; 59:393–397.
13. Paick JS. Transurethral resection of the ejaculatory duct. Int J Urol 2000; 7(suppl):S42–S47.
14. Weintraub MP, De Mouy E, Hellstrom WJ. Newer modalities in the diagnosis and treatment of ejaculatory duct obstruction. J Urol 1993; 150:1150–1154.
15. Nagler HM, Rotman M, Zoltan E, et al. The natural history of partial ejaculatory duct obstruction. J Urol 2002; 167:253–254.
16. Meacham RB, Townsend RR, Drose JA. Ejaculatory duct obstruction: diagnosis and treatment with transrectal sonography. AJR Am J Roentgenol 1995; 165:1463–1466.
17. Kuligowska E, Baker CE, Oates RD. Male infertility: role of transrectal US in diagnosis and management. Radiology 1992; 185:353–360.
18. Carter SS, Shinohara K, Lipshultz LI. Transrectal ultrasonography in disorders of the seminal vesicles and ejaculatory ducts. Urol Clin North Am 1989; 16:773–790.
19. Jarow JP. Transrectal ultrasonography of infertile men. Fertil Steril 1993; 60:1035–1039.
20. Philip J, Manikandan R, Lamb GH, et al. Ejaculatory-duct calculus causing secondary obstruction and infertility. Fertil Steril 2007; 88:706.e9–706.e11.
21. Jarow JP. Seminal vesicle aspiration in the management of patients with ejaculatory duct obstruction. J Urol 1994; 152:899–901.
22. Farley S, Barnes R. Stenosis of ejaculatory ducts treated by endoscopic resection. J Urol 1973; 109:664–666.
23. Fisch H, Lambert SM, Goluboff ET. Management of ejaculatory duct obstruction: etiology, diagnosis, and treatment. World J Urol 2006; 24:604–610.
24. Netto NR Jr, Esteves SC, Neves PA. Transurethral resection of partially obstructed ejaculatory ducts: seminal parameters and pregnancy outcomes according to the etiology of obstruction. J Urol 1998; 159:2048–2053.
25. Goldstein M. Vasography. In: Goldstein M, ed. Surgery of Male Infertility. Philadelphia, PA: Saunders, 1995: 26–32.
26. Schroeder-Printzen I, Ludwig M, Kohn F, et al. Surgical therapy in infertile men with ejaculatory duct obstruction: technique and outcome of a standardized surgical approach. Hum Reprod 2000; 15:1364–1368.
27. Goluboff ET, Stifelman MD, Fisch H. Ejaculatory duct obstruction in the infertile male. Urology 1995; 45:925–931.
28. Goluboff ET, Kaplan SA, Fisch H. Seminal vesicle urinary reflux as a complication of transurethral resection of ejaculatory ducts. J Urol 1995; 153:1234–1235.
29. Jarow JP, Zagoria RJ. Antegrade ejaculatory duct recanalization and dilation. Urology 1995; 46:743–746.
30. Schlegel PN. Management of ejaculatory duct obstruction. In: Lipshultz LI and Howards SS, eds. Infertility in the Male (3rd ed). St Louis, MO: Mosby, 1997:385–394.
31. Schoor RA, Elhanbly S, Niederberger CS, et al. The role of testicular biopsy in the modern management of male infertility. J Urol 2002; 167:197–200.
32. Kim ED, Winkel E, Orejuela F, et al. Pathological epididymal obstruction unrelated to vasectomy: results with microsurgical reconstruction. J Urol 1998; 160:2078–2080.
33. Silber SJ, Grotjan HE. Microscopic vasectomy reversal 30 years later: a summary of 4010 cases by the same surgeon. J Androl 2004; 25:845–859.
34. Dohle GR. Inflammatory-associated obstructions of the male reproductive tract. Andrologia 2003; 35:321–324.
35. Goldstein M, Tanrikut C. Microsurgical management of male infertility. Nat Clin Pract Urol 2006; 3:381–391.
36. McVicar CM, O'Neill DA, McClure N, et al. Effects of vasectomy on spermatogenesis and fertility outcome after testicular sperm extraction combined with ICSI. Hum Reprod 2005; 20:2795–2800.
37. Carbone DJ Jr, Shah A, Thomas AJ Jr ,et al. Partial obstruction, not antisperm antibodies, causing infertility after vasovasostomy. J Urol 1998; 159:827–830.
38. Schiff JD, Ramirez ML, Bar-Chama, N. Medical and surgical management male infertility. Endocrinol Metab Clin North Am 2007; 36:313–331.
39. Shin D, Lipshultz LI, Goldstein M, et al. Herniorrhaphy with polypropylene mesh causing inguinal vasal obstruction: a preventable cause of obstructive azoospermia. Ann Surg 2005; 241:553–558.
40. Sheynkin YR, Hendin BN, Schlegel PN, et al. Microsurgical repair of iatrogenic injury to the vas deferens. J Urol 1998; 159:139–141.
41. Belker AM, Thomas AJ Jr, Fuchs EF, et al. Results of 1,469 microsurgical vasectomy reversals by the Vasovasostomy Study Group. J Urol 1911; 145:505–511.
42. Silber SJ. Microscopic technique for reversal of vasectomy. Surg Gynecol Obstet 1976; 143:631.
43. Goldstein M, Li PS, Matthews, GJ. Microsurgical vasovasostomy: the microdot technique of precision suture placement. J Urol 1998; 159:188–190.
44. ASRM Practice Committee. Report on management of obstructive azoospermia. Fertil Steril 2006; 86:S259–S263.
45. Schlegel PN, Goldstein M. Microsurgical vasoepididymostomy: refinements and results. J Urol 1993; 150:1165–1168.

46. Marmar JL. Modified vasoepididymostomy with simultaneous double needle placement, tubulotomy and tubular invagination. J Urol 2000; 163:483–486.
47. Chan PT, Li PS, Goldstein M. Microsurgical vasoepididymostomy: a prospective randomized study of 3 intussusception techniques in rats. J Urol 2003; 169:1924–1929.
48. Schiff J, Chan P, Li PS, et al. Outcome and late failures compared in 4 techniques of microsurgical vasoepididymostomy in 153 consecutive men. J Urol 2005; 174:651–655; quiz 801.
49. Gerrard ER Jr, Sandlow JI, Oster RA, et al. Effect of female partner age on pregnancy rates after vasectomy reversal. Fertil Steril 2007; 87:1340–1344.
50. Kuhnert B, Nieschlag E. Reproductive functions of the ageing male. Hum Reprod Update 2004; 10:327–339.
51. Chan PT, Goldstein M. Superior outcomes of microsurgical vasectomy reversal in men with the same female partners. Fertil Steril 2004; 81:1371–1374.
52. Kim SW, Ku JH, Park K, et al. A different female partner does not affect the success of second vasectomy reversal. J Androl 2005; 26:48–52.
53. Chamley LW, Clarke GN. Antisperm antibodies and conception. Semin Immunopathol 2007; 29:169–184.
54. Matthews GJ, Schlegel PN, Goldstein M. Patency following microsurgical vasoepididymostomy and vasovasostomy: temporal considerations. J Urol 1995; 154:2070–2073.
55. Matthews GJ, McGee KE, Goldstein M. Microsurgical reconstruction following failed vasectomy reversal. J Urol 1997; 157:844–846.
56. Palermo G, Joris H, Devroey P, et al. Pregnancies after intracytoplasmic injection of single spermatozoon into an oocyte. Lancet 1992; 340:17–18.
57. Pavlovich CP, Schlegel PN. Fertility options after vasectomy: a cost-effectiveness analysis. Fertil Steril 1997; 67:133–141.
58. Lee R, Li PS, Goldstein M, et al. A decision analysis of treatments for obstructive azoospermia. Hum Reprod 2008; 23:2043–2049.

12 Surgery for male infertility: Surgical sperm retrievals

Giovanni M. Colpi, Guido Piediferro, Fabrizio I. Scroppo, Elisabetta M. Colpi, and Patrizia Sulpizio

Surgical sperm retrieval techniques are performed in view of intracytoplasmic sperm injection (ICSI) procedures. Mainly based upon when they were introduced into clinical practice, they may be classified as follows:

- From the epididymis: artificial spermatocele, microsurgical epididymal sperm aspiration, percutaneous epididymal sperm aspiration
- From the distal seminal tract: seminal tract washout, microsurgical vas deferens sperm aspiration
- From the testis: percutaneous testicular sperm aspiration or testicular fine needle aspiration, testicular sperm extraction, microsurgical testicular sperm extraction

Nowadays, sperm retrieval from the distal seminal tract is virtually no longer used, and retrieval techniques from the epididymis are indicated only for certain cases of obstructive azoospermia.

However, in all cases of azoospermia, testicular sperm retrievals are strongly preferred, even though each procedure has its correct indications.

SURGICAL SPERM RETRIEVALS FROM THE SEMINAL TRACT

Microepididymal Sperm Aspiration

Introduction

Temple-Smith et al. (1) were the first to use microsurgically aspirated spermatozoa from the epididymis for in vitro fertilization (IVF) as a therapeutic option in patients with irreparable Obstructive Azoospermia (OA). The use of these spermatozoa with ICSI led to increased fertilization and pregnancy rates compared to their use with conventional IVF. Today, microepididymal sperm aspiration (MESA) with ICSI is an established treatment for OA, especially in congenital bilateral aplasia of the vas deferens (CBAVD), in inoperable obstruction of the seminal tract, in ejaculatory disorders where conservative therapy was unsuccessful, and in cases of failed vaso-vasostomy and/or vaso-epididymostomy (2).

Technique

MESA consists of microscopically guided aspiration of spermatozoa under general or spinal anesthesia (3,4). The technique involves incising the scrotum, opening the tunica vaginalis, and exploring the scrotal content. The epididymal tunica is incised under the operating microscope and a dilated epididymal tubule (preferably in an avascular area) is selected, isolated, and incised longitudinally using microscissors or a microknife. The tubule opening must be clean; therefore, a thorough hemostasis must be performed, using a bipolar thermal device, to avoid contamination with blood cells that may affect in vitro sperm fertilizing capacity. Spermatozoa in the fluid emerging from the open tubule are checked by touching it to a glass slide, adding a drop of Ringer's solution, covering it with a coverslip, and examining it fresh in the operating room using a phase contrast microscope (400× magnification); alternatively, a 10 μL drop of epididymal fluid is aspirated and put into a Makler™ chamber to check for motile spermatozoa. Once sperm has been found, actual aspiration from the open epididymal tubule is performed using either a 24-G cannula mounted onto a 1-mL syringe and containing gamete culture medium or a glass micropipette with 350 μ ground tip (according to Schlegel). Some authors prefer to use a dry micropipette that allows retrieval of an adequate amount of sperm simply due to a capillary effect aided by gentle pressure on the epididymis (3). The aspirated spermatozoa are then diluted in 2 to 3 mL of suitable medium—usually buffered Earle's medium or human tubular fluid medium (HTFM) (5)—in a pre-filled Eppendorf chamber. The epididymal tubule is closed using 9-0, 10-0, or 11-0 monofilament nylon sutures. If the attempt to retrieve motile spermatozoa is unsuccessful, further attempts may be made in a cranial direction, if necessary, as far as the efferent ductules. The most motile spermatozoa are usually found either inside the tubules of the proximal portion of the caput epididymis or inside the vasa efferentia, and therefore some authors prefer to use epididymal sperm obtained by MESA from the caput tubules, which is thought to provide better results as for the delivery rates (6). The space between the two folds of the tunica vaginalis may be filled with heparinized saline and the scrotum closed with 3-0 Vicryl™ uninterrupted suture. Once the sperms have been collected, they may be utilized either fresh or cryopreserved for subsequent use in order to avoid repeating the procedure. Fresh or frozen–thawed epididymal spermatozoa are applied to a two-layer Percoll gradient and then processed like ejaculated semen.

To minimize the costs and morbidity of MESA, some authors modified the original technique, devising mini-microepididymal sperm aspiration: under local anesthesia, a 1-cm scrotal incision is performed and the dilated tubules suitable for aspiration are exposed and identified under 25× magnification (7).

Complications and Caveat

Complications of MESA are extremely rare and similar to those related to any scrotal exploration, such as pain, hematoma, and infection. Antibiotic prophylaxis may be advisable. In addition, when MESA is performed in patients with cystic fibrosis or CBAVD, transmission of a mutated Cystic Fibrosis Transmembrane conductance Regulator (CFTR) gene is inevitable; genetic counselling must therefore be offered to men with CF (and CBAVD) and to their partners before performing assisted reproductive techniques.

Results

In OA patients, MESA is effective in retrieving sperms in over 90% of cases, and success rates (mainly in terms of pregnancy rates per cycle) are not related to the cause of obstruction (2,8). Regarding fertilization and pregnancy rates per cycle, results are comparable to those obtained with ejaculated sperm, with clinical pregnancy rates about 40%, and up to over 60% in some surveys. In addition, no significant differences in these rates emerge using fresh as opposed to frozen material (9,10). Sperm cryopreservation facilitates organization of the procedure, avoiding the need to proceed simultaneously with oocyte retrieval, with obvious advantages for the couple and the medical team.

PERCUTANEOUS EPIDIDYMAL SPERM ASPIRATION

Introduction

An alternative to MESA is percutaneous epididymal sperm aspiration (PESA) (11), aimed at reducing the technical difficulty, invasiveness, time, and cost of MESA. As it requires specific training in microsurgery, the use of MESA is restricted to a limited number of Centers. PESA has the same indications as MESA and may also be used as a diagnostic technique to confirm sperm production; its use must be limited to those Obstructive Azoospermia (OA) patients where a microsurgical recanalization was excluded a priori.

Technique

A PESA procedure is relatively simple. Following anesthetic infiltration of the spermatic chord at the external inguinal ring, the caput epididymis is held between the surgeon's fingers and a 21G Butterfly™ needle is inserted into the epididymis. Negative pressure is applied by drawing back the plunger of an attached 20-mL syringe. The needle tip is moved gently inwards and outwards within the epididymis until a column of opalescent fluid rises in the needle tubing. When a sufficient quantity has been aspirated, the needle is extracted and the content of the syringe is flushed into a sterile Eppendorf tube containing the same culture medium used for the syringe (11,12).

Complications

PESA is a relatively safe procedure, but it is not entirely free from complications such as epididymal fibrosis, localized pain, and intrascrotal hematomas. The risk of the latter is potentially greater than with MESA, as PESA is a "blind" procedure (13).

The considerations made earlier about MESA also apply to patients with CF and CBAVD undergoing PESA.

Results

Despite its extreme simplicity, repeatability, and inexpensiveness, the results with PESA are overall inferior to those obtained with MESA. Actually, in 10% of cases no spermatozoa can be retrieved and their number is often inadequate for cryopreservation (14). In addition, pregnancy rates per cycle (19–34%) are found to be overall lower than with MESA (12). Repetition of PESA procedures in the same patients can still be successful (12), and motile spermatozoa are retrieved in about one-third of cases, when a new procedure is performed following a first unsuccessful attempt (15).

ARTIFICIAL SPERMATOCELE

General

In the era before ICSI, artificial spermatocele for subsequent percutaneous sperm retrieval was a therapeutic option for treating OA due to obstruction or congenital absence of the vasa deferentia. The theoretical advantages of artificial spermatocele would appear to be evident, as a couple could autonomously aspirate the spermatocele and perform intravaginal insemination at home, but in clinical practice, the use of alloplastic spermatoceles has resulted in unacceptably low pregnancy rates.

Results

Brindley et al. (16) reported two full term pregnancies after artificial insemination in 12 patients treated by vas cannulation and implanted sperm reservoirs. Belker et al. (17) reported 7 pregnancies (4 of which were full term) in 91 partners of patients treated with implantation of an alloplastic spermatocele, while one decade later artificial spermatocele implantation resulted in successful sperm retrieval from the aspirated fluid in one third of the patients.

Conclusions

Over time, poor results have led to abandoning this technique despite some successful pregnancies (18). However, it should be noted that spermatocele implantation is mostly free from complications, and that the relative quality of the obtained sperm samples could have a totally different clinical impact with modern seminal preparations and ICSI techniques.

OTHER SURGICAL SPERM RETRIEVAL PROCEDURES

Introduction

They include seminal tract washout (STW) and microsurgical vas deferens sperm aspiration (MVSA). Both these techniques were originally devised to treat anejaculation due to spinal cord injury (19,20). Their use was subsequently extended to include the treatment of voiding disturbances of the ampullovesicular tract due to extended retroperitoneal lymph node dissection for testicular cancer, neurogenic and psychogenic anejaculation, and all cases of untreatable anejaculation (21).

Techniques

STW

Under a local anesthetic, when necessary, a small scrotal incision is performed, the vas deferens is exposed either mono- or bilaterally and denuded of the surrounding tunicae for a short tract, and a short 25-G Butterfly™ needle is inserted into its lumen. The bladder, which has been previously voided of urine by a catheter, is refilled with 20 mL of an appropriate medium, such as Ham's solution. The seminal tract downstream is then washed through the needle with 20 mL of the same medium. Sperm-containing medium is immediately recovered from the bladder, centrifuged, and the pellet prepared according to the mini-Percoll technique, which is then resuspended with swim-up procedure in 0.5 mL of 10% T6 medium (22).

MVSA

This technique is more complex because it requires microsurgical half-transection of the vas deferens, direct aspiration of spermatozoa from the vas lumen, and microsurgical repair of the sectioned vas wall.

Results

In cases of untreatable anejaculation, both STW and MVSA allow retrieval of great amounts of good quality spermatozoa that can be cryopreserved and used even for conventional IVF, with a total sperm count in the range of 1×10^6 to $2{,}430 \times 10^6$ for STW and of 0.5×10^6 to 252×10^6 for MVSA (22,23). Using STW, reported pregnancy rates are 25% per cycle and 33% per couple, while for MVSA the reported pregnancy rates are 37% for aspiration and 37% for embryo transfer (21,22).

SURGICAL SPERM RETRIEVALS FROM THE TESTIS

Testicular Fine Needle Aspiration

Introduction and Indications

Testicular fine needle aspiration (TeFNA) is indicated in cases of OA, especially when no recanalization surgery is planned. It provides almost certain retrieval of sperm for utilization in ICSI, which, however, is quantitatively inferior and has greater blood contamination (therefore is less suitable for cryopreservation) compared to TESE, and it can be easily repeated with success at each cycle (24).

Technique

TeFNA is performed using a 21-G Butterfly™ needle attached to a 20-mL plastic syringe, used as an aspiration device. Under local anesthesia, the needle is directly inserted into the testicular tissue various times. Once aspiration has been completed, the needle is flushed with culture medium into one well of a four-well plate. The procedure may be repeated several times (25). After needle removal, maintaining a moderate pressure where the needle was inserted is advisable, in order to facilitate hemostasis.

Results

Sperm retrieval is routinely possible in OA, but the conventional freezing procedure is not appropriate for spermatozoa obtained by TeFNA because of their very low number and poor in situ motility (26). In cases of NOA, TeFNA results in very low retrieval rates, such as 21.1% (median) in a review (27) and 10% in a recent study (28); it is successful almost exclusively in cases of severe hypospermatogenesis (29,30). In addition, TeFNA only allows a cytological examination, therefore it is not suitable for detecting carcinomas in situ and testicular malignancies (31).

Case Report 1

A 35-year-old Caucasian man who has been trying to have children with a 30-year-old, gynecologically normal woman since 5 years. He had a left varicocelectomy at the age of 20; postoperative semen analyses showed mild oligozoospermia. At the age of 33, he had consistent findings of cryptoazoospermia, with normal gonadotropins and karyotype, and no Y chromosome microdeletions. The couple underwent the first ICSI cycle with fresh sperm from TeFNA at an infertility center: fertilization occurred, one embryo was transferred, no pregnancy. In a second Center, a further ICSI cycle from fresh TeFNA was carried out after HMG treatment: no fertilization of any oocyte. The man came to our observation two months later. Clinical examination: right and left orchidometry 12 and 10 mL, respectively; normal testicular consistency; normal epididymes, vasa, penis, and prostate. Semen analysis: volume 4 mL; cryptozoospermia. Slightly increased FSH. Testis sonography: rare microcalcifications on the right side. Normal TRUS. The patient underwent scrotal exploration, testis biopsy, and TESE with sperm cryopreservation. Sperms were found in both the right and left TESE samples, where histology showed a hypospermatogenesis pattern on both sides (6.5 and 8 mature spermatids/tubule, respectively) and carcinoma in situ areas in the right biopsy.

Considerations & Conclusions: All infertile males should undergo appropriate diagnostic screening, in particular in case of poor and continuously worsening semen quality. Surgery coupling TESE and biopsy led to detecting a carcinoma in situ, which had remained undiagnosed with two successive TeFNAs.

In (cryptoazoospermia)NOA patients, resorting to TESE is strongly recommended, not only because of the higher successful retrieval rate but also for an appropriate histological examination, given their nonnegligible risk of testicular carcinoma in situ. (Presented at the XXI Congress of the Italian Society of Andrology, Trieste, 2004)

Complications

The (rare) complications of TeFNA, a simple but "blind" technique, include hematocele, intratesticular hematoma, and accidental puncture of the epididymis that might jeopardize the success of any subsequent surgical recanalization.

In an animal model (rat), TeFNA involved severe, progressive, and irreversible damage of tubules along the needle's path, and caused extensive tubular atrophy; on the contrary, TESE caused localized scar fibrosis, with decreased tubular volume and increased interstitial tissue in the adjacent parenchyma, but left the rest of the testis unharmed (33).

TESTICULAR SPERM EXTRACTION

Introduction and Indications

Testicular sperm extraction (TESE) was first introduced by Silber et al. (34) as a sperm retrieval method for ICSI in cases of OA where MESA had failed. It was subsequently also used in NOA.

Ideally, when an invasive diagnostic procedure is to be performed on the testis (i.e., testicular biopsy, and scrotal exploration and vasography), TESE should also be carried out for sperm cryopreservation (35,36) in order to avoid unnecessary repetition of the procedure in OA cases, or unnecessary ovarian stimulation for ICSI for women with an NOA partner (see technique: TESE).

Technique

TESE—either as a single extraction (single TESE) or as multiple extractions from different areas of the testis surface (multiple TESE) (30)—may be performed under a local anesthetic using one of the following techniques:

- Exposing the testicle completely, along with scrotal exploration in case of suspected OA, to evaluate the presence of dilated epididymal tubules and the possibility of surgical recanalization (tubulovasostomy) to be performed at the same time;
- Using the "window" technique, i.e., performing a very small longitudinal or transversal incision of the scrotum.

In both cases the surgical steps are: opening the tunica vaginalis, performing a transverse albugineotomy of about 5 to 10 mm, forcing out and excising a small quantity of testicular tissue, controlling hemostasis (bleeding mainly comes from the subalbugineal tiny vessels), closing the albugineotomy, the tunica vaginalis, the dartos, and the skin.

Avoiding touching the testis surface with gauze and infusing 1.5 mg of betamethasone solution inside the vaginal cavity, while ending its reconstruction, prevents adhesions with the albuginea from forming, making repetition of the procedure or subsequent surgical recanalization easier.

Biological preparation of the removed tissue is the same as for MicroTESE (see Microdissection of Testicular Tissue).

Results

The retrieval of testicular spermatozoa in cases of NOA is significantly better—quantitatively and qualitatively—with TESE than with TeFNA (37,38). TESE is the recommended procedure to retrieve spermatozoa in NOA patients (39), yielding sperm for ICSI in 49.5% (40), and in 52.2% compared to 23.0% by TeFNA (38) (see also Table 1). In these patients a high sperm recovery rate is achieved even when repeating TESE (41). Multiple TESE would appear to improve the success rate compared to single TESE (52.5%) [review by Colpi et al. (27)].

Table 1 Successful Sperm Retrieval by Single TESE in NOA Patients from Literature

References	No. of TESE	Sperm +	%Success
42	29	14	48.2
43	30	21	70
44	16	10	62
45	37	16	43
46	64	49	77
47	81	23	28
30	35	22	63
48	250	157	62.8
49	216	71	37.5
50	55	33	60
51	81	47	58
52	26	12	46.2
53	44	32	72.7
54	83	32	39
55	23	15	65.2
56	12	5	41.6
57	107	53	49.5
41	784	384	49.0
58	40	21	52.5
Total	2013	1017	50.5

Complications

The very rare complications of TESE are those common to any small surgical procedure: infection and bleeding with scrotal hematomas that rarely require surgical drainage. In cases of NOA patients with very small testes, testosterone deficiency following surgery must be considered (59,60).

MICRODISSECTION OF TESTICULAR TISSUE

Introduction and Indications

In an effort to increase the chances of finding islands of spermatogenesis in sampled tissue, Schlegel (46) devised microdissection of testicular tissue (MicroTESE). This technique, involving book-like opening of the testis followed by a careful search for suitable tubules using an operating microscope, allows the surgeon to recover sperms in some "difficult" cases of NOA.

Technique

MicroTESE (46) involves "bivalve" opening of the testicle by means of an equatorial or longitudinal incision under general or spinal anesthesia and removal of single tubules observed to have the largest diameter under an operating microscope or, in the absence of larger tubules, of those closest to vessels and at different depths in the pulp (testicular mapping) (27).

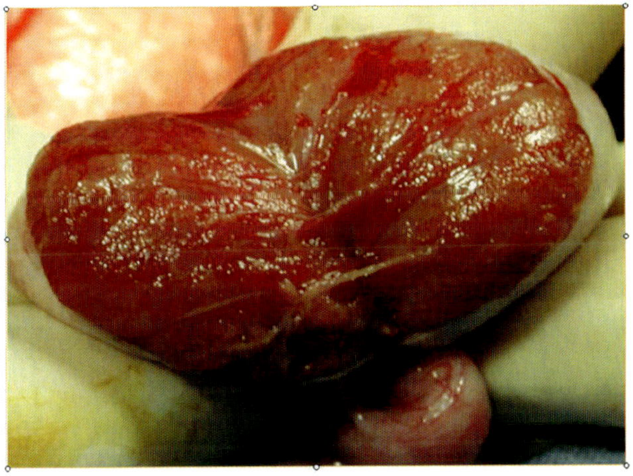

Figure 1 MicroTESE: Bivalve transversal opening of the testis, obtained by careful and gentle separation of the lobules by means of a spatula. The exposed surfaces of the testicular pulp are then observed at 18× to 24× optical magnification. See also color insert.

The surgical steps are as follows:

1. An equatorial incision is performed under general anesthesia along three-fourths of the circumference. A relatively avascular albugineal line is selected for this purpose. Microcoagulation of the few bleeding subalbugineal vessels is performed by a bipolar thermal device.
2. Testicular lobules are carefully separated (Fig. 1). Individual seminiferous tubules are then extracted from either side. About 30 testicular draws are usually obtained from each testis. Microdissection is performed with 18× to 24× optical magnification.
3. At the end, testicular pulp is gently compressed by gauze for 2′ to ensure hemostasis. The tunica albuginea is then closed with a Vicryl 5-0 continuous suture, followed by closure of the tunica vaginalis and infusion of a corticosteroid solution inside its cavity, and by dartos skin closing.

The fragments of testicular tissue (TESE) or extracted tubules (MicroTESE) are put into a Petri dish, in 2 mL HTF medium. Careful fragmentation of the tubules by tiny scissors is performed, and the fluid is passed through a 24-G angiocatheter several times, until a cloudy suspension is obtained. At the end, the fluid is microscopically examined to detect spermatozoa and other germ cells.

Results

MicroTESE may increase positive retrievals in NOA subjects (54–63.4%) (28,46,65), and a previous failure with TESE does not exclude a successful MicroTESE (61). In fact, successful MicroTESE retrievals were reported even in the worst histological conditions, such as Sertoli cell-only syndrome (SCOS) (28,62). Compared with TESE, MicroTESE was reported to achieve higher success rates (54.6% versus 35.7% in a meta-analysis (38); see also Table 2) and had significantly more effective results in patients with high follicle stimulating hormone (FSH) levels (62,63); therefore, at least in these patients, MicroTESE should be the preferred choice.

Complications

With MicroTESE, less testicular tissue is removed (46), thus greatly reducing the risk of endocrine deprivation (69,70). Moreover, there appear to be significantly fewer vascular complications than with TESE (71); at six-month ultrasound follow-up no parenchymal or vascularization abnormalities were reported (27).

PREDICTIVE FACTORS OF SPERM RETRIEVAL IN NONOBSTRUCTIVE AZOOSPERMIA

The only good predictor of successful retrieval is testicular histology (72), which is unfortunately the least useful predictor for clinicians, since the histological sample is usually obtained at the same time as TESE.

No clear relation was found between successful sperm retrieval and serum FSH levels or serum inhibin-B levels or testicular volume (73); seminal plasma inhibin-B was reported as an independent predictor of a positive TESE (74). Even formulas to calculate the predictivity rates with these data, crossed with other clinical (age, duration of fertility) and hormonal

Table 2 Successful retrievals with TESE Vs. MicroTESE

References	No. of TESE	Sperm +	%Success	MicroTESE	Sperm +	%Success
46	10	22	45	17	27	63
64	30	100	30	47	100	47
65	9	22	40.9	14	22	63.6
66	4	17	24	8	17	48
67	4	24	16.7	33	74	44.6
68	13	37	35.1	24	56	42.9
69	26	83	32	262	460	57
62: only SCOS	5	40	12.5	11	40	27.5
62: other histology	24	29	82.7	25	29	86.2

(LH, testosterone, prolactin) parameters turned out unhelpful. In fact, a very high FSH value and a very low testicular volume do not completely exclude the possibility of successful retrieval of testicular spermatozoa (62).

Case Report 2

A 42-year-old Caucasian man who at the age of nine underwent orchiopexy for bilateral cryptorchidism. He had left orchidectomy at the age of 11 due to testicular atrophy. Has been trying to have children for two years: all semen analyses showed normal semen volume and pH, but azoospermia. Genetic investigations were normal. Scrotal color Doppler ultrasound: Testis of 5.5 mL volume, with a homogeneously hypoechoic pattern and poor vascularization. Serum FSH higher than 6.5 times the maximum normal range value. Owing to the very poor prognosis for retrieval, the patient underwent MicroTESE and testicular biopsy. Sperm retrieval was successful (75 sperms/mm^3 in the fluid after tubular fragmentation). Histology showed severe hypospermatogenesis (mean: 4 mature spermatids per tubule).

Conclusions: Not even a small testicular volume coupled with a very high serum FSH level can exclude an outright successful sperm retrieval. In the worst prognosis cases, MicroTESE should be the choice.

Finally, in patients with AZFa and AZFb microdeletions, no spermatozoa can be retrieved (75).

ICSI RESULTS IN CASES OF AZOOSPERMIA

ICSI results from surgically retrieved spermatozoa are significantly worse in cases of NOA compared to OA (76). The fertilization rate is 57.0% versus 80.5% (77), and the birth rate is 19% versus 28% (78) with a higher miscarriage rate (11.5% versus 2.5%) (79). A meta-analysis confirmed these data (80).

In an extensive study on NOA and OA couples, Vernaeve et al. (81) reported that multiple birth rates were respectively 21% versus 27%, overall preterm delivery rates were 38% versus 26%, and prematurity rates were 24% versus 13% for singletons and 86% versus 54% for twins (relative risk, 1.59; 95% confidence interval, 1.04–2.42); early perinatal mortality rate was 6.6% versus 1.5%, major birth defects were observed in 4% versus 3% of liveborn babies; prenatal karyotypes showed 7% de-novo abnormalities in the NOA group versus 1% in the OA group; however, the differences were not statistically significant.

Literature does not currently show any significant differences in ICSI results from fresh compared to frozen–thawed spermatozoa (78,82–84), though conflicting results have also been reported (85).

A meta-analysis (80) carried out on 17 heterogeneous, uncontrolled, retrospective studies did not show any statistically significant differences between frozen–thawed versus fresh spermatozoa from TESE with respect to fertilization rate and evolutive pregnancy rate, while implantation rate and clinical pregnancy rate from fresh spermatozoa were significantly higher.

In cases of NOA, spermatozoa for cryopreservation should precautionarily be retrieved with TESE/MicroTESE, to avoid the risk of unnecessary ovarian stimulation in case of unsuccessful sperm retrieval. This should be considered especially in countries where heterologous insemination is illegal. However, diagnostic testicular biopsy and a TESE/MicroTESE procedure with cryopreservation should be performed at the same time (86).

In OA patients, ICSI results from testicular or epididymal spermatozoa do not show any significant differences (80,82,87).

To date, there is insufficient evidence to recommend any specific sperm retrieval technique for azoospermic men undergoing ICSI. Therefore, the least invasive technique that can guarantee the highest successful sperm retrieval rate must be used in azoospermic patients (88): specifically, TESE or MicroTESE for cases of NOA, and TeFNA, TESE, or MESA for OA. MESA and TESE have become the most popular sperm retrieval techniques over the years. If these techniques are performed together with cryopreservation of extracted spermatozoa, a single surgical intervention can provide spermatozoa for several ICSI attempts (89).

CONCLUSIONS: THE THERAPEUTIC APPROACH IN AZOOSPERMIA

Sometimes, differential diagnosis between OA and NOA may still remain unclear despite careful clinical history and examination, even coupled with noninvasive diagnostic investigations (hormones, genital sonographies, etc.) (90). In this case, testicular biopsy and scrotal exploration are useful and should be performed at the same time as TESE, cryopreserving retrieved sperm to avoid unnecessary repetition of surgery.

Only when reconstructive surgery is unfeasible in some OA patients (i.e., bilateral vas agenesis) should TeFNA (timed at pick-up for ICSI) be resorted to, anticipating the possibility of performing also TESE (and possibly MESA) in the rare case of unsuccessful retrieval due to technical problems, or TESE in the very rare case of concomitant spermatogenic damage. MESA provides best sperm retrieval quantitatively and qualitatively and allows cryopreservation (which is almost always impossible with TeFNA), thus avoiding repetition of the procedure in subsequent ICSI cycles. In OA cases where microsurgical tubulovasostomy or vaso-vasostomy cannot be excluded, precautionary TESE, just for cryopreservation (which is useful in case of failure of reconstructive surgery), should be performed at the same time as reconstructive microsurgery; in fact, TeFNA, PESA, and MESA may damage the epididymis and jeopardize the recanalization outcome.

On the contrary, in NOA cases resorting to TESE (or MicroTESE, especially in cases with a more unfavorable retrieval prognosis) for cryopreservation is mandatory, before beginning ovarian stimulation of the partner for ICSI procedure.

Figure 2 summarizes a flowchart for treating azoospermia.

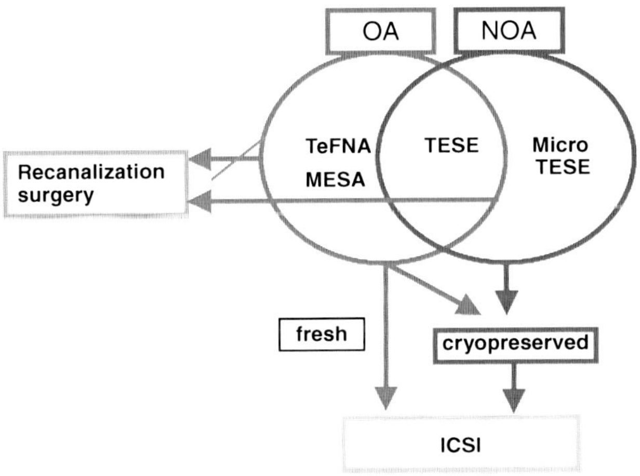

Figure 2 A flowchart for treatment of azoospermia.

Recommendations

A testis biopsy aimed to differentiate OA from NOA is indicated only in azoospermic patients with normal orchidometry and normal FSH (grade B recommendation).

In OA due to epididymal obstruction (CBAVD excluded), MESA and/or TESE and sperm cryopreservation should be carried out together with a microsurgical seminal tract recanalization (grade B recommendation).

In NOA, TESE (either single, multiple, or microsurgical) should be used rather than TeFNA, due to their quite different chances of successful sperm retrieval.

In NOA with very high FSH, microsurgical TESE should be preferred (grade A recommendation).

In NOA, sperm cryopreservation should follow any successful TESE procedure (grade B recommendation).

REFERENCES

1. Temple-Smith PD, Southwick GJ, Yates CA, et al. Human pregnancy by in vitro fertilization (IVF) using sperm aspirated from the epididymis. J In Vitro Fertil Embryo Transfer 1985; 2:119–122.
2. Belker AM and the Sperm Microaspiration Retrieval Techniques Study Group. Results in the United States with sperm microaspiration retrieval techniques and assisted reproductive technologies. J Urol 1994; 151(5):1255–1259.
3. Goldstein M, Tanrikut C. Microsurgical management of male infertility. Nat Clin Pract Urol 2006; 3(7):381–391.
4. Tournaye H, Devroey P, Liu J, et al. Microsurgical epididymal sperm aspiration and intracytoplasmic sperm injection: a new effective approach to infertility as a result of congenital bilateral absence of the vas deferens. Fertil Steril 1994; 61(6):1045–1051.
5. Hovatta O, Moilanen J, von Smitten K, et al. Testicular needle biopsy, open biopsy, epididymal aspiration and intracytoplasmatic sperm injection in obstructive azoospermia. Hum Reprod 1995; 10(10):2595–2599.
6. Silber SJ, Ord T, Balmaceda J, et al. Congenital absence of the vas deferens. The fertilizing capacity of human epididymal sperm. N Engl J Med 1990; 323(26):1788–1792.
7. Nudell DM, Conaghan J, Pedersen RA, et al. The mini-micro-epididymal sperm aspiration for sperm retrieval: a study of urological outcomes. Hum Reprod 1998; 13(5):1260–1265.
8. Pasqualotto FF, Rossi LM, Guilherme P, et al. Etiology-specific outcomes of intracytoplasmic sperm injection in azoospermic patients. Fertil Steril 2005; 83(3):606–611.
9. Cayan S, Lee D, Conaghan J, et al. A comparison of ICSI outcomes with fresh and cryopreserved epididymal spermatozoa from the same couples. Hum Reprod 2001; 16(3):495–499.
10. Tournaye H, Merdad T, Silber S, et al. No differences in outcome after intracytoplasmic sperm injection with fresh or with frozen-thawed epididymal spermatozoa. Hum Reprod 1999; 14(1):90–95.
11. Craft I, Tsirigotis M, Bennett V, et al. Percutaneous epididymal sperm aspiration and intracytoplasmic sperm injection in the management of infertility due to obstructive azoospermia. Fertil Steril 1995; 63(5):1038–1042.
12. Meniru GI, Gorgy A, Batha S, et al. Studies of percutaneous epididymal sperm aspiration (PESA) and intracytoplasmic sperm injection. Hum Reprod Update 1998; 4(1):57–71.
13. Goldstein M. Surgical management of male infertility and other scrotal disorders. In: Walsh PC et al, eds. Campbell's Urology, (8th ed). Philadelphia, PA: WB Saunders, 2002:1533–1587.
14. Levine LA, Lisek EW. Successful sperm retrieval by percutaneous epididymal and testicular sperm aspiration. J Urol 1998; 159(2):437–440.
15. Pasqualotto FF, Rossi-Ferragut LM, Rocha CC, et al. The efficacy of repeat percutaneous epididymal sperm aspiration procedures. J Urol 2003; 169(5):1779–1781.
16. Brindley GS, Scott GI, Hendry WF. Vas cannulation with implanted sperm reservoirs for obstructive azoospermia or ejaculatory failure. Br J Urol 1986; 58(6):721–723.
17. Belker AM, Jimenez-Cruz DJ, Kelâmi A, et al. Alloplastic spermatocele: poor sperm motility in intraoperative epididymal fluid contraindicates prosthesis implantation. J Urol 1986; 136(2):408–409.
18. Schoysman R, Segal L, Van der Zwalmen P, et al. Assisted fertilization with epididymal spermatozoa. Acta Eur Fertil 1993; 24(1):7–12.
19. Colpi GM, Negri L, Stamm J, et al. Full-term pregnancy obtained with sperm recovered by seminal tract washout from an anejaculating, spinal cord injury man. J Urol 1992; 148(4):1266–1267.
20. Hirsh AV, Mills C, Tan SL, et al. Pregnancy using spermatozoa aspirated from the vas deferens in a patient with

ejaculatory failure due to spinal injury. Hum Reprod 1993; 8(1):89–90.

21. Hovatta O, von Smitten K. Sperm aspiration from vas deferens and in-vitro fertilization in cases of non-treatable anejaculation. Hum Reprod 1993; 8(10):1689–1691.
22. Colpi GM, Negri L, Grugnetti C, et al. Seminal tract washout: a new tool for assisted conception. In: Colpi GM, Balerna M, eds. Treating Male Infertility, Basel: Karger, 1994: 225–232.
23. Levine LA, Fakouri BJ. Experience with vasal sperm aspiration. J Urol 1998; 159(5):1551–1553.
24. Tournaye H, Clase K, Aytoz A, et al. Fine needle aspiration versus open biopsy for testicular sperm recovery: a controlled study in azoospermic patients with normal spermatogenesis. Hum Reprod 1998; 13:901–904.
25. Bourne H, Watkins W, Speirs A, et al. Pregnancy after intracytoplasmic sperm injection of sperm collected by fine needle biopsy of the testis. Fertil Steril 1995; 64:433–436.
26. Sereni E, Bonu MA, Fava L, et al. Freezing spermatozoa obtained by testicular fine needle aspiration: a new technique. Reprod Biomed Online 2008; 16(1):89–95.
27. Colpi GM, Piediferro G, Nerva F, et al. Sperm retrieval for intra-cytoplasmic sperm injection in non-obstructive azoospermia. Min Urol Nefrol 2005; 57:99–107.
28. El-Haggar S, Mostafa T, Abdel Nasser T, et al. Fine needle aspiration vs. mTESE in non-obstructive azoospermia. Int J Androl 2008; 31(6):595–601.
29. Aridogan IA, Bayazit Y, Yaman M, et al. Comparison of fine-needle aspiration and open biopsy of testis in sperm retrieval and histopathologic diagnosis. Andrologia 2003; 35:121–125.
30. Ezeh UI, Moore HD, Cooke ID. A prospective study of multiple needle biopsies versus a single open biopsy for testicular sperm extraction in men with non-obstructive azoospermia. Hum Reprod 1998; 13:3075–3080.
31. Bergmann M. Evaluation of testicular biopsy samples from the clinical perspective. In: Schill WB, Comhaire FH, Hargreave TB, eds. Andrology for the Clinician, Berlin, Heidelberg: Springer-Verlag, 2006:454–461.
32. Piediferro G, Contalbi G, Nerva F, et al. Carcinoma in situ in azoospermia non-ostruttiva sfuggito alla TeFNA e diagnosticato con TESE: case report. Atti XXI Congr Naz Soc It Androl, Trieste, 23–26 settembre 2004, P52.
33. Shufaro Y, Prus D, Laufer N, et al. Impact of repeated fine needle aspiration (TEFNA) and testicular sperm extraction (TESE) on the microscopic morphology of the testis: an animal model. Human Reprod 2002; 17:1795–1799.
34. Silber SJ, Nagy Z, Liu J, et al. The use of epididymal and testicular spermatozoa for intracytoplasmic sperm injection: the genetic implications for male infertility. Hum Reprod 1995; 10:2031–2043.
35. Jezeh D, Knuth UA, Schulze W. Successful testicular sperm extraction (TESE) in spite of high serum follicle stimulating hormone and azoospermia: correlation between testicular morphology, TESE results, semen analysis and serum hormone values in 103 infertile men. Hum Reprod 1998; 13:1230–1234.
36. Prins GS, Dolgina R, Studney P, et al. Quality of cryopreserved testicular sperm in patients with obstructive and nonobstructive azoospermia. J Urol 1999; 161:1504–1506.
37. Hauser R, Yogev L, Paz G, et al. Comparison of efficacy of two techniques for testicular sperm retrieval in nonobstructive azoospermia: multifocal testicular sperm extraction versus multifocal testicular sperm aspiration. J Androl 2006; 27:28–33.
38. Yang J, Liu JH, Zou XF, et al. Sperm retrieval and the predictive parameter of non-obstructive azoospermia: a meta-analysis of literatures 1990 to 2008. Zhonghua Yi Xue Za Zhi 2008; 88(30):2131–2135.
39. Dohle GR, Jungwirth A, Colpi GM, et al. Guidelines on Male Infertility. European Association of Urology Guidelines, 2007.
40. Donoso P, Tournaye H, Devroey P. Which is the best sperm retrieval technique for non-obstructive azoospermia? A systematic review. Hum Reprod Update 2007; 13(6):539–549.
41. Vernaeve V, Verheyen G, Goossens A, et al. How successful is repeat testicular sperm extraction in patients with azoospermia? Hum Reprod 2006; 21:1551–1554.
42. Kahraman S, Ozgur S, Alatas C, et al. Fertility with testicular sperm extraction and intracytoplasmic sperm injection in non-obstructive azoospermic men. Hum Reprod 1996; 11:765–760.
43. Mulhall JP, Burgess CM, Cunningham D, et al. Presence of mature sperm in testicular parenchyma of men with nonobstructive azoospermia: prevalence and predictive factors. Urology 1997; 49:91–95.
44. Schlegel PN, Palermo GD, Goldstein M, et al. Testicular sperm extraction with intracytoplasmic sperm injection for nonobstructive azoospermia. Urology 1997; 49:435–440.
45. Friedler S, Raziel A, Strassburger D, et al. Testicular sperm retrieval by percutaneous fine needle sperm aspiration compared with testicular sperm extraction by open biopsy in men with non-obstructive azoospermia. Hum Reprod 1997; 12:1488–1493.
46. Jezek D, Knuth UA, Schulze W. Successful testicular sperm extraction (TESE) in spite of high serum follicle stimulating hormone and azoospermia: correlation between testicular morphology, TESE results, semen analysis and serum hormone values in 103 infertile men. Hum Reprod 1998; 13:1230–1234.
47. Ostad M, Liotta D, Ye Z, et al. Testicular sperm extraction for nonobstructive azoospermia: results of a multibiopsy approach with optimized tissue dispersion. Urology 1998; 52:692–696.
48. Schulze W, Thoms F, Knuth UA. Testicular sperm extraction: comprehensive analysis with simultaneously

performed histology in 1418 biopsies from 766 subfertile men. Hum Reprod 1999; 14:82–96.
49. Amer M, Haggar SE, Moustafa T, et al. Testicular sperm extraction: impact to testicular histology on outcome, number of biopsies to be performed and optional time for repetition. Hum Reprod 1999; 14:3030–3034.
50. Ben Yosef D, Yogev L, Hauser R, et al. Testicular sperm retrieval and cryopreservation prior to initiating ovarian stimulation as the first line approach in patients with non-obstructive azoospermia. Hum Reprod 1999; 14:1794–1801.
51. Su LM, Palermo GD, Goldstein M, et al. Testicular sperm extraction with intracytoplasmic sperm injection for non-obstructive azoospermia: testicular histology can predict success of sperm retrieval. J Urol 1999; 161:112–116.
52. Ng HY, Lau YL, Yeung SB, et al. Testicular sperm extraction and intracytoplasmic sperm injection in non-obstructive azoospermia. Chin Med J (Engl) 2000; 113:246–250.
53. Kitamura M, Nishimura K, Miura H, et al. Predictor factor for TESE-ICSI for nonobstructive azoospermia. Nippon Hinyokika Gakkai Zasshi 2000; 91:589–594.
54. Friedler S, Raziel A, Schachter M, et al. Outcome of first and repeated testicular sperm extraction and ICSI in patients with non-obstructive azoospermia. Hum Reprod 2002; 17:2356–2361.
55. Damani MN, Master V, Meng MV, et al. Postchemotherapy ejaculatory azoospermia: fatherhood with sperm from testis tissue with intracytoplasmic sperm injection. J Clin Oncol 2002; 15:930–936.
56. Meseguer M, Garrido N, Remohi J, et al. Testicular sperm extraction (TESE) and ICSI in patients with permanent azoospermia after chemotherapy. Hum Reprod 2003; 18:1281–1285.
57. Negri L, Albani E, Di Rocco M, et al. Testicular sperm extraction in azoospermic men submitted to bilateral orchipexy. Hum Reprod 2003; 18: 2534–2539.
58. Mostafa T, Amer MK, Abdel-Malak G, et al. Seminal plasma anti-Müllerian hormone level correlates with semen parameters but does not predict success of testicular sperm extraction (TESE). Asian J Androl 2007; 9(2):265–270.
59. Pantke P, Diemer T, Marconi M, et al. Testicular sperm retrieval in azoospermic men. Eur Urol 2008; S7:703–714.
60. Takada S, Tsujimura A, Ueda T, et al. Androgen decline in patients with nonobstructive azoospemia after microdissection testicular sperm extraction. Urology 2008; 72(1):114–118.
61. Ramasamy R, Schlegel PN. Microdissection testicular sperm extraction: effect of prior biopsy on success of sperm retrieval. J Urol 2007; 177(4):1447–1449.
62. Colpi GM, Colpi EM, Piediferro G, et al. Microsurgical TESE versus conventional TESE for ICSI in non-obstructive azoospermia: a randomized controlled study. Reprod Biomed Online 2009; 18(3):315–319.
63. Ramasamy R, Lin K, Gosden LV, et al. High serum FSH levels in men with nonobstructive azoospermia does not affect success of microdissection testicular sperm extraction. Fertil Steril 2009; 92(2):590–593.
64. Amer M, Ateyah A, Hany R, et al. Prospective comparative study between microsurgical and conventional testicular sperm extraction in non-obstructive azoospermia: follow-up by serial ultrasound examinations. Hum Reprod 2000; 15, 653–656.
65. Colpi GM, Piediferro G, Nerva F, et al. TESE microchirurgica nelle azoospermie non ostruttive. Giorn It Andr 2001; 8:133.
66. Okubo K, Ogura K, Ichioka K, et al. Testicular sperm extraction for non-obstructive azoospermia: results with conventional and microsurgical techniques. Hinyokika Kiyo 2002; 48, 275–280.
67. Okada H, Dobashi M, Yamazaki T, et al. Conventional versus microdissection testicular sperm extraction for non-obstructive azoospermia. J Urol 2002; 168, 1063–1067.
68. Tsujimura A, Matsumiya K, Miyagawa Y, et al. Conventional multiple or microdissection testicular sperm extraction: a comparative study. Hum Reprod 2002; 17, 2924–2929.
69. Ramasamy R, Yagan N, Schlegel PN. Structural and functional changes to the testis after conventional versus microdissection testicular sperm extraction. Urology 2005; 65:1190–1194.
70. Ishikawa T, Yamaguchi K, Chiba K, et al. Serum hormones in patients with nonobstructive azoospermia after microdissection testicular sperm extraction. J Urol 2009; 182(4):1495–1499.
71. Dardashti K, Williams RH, Goldstein M. Microsurgical testis biopsy: a novel model technique for retrieval of testicular tissue. J Urol 2000; 163:1206–1207.
72. Tournaye H, Liu J, Nagy PZ, et al. Correlation between testicular histology and outcome after intracytoplasmic sperm injection using testicular spermatozoa. Hum Reprod 1996; 11(1):127–132.
73. Seo JT, Ko WJ. Predictive factors of successful testicular sperm recovery in non-obstructive azoospermia patients. Int J Androl 2001; 38:306–310.
74. Nagata Y, Fujita K, Banzai J, et al. Seminal plasma inhibin-B level is a useful predictor of the success of conventional testicular sperm extraction in patients with non-obstructive azoospermia. J Obstet Gynaecol Res 2005; 31(5):384–388.
75. Hopps CV, Mielnik A, Goldstein M, et al. Detection of sperm in men with Y chromosome microdeletions of the AZFa, AZFb, and AZFc regions. Hum Reprod 2003; 18:1660–1665.
76. Vernaeve V, Tournaye H, Osmanagaoglu K, et al. Intracytoplasmic sperm injection with testicular spermatozoa is less successful in men with nonobstructive azoospermia than in men with obstructive azoospermia. Fertil Steril 2003; 79:529–533.

77. Palermo GD, Schlegel PN, Hariprashad JJ, et al. Fertilization and pregnancy outcome with intracytoplasmic sperm injection for azoospermic men. Hum Reprod 1999; 14:741–748.
78. Sousa M, Cremades N, Silva J, et al. Predictive value of testicular histology in secretory azoospermic subgroups and clinical outcome after microinjection of fresh and frozen-thawed sperm and spermatids. Hum Reprod 2002; 17:1800–1810.
79. Borges E Jr, Rossi-Ferragut LM, Pasqualotto FF, et al. Testicular sperm results in elevated miscarriage rates compared to epididymal sperm in azoospermic patients. Sao Paolo Med J 2002; 120:122–126.
80. Nicopullos JD, Gilling-Smith C, Almeida PA, et al. Use of surgical sperm retrieval in azoospermic men: a meta-analysis. Fertil Steril 2004; 82:691–701.
81. Vernaeve V, Bonduelle M, Tournaye H, et al. Pregnancy outcome and neonatal data of children born after ICSI using testicular sperm in obstructive and non-obstructive azoospermia. Hum Reprod 2003; 18:2093–2097.
82. Gil Salom M. Spermatic recovery techniques for intracytoplasmic spermatozoid injection (ICSI) in male infertility. Arch Esp Urol 2004; 57:1035–1046.
83. Schwarzer JU, Fiedler K, Hertwig I, et al. Sperm retrieval procedures and intracytoplasmatic spermatozoa injection with epididymal and testicular sperms. Urol Int 2003; 70:119–123.
84. Verheyen G, Vernaeve V, Van Landuyt L, et al. Should diagnostic testicular sperm retrieval followed by cryopreservation for later ICSI be the procedure of choice for all patients with non-obstructive azoospermia? Hum Reprod 2004; 19:2822–2830.
85. Wald M, Ross LS, Prins GS, et al. Analysis of outcomes of cryopreserved surgically retrieved sperm for IVF/ICSI. J Androl 2006; 27:60–65.
86. Weidner W, Colpi GM, Hargreave TB, et al. The EAU Working Group on Male Infertility. EAU guidelines on male infertility. Eur Urol 2002; 42:313–322.
87. Moghadam KK, Nett R, Robins JC, et al. The motility of epididymal or testicular spermatozoa does not directly affect IVF/ICSI pregnancy outcomes. J Androl 2005; 26:619–623.
88. Van Peperstraten A, Proctor ML, Johnson NP, et al. Techniques for surgical retrieval of sperm prior to ICSI for azoospermia. Cochrane Database Syst Rev 2006; 3:CD002807.
89. Diemer T, Schroeder-Printzen I, Weidner W. Surgical sperm retrieval. Urologe A 2007; 46:789–798.
90. Colpi GM, Negri L, Benaglia R, et al. Only a full diagnostic surgery allows a correct classification of azoospermic men entering a TESE-ICSI programme. Hum Reprod 2000; 15(suppl 1):245.

0.5 mm. The vasal veins usually are preserved to provide venous return; however, if greater than 3 mm in diameter, they are dissected free of the vasal artery and ligated. The vas deferens is always accompanied by two sets of vessels. As long as at least one set of vasal veins remains intact, venous return will be adequate. At the completion of the dissection, the cord is run over the index finger and inspected to verify that all veins have been identified and ligated. Only the testicular artery, lymphatics, and vas deferens with its vessels should be intact [Fig. 3(J)].

Delivery of the testis into the operative field enables visual inspection of all possible avenues of testicular venous drainage. Delivery of only the cord allows access to most external spermatic collaterals but may miss those close to the testis. In addition, only delivery of the testis will reveal scrotal or gubernacular collaterals, which have been demonstrated radiographically to be the cause of 10% of recurrent varicoceles (48). The testis is delivered with gentle upward traction on the cord and upward pressure on the testis through the invaginated scrotum. All external spermatic veins are divided with hemoclips. All gubernacular veins are cauterized or divided with hemoclips [Fig. 3(K)].

After adequate hemostasis is achieved, the testis and the spermatic cord are returned to their native positions. The external oblique aponeurosis, if opened, is reapproximated with continuous suturing using the previously placed 3–0 suture. Scarpa's and Camper's fascia are closed with a few interrupted monofilament absorbable stitches of 3–0 and 4–0, respectively. The skin is reapproximated with a 5–0 monofilament absorbable subcuticular suture reinforced by two to three Steri-Strips [Fig. 3(L)]. A scrotal supporter is applied and stuffed with fluff-type dressings. The patient is discharged the same day with a prescription for dihydrocodeinone with paracetamol. Light work may be resumed in two or three days.

Laparoscopic Approach

Laparoscopy varicocelectomies have been performed since the late 1980s (49). Laparoscopic varicocele ligation is essentially

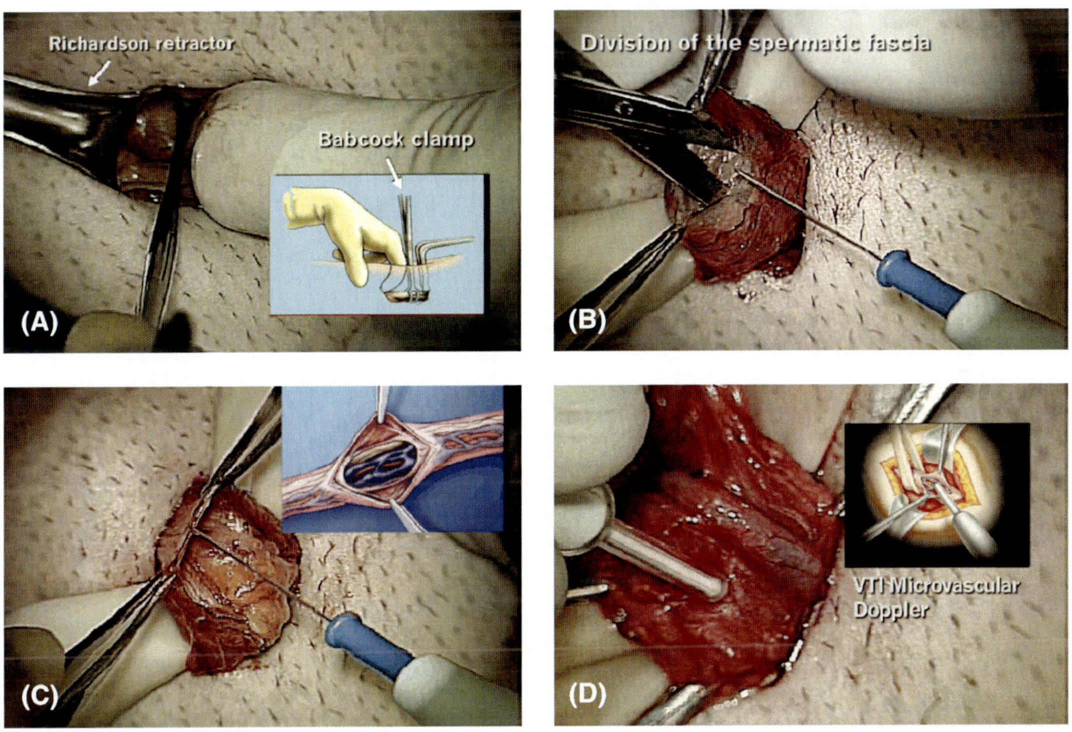

Figure 3 Microsurgical inguinal/subinguinal varicocelectomy. (**A**) An index finger and small Richardson retractor are used to expose the spermatic cord, which is grasped with a Babcock clamp. (**B**) A Penrose drain is placed around the spermatic cord (**C**). The external and internal spermatic fasciae are opened. (**D**) A micro-Doppler probe aids in the identification of the testicular artery(ies). (**E**) A vessel loop is placed around the testicular artery. (**F**) The confirmation test to distinguish an artery from a vein. (**G**) An example of lymphatics. (**H**) One black and one white silk suture ligatures are used to ligate veins near the artery. (**I**) Surgical clips are used to ligate veins a safe distance away from the artery. (**J**) A diagram depicting complete internal spermatic vein ligation, with sparing of the testicular artery and lymphatics (and nerves). (**K**) A diagram of possible collateral drainage via external spermatic and gubernacular veins. (**L**) Completed skin closure with Steri-Strip reinforcement. *Source: Courtesy of Marc Goldstein, M.D., and Philip S. Li, M.D.*

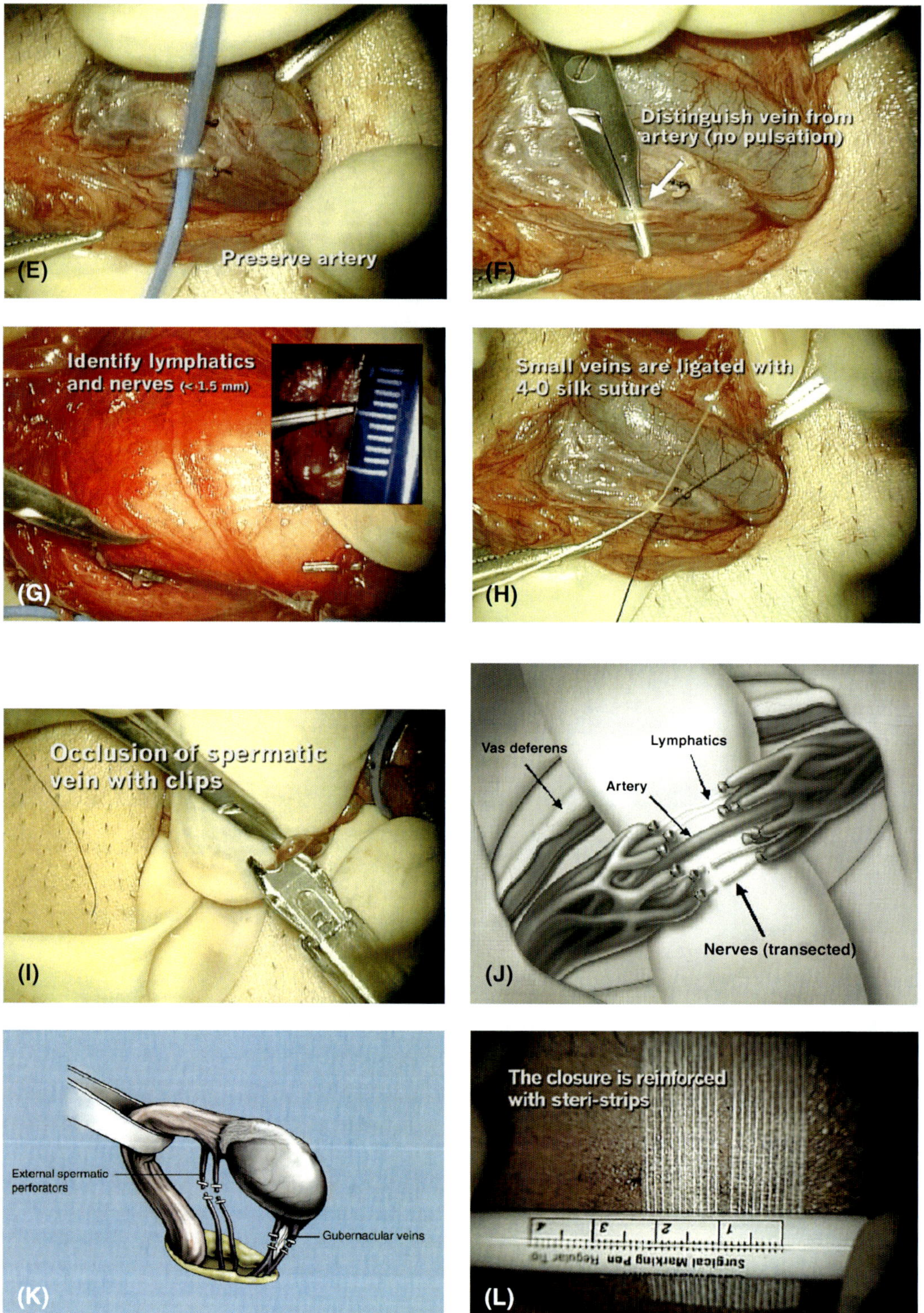

Figure 3 *(Continued).*

63. Tauber R, Johnsen N. Antegrade scrotal sclerotherapy for the treatment of varicocele: technique and late results. J Urol 1994; 151(2):386–390.
64. Ferguson JM, Gillespie IN, Chalmers N, et al. Percutaneous varicocele embolization in the treatment of infertility. Br J Radiol 1995; 68(811):700–703.
65. Morag B, Rubinstein ZJ, Goldwasser B, et al. Percutaneous venography and occlusion in the management of spermatic varicoceles. AJR Am J Roentgenol 1984; 143(3):635–640.
66. Matthews RD, Roberts J, Walker WA, et al. Migration of intravascular balloon after percutaneous embolotherapy of varicocele. Urology 1992; 39(4):373–375.
67. Verhagen P, Blom JM, van Rijk PP, et al. Pulmonary embolism after percutaneous embolization of left spermatic vein. Eur J Radiol 1992; 15(3):190–192.
68. Lenz M, Hof N, Kersting-Sommerhoff B, et al. Anatomic variants of the spermatic vein: importance for percutaneous sclerotherapy of idiopathic varicocele. Radiology 1996; 198(2):425–431.
69. Zorgniotti AW, Sealfon AI. Scrotal hypothermia: new therapy for poor semen. Urology 1984; 23(5):439–441.
70. Zorgniotti AW, Cohen MS, Sealfon AI. Chronic scrotal hypothermia: results in 90 infertile couples. J Urol 1986; 135(5):944–947.
71. Misseri R, Gershbein AB, Horowitz M, et al. The adolescent varicocele. II: the incidence of hydrocele and delayed recurrent varicocele after varicocelectomy in a long-term follow-up. BJU Int 2001; 87(6):494–498.
72. Marmar JL, Kim Y. Subinguinal microsurgical varicocelectomy: a technical critique and statistical analysis of semen and pregnancy data. J Urol Oct 1994; 152(4):1127–1132.
73. Goldstein M, Gilbert BR, Dicker AP, et al. Microsurgical inguinal varicocelectomy with delivery of the testis: an artery and lymphatic sparing technique. J Urol 1992; 148(6):1808–1811.
74. Penn I, Mackie G, Halgrimson CG, et al. Testicular complications following renal transplantation. Ann Surg 1972; 176(6):697–699.
75. Madgar I, Weissenberg R, Lunenfeld B, et al. Controlled trial of high spermatic vein ligation for varicocele in infertile men. Fertil Steril 1995; 63(1):120–124.
76. O'Brien JH, Bowles B, Kamal KM, et al. Microsurgical varicocelectomy for infertile couples with advanced female age: natural history in the era of ART. J Androl 2004; 25(6):939–943.
77. Matthews GJ, Matthews ED, Goldstein M. Induction of spermatogenesis and achievement of pregnancy after microsurgical varicocelectomy in men with azoospermia and severe oligoasthenospermia. Fertil Steril 1998; 70(1):71–75.
78. Gat Y, Bachar GN, Everaert K, et al. Induction of spermatogenesis in azoospermic men after internal spermatic vein embolization for the treatment of varicocele. Hum Reprod 2005; 20(4):1013–1017.
79. Evers JL, Collins JA. Surgery or embolisation for varicocele in subfertile men. Cochrane Database Syst Rev 2004; (3): CD000479.
80. Ficarra V, Cerruto MA, Liguori G, et al. Treatment of varicocele in subfertile men: The Cochrane Review—a contrary opinion. Eur Urol 2006; 49(2):258–263.
81. Marmar JL, Agarwal A, Prabakaran S, et al. Reassessing the value of varicocelectomy as a treatment for male subfertility with a new meta-analysis. Fertil Steril 2007; 88(3):639–648.
82. Cook DJ, Sackett DL, Spitzer WO. Methodologic guidelines for systematic reviews of randomized control trials in health care from the Potsdam Consultation on Meta-Analysis. J Clin Epidemiol 1995; 48(1):167–171.
83. Gat Y, Gornish M, Belenky A, et al. Elevation of serum testosterone and free testosterone after embolization of the internal spermatic vein for the treatment of varicocele in infertile men. Hum Reprod 2004; 19(10):2303–2306.
84. Su LM, Goldstein M, Schlegel PN. The effect of varicocelectomy on serum testosterone levels in infertile men with varicoceles. J Urol 1995; 154(5):1752–1755.
85. Cozzolino DJ, Lipshultz LI. Varicocele as a progressive lesion: positive effect of varicocele repair. Hum Reprod Update 2001; 7(1):55–58.
86. Tanrikut C, Choi JM, Lee RK, et al. Varicocele is a risk factor for androgen deficiency. American Society for Reproductive Medicine 63rd Annual Meeting; Washington, D.C., 2007.
87. Tanrikut C, Choi JM, Rosoff JS, et al. Improvement in serum testosterone levels after varicocelectomy. American Society for Reproductive Medicine 63rd Annual Meeting; Washington, D.C., 2007.
88. Skoog SJ, Roberts KP, Goldstein M, et al. The adolescent varicocele: what's new with an old problem in young patients? Pediatrics 1997; 100(1):112–121.
89. Kass EJ, Belman AB. Reversal of testicular growth failure by varicocele ligation. J Urol 1987; 137(3):475–476.
90. Okuyama A, Nakamura M, Namiki M, et al. Surgical repair of varicocele at puberty: preventive treatment for fertility improvement. J Urol. 1988; 139(3):562–564.
91. Steeno O, Knops J, Declerck L, et al. Prevention of fertility disorders by detection and treatment of varicocele at school and college age. Andrologia 1976; 8(1):47–53.
92. Schiff J, Kelly C, Goldstein M, et al. Managing varicoceles in children: results with microsurgical varicocelectomy. BJU Int 2005; 95(3):399–402.

14 Assisted reproduction with surgically retrieved sperm

Valérie Vernaeve and Herman Tournaye

INTRODUCTION

Azoospermia, defined as the complete absence of spermatozoa in the ejaculate, in at least two semen samples after extended preparation including centrifugation (1,2), is the most common indication for surgical retrieval of sperm. Other indications are complete astheno and/or necrozoospermia and ejaculatory disorders.

Azoospermia is present in 1% of the general population and in 10% to 15% of infertile men (3). It is caused by genital tract obstruction, deficient spermatogenesis, or a hypogonadotrophic hypogonadism. The latter category is extremely rare and can be treated medically (2). Although not completely accurate, azoospermic patients are therefore often classified as either obstructive (OA) or nonobstructive (NOA).

In OA, complete spermatogenesis is found at histology (4), whereas in NOA, testicular histology may show maturation arrest with or without focal spermatogenesis, germ-cell aplasia (Sertoli cell-only syndrome or SCO) with or without focal spermatogenesis, or tubular sclerosis and atrophy. A newer classification of the histological pattern of testicular biopsies has been recently proposed: (*i*) normal testicular biopsy, (*ii*) hypospermatogenesis, (*iii*) germ cell arrest, (*iv*) SCO appearance, (*v*) seminiferous tubule hyalinization, (*vi*) carcinoma in situ, and (*vii*) immature testis (5).

To differentiate both types of azoospermia, clinical and endocrinological findings must be combined with the histopathology of the testes. The study by Matsumiya et al. illustrates this very well. This study on 102 men with azoospermia showed that 46% had a primary testicular failure with no evidence of obstruction at clinical work-up, 13% had a primary testicular failure because of 47,XXY Klinefelter's syndrome, 14% had OA azoospermia with evidence of obstruction and normal spermatogenesis at testicular biopsy. But 27% of men had no clinical signs of obstruction according to their work-up even including vasography; however, these men showed normal spermatogenesis and thus per definition had an obstruction (6). If no histology had been carried out, these men may have been wrongly classified as NOA. Therefore, the WHO advises performing a testicular biopsy in order to make an appropriate diagnosis in azoospermic men (7). The finding by Matsumiya et al. is an important issue, since it may explain differences in the retrieval rates after sperm extraction and even pregnancy rates among different studies in the literature.

RETRIEVING SPERM IN PATIENTS WITH OBSTRUCTIVE AZOOSPERMIA (OA)

Case: A couple is attending the fertility outpatient clinic. The wife is G0P0, 32 years old, has a normal hysterosalpingography and no other gynecologic pathology. Her husband is 45-years old man and has had a vasectomy three years ago after having three children from a previous relationship.

In this case, a reconstructive surgery (vasovasostomy) would be indicated, with simultaneous cryopreservation of sperm either obtained from the vas deferens or from a testicular biopsy to be used in case the reconstructive surgery would be unsuccessful.

If the wife would have a concomitant problem, for example, severe endometriosis, reconstructive surgery in the man would not be indicated and a simple surgical sperm retrieval for ICSI (intracytoplasmic sperm injection) should be performed.

In other cases of OA, when the cause or the site of suspected obstruction is unknown, a scrotal exploration is recommended. This procedure is of diagnostic value and offers an opportunity to perform reconstructive surgery such as vasovasostomy or epididymovasostomy (8). If reconstruction is not feasible, microsurgical epididymal sperm aspiration (MESA) can still be performed during the exploration and high numbers of retrieved epididymal spermatozoa can be frozen for later use.

Case: A woman (30 years old) and her husband, diagnosed with a congenital bilateral agenesis of the vas deferens (CBAVD), are referred for treatment.

Here, an IVF–ICSI cycle will be proposed right away, because a microsurgical reconstruction is not possible in this case.

In order to retrieve sperm, a percutaneous epididymal sperm aspiration (PESA) can be performed the day of the egg retrieval. This procedure is less invasive than MESA and can be repeatedly performed under local anesthesia (9). Theoretically, PESA may cause more epididymal damage and fibrosis than MESA, but this issue is not relevant where reconstruction is not possible. The quantity of spermatozoa recovered may be lower than with MESA, and at least 20% of attempts are unsuccessful and may require MESA or testicular sperm retrieval [(10); level of evidence 3].

In OA, the epididymis is the preferred site for sperm retrieval. Motile epididymal sperm shows very low levels of DNA damage and can be retrieved in sufficient numbers to ensure cryopreservation (11). There are no differences in the outcome after ICSI using either fresh or frozen-thawed epididymal spermatozoa

[(12); level of evidence 2b]. Testicular sperm can also be easily obtained with testicular fine-needle aspiration, with a high sperm retrieval rate (SRR) in men with normal spermatogenesis [(13); level of evidence 2a].

Nevertheless, even in cases of OA, testicular sperm extraction (TESE) may be preferred over FNA whenever cryopreservation is an option and motile epididymal sperm has not been obtained. If testicular aspiration is performed with a needle of a larger diameter, tissue cylinders may be obtained facilitating cryopreservation (14). Unfortunately, these alternative methods are less patient-friendly than fine-needle aspiration and require locoregional anesthesia.

SURGICAL METHODS FOR RETRIEVING SPERM IN PATIENTS WITH NON-OBSTRUCTIVE AZOOSPERMIA (NOA)

NOA results from a testicular failure. This problem affects 10% of infertile men and is diagnosed in 60% of azoospermic men (3,6). Etiologies for testicular failure include genetic disorders such as sexual chromosomal abnormalities, translocations and microdeletions of the Y chromosome, cryptorchidism, testicular torsion, and exposure to irradiation and gonadotoxins (3).

How to Predict Successful Sperm Retrieval?

Case: A couple attends the outpatient clinic; the wife is 33 years old and her husband aged 36. None of them had children before. The man has a suspicion of NOA [history of orchidopexy for cryptorchidism, testicular volume of 10 mL, follicle-stimulating hormone (FSH) of 26 IU/L], and he would like to know if you will be able to retrieve sperm in his particular case, as he is concerned about the side effects of the hormonal treatment his wife will need to undergo for an ICSI treatment.

Overall, according to large series on unselected patients with NOA, the TESE sperm retrieval rate will be approximately 50% [(15); level of evidence 3]. Testicular spermatozoa can be retrieved in NOA men despite the absence of ejaculated spermatozoa in their semen, because of the existence of isolated foci of active spermatogenesis.

An ICSI using testicular spermatozoa involves treatment for both partners, that is, the husband undergoes surgery for testicular sperm recovery and his wife undergoes ovarian stimulation and eventually oocyte retrieval. An unsuccessful sperm recovery procedure has thus important emotional and financial implications. Objective counseling based on predictive factors may offer realistic expectations for both the couple and the physician. Tournaye et al. investigated different potential predictive parameters, that is, the presence of at least one single spermatozoon in at least one preliminary semen analysis, the maximum testicular volume, serum FSH, and the presence of spermatozoa in the histology of a randomly taken testicular biopsy [(16); level of evidence 3]. It was found that none of these parameters could be used to predict the outcome of a TESE procedure in the NOA subgroup of patients. The findings from semen analysis turned out to be the weakest predictor, and the presence of spermatozoa in histology to be the only parameter that had a limited clinical value in predicting sperm recovery during TESE. The study performed by Ezeh et al. corroborated these findings and added that neither the age of the men nor the body mass index could be used to predict successful TESE (17). They also found that the presence of spermatids at testicular histopathology was the best predictor. Several other studies too corroborate these initial reports. The predictive value of serum inhibin B, a direct product of the Sertoli cells, has been investigated too [(18,19); level of evidence 3]. This hormone too failed, alone or in combination with serum FSH, to predict the retrieval of sperm by TESE in men with NOA. Brandell et al. investigated the predictive power of genetic markers (20). They reported on a limited series of patients, in which the presence of AZFb microdeletions of the Y chromosome indicated an unsuccessful TESE. Unfortunately, only approximately 5% of NOA patients show Yq microdeletions, mostly in the AZFc region.

Thus, we can inform this couple that with some of the currently available parameters, the probability for successful sperm retrieval may not be predicted accurately enough for an individual patient. The chance for retrieving sperm by TESE in this couple would be around 50%.

How to Perform a Sperm Retrieval in NOA Patients?

Case: A man with a NOA, because of a nonmosaic Klinefelter syndrome, needs sperm retrieval for ICSI. He would like to know how the procedure will be performed and what his chances are that spermatozoa will be recovered.

In the case of NOA (included in nonmosaic Klinefelter patients), sperm will be recovered in about half of the patients by open TESE [(15,21–23); level of evidence 3).

An ideal surgical technique would enable the retrieval of a sufficient amount of motile spermatozoa to inject all available oocytes and to cryopreserve the remainder in case if a further attempt is needed, and this with a minimal trauma to the testis. Nevertheless, none of the currently available techniques fulfills these criteria.

Three techniques are currently available for testicular sperm retrieval in NOA patients: fine needle aspiration (FNA), open testicular biopsy (TESE), and microdissection (MD) TESE.

FNA may limit the adverse effects of the sperm retrieval, including hematoma, inflammation and devascularization [(24–26); level of evidence 3). Different techniques have been described with variations in the needle diameter (18–21 gauge) and the number of testicular punctures. The main advantages of this technique are its simplicity, low cost, minimally invasive character, and that it produces less postoperative pain compared with TESE under local anesthesia (27). Initially, some studies showed that performing FNA in NOA patients may possibly increase the chance of finding a site of active spermatogenesis by reaching deeper testicular sites (9,28). However, other groups failed to corroborate these results. A controlled study by Friedler et al. shows that sperm retrieval by FNA is a less-efficient method than the open biopsy in NOA, with a SRR of

11% achieved by FNA versus 43% by TESE (29). Two other controlled studies also reported a significantly lower recovery rate by retrieval with multiple needle biopsies compared to open biopsies (27,30). Differences in the definition of NOA, that is, defined on a clinical basis only without histopathology, the subselection of patients or the inclusion of patients with hypospermatogenesis may account for these contradictory findings. An additional disadvantage is that frequently there are no supernumerary spermatozoa to cryopreserve because of the limited numbers being retrieved (29,31). Larger needle diameters and the use of a testicular gun biopsy have also been proposed (14), but these techniques are more painful and often require locoregional anesthesia.

Because open TESE yields a higher sperm recovery than FNA, it is currently the most frequently used technique in NOA men with a mean retrieval rate of around 50% according to review papers [(21,22); level of evidence 3]. In cases associated with cryptorchidism, a significantly higher retrieval rate than in unexplained NOA has been reported in two studies: 74% versus 58% (32), and 51.9% (95%CI: 40.9–62.6) versus 33.3% (95%CI: 27.0–39.7) (33), which could, however, be a consequence of the inclusion of patients with retractile testis rather than with cryptorchidism.

The most appropriate number of biopsies to be taken remains controversial. On the basis of the assumption that multifocal distribution of spermatogenesis throughout the entire testis is present in many patients with NOA, some authors advocate taking only a single biopsy to control the adverse effects on testicular function (34), as the removal of large samples of testicular tissue may lead in some cases to testicular atrophy (25). The absence of spermatozoa in one single testicular biopsy, however, does not preclude the presence of some spermatozoa in the rest of the testes (35). Therefore, multiple biopsies may be recommended for achieving high recovery rates (36,37).

The evidence provided by observational studies favors multiple biopsies. Hauser et al. showed that in approximately 46% of the NOA patients, spermatozoa could only be recovered by multiple biopsies [(38); level of evidence 2b]. A larger observational study including 316 NOA men and comparing single bilateral biospy with multiple biospy also showed that the multiple biopsy approach enabled a significantly higher SRR compared with single biopsy (49% vs. 37.5%) [(36); level of evidence 3].

Two descriptive studies compared SRR according to the location of the biopsy reporting contradictory results: Hauser et al. (38) found no advantage of any particular site of the testis after performing biopsies at the upper pole, midline, and proximal pole, whereas Witt et al. (39) concluded from a smaller series (20 testicles) that the midline portion of the testis ensured the highest SRR (level of evidence 3).

Microdissection (MD) TESE was developed to combine the advantages of a less-invasive approach with an open excisional biopsy, hence minimizing testicular trauma by identifying the zones of active spermatogenesis through optical magnification, and therefore facilitating the removal of smaller amount of testicular tissue [(40–42); level of evidence 3). Furthermore, the identification of avascular regions for the opening of the tunica albuginea could minimize the risk for vascular injury. The results of this technique, in terms of recovery and complication rate, are encouraging in cases where enlarged spermatozoa-containing tubules can be identified, that is, when a Sertoli cell-only pattern predominates throughout the testis (40,42,43). The largest study on MD reported the results of 684 procedures in 563 men achieving an SRR of 61% [(44); level of evidence 3]. However, it is not evident whether these techniques will improve recovery rates when enlarged tubules are not present, such as in cases with maturation arrest. Okada et al. (45) found a significantly higher SRR after MD compared to conventional TESE only in patients having SCO (33.9% vs. 6.3%; $p = 0.04$) but not in men with maturation arrest (75% vs. 37.5%; $p = 0.2$) (level of evidence 3). In addition to histopathology, testicular volume has also shown a correlation with MD SRR. A retrospective study found that only men with a testicular volume lower than 10 mL had a better recovery rate with MD compared with TESE (42% vs. 27%) [(41); level of evidence 3]. In contrast to these results, Tsujimura et al. [(46); level of evidence 3] reported comparable results with conventional and MD techniques. Clearly, more prospective randomized studies, in well-defined large and unselected populations of NOA patients, should be conducted before recommending this strategy as the gold standard.

In recent years, the addition of noninvasive tests such as color Doppler ultrasound to guide FNA or TESE through the identification of regions with higher vascularization showing active spermatogenesis has been investigated (47). Several authors found a higher SRR in areas with a good vascularity compared with a poor vascularity (48). Hence, these techniques could reduce the number of biopsies required to retrieve sperm, thus minimizing testicular damages. Nevertheless, again more studies are required to establish the added value of these noninvasive tests.

We can therefore inform our patient that in his case (as in most other NOA patients), performing multiple biopsies will yield the highest sperm recovery rate and that the addition of the use of an operation microscope may be beneficial whenever enlarged tubuli can be visualized (SCO patients).

How to Schedule the TESE Procedure?

Case: The male partner of the couple described in the section "how to predict successful sperm retrieval" is very concerned about the treatment his young wife will need to undergo because of his problem of azoospermia. In case of unsuccessful TESE, they are not willing to use donor sperm.

As TESE will not be successful in all NOA patients, a preliminary testicular biopsy with freezing of the tissue for later use may avoid pointless ovarian stimulation in the female partner in many NOA couples and may theoretically render repeated biopsies unnecessary.

A study evaluated the outcome of 97 ICSI cycles scheduled with frozen-thawed testicular sperm in 69 histologically defined NOA patients (49). Results were comparable to those of ICSI with fresh testicular sperm (level of evidence 3): clinical pregnancy rate per ET of 25% and 17.9%, respectively, in cycles using frozen-thawed and fresh testicular sperm. The implantation rate per replaced embryo was 11.3% compared to 8.6% using fresh testicular sperm. The observed tendency toward better results with frozen-thawed spermatozoa may be explained by patient selection: the frozen-thawed group represents a subgroup of patients where the quality of testicular biopsies was adequate enough to allow cryopreservation. However, this approach involving preliminary freezing of the testicular samples has an important disadvantage when all tissue samples with at least one spermatozoon observed are frozen: in approximately 20% of these patients no spermatozoa can be recovered for ICSI after thawing. Yet, a successful back-up fresh retrieval can be performed in most of these couples (49).

Thus, we need to inform our patient about the advantages and disadvantages of performing a preliminary biopsy followed by cryopreservation whenever spermatozoa are successfully recovered. A pointless stimulation can be avoided with a similar pregnancy rate as after the use of fresh testicular sperm, but in 20% of the cases, no sperm will be found after thawing and a new TESE will need to be performed on the day of egg retrieval.

How Many TESE Procedures to Perform?

Case: A couple in which the husband has an NOA because of a chromosomal translocation had already one successful TESE procedure, but, unfortunately, his wife was not pregnant after this ICSI cycle and no testicular sperm has been frozen. They would like to know which probability they have of having again a successful TESE and when the next procedure should be performed.

Repeated TESE procedures yield high recovery rates even in NOA men [(50,51); level of evidence 3]. A retrospective study including only men in whom sperm had been found on a first TESE reported an SRR of 74.7% and 82.3% after the second and third attempt, respectively (51). The best moment to perform a second biopsy in patients that require a repeated TESE remains controversial. Schlegel and Su recommended that TESE should be repeated at an interval of ≥6 months, because the chances of retrieving sperm went up to 80% compared with 25% when TESE was repeated after a shorter interval [(52); level of evidence 3). Amer et al. also found a higher sperm recovery rate (94.7%) if the sperm recovery procedure was performed ≥3 months compared to 75% when performed <3 months (36). However, in a larger series (156 biopsies), similar SRR was present when the second TESE was performed before or after six months from the first procedure (82% vs. 76.5%) (51).

We can therefore inform our couple that after a first successful TESE, there is a very high probability of finding sperm again in a next procedure and that the time interval between the two procedures may influence the result. For the problem of translocation, a preimplantation genetic diagnosis may improve the implantation rate by selecting unaffected embryos.

COMPLICATIONS OF TESTICULAR SPERM EXTRACTIONS

Case: A 48-year-old men with an idiopathic NOA, showing a SCOS at histology, would like to know if there are some complications after performing a testicular sperm extraction.

Performing a sperm extraction may lead to testicular damage secondary to anoxia either as the consequence of the interference of the vascular supply to the seminiferous tubules or as an increased intratesticular pressure secondary to bleeding enclosed within the tunica albuginea. According to Schlegel and Su, 82% of patients who had testicular biopsy show intratesticular abnormalities on a scrotal ultrasound, suggesting persistent hematoma and/or inflammation even as long as three months after TESE (52). The majority of these ultrasound abnormalities are resolved within six months after TESE, leaving linear scars or calcifications [(24,25,52); level of evidence 3]. There is little evidence that multiple, blind testicular needle aspirations carry any less risk of testicular injury than an open biopsy with identification of testicular vessels. Only few papers are available on this subject, and they all report very few vascular complications after FNA [(29,53); level of evidence 3].

The use of microsurgical sperm retrieval procedures may even further minimize the risk of inadvertent vascular injury to the testis [(40,43,45); level of evidence 3]. Nevertheless, MD requires special surgical skills along with the need of magnification equipment, thus making it less accessible to all IVF centers.

Multiple studies have shown ultrasonographic changes after TESE, which have been attributed to the development of scar tissue [(15,24,40,52); level of evidence 3]. Although FNA has been associated with a lesser trauma to the testis, Shufaro et al. (54) found in an animal model extensive architectural distortion of the tubules, chronic inflammation, necrosis, and degenerative changes associated with the puncture but not related to the inflicted negative suction. On the other hand, TESE showed only local chronic inflammation and degenerative cells on the biopsied area. Only two studies compared the incidence of fibrosis at six months after TESE and MD. Both found significantly less scar tissue after MD compared to conventional TESE (40,45).

Another concern is the decrease in serum testosterone after testicular sperm extraction, particularly in severely oligozoospermic men showing already a significantly lower serum testosterone levels than fertile men (55). A further decrease in Leydig cell function after testicular biopsy can further reduce serum testosterone output. Therefore, NOA men should be considered to be at high risk of developing androgen deficiency and hypogonadism after TESE [(26,56); level of evidence 3].

Although after MD a lesser amount of testicular tissue is removed, this decline in serum testosterone also seems to be present using this approach (45,57). Komori et al., however, did not found such a decrease in serum testosterone neither after conventional TESE nor after MD (58). As all these studies concern a limited number of patients, further studies on this subject are needed.

Another concern is the occurrence of antigenic stimulation after testis biopsy. Hjort et al. found the presence of antisperm antibodies in 31% of the patients who had undergone a previous testicular biopsy 10 days to 5 weeks before analysis of their sera (59). However, Komori et al. evaluated the presence of antisperm antibodies before and one year after TESE in patients with NOA azoospermia and found no incidence of new antisperm antibody formation (58).

We may therefore inform our patient that the performance of a testicular sperm extraction is not without complications. In his case, although getting the lowest complication rates, an FNA is not indicated because of the low recovery rate. If the center disposes of an operative microscope, an MD can be performed, as in his case we probably will be able to visualize the enlarged tubules and therefore retrieve a smaller amount of testicular tissue.

ICSI OUTCOME AFTER THE USE OF TESTICULAR SPERM

Case: A 44-year-old man with a congenital absence of the vas deferens (CBAVD) would like to know whether there is a different outcome between the use of epididymal and testicular sperm and whether the use of frozen sperm may influence the results.

In patients with OA azoospermia, fertilization rate and pregnancy outcome after the use of epididymal spermatozoa compare favorably with those of ICSI using ejaculated spermatozoa [(60); level of evidence 3]. Furthermore, a review has shown that pregnancy rates after ICSI using testicular spermatozoa from patients with normal spermatogenesis are comparable to those obtained after ICSI using epididymal spermatozoa [(61); level of evidence 2a].

The ICSI outcome after the use of frozen-thawed epididymal spermatozoa too is comparable to that after using freshly retrieved spermatozoa [(12,61); level of evidence 2a).

As for epididymal spermatozoa, the outcome after ICSI with either fresh or frozen-thawed testicular spermatozoa is comparable as well [(62); level of evidence 2a].

We may thus inform our patient that in his case both epididymal and testicular sperm can be used with the same success rate, but that a PESA should be attempted as the first-line approach. The choice between fresh or frozen epididymal or testicular sperm will be based on convenience rather than on conclusive medical grounds.

Case: A man of 28 years having an idiopathic NOA would like to know the pregnancy rate if sperm is recovered by TESE. His wife is 24 years old.

Initial publications, mostly dealing with small series, reported contradictory results on fertilization and pregnancy rates in patients in whom azoospermia results from a primary testicular failure. A meta-analysis showed a significantly improved fertilization rate [relative risk (RR) 1.18; 95%CI: 1.13–1.23] and clinical pregnancy rate (RR 1.36; 95% CI: 1.10–1.69) in men with OA as compared to NOA with a nonsignificant increase in ongoing pregnancy rate (61). This meta-analysis did not find any difference in either implantation rate or miscarriage rate between the two groups. These differences among the published reports can easily be explained by the heterogeneity of the patient population examined. In many of these reports, patient selection is performed after a preliminary biopsy. In some series, a large group of patients with NOA show hypospermatogenesis at testicular histology, whereas other publications only deal with small case-series. The definition of NOA is often unclear and based only on clinical parameters, while no proper histological diagnosis is present. A large study, not included in the meta-analysis of Nicopoulos, analyzed the outcome of a consecutive series of 306 cycles in 235 patients with a well-defined (clinically and histologically) NOA (63). The control group comprised 605 cycles performed in 360 azoospermic men with normal spermatogenesis. In this large series, a significantly lower fertilization rate was observed in men with NOA compared to men with OA (48.5% vs. 59.7%). Both the clinical implantation rate and clinical pregnancy rate per cycle were significantly lower in the NOA group compared to the OA group: 8.6% versus 12.5%, and 15.4% versus 24%, respectively (level of evidence 2b). Whenever this series would have been included in the meta-analysis, the conclusion would probably be different given that this study outnumbers all the other series included. Moreover, the above-mentioned meta-analysis includes different papers relating to the same patient population (repeated publications from the same group on extended patient series).

In order to counsel patients more adequately, Osmanagaoglu et al. calculated life-table statistics in couples undergoing ICSI with testicular sperm from azoospermic men with NOA (64). It was observed that after three cycles, the expected chance of fathering a child was 31% in the NOA group compared to 48% in the OA group. Again, these data corroborate the finding that NOA patients perform less than OA patients after ICSI.

We may therefore inform this couple that in their case we are facing two problems: (i) the probability of finding sperm of approximately 50% (without being able to predict the retrieval rate) and (ii) the lower pregnancy rate compared to patients showing normal spermatogenesis.

In order to enhance the pregnancy rate in NOA patients, some authors have proposed the use of preimplantation genetic diagnosis (PGD) because an increased incidence of aneuploid embryos has been described (65,66). However, this approach needs to be confirmed by prospective randomized studies.

PREGNANCIES AND CHILDREN OBTAINED AFTER TESE–ICSI

Case: A couple from the Netherlands is very concerned about the well-being of children born after the use of testicular sperm, as in their country the use of testicular spermatozoa from men with NOA has been restricted. They would like to know if there is a reason to be concerned.

A possible explanation for the observed lower fertilization and pregnancy rate in patients with severe testicular failure may be the use of immature gametes. As a result, there have been concerns regarding possible adverse effects on children born after TESE–ICSI, especially in NOA. The spermatozoa from

NOA men are known to show higher chromosomal aneuploidy rates (67). Furthermore, The aneuploidy frequency in embryos obtained from NOA as well as OA is very high, 53% versus 60%, respectively (66). It is also assumed that genomic imprinting may be incomplete or deficient (68).

So far, few publications have focused on the obstetrical and neonatal outcome of children born after ICSI using testicular sperm and registries on the outcome of ICSI pregnancies obtained with testicular sperm do not differentiate between OA and NOA. We therefore examined the outcome of 70 pregnancies and neonatal data concerning 61 children born after ICSI using testicular sperm from men with clinically and histologically defined NOA (69). The results were compared with 204 pregnancies and 196 children born after TESE–ICSI in OA men. There were no statistical significant differences with respect to the outcome of the pregnancies between the two groups studied. No differences were observed between the two groups regarding the birth weight of the children or the early perinatal mortality rate. Major malformations were present in 4% of the liveborn children obtained with testicular sperm of NOA men versus 3% in children of OA men (level of evidence 3). These rates are comparable to the rates observed in ICSI children after the use of ejaculated sperm, using the same methodology and definitions as in this study, where a 3.4% major malformation rate was found (70). Other groups did not report an increased malformation rate after the use of testicular sperm either (71–73). In these studies, however, the subgroups of testicular sperm were also small and, unfortunately, no distinction was made between OA and NOA azoospermia. Only the report by Palermo et al. made this distinction, although it is not clear whether this was based on a histopathological basis, which is an important prerequisite for categorizing the type of azoospermia (74).

We may thus inform our couple that so far, from these limited data, we may conclude that the results in terms of pregnancy and child outcome are rather reassuring. But since the published studies only comprise a small number of patients, further study is certainly recommended.

REFERENCES

1. Ron-El R, Strassburger D, Friedler S, et al. Extended sperm preparation: an alternative to testicular sperm extraction in non-obstructive azoospermia. Hum Reprod 1997; 12:1222–1226.
2. World Health Organisation. Towards more objectivity in diagnosis and management of male infertility. Results of a World Health Organisation Multicentre Study. Int J Androl 1987; (suppl 7):1–53.
3. Jarow JP, Espeland MA, Lipshultz LI. Evaluation of the azoospermic patients. J Urol 1989; 142:62.
4. Jow WW, Steckel J, Schlegel PN, et al. Motile sperm in human testis biopsy specimens. J Androl 1993; 14:194–198.
5. Mc Lachlan RI, Rajpert-De Meyts E, Hoei-Hansen CE, et al. Histological evaluation of the human testis—approaches to optimizing the clinical value of the assessment: mini review. Hum Reprod 2007; 22:2–16.
6. Matsumiya K, Namiki M, Takahara S, et al. Clinical study of azoospermia. Int J Androl 1994; 17:140–142.
7. Tournaye H. Gamete source and manipulation. In: Vayena E, Rowe PJ, Griffin PD, eds. Current Practices and Controversies in Assisted Reproduction: Report of a Meeting on "Medical, Ethical and Social Aspects of Assisted. Reproduction" held at WHO Headquarters in Geneva, Switzerland, September 17–21, 2001. Oxford University Press, 2002.
8. Heidenreich A, Altmann P, Engelmann UH. Micorsurgical vasovasostomy versus microsurgical epididymal sperm aspiration/testicular extraction of sperm combined with intracytoplasmic sperm injection. A cost-benefit analysis. Eur Urol 2000; 37:609–614.
9. Rosenlund B, Kvist U, Ploen L, et al. A comparison between open and percutaneous needle biopsies in men with azoospermia. Hum Reprod 1998; 13:1266–1271.
10. Lin YM, Hsu CC, Kuo TC, et al. Percutaneous epididymal sperm aspiration versus microsurgical epididymal sperm aspiration for irreparable obstructive azoospermia—experience with 100 cases. J Formos Med Assoc 2000; 99: 459–465.
11. Ramos L, Kleingeld P, Meuleman E, et al. Assessment of DNA fragmentation of spermatozoa that were surgically retrieved from men with obstructive azoospermia. Fertil Steril 2002; 77:233–237.
12. Tournaye H, Merdad T, Silber S, et al. No differences in outcome after intracytoplasmic sperm injection with fresh or with frozen-thawed epididymal spermatozoa. Hum Reprod 1999; 14:90–94.
13. Tournaye H, Clasen K, Aytoz A, et al. Fine needle aspiration versus open biopsy for testicular sperm recovery: a controlled study in azoospermic patients with normal spermatogenesis. Hum Reprod 1998; 13:901–904.
14. Carpi A, Menchini Fabris FG, Todeschini G, et al. Large-needle percutaneous aspiration biopsy of the testis in men with non obstructive azoospermia. Fertil Steril 2006; 86:464–465.
15. Tournaye H, Camus M, Vandervorst M, et al. Surgical sperm retrieval for intracytoplasmic sperm injection. Int J Androl 1997; 20(suppl 3):69–73.
16. Tournaye H, Verheyen G, Nagy P, et al. Are there any predictive factors for successful testicular sperm recovery in azoospermic patients? Hum Reprod 1997; 12:80–86.
17. Ezeh UI, Taub NA, Moore HD, et al. Establishment of predictive variables associated with testicular sperm retrieval in men with non-obstructive azoospermia. Hum Reprod 1999; 14:1005–1012.
18. Tunc L, Kirac M, Gurocak S, et al. Can serum inhibin B and FSH levels, testicular histology and volume predict the outcome of testicular sperm extraction in patients with non-obstructive azoospermia? Int Urol Nephrol 2006; 38:629–635.

19. Vernaeve V, Tournaye H, Schiettecatte J, et al. Serum inhibin B cannot predict testicular sperm retrieval in patients with non-obstructive azoospermia. Hum Reprod 2002; 17:971–976.
20. Brandell RA, Mielnik A, Liotta D, et al. AZFb deletions predict the absence of spermatozoa with testicular sperm extraction: Preliminary report of a prognostic genetic test. Hum Reprod 1998; 13:2812–2815.
21. Colpi GM, Piediferro G, Nerva F, et al. Sperm retrieval for intracytoplasmic sperm injection in non-obstructive azoospermia. Minerva Urol Nefrol 2005; 57:99–107.
22. Donoso P, Tournaye H, Devroey H. Which is the best sperm retrieval technique for non-obstructive azoospermia? A systematic review. Hum Reprod Update 2007; 13:539–549.
23. Vernaeve V, Staessen C, Verheyen G, et al. Can biological or clinical parameters predict testicular sperm recovery in 47,XXY Klinefelter's patients? Hum Reprod 2004; 19:1135–1139.
24. Ron-El R, Strauss S, Friedler S, et al. Serial sonography and colour flow Doppler imaging following testicular and epididymal sperm extraction. Hum Reprod 1998; 13:3390–3393.
25. Schlegel PN, Palermo GD, Goldstein M, et al. Testicular sperm extraction with intracytoplasmic sperm injection for non-obstructive azoospermia. Urology 1997; 49:435–440.
26. Schill T, Bals-Pratsch M, Küpker W, et al. Clinical and endocrine follow-up of patients after testicular sperm extraction. Fertil Steril 2003; 79:281–286.
27. Tournaye H. Surgical sperm recovery for intracytoplasmic sperm injection: which method is to be preferred? Hum Reprod 1999; 14:71–81.
28. Westlander G, Rosenlund B, Söderlund B, et al. Sperm retrieval, fertilization, and pregnancy outcome in repeated testicular sperm aspiration. J Assist Reprod Genet 2001; 18:171–177.
29. Friedler S, Raziel A, Strassburger D, et al. Testicular sperm retrieval by percutaneous fine needle sperm aspiration compared with testicular sperm extraction by open biopsy in men with non-obstructive azoospermia. Hum Reprod 1997; 12:1488–1493.
30. Ezeh UI, Moore HD, Cooke ID. A prospective study of multiple needle biopsies versus a single open biopsy for testicular sperm extraction in men with non-obstructive azoospermia. Hum Reprod 1998; 13:3075–3080.
31. Hauser R, Yogev L, Paz G, et al. Comparison of efficacy of two techniques for testicular sperm retrieval in nonobstructive azoospermia: multifocal testicular sperm extraction versus multifocal testicular sperm aspiration. J Androl 2006; 27:28–33.
32. Raman JD, Schlegel P. Testicular sperm extraction with intracytoplasmic sperm injection is successful for the treatment of nonobstructive azoospermia associated with cryptorchidism. J Urol 2003; 170:1287–1290.
33. Vernaeve V, Tournaye H, Osmanagaoglu K, et al. Testicular sperm recovery and ICSI in patients with non-obstructive azoospermia with a history of orchidopexia. Hum Reprod 2004b; 19:2307–2312.
34. Silber SJ, Nagy Z, Devroey P, et al. Distribution of spermatogenesis in the testicles of azoospermic men: the presence or absence of spermatids in the testes of men with germinal failure. Hum Reprod 1997; 12:2422–2428.
35. Gottschalk-Sabag S, Weiss DB, Folb-Zacharow N, et al. Is one testicular specimen sufficient for quantitative evaluation of spermatogenesis? Fertil Steril 1995; 64:399–402.
36. Amer M, Haggar SE, Moustafa T, et al. Testicular sperm extraction: impact of testicular histology on outcome, number of biopsies to be performed and optimal time for repetition. Hum Reprod 1999; 14:3030–3034.
37. Tournaye H, Camus M, Goosens A, et al. Recent concepts in the management of infertility because of non-obstructive azoospermia. Hum Reprod 1995; 10(suppl 1):115–119.
38. Hauser R, Botchan A, Amit A, et al. Multiple testicular sampling in non-obstructive azoospermia: is it necessary? Hum Reprod 1998; 13:3081–3085.
39. Witt MA, Richard JR, Smith SE, et al. The benefit of additional biopsy sites when performing testicular sperm extraction on non-obstructive azoospermia. Fertil Steril 1997; 67:S79–S80.
40. Amer M, Ateyah A, Hany R, et al. Prospective comparative study between microsurgical and conventional testicular sperm extraction in non-obstructive azoospermia: follow-up by serial ultrasound examinations. Hum Reprod 2000; 15:653–656.
41. Mulhall JP. The utility of optical loupe magnification for testis sperm extraction in men with nonobstructive azoospermia. J Androl 2005; 26:178–181.
42. Schlegel P. Testicular sperm extraction: microdissection improves sperm yield with minimal tissue excision. Hum Reprod 1999; 14:131–135.
43. Ramasamy R, Yagan N, Schlegel PN. Structural and functional changes to the testis after conventional versus microdissection testicular sperm extraction. Urology 2005; 65:1190–1194.
44. Schlegel PN, Tanrikut A, Li PS. Microdissection testicular sperm extraction (TESE) in non-obstructive azoospermia. Fertil Steril 2006; 86:S519.
45. Okada H, Dobashi M, Yamazaki T, et al. Conventional versus microdissection testicular sperm extraction for nonobstructive azoospermia. J Urol 2002; 168:1063–1067.
46. Tsujimura A, Matsumiya K, Miyagawa Y, et al. Conventional multiple or microdissection testicular sperm extraction: a comparative study. Hum Reprod 2002; 17:2924–2929.
47. Herwig R, Tosun K, Pinggera GM, et al. Tissue perfusion essential for spermatogenesis and outcome of testicular sperm extraction (TESE) for assisted reproduction. J Assist Reprod Genet 2004; 21:175–180.

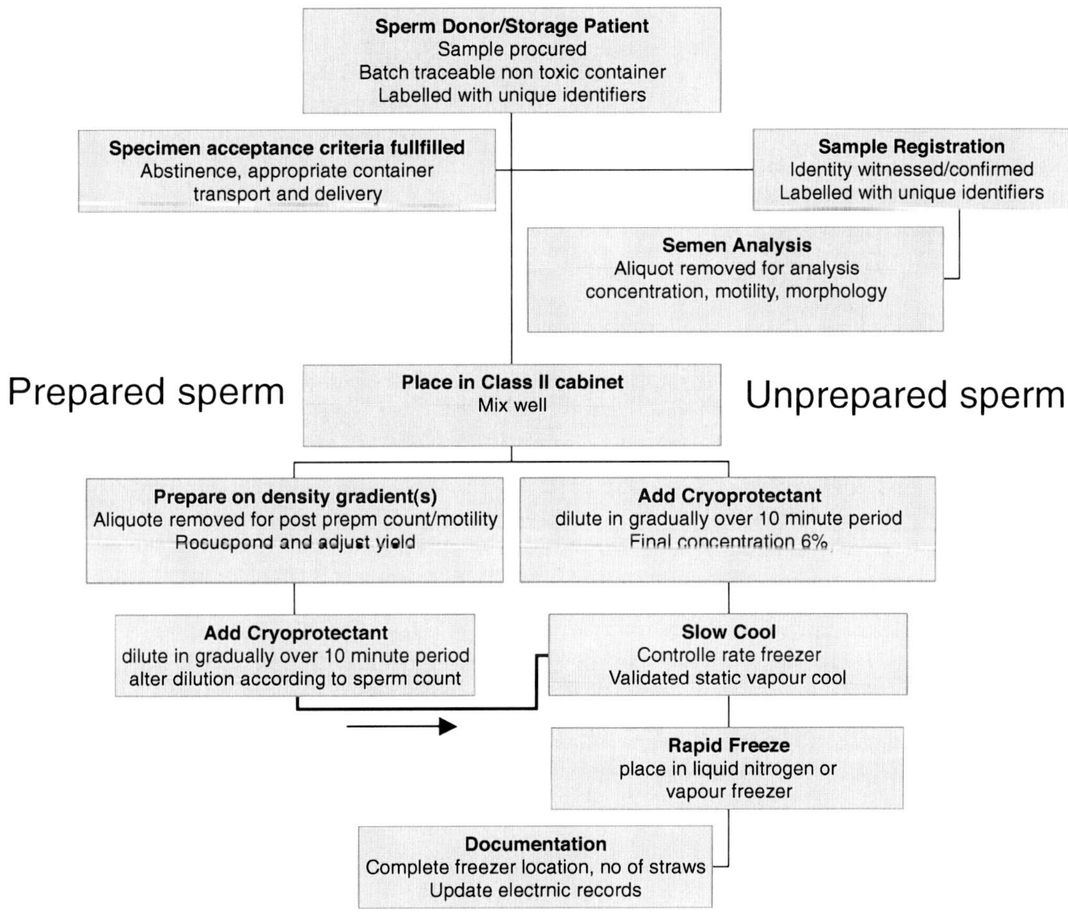

Figure 1 Flow diagram showing the sperm cryopreservation process.

without breakage. Unfortunately for the sperm banking industry, very few options satisfy all of the above. The commonly used plastic cryovials provide a convenient method for packaging sperm and can be conveniently stored to make economic use of freezer space. However, as Mortimer illustrates, cryovials are not the ideal environment for heat exchange during sperm cooling, with temperatures toward the center of the vial lagging behind those at the outer vial edge (30). Furthermore, with an ineffective seal, plastic cryovials (Fig. 2) are unsuitable for use in the majority of current sperm storage banks that tend to consist of liquid phase nitrogen dewars (see later in this chapter). Liquid ingress is a common occurrence and represents a potential explosion risk as the vial is removed from storage and begins to warm. Technicians have been severely injured when removing cryovials containing liquid nitrogen, yet surprisingly their large-scale use in the liquid phase continues (35). An ineffective seal not only poses a clear danger to the staff using them but also represents a potential cross-contamination risk, if liquid nitrogen is free to move between vials (36).

The most effective packaging in terms of uniform cooling is the pailette or straw and the modern version, the ionomeric resin straw (CBS, France), has the additional benefits of increased tensile strength at low temperatures and a more effective seal. These so-called high security straws are conveniently packaged in sterile units; after filling they can be effectively "welded" (thermosoldered) at either end. Labeling is in the form of a colored labeling collar that is affixed prior to final sealing (Fig. 3). Filling is also improved and rendered virtually contamination-free by virtue of a sterile filling nozzle that prevents contact between the material to be frozen and outside of the straw while providing a convenient "air gap" for expansion of contents on cooling. It is important that any contamination on the outside of each straw be removed before immersing straws into liquid nitrogen. Although a vast improvement on other sperm packaging systems and undoubtedly currently the best available, users should never view them as totally "risk free." CBS straws are indeed more robust and leakproof than any predecessor; however, cooling any material to ultralow

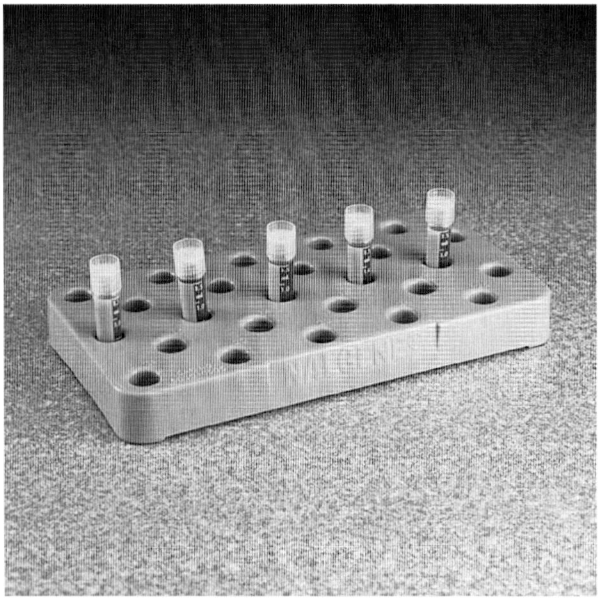

Figure 2 Cryovials with external threaded lid.

(liquid nitrogen) temperatures will alter its characteristics. The flattened sealed ends of a CBS straw may be broken off and the straw itself can break (albeit with more force than a polyterepthalate glycol (PTEG) or polyvinyl chloride (PVC) straw). Reliance on the Symms sealer (Fig. 4) to thermosolder the straw ends must be accounted for during risk analysis and a spare machine should be made available if necessary.

Cooling

The optimal cooling rates for human sperm are thought to be between 1°C and 10°C/min (15) and cooling significantly outside of these margins appears to result in cell damage. Those cooled too quickly will be killed by intracellular ice and those

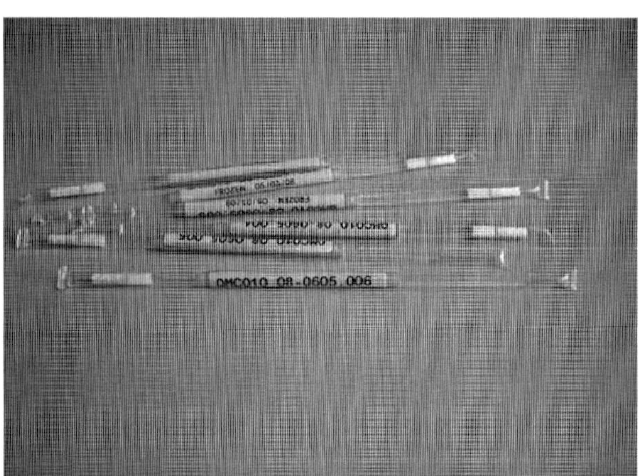

Figure 3 CBS straws.

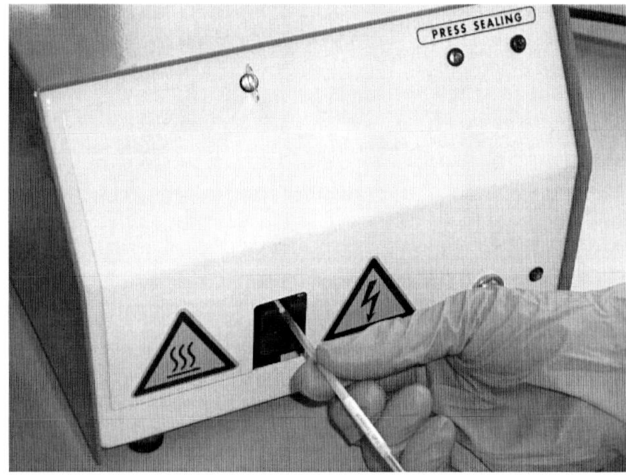

Figure 4 The Symms sealer.

cooled too slowly will undergo excessive osmotic stresses and solute toxicity (9). Cooling protocols vary enormously from center to center and in some cases validation appears to be nonexistent. This situation must be remedied in the very near future as in an accredited and regulated center, validation of all methods is mandatory. Practices vary with some centers using controlled rate freezing (CRF) and others using various static vapor cooling methods, suspending sperm above either a liquid nitrogen reservoir or a vapor shipper. For sperm freezing there is little evidence to suggest superiority of one over the other. Ragni and colleagues (37) suggested that CRF limited cryodamage, particularly for abnormal samples from oncology patients. McLaughlin and colleagues (38) (1990) compared CRF with their standard vapor freezing protocol and showed that the vapor cooling rates inside 0.25-mL straws varied from the bottom of the straw to the top and there was considerable variation between replicates. Interestingly, they suggested that more motile spermatozoa survived the CRF freezing procedure, although the percentage of intact spermatozoa and their velocity was very similar after both procedures. A similar study by Paras and coworkers (39) found no obvious differences in either motility or viability after comparing CRF with vapor freezing. This may be partly explained by the relative resistance of sperm to variation in cooling rate but will depend on the center using a vapor method that provides a cooling rate that approximates to the optimum.

It is clear however from some reports that the static vapor cooling procedure in one center may be very different from that of another. The description of a cooling protocol as "suspension" in nitrogen vapor can be highly misleading as there is often huge variation in the distance from the coolant (liquid nitrogen) and therefore the resulting temperature of the vapor and the subsequent cooling rate. Figure 5 shows the difference in cooling rates achieved in a nitrogen vessel when a thermocouple is placed inside a sample and at various heights from

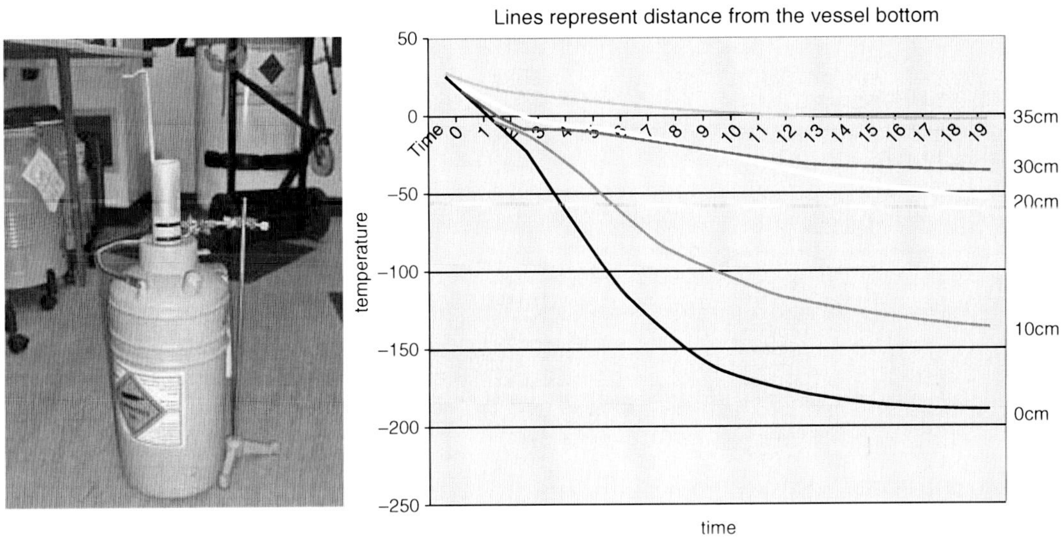

Figure 5 Dry shipper cooling method showing the rates of cooling at different heights of the vessel.

the bottom of a dry shipper. Not only does the cooling rate slow down with increasing distance but cooling is far from linear, which means that to achieve a consistent cooling rate of, for example, −10° per minute, specimens must be moved to different heights at specified times during the cooling process. Therefore, authors/centers describing cryopreservation practice as suspending sperm 5, 10, or 15 cm from the liquid nitrogen source could easily be misinterpreted (30,40,41) as they will clearly have profoundly different cooling rates.

Translation from the current literature by other centers may not be straightforward. Mortimer (2004) illustrates this by showing delayed cooling in increased sample volumes and suggests that only plastic straws provide an environment for optimum cooling of sperm, particularly when compared to that provided by larger plastic cryovials (30). This has been confirmed by studies in our own laboratory, which have clearly shown that the cooling rate of sample frozen in the center of a cryovial is 1°C to 2°C slower than that of the sample adjacent to the inner vial wall. Validation of a cooling rate should therefore examine the cooling fluid itself and not the temperature of the cooling chamber, and this would apply equally to computer controlled freezing and static vapor cooling.

Storage

Sperm can be successfully stored at temperatures even as high as −80°C for a limited period and indeed some commercial sperm donor banks transport samples on dry ice at approximately −79°C over several days. However, it has been shown that storage for long periods at this temperature will result in a progressive decline in postthaw sperm quality (42,43). Therefore, for convenience more than any other reason, liquid nitrogen has become the coolant of choice as it is relatively inert, is liquid at −196°C, and can be conveniently stored with care at relatively low pressures.

The majority of laboratories storing sperm have tended to do so in medium-sized liquid nitrogen vessels or dewars, which are essentially large metal vacuum flasks with the capacity for between 2000 and 8000 straws depending on their volume and how they are arranged (Fig. 6). The advantage of the liquid nitrogen dewar is in its simplicity, being a very basic piece of equipment with no moving parts, requiring little or no servicing, and having a relatively good history in terms of catastrophic failure. By ensuring that samples are immersed in liquid nitrogen, we can be assured that they will be maintained at a suitable temperature. Some larger sperm banks however, particularly those storing for cancer patients for some 20 years or more,

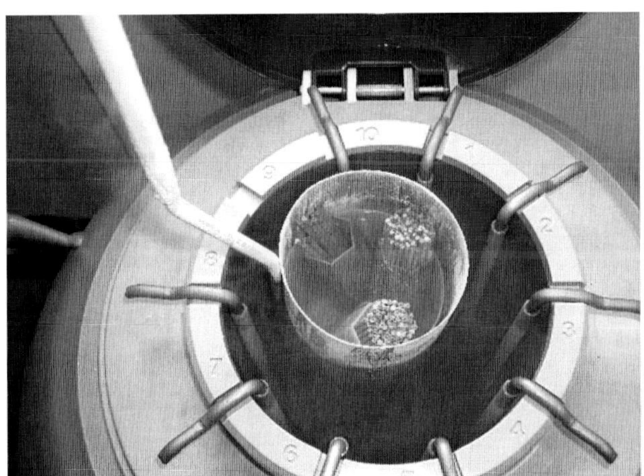

Figure 6 Standard liquid nitrogen dewar.

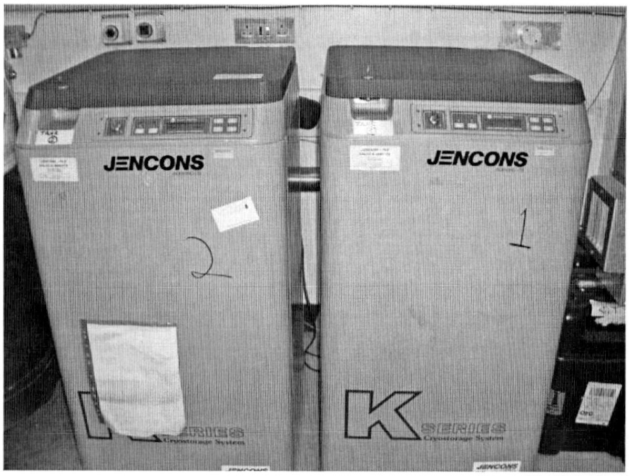

Figure 7 Nitrogen vapor refrigerators.

have reached such a size that warrants the use of bulk refrigerators that can be used either for liquid or vapor phase storage (Fig. 7). In contrast to the dewar, the technology and monitoring associated with an automated vapor storage system is considerable, and relates largely to the sensing of liquid level and temperatures and a considerable reliance on autofilling systems. Faulty liquid level sensing can lead to failure to fill, or indeed overfilling, either of which can be extremely hazardous for the operator or the specimens (44). To keep specimens in the vapor phase, running costs are significantly higher, using on average four times the quantities of liquid nitrogen and are related to the poor thermal properties of a freezer with a relatively large diameter opening.

The number of reproductive storage laboratories following a vapor storage route has been limited, which may be because many centers store considerably less material than do those facilities involved in blood and tissue banking. Moreover, there has also been a long-held suspicion that vapor phase storage cannot achieve suitable temperatures and may not be inherently any safer than liquid storage. To an extent the latter may be partly true in that the evidence supporting the relative safety of vapor storage is unconvincing and a move over to bulk storage in automated refrigerators should be viewed with caution. In their support, a well-designed vapor system with a highly conductive aluminum inventory (racking) system will easily achieve appropriately low temperatures, even just under the freezer lid (44). Operator safety is indeed improved by virtue of the ability to retrieve samples without the need to handle large volumes of liquid nitrogen. The question over sample safety and whether storage in vapor reduces the (already small) risk of microbial transmission is difficult to answer but would certainly depend upon assurances over the integrity of the packaging material in use and whether its seal can be guaranteed.

The choice of storage vessel is an individual one and ultimately should be made to suit the center based on a number of criteria including the number of specimens likely to be stored at any given time, the packaging material used, the choice of inventory (racking), and indeed the available facilities including floor space. Centers storing cryovials, as previously mentioned, should be storing in vapor phase refrigerators only, regardless of other factors. Sperm banks of any more than 20,000 (0.5 mL) straws should be looking toward bulk storage as floor space is taken over by many dewars and this in itself may become hazardous.

Storage Inventory (Racking)

The design of the freezer furniture or racking is largely governed by the packaging system used and the size of the vessel in use and to a degree by whether storage is carried out in the liquid or vapor phase of nitrogen. It must fulfil some basic needs with regard to minimizing sample losses, keeping them at an appropriate temperature (particular during vapor storage), and allowing easy access to individual sample units. Centers using straws tend to store them in individual freezing goblets stacked in a circular canister in a standard liquid phase dewar. If storing plastic goblets in a large vapor refrigerator, these may be stacked up to 4 deep, in which case metal dividers should be inserted into each goblet to improve conductance and keep samples at the top of the inventory at temperatures similar to those at the bottom.

Storage in the vapor phase requires racking to be highly conductive to ensure the maintenance of an appropriate temperature toward the top of the inventory. Plastic tubes or towers are therefore inappropriate. Either towers with individual drawers (for vial storage) or a large canister system can be employed, the latter being particularly useful if, like some older sperm banks, there is a mixture of packaging types, that is, straws and vials, in which case straws can be placed in goblets within visotubes and stacked toward the lower end of the freezer where it is colder. Vials clipped onto aluminum canes will improve thermal conductivity and help the freezer achieve very low temperatures toward the top of the inventory.

RISK MEASURES DURING CRYOPRESERVATION

The risk or potential hazards associated with cryopreservation in a clinical setting are considerable, particularly if the stored material in question represents the patient's only chance of fatherhood. Apart from the more obvious health and safety measures required for working with liquid nitrogen, centers must pay attention to the risk of loss of, or misidentification of, patient material; premature thaw; and contamination damage to material and breaches of containment. Risk management must be viewed as integral to the total quality management system (Table 2) now required for accreditation and licensing of storage banks across the EU. Loss of, or misidentification of, material and donor/patient recipient errors have all occurred and the consequences are extremely damaging and costly both to the affected parties and the reputation of the center providing the service. The additional processing steps required for cryopreservation and movement of material from specimen

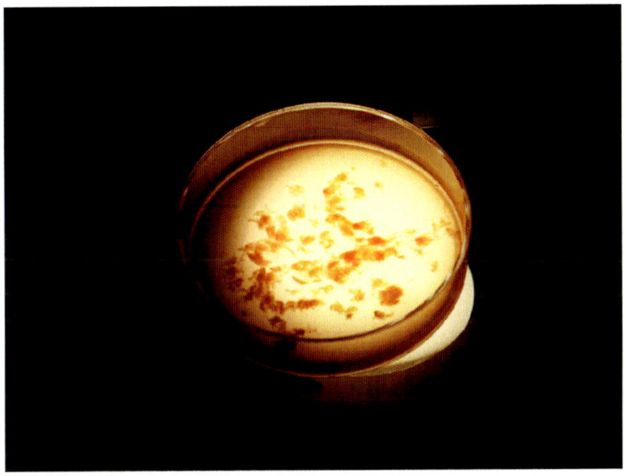

Figure 2 Shredded testicular biopsy fractions in suspension from a patient with obstructive azoospermia.

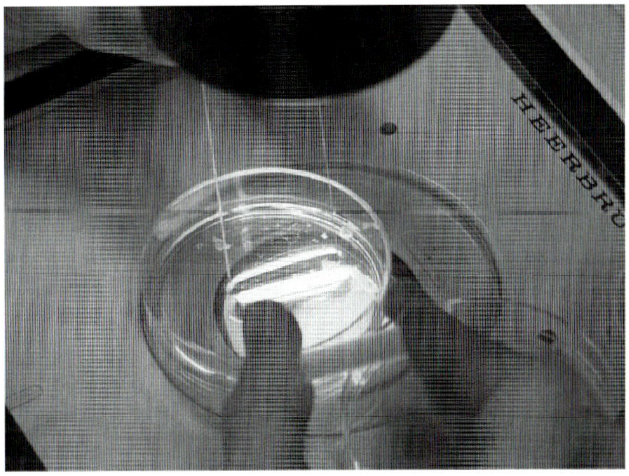

Figure 4 Mechanical shredding of testicular biopsies by means of microscopic glass slides from a patient with nonobstructive azoospermia.

have successfully been used in clinical practice (LOE II). In Brussels, collagenase type IV, a specific protease that degrades collagen type IV present in the basement membrane and the extracellular matrix, is used since 1997, aiming to reduce the proportion of sperm recovery failures in patients with nonobstructive azoospermia (Table 4) (14,15). In 26% of negative cases after mechanical treatment of the testicular biopsies, spermatozoa for ICSI were retrieved after enzymatic dissociation of the tissue. Nevertheless, the procedure of searching for adequate sperm in the final fraction can still be cumbersome and time consuming. The required time period to find the sperm depends on

1. the severity of the NOA cases allocated in the specific IVF clinic,
2. the degree of impaired spermatogenesis, and
3. the number of mature oocytes retrieved from the female partner.

On the basis of a 10-years' experience, it may be stated that the probability to find sperm in droplets of the prepared testicular fraction is extremely low if no single spermatozoon or elongated spermatid has been observed after 30-minute observation (LOE IV). In extreme situations, the procedure may require several hours.

In 2004, Kamal et al. (16) suggested **dissection of the biopsy** with isolation of the most dilated tubules under the stereomicroscope in order to maximize sperm retrieval and found

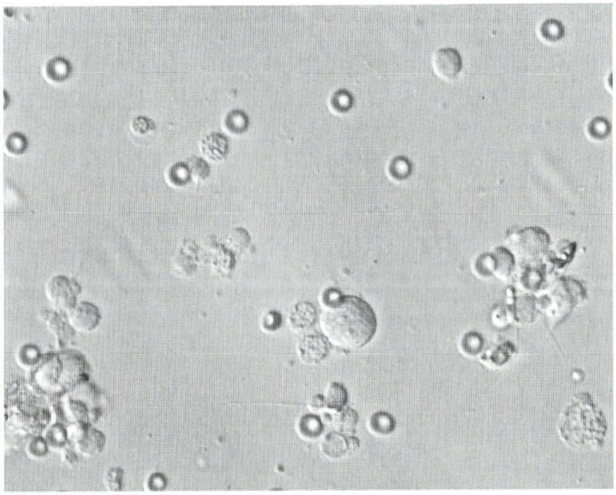

Figure 3 Suspension of testicular cells from a patient with obstructive azoospermia, under the inverted microscope.

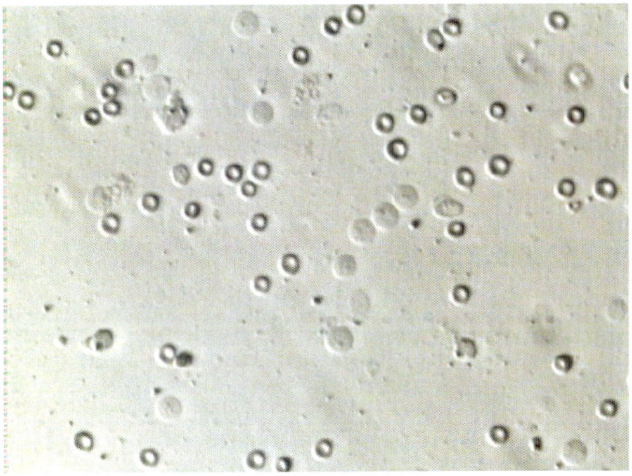

Figure 5 Testicular biopsy suspension with Sertoli cell nuclei (and red blood cells) from a patient with nonobstructive azoospermia (Sertoli-cell–only syndrome), under the inverted microscope.

Table 3 Erythrocyte-lysing Buffer (ELB) (adapted from Ref. 11)

Material
NH_4Cl 155 mM
$KHCO_3$ 10 mM
EDTA 2 mM
ELB solution
For 250 mL: take 20.7 g NH_4Cl + 0.25 g $KHCO_3$ + 0.146 g EDTA
Dissolve in Milli-Q water
Adjust the pH to 7.2 with 0.1M NaOH
Adjust the volume to 250 mL with milli-Q water
Filter the solution
Aliquot in 10 mL fractions and store at $-20°C$
Procedure
Centrifuge the minced tissue at 750×g for 5 min
Remove the supernatant
Add 1–2 mL of ELB solution and mix by shaking
Incubate at room temperature for 5 min
Add excess sperm buffer to dilute the ELB
Centrifuge at 750×g for 5 min
Remove the supernatant and resuspend the pellet in 0.5–1 mL of fresh sperm buffer
Smear droplets on the bottom of a petri dish and overlayer with paraffin oil for sperm searching

a higher sperm recovery rate than in conventionally treated specimens. Very recently, Zohdy et al. (17) developed a new concept—**biopsy freezing + crushing**—for the extraction of testicular spermatozoa from men with NOA. Immediately after the retrieval procedure, the biopsy was quickly frozen in liquid nitrogen vapor for two minutes and plunged in LN_2 for only seven seconds. The tissue was immediately crushed gently before melting, washed, and examined under the microscope. Spermatozoa were identified more easily in the crushed fractions than in the minced suspensions and immediate interaction with the surgeon performing the retrieval was possible, leading to a reduction of biopsies harvested and reduced pathological consequences (LOE IV). Larger studies are needed to verify the value of this new technique.

In vitro Culture of Testicular Tissue

On the basis of the knowledge that testicular sperm are functionally/morphologically immature and obtain their final maturity only during passage through the epididymis, the effect of in vitro culture of testicular sperm up to 120 hours has been tested. It has been demonstrated in cases with OA that, without the need of specific culture media, the rate of spermatozoa with normal morphology improved after in vitro culture up to 72 hours, mainly associated with the loss of residual cytoplasm from the neck region (18). Also the quality of motility (progressive motility) increased while the total proportion of motile cells remained unchanged. In NOA cases, however, the outcome of in vitro culture seemed unpredictable and was considered unsuccessful, as

Table 4 Enzymatic Treatment of Testicular Tissue (adapted from Ref. 14)

Material
Isotonic sperm buffer
Collagenase type IV-S (Sigma C1889)
$CaCl_2$ stock solution: 0.125 g/50 mL
DNase (Sigma D5025)
Enzyme solution
Make the solution freshly, the volume according to the amount of tissue (20–30 mg/mL)
Final activity of the enzyme solution is 1000 IU/mL
Solubilize the enzyme powder in the buffer
Add 5 μL $CaCl_2$ solution per mL enzyme solution
Add a knife-tip DNase to avoid sticking by free DNA
Mix well by vortexing
Procedure
Centrifuge the tissue suspension and remove the supernatant
Add the enzyme solution to the pellet
Mix well by shaking
Incubate at 37°C for 1 hr
Mix each 10 min by shaking in order to facilitate dissociation
Stop the reaction by adding excess buffer solution
Centrifuge at 50×g for 2–3 min to remove undigested fractions
Transfer the supernatant to a conical centrifuge tube
Centrifuge at 1000×g for 5 min
Remove the supernatant and resuspend the pellet in 10 mL buffer
Wash again at 1000×g for 5 min
Resuspend the pellet in 50–100 μL buffer
Smear droplets on the bottom of a petri dish and overlayer with paraffin oil for sperm searching

nonmotile sperm remained immotile after incubation (LOE III). This indicated that in NOA patients, testicular spermatozoa should preferably be extracted (or thawed) and injected without delay on the same day (LOE IV). This recommendation is strengthened by the observation that DNA fragmentation in testicular sperm is increased by 4-hour and 24-hour incubation (LOE III) (19).

SELECTION OF TESTICULAR SPERMATOZOA FOR ICSI

Maturational Stages Used for ICSI

Basically, the most mature stage of the male gamete in the testis and the end product of spermiogenesis is the fully elongated spermatid (mostly referred to as spermatozoon). Only during passage through the epididymis, the sperm cells are functionally and morphologically completing maturation and becoming fully mature spermatozoa. In all cases of obstructive azoospermia, a sufficient number of mature-looking spermatozoa can be selected to inject all the mature oocytes. In nonobstructive azoospermia, however, recovery of fully elongated spermatids or spermatozoa fails in approximately 50% of the cases, and less mature stages of spermiogenesis (elongated/elongating spermatids) are frequently used for ICSI. On the basis of experiments

- ⇨ After communication of this result by the embryologist to the clinician, it was decided to perform a fresh TESE under general anesthesia
- ⇨ After enzymatic digestion of the fresh biopsies, seven motile (type C) spermatozoa for ICSI were found after three hours
- ⇨ The rest of the suspension was not frozen
- ⇨ Histological examination revealed Sertoli-cell–only syndrome

Recommendations

1. Careful clinical work-up of the azoospermic patient is essential for the diagnosis of obstructive (OA) or nonobstructive azoospermia (NOA).
2. In case of OA, different sperm retrieval procedures lead to successful sperm recovery and successful outcome of ICSI cycles.
   - TESA or FNA, fresh/frozen
   - Open excisional biopsy (TESE), fresh/frozen
   - Percutaneous epididymal sperm aspiration
3. In case of NOA, open testis biopsy (TESE) is the preferred sperm retrieval procedure. If the use of frozen material for ICSI is planned, scheduling a fresh biopsy retrieval on the day of oocyte pickup is advocated if the frozen quality is doubtful.
4. Each IVF center should define its strategy considering the use of fresh or frozen–thawed testicular sperm for ICSI.
5. Especially in NOA, the criteria for patient allocation should be defined.
6. Injection of motile (twitching) sperm is an important condition for successful outcome of ICSI.

REFERENCES

1. Palermo G, Joris H, Devroey P, et al. Pregnancies after intracytoplasmic injection of single spermatozoon into an oocyte. Lancet 1992; 340:17–18.
2. Schoysman R, Vanderzwalmen P, Nijs M, et al. Successful fertilization by testicular spermatozoa in an in-vitro fertilization programme? Hum Reprod 1993; 8:1339–1340.
3. World Health Organization. Laboratory Manual for the Examination of Human Semen and Sperm-Cervical Mucus Interaction, 4th ed. Cambridge University Press, UK, 1999.
4. Tournaye H, Verheyen G, Nagy P, et al. Are there any predictive factors for successful testicular sperm recovery in azoospermic patients? Hum Reprod 1997; 12:80–86.
5. Vernaeve V, Tournaye H, Schiettecatte J, et al. Serum inhibin B cannot predict testicular sperm retrieval in patients with non-obstructive azoospermia? Hum Reprod 2002; 17:971–976.
6. Amer M, Haggar SE, Moustafa T, et al. Testicular sperm extraction: Impact of testicular histology on outcome, number of biopsies to be performed and optimal time for repetition. Hum Reprod 1999; 14:3030–3034.
7. Donoso P, Tournaye H, Devroey P. Which is the best sperm retrieval technique for non-obstructive azoospermia? A systematic review. Hum Reprod Update 2007; 13: 539–549.
8. Schlegel PN, Su LM. Physiological consequences of testicular sperm extraction. Hum Reprod 1997; 12:1688–1692.
9. Ron-El R, Strauss S, Friedler S, et al. Serial sonography and colour flow Doppler imaging following testicular and epididymal sperm extraction. Hum Reprod 1998; 13:3390–3393.
10. Verheyen G, Nagy Z, Joris H, et al. Quality of frozen-thawed testicular sperm and its preclinical use for intracytoplasmic sperm injection into in vitro-matured germinal-vesicle stage oocytes. Fertil Steril 1997; 67:74–80.
11. Verheyen G, De Croo I, Tournaye H, et al. Comparison of four mechanical methods to retrieve spermatozoa from testicular tissue. Hum Reprod 1995; 10:2956–2959.
12. Nagy ZP, Verheyen G, Tournaye H, et al. An improved treatment procedure for testicular biopsy specimens offers more efficient sperm recovery: Case series. Fertil Steril 1997; 68:376–379.
13. Salzbrunn A, Benson DM, Holstein AF, et al. A new concept for the extraction of testicular spermatozoa as a tool for assisted fertilization (ICSI). Hum Reprod 1996; 11:752–755.
14. Crabbé E, Verheyen G, Tournaye H, et al. The use of enzymatic procedures to recover testicular germ cells. Hum Reprod 1997; 12:1682–1687.
15. Crabbé E, Verheyen G, Silber S, et al. Enzymatic digestion of testicular tissue may rescue the intracytoplasmic sperm injection cycle in some patients with non-obstructive azoospermia. Hum Reprod 1998; 13:2791–2796.
16. Kamal A, Fahmy I, Mansour RT, et al. Selection of individual testicular tubules from biopsied testicular tissue with a stereomicroscope improves sperm retrieval rate. J Androl 2004; 25:123–127.
17. Zohdy W, Abbas S, Abdel Jalil AK. Freezing and crushing technique: A new concept for the extraction of testicular spermatozoa from men with nonobstructive azoospermia. Fertil Steril 2009; 91:653–655.
18. Liu J, Tsai YL, Katz E, et al. Outcome of in-vitro culture of fresh and frozen-thawed human testicular spermatozoa. Hum Reprod 1997; 12:1667–1672.
19. Dalzell LH, McVicar CM, McClure N, et al. Effects of short and long incubations on DNA fragmentation of testicular sperm. Fertil Steril 2004; 82: 1443–1445.
20. Edwards RG, Tarin JJ, Dean N, et al. Are spermatid injections into human oocytes now mandatory? Hum Reprod 1994; 9:2217–2219.
21. Tesarik J, Mendoza C, Testart J. Viable embryos from injection of round spermatids into oocytes, N Engl J Med 1995; 24;333(8):525.
22. Tesarik J, Rolet F, Brami C, et al. Spermatid injection into human oocytes. II. Clinical application in the treatment

of infertility due to non-obstructive azoospermia. Hum Reprod 1996; 11:780–783.
23. Tesarik J, Mendoza C. Spermatid injection into human oocytes. I. Laboratory techniques and special features of zygote development. Hum Reprod 1996; 11:772–779.
24. Verheyen G, Crabbé E, Joris H, et al. Simple and reliable identification of the human round spermatid by inverted phase-contrast microscopy, Hum Reprod 1998; 13:1570–1577.
25. Schulze W, Thoms F, Knuth UA. Testicular sperm extraction: Comprehensive analysis with simultaneously performed histology in 1418 biopsies from 766 subfertile men. Hum Reprod 1999; 14(suppl 1):82–96.
26. Silber SJ, Johnson L, Verheyen G, et al. Round spermatid injection. Fertil Steril 2000; 73:897–900.
27. Nagy ZP, Joris H, Verheyen G, et al. Correlation between motility of testicular spermatozoa, testicular histology and the outcome of intracytoplasmic sperm injection. Hum Reprod 1998; 13:890–895.
28. Tournaye H, Liu J, Nagy Z, et al. The use of testicular sperm for intracytoplasmic sperm injection in patients with necrozoospermia. Fertil Steril 1996; 66(2):331–334.
29. Nijs M, vanderzwalmen P, Vandamme B, et al. Fertilizing ability of immotile spermatozoa after intracytoplasmic sperm injection. Hum Reprod 1996; 11:2180–2185.
30. Tournaye H, Liu J, Nagy PZ, et al. Correlation between testicular histology and outcome after intracytoplasmic sperm injection using testicular spermatozoa. Hum Reprod 1996; 11(1):127–132.
31. Verheyen G, Vernaeve V, Van Landuyt L, et al. Should diagnostic testicular sperm retrieval followed by cryopreservation for later ICSI be the procedure of choice for all patients with non-obstructive azoospermia? Hum Reprod 2004; 19:2822–2830.
32. Dafopoulos K, Griesinger G, Schultze-Mosgau A, et al. Factors affecting outcome after ICSI with spermatozoa retrieved from cryopreserved testicular tissue in non-obstructive azoospermia, Reprod Biomed Online 2005; 10(4):455–460.
33. Verheyen G, Joris H, Crits K, et al. Comparison of different hypo-osmotic swelling solutions to select viable immotile spermatozoa for potential use in intracytoplasmic sperm injection. Hum Reprod Update 1997; 3(3):195–203.
34. Tsai YL, Liu J, Garcia JE, et al. Establishment of an optimal hypo-osmotic swelling test by examining single spermatozoa in four different hypo-osmotic solutions. Hum Reprod 1997; 12(5):1111–1113.
35. Liu J, Tsai YL, Katz E, et al. High fertilization rate obtained after intracytoplasmic sperm injection with 100% non-motile spermatozoa selected by using a simple modified hypo-osmotic swelling test. Fertil Steril 1997; 68(2):373–375.
36. Sallam H, Farrag A, Agameya A, et al. The use of a modified hypo-osmotic swelling test for the selection of viable ejaculated and testicular immotile spermatozoa in ICSI. Hum Reprod 2001; 16(2):272–276.
37. Sallam HN, Farrag A, Agameya AF, et al. The use of the modified hypo-osmotic swelling test for the selection of immotile testicular spermatozoa in patients treated with ICSI: A randomized controlled study. Hum Reprod 2005; 20(12):3435–3440.
38. de Oliveira NM, Vaca Sánchez R, Rodriguez Fiesta S, et al. Pregnancy with frozen-thawed and fresh testicular biopsy after motile and immotile sperm microinjection, using the mechanical touch technique to assess viability. Hum Reprod 2004; 19(2):262–265.
39. Aktan TM, Montag M, Duman S, et al. Use of a laser to detect viable but immotile spermatozoa. Andrologia 2004; 36(6):366–369.
40. Balaban B, Urman B, Sertac A, et al. In-vitro culture of spermatozoa induces motility and increases implantation and pregnancy rates after testicular sperm extraction and intracytoplasmic sperm injection. Hum Reprod 1999; 14:2808–2811.
41. Terriou P, Hans E, Giorgetti C, et al. Pentoxifylline initiates motility in spontaneously immotile epididymal and testicular spermatozoa and allows normal fertilization, pregnancy, and birth after intracytoplasmic sperm injection. J Assist Reprod Genet 2000; 17(4):194–199.
42. Kovacic B, Vlaisavljevic V, Reljic M. Clinical use of pentoxifylline for activation of immotile testicular sperm before ICSI in patients with azoospermia. J Androl 2006; 27(1):45–52.
43. Mansour RT, Aboulghar MA, Serour GI, et al. The effect of sperm parameters on the outcome of intracytoplasmic sperm injection. Fertil Steril 1995; 64:982–986.
44. Nagy ZP, Liu J, Joris H, et al. The result of intracytoplasmic sperm injection is not related to any of the three basic sperm parameters. Hum Reprod 1995; 10(5):1123–1129.
45. Svalander P, Jakobsson AH, Forsberg AS, et al. The outcome of intracytoplasmic sperm injection is unrelated to 'strict criteria' sperm morphology. Hum Reprod 1996; 11(5):1019–1022.
46. De Vos A, Van De Velde H, Joris H, et al. Influence of individual sperm morphology on fertilization, embryo morphology, and pregnancy outcome of intracytoplasmic sperm injection. Fertil Steril 2003; 79(1):42–48.
47. Yavetz H, Yogev L, Kleiman S, et al. Morphology of testicular spermatozoa obtained by testicular sperm extraction in obstructive and nonobstructive azoospermic men and its relation to fertilization success in the in vitro fertilization-intracytoplasmic sperm injection system. J Androl 2001; 22(3):376–381.
48. Bartoov B, Berkovitz A, Eltes F. Selection of spermatozoa with normal nuclei to improve the pregnancy rate with intracytoplasmic sperm injection. N Engl J Med 2001; 345(14):1067–1068.

49. Bartoov B, Berkovitz A, Eltes F, et al. Pregnancy rates are higher with intracytoplasmic morphologically selected sperm injection than with conventional intracytoplasmic injection. Fertil Steril 2003; 80(6):1413–1419.
50. Berkovitz A, Eltes F, Yaari S, et al. The morphological normalcy of the sperm nucleus and pregnancy rate of intracytoplasmic injection with morphologically selected sperm. Hum Reprod 2005; 20:185–190.
51. Berkovitz A, Eltes F, Lederman H, et al. How to improve IVF-ICSI outcome by sperm selection. Reprod Biomed Online 2006; 12(5):634–638.
52. Crabbé E, Verheyen G, Tournaye H, et al. Freezing of testicular tissue as a minced suspension preserves sperm quality better than whole-biopsy freezing when glycerol is used as cryoprotectant. Int J Androl 1999; 22(1):43–48.
53. Steele EK, McClure N, Lewis SE. Comparison of the effects of two methods of cryopreservation on testicular sperm DNA. Fertil Steril 2000; 74: 450–453.
54. Craft I, Tsirigotis M. Simplified recovery, preparation and cryopreservation of testicular spermatozoa. Hum Reprod 1995; 10(7):1623–1626.
55. Cohen J, Garrisi GJ, Congedo-Ferrara TA, et al. Cryopreservation of single human spermatozoa. Hum Reprod 1997; 12(5):994–1001.
56. Walmsley R, Cohen J, Ferrara-Congedo T, et al. The first births and ongoing pregnancies associated with sperm cryopreservation in evacuated egg zonae. Hum Reprod 1998; 13(suppl 4):61–70.
57. Hsieh Y, Tsai H, Chang C, et al. Cryopreservation of human spermatozoa within human or mouse empty zona pellucidae. Fertil Steril 2000; 73:694–698.
58. Keros V, Rosenlund B, Hultenby K, et al. Optimizing cryopreservation of human testicular tissue: Comparison of protocols with glycerol, propanediol and dimethylsulphoxide as cryoprotectants. Hum Reprod 2005; 20(6):1676–1687.
59. Devroey P, Liu J, Nagy Z, et al. Normal fertilization of human oocytes after testicular sperm extraction and intracytoplasmic sperm injection. Fertil Steril 1994; 62:639–641.
60. Nagy Z, Liu J, Cecile J, et al. Using ejaculated, fresh, and frozen-thawed epididymal and testicular spermatozoa gives rise to comparable results after intracytoplasmic sperm injection. Fertil Steril 1995; 63(4):808–815.
61. Silber SJ, Van Steirteghem AC, Liu J, et al. High fertilization and pregnancy rate after intracytoplasmic sperm injection with spermatozoa obtained from testicle biopsy. Hum Reprod 1995; 10:148–152.
62. Kahraman S, Ozgur S, Alatas C, et al. High implantation and pregnancy rates with testicular sperm extraction and intracytoplasmic sperm injection in obstructive and non-obstructive azoospermia. Hum Reprod 1996; 11:673–676.
63. Mansour RT, Kamal A, Fahmy I, et al. Intracytoplasmic sperm injection in obstructive and non-obstructive azoospermia. Hum Reprod 1997; 12:1974–1979.
64. Van Steirteghem A, Nagy P, Joris H, et al. Results of intracytoplasmic sperm injection with ejaculated, fresh and frozen-thawed epididymal and testicular spermatozoa. Human Reprod 1998; 13(suppl 1):134–142.
65. De Croo I, Van der Elst J, Everaert K, et al. Fertilization, pregnancy and embryo implantation rates after ICSI in cases of obstructive and non-obstructive azoospermia. Hum Reprod 2000; 15:1383–1388.
66. Devroey P, Nagy P, Tournaye H, et al. Outcome of intracytoplasmic sperm injection with testicular spermatozoa in obstructive and non-obstructive azoospermia. Hum Reprod 1996; 11:1015–1018.
67. Silber SJ, van Steirteghem A, Nagy Z, et al. Normal pregnancies resulting from testicular sperm extraction and intracytoplasmic sperm injection for azoospermia due to maturation arrest. Fertil Steril 1996; 66:110–117.
68. Schlegel PN, Palermo GD, Goldstein M, et al., Testicular sperm extraction with intracytoplasmic sperm injection for nonobstructive azoospermia. Urology 1997; 49:435–440.
69. Madgar I, Hourvitz A, Levron J. Outcome of in vitro fertilization and intracytoplasmic injection of epididymal and testicular sperm extracted from patients with obstructive and nonobstructive azoospermia. Fertil Steril 1998; 69:1080–1084.
70. Palermo GD, Schlegel PN, Hariprashad JJ, et al. Fertilization and pregnancy outcome with intracytoplasmic sperm injection for azoospermic men. Hum Reprod 1999; 14:741–748.
71. Balaban B, Urman B, Isiklar A, et al. Blastocyst transfer following intracytoplasmic injection of ejaculated, epididymal or testicular spermatozoa. Hum Reprod 2001; 16: 125–129.
72. Windt ML, Coetzee K, Kruger TF, et al. Intracytoplasmic sperm injection with testicular spermatozoa in men with azoospermia. J Assist Reprod Genet 2002; 19:53–59.
73. Vernaeve V, Tournaye H, Osmanagaoglu K, et al. Intracytoplasmic sperm injection with testicular spermatozoa is less successful in men with nonobstructive azoospermia than in men with obstructive azoospermia. Fertil Steril 2003; 79:529–533.
74. Nicopoullos JD, Gilling-Smith C, Almeida PA, et al. Use of surgical sperm retrieval in azoospermic men: A meta-analysis. Fertil Steril 2004; 82:691–701.
75. Romero J, Remohi J, Minguez Y, et al. Fertilization after intracytoplasmic sperm injection with cryopreserved testicular spermatozoa. Fertil Steril 1996; 65:877–879.
76. Gil-Salom M, Romero J, Minguez Y, et al. Pregnancies after intracytoplasmic sperm injection with cryopreserved testicular spermatozoa. Hum Reprod 1996; 11:1309–1313.
77. Gil-Salom M, Romero J, Rubio C, et al. Intracytoplasmic sperm injection with cryopreserved testicular spermatozoa. Mol Cell Endocrinol 2000; 169:15–19.
78. De Croo I, Van der Elst J, Everaert K, et al. Fertilization, pregnancy and embryo implantation rates after ICSI

with fresh or frozen-thawed testicular spermatozoa. Hum Reprod 1998; 13:1893–1897.

79. Prins GS, Dolgina R, Studney P, et al. Quality of cryopreserved testicular sperm in patients with obstructive and nonobstructive azoospermia. J Urol 1999; 161:1504–1508.

80. Huang FJ, Chang SY, Tsai MY, et al. Clinical implications of intracytoplasmic sperm injection using cryopreserved testicular spermatozoa from men with azoospermia. J Reprod Med 2000; 45:310–316.

81. Wood S, Thomas K, Schnauffer K, et al. Reproductive potential of fresh and cryopreserved epididymal and testicular spermatozoa in consecutive intracytoplasmic sperm injection cycles in the same patients. Fertil Steril 2002; 77:1162–1166.

82. Friedler S, Raziel A, Soffer Y, et al. Intracytoplasmic injection of fresh and cryopreserved testicular spermatozoa in patients with nonobstructive azoospermia—A comparative study. Fertil Steril 1997; 68:892–897.

83. Oates RD, Mulhall J, Burgess C, et al. Fertilization and pregnancy using intentionally cryopreserved testicular tissue as the sperm source for intracytoplasmic sperm injection in 10 men with non-obstructive azoospermia. Hum Reprod 1997; 12:734–739.

84. Ben-Yosef D, Yogev L, Hauser R, et al. Testicular sperm retrieval and cryopreservation prior to initiating ovarian stimulation as the first line approach in patients with nonobstructive azoospermia. Hum Reprod 1999; 14:1794–1801

85. Habermann H, Seo R, Cieslak J, et al. In vitro fertilization outcomes after intracytoplasmic sperm injection with fresh or frozen-thawed testicular spermatozoa. Fertil Steril 2000; 73:955–960.

86. Kupker W, Schlegel PN, Al-Hasani S, et al. Use of frozen-thawed testicular sperm for intracytoplasmic sperm injection. Fertil Steril 2000; 73:453–458.

87. Brinster RL, Avarbock MR, Germline transmission of donor haplotype following spermatogonial transplantation. Proc Natl Acad Sci U S A 1994; 91:11303–11307.

88. Brinster RL, Zimmerman JW. Spermatogenesis following male germ-cell transplantation. Proc Natl Acad Sci U S A 1994; 91:11289–11302.

89. Ogawa T, Arechnaga GM, Avarbock MR, et al. Transplantation of testis germinal cells into mouse seminiferous tubules. Int J Dev Biol 1997; 41:111–122.

90. Russell LD, Nagano M, Brinster RL. Spermatogonial transplantation. In: Stefanini et al., eds. Testicular Function: From Gene Expression to Genetic Manipulation. Berlin, Germany: Springer, 1998:41–57.

91. Schlatt S, Rosiepen G, Weinbauer GF, et al. Germ cell transfer into rat, bovine, monkey and human testes. Hum Reprod 1999; 14:144–150.

92. Kvist K, Thorup J, Byskov AG, et al. Cryopreservation of intact testicular tissue from boys with cryptorchidism. Hum Reprod 2006; 21:484–491.

93. Keros V, Hultenby K, Borgstrom B, et al. Methods of cryopreservation of testicular tissue with viable spermatogonia in pre-pubertal boys undergoing gonadotoxic cancer treatment. Hum Reprod 2007; 22:1384–1395.

94. Goossens E, Frederickx V, Geens M, et al. Cryosurvival and spermatogenesis after allografting prepubertal mouse tissue: Comparison of two cryopreservation protocols. Fertil Steril 2008; 89:725–727.

95. Jahnukainen K, Ehmcke J, Hergenrother SD, et al. Effect of cold storage and cryopreservation of immature nonhuman primate testicular tissue on spermatogonial stem cell potential in xenografts. Hum Reprod 2007; 22:1060–1067.

96. Geens M, De Block G, Goossens E, et al. Spermatogonial survival after grafting human testicular tissue to immunodeficient mice. Hum Reprod 2007; 21:390–396.

97. Geens M, Van de Velde H, De Block G, et al. The efficiency of magnetic-activated cell sorting and fluorescence-activated cell sorting in the decontamination of testicular cell suspensions in cancer patients. Hum Reprod 2008; 22: 733–742.

17 Donor insemination: Past, present, and future challenges

Vanessa J. Kay and Christopher L. R. Barratt

In the last 20 years, concomitant with the development of intracytoplasmic sperm injection (ICSI), donor insemination (DI) has undergone a radical number of changes, for example, exclusive use of cryopreserved semen, removal of the anonymity of sperm donors, widespread development of commercial sperm banking, increasing treatment of single and lesbian women, changes in societies' attitudes to the use of donor gametes—to name but a few. The purpose of this chapter is to discuss a number of these issues in the context of the history of DI and to look to the future of this treatment regimen.

There have been a number of landmarks in the development of DI but three in particular stand out. First, the advances in sperm storage and cryopreservation techniques that resulted in the first human pregnancy from cryopreserved semen—reported in 1953 (1). This allowed the universal shipment and storage of semen and facilitated the development of DI as a treatment for male infertility. The second landmark was the report by John Tyler and colleagues from Sydney, Australia, of the transmission of HIV via DI to four of eight recipients of donor semen from a man who was HIV seropositive (2). This added further evidence that HIV was transmitted via semen–at the time a debatable point in some arenas—but, for DI, it had a profound impact on the recruitment, selection, and screening of donors. Until this time there was significant use of fresh semen that produced on average superior pregnancy rates compared with cryopreserved semen. As cryopreserved semen allowed for the storage of samples and the retesting of the donors for HIV serum antibodies up to six months later, the exclusive use of cryopreserved semen became inevitable. The third significant landmark was dramatic changes in the regulatory framework in a number of countries, for example, Sweden, Australia, the Netherlands, and the United Kingdom. The regulatory framework was accompanied by a change in the attitudes to DI. This is exemplified by the clear trend in removal of anonymity of semen donors—first initiated in Sweden in 1985.

As a result of the above, DI operates in a very different framework to what it has in the past and faces a number of challenges.

IS DONOR INSEMINATION A TREATMENT IN CONTINUAL DECLINE?

Unlike IVF/ICSI, where there is a plethora of worldwide information, comprehensive national data on the use of DI are not widely available; thus, it is difficult to accurately determine regional and worldwide trends. In the United Kingdom, which has a well-regulated assisted conception sector, the Human Fertilisation and Embryology Authority (HFEA) publish annual statistics on each and every treatment cycle in assisted conception. As such, at least since 1992, we can see a trend in the use of DI (Fig. 1 and Tables 1 and 2). It is clear that there is a noticeable decline in the use of DI. A similar picture is observed in Australia and New Zealand, where there has been a decline from 5425 cycles in 1998 to 3356 cycles in 2005 (3). Interestingly, in parallel, there has been a dramatic rise in the number of ICSI cycles, the number of which is still rising. In the United Kingdom, for example, there was an 18% increase in the number of patients receiving ICSI treatment between 2004 and 2006 (16,698 vs. 19,506) (Table 1). This trend is mirrored by the experience throughout the world [39.6% of assisted reproductive techniques (ART) cycles were ICSI in 1997, which has risen to 58.9% in 2004] (4).

It is not possible to accurately quantify the reasons for the decline in DI treatment, but an overriding factor is the availability of alternative therapy to treat the male, that is, ICSI. As such, the decline in the use of DI was predictable. However, in the United Kingdom, as with a number of other countries (please refer to the following section), there has been a significant number of changes in the regulatory framework, for example, removal of anonymity and changes in guidelines for expenses of gamete donors, which have exacerbated the decline in the availability of the service, hence restricting the possibility of treatment. It is, therefore, not possible to determine whether the decline in DI is entirely due to the use of ICSI and/or a combination of other factors.

PREVALENCE OF LOW PREGNANCY RATES FROM DONOR INSEMINATION

Unfortunately, at least in the United Kingdom, there has been no notable increase in the success rates of DI (livebirths/treatment cycle) (Table 2). Since 1994 the success rates have not noticeably increased (approximately 10% LRB/cycle). This is remarkable and we would say unacceptable. David and colleagues were achieving this standard of success nearly 40 years ago--in 1970s using cryopreserved semen (5). Bearing in mind the technological advances in assisted conception, which have undoubtedly facilitated the increase in success of IVF/ICSI, it is very surprising that our success in DI remains so low. DI is a very simple treatment and as long as the female has no significant pathology, semen is inseminated at roughly the correct time, success rates greater than 10% should easily be achieved. Why, then, are success rates so poor? They are a plethora of reasons (possible excuses), which are included in the following sections.

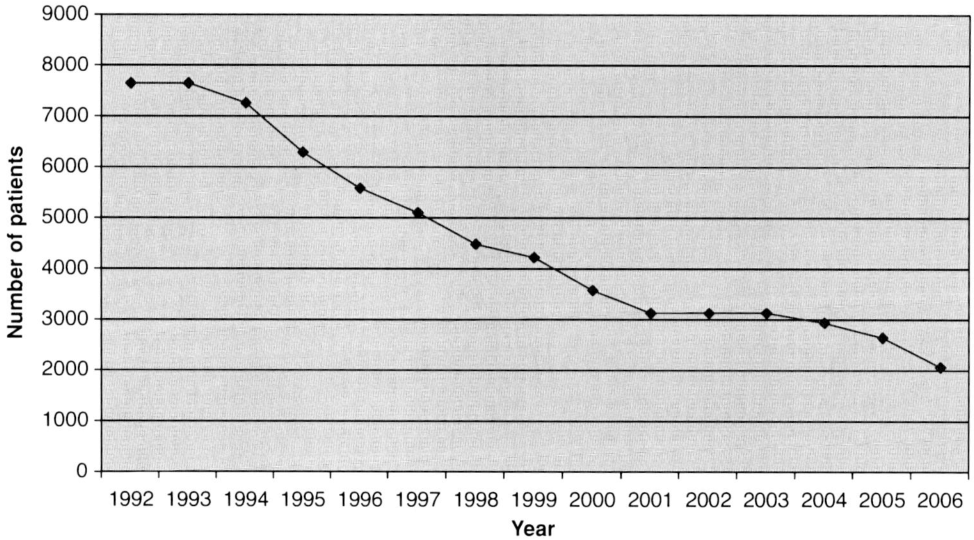

Figure 1 Number of DI patients per year in the UK, 1992–2006.

The Quality of the Semen Is Poorer Than in the Past

In order to compensate for the increasing difficulty in recruiting donors, it is possible that the normally high standards/threshold for acceptable semen parameters have been reduced. This would allow more donors to be accepted into a program and thus, at first glance, maintain the number of active donors. However, the semen quality would be reduced. At least from our clinical experience in obtaining semen from U.K. suppliers (sperm banks), this is the case. This is inappropriate and represents a false economy. There is a plethora of data showing that semen quality is critical for success in DI; for example, data from CECOS show that the mean fecundity is doubled if the number of motile sperms per straw (insemination) is increased from <5 to >10 million motile cells. Recruiting semen donors has always been challenging, time consuming, and difficult (6). There is a very high attrition rate throughout the recruitment, screening, and

Table 1 Treatment Cycles Per Year for DI, IVF, and ICSI in the U.K., HFEA Data, 2006

Year	DI	IVF	ICSI	Total
1992	26,078	18,201	128	44,407
1993	24,230	21,239	578	46,047
1994	21,484	23,517	1,284	46,285
1995	18,001	25,414	3,822	47,237
1996	14,913	27,203	6,176	48,292
1997	13,305	25,033	8,917	47,255
1998	11,579	23,551	11,906	47,036
1999	10,207	22,737	12,077	45,021
2000	8,354	22,722	12,728	43,804
2001	7,580	22,344	13,858	43,782
2002	7,323	22,479	14,921	44,743
2003	7,322	21,899	15,521	44,742
2004	6,888	23,283	16,698	46,869
2005	5,839	23,704	17,523	47,066
2006	4,001	22,076	19,506	45,583

Abbreviations: DI, donor insemination; IVF, in vitro fertilization; ICSI, intracytoplasmic sperm injection; HFEA, Human Fertilisation and Embryology Authority.

Table 2 Trends in Donor Insemination in the United Kingdom, 1992–2006

Year	Number of patients	Number of treatment cycles[a]	% Low Birth Rate (LBR)	Number of IVF cycles with donor sperm	% IVF cycle using donor sperm
1992	7,642	26,078	5.2	1,252	8.8
1993	7,634	24,230	6.4	1,657	10.1
1994	7,258	21,484	8.0	1,634	9.3
1995	6,296	18,001	8.8	1,527	8.3
1996	5,583	14,913	9.7	1,363	7.6
1997	5,106	13,305	9.6	1,150	7.3
1998	4,496	11,579	10.0	1,021	6.5
1999	4,224	10,207	10.7	929	6.4
2000	3,575	8,354	10.4	873	5.8
2001	3,138	7,580	10.5	781	5.7
2002	3,134	7,323	11.3	814	5.6
2003	3,113	7,322	10.7	802	5.4
2004	2,951	6,888	10.3	798	5.1
2005	2,639	5,839	[b]	807	5.0
2006	2,054	4,001	[b]	524	3.8

[a]Excludes IVF.
[b]Data not available.
Abbreviations: LBR, live birth rate; IVF, in vitro fertilization.

selection process. Often, fewer than 5% of men who enquire about being a semen donor actually end up being accepted for use in treatment (7). So while it is difficult to recruit donors, and it is easier to reduce standards, there is nothing to be gained and everything to lose by reducing the threshold for acceptance.

Cryopreservation Reduces Semen Fertilizing Ability

This is undoubtedly correct. Historical controls provide ample evidence that, in comparable doses, cryopreserved semen produces fewer pregnancies (52% cumulative pregnancy rate vs. 83% cumulative pregnancy rate for cryopreserved vs. fresh semen, respectively) (8). However, as a result of the need to screen donors for HIV, there is an absolute necessity to use cryopreserved semen. Since the original methods of vapor freezing with glycerol, there have been many improvements in cryopreservation regimes, which significantly enhance the preservation of the functional ability of cryopreserved cells (9). Therefore, it is our premise that as 10% per cycle success rates were being achieved using intracervical insemination with cryopreserved semen in the 1970s, with our enhanced knowledge base, we should be able to double these.

Optimal Timing and Site of Insemination Remains Unresolved

In spite of improvements in cryopreservation methods, spermatozoa survival in a functional state in the female reproductive tract will be reduced. As such it is important to inseminate the spermatozoa in the preovulatory period to account for the limited (reduced) fertile window of the cryopreserved spermatozoon. A variety of papers have discussed the "best" methods to do this: basal body temperature, ultrasound follicle tracking, luteinizing hormone dipsticks, etc., but accurate timing of inseminations, taking into account the considerable variations between and within patients in ovulatory patterns (Table 3), is absolutely necessary.

Perhaps because of the reduced fertilizing potential of cryopreserved sperm, a number of authors have suggested that two inseminations per treatment cycle are necessary. The evidence to support the use of two rather than one well-timed insemination remains inconsistent and thus, in view of the potential shortage of semen, one well-timed insemination with high quality semen should be sufficient.

The main method of insemination of CECOS is intracervical (11), with intrauterine insemination (IUI) being used, following unsuccessful intracervical insemination, for example, after 12 failed cycles. However, the trend in the United States is for first-line treatment using IUI (12), often using IUI-ready preparations. It is difficult to assess whether IUI is really necessary as a first choice, as often when studies have compared the use of IUI with intracervical inseminations, the conception rates in the latter have been very poor compared with those in normal practice (13).

Table 3 Distribution of the Day of the Onset of the LH Surge in 250 Regularly Cycling Women, Attending from Day 8 or 9 of the Cycle for Daily LH Monitoring

Day of cycle	Number of subjects	% Starting LH rise	Cumulative %
<9	13	5.2	5.2
10	26	10.4	15.6
11	41	16.4	32.0
12	45	18.0	50.0
13	39	15.6	65.6
14	27	10.8	76.4
15	23	9.2	85.6
16	21	8.4	94.0
17	1	0.4	94.4
18	7	2.8	97.2
19	6	2.4	99.6
20	1	0.4	100

Abbreviations: LH, luteinizing hormone.
Source: Adapted from Ref 10.

The Effective Screening of Recipients

Clearly, an important factor in outcome with DI is the fertility of the female partner. There are various factors that may result in decreased female fertility. It is well established that the age at which women decide to start a family is increasing; for example, the mean age of childbearing has increased in England and Wales from 26.4 years in 1978 to 28.9 years by 1998 (14). Female age is known to be an important prognostic factor in all fertility treatments. Ferrara et al. (15) confirmed that IUI with DI is a poor treatment option for women older than 40 years (overall pregnancy rate in those aged <35 years is 18.5% and in those aged >40 years is 5.4%).

Another issue that adversely affects female fertility is obesity, which has been increasing by 10% to 40% in Europe in the last 10 years (16). Women who are overweight are more likely to be infertile and have lower success rates with all fertility treatments, including assisted conception (17). While it is known that obesity may cause infertility due to anovulation, there is increasing evidence that even when anovulation has been excluded, obesity affects the chance of spontaneous pregnancy, with a linear decrease in pregnancy once body mass index is more than 29 kg/m^2 (18). This is of particular relevance in DI, when ovulatory dysfunction should be excluded or corrected with appropriate therapy before commencing treatment. In a study on DI by Zaadstra et al. (19), a 0.1 unit increase in waist-to-hip ratio led to a 30% decrease in probability of conception per cycle. There is little doubt that success rates with DI can be improved by rationing access to treatment by female age and weight. However, there remains contention as to the precise criteria at which these restrictions should apply.

The rate of pelvic infection with *Chlamydia* is known to be rising rapidly, with an increase of 61% in U.K. clinics from 1996 to 1999 and being highest in women younger than 20 years

(20). It is well established that *Chlamydia trachomatis*, even when asymptomatic, causes pelvic inflammatory disease leading to tubal infertility (21). Tubal disease will decrease pregnancy rates from DI (22). Moreover, with the advancing age of recipients, other pelvic pathologies that reduce fertility, such as endometriosis and uterine fibroids, will become increasingly common.

Previous studies have reported that asymptomatic ovulatory women with no history of pelvic disease have a low incidence of abnormal findings at hysterosalpingogram [HSG; 2.8% (23)]. Moreover, the probability of finding pelvic pathology is only 1.8% in couples with severe male factor infertility willing to undergo ICSI (24). It has been established in DI recipients that pelvic pathology is less common in women with azoospermic partners, compared to those with oligoasthenoteratozoospermic partners (25). A likely explanation is that in men with poor semen quality, there is more likely to be coexisting female factors, as the highly fertile women have already conceived spontaneously.

Given this low rate of pelvic disease, it has been advised that tubal assessment should be performed only in women with a history suggestive of tubal damage or only after three unsuccessful treatment cycles (26). However, in view of this increasing prevalence of *Chlamydia* infection, the rising maternal age, and the shortage of donor sperm, it may be reasonable to consider offering tubal assessment prior to DI treatment.

Another issue to consider is the optimal method to assess for pelvic pathology. Laparoscopy and HSG are currently the two most widely used methods. Laparoscopy is more invasive, but it has been shown to detect more pelvic pathology and, if required, treatment can be performed during the procedure. In women undergoing IUI with a normal HSG, laparoscopy demonstrated severe pelvic disease in 4% that resulted in a change of treatment to in vitro fertilization (IVF) or open surgery. A further 21% had less severe pelvic disease (endometriosis and adhesions), which was treated laparoscopically followed by IUI (27). However, prospective studies are required to evaluate the cost-effectiveness and whether the changes that resulted from the laparoscopy led to improved overall pregnancy. As such, it has been recommended that HSG be used to screen for tubal disease and laparoscopy be reserved for women with a history or clinical findings suggestive of pelvic disease (26).

RECRUITMENT AND SCREENING OF SEMEN DONORS

Recruitment of Donors

There have been dramatic developments in the regulations surrounding the recruitment and use of semen donors. There is a strong trend to remove anonymity. Sweden was the first country to effectively remove anonymity. On March 18, 1985, the Swedish Parliament enacted legislation providing the child with the right "when sufficiently mature" to receive identifying information about the semen provider (28). The reasons for the removal of anonymity include the principle that children have a right for information regarding their genetic parents. There are various factors that have influenced this principle, including evidence that an increasing number of diseases have a genetic origin, more accurate DNA testing allowing children to identify their genetic origins, allowing donor offspring to identify genetically related partners, and increasing use of family donors for organ donation. Following the example of Sweden, a number of countries have removed the use of anonymous sperm donors, for example, the Netherlands and the United Kingdom, while other counties have a mixed system (dual track) with identifiable and anonymous donation, for example, the United States and Australia (29).

Infertility service providers expressed considerable reservations that the change in policy, that is, removal of anonymity, would result in a decline in the availability of donors. This was supported by research in both the United Kingdom and Sweden that showed that 63% to 70% of donors would not donate if tracing was possible (30,31). However, in the United Kingdom, following extensive discussion including consultation with the public, the law was changed (32,33). In order to alleviate concerns over the perceived increased challenges of recruiting semen donors, that is, a shortage of donors, an interim period (12 months) was allowed whereby a dual-track system operated—anonymous and identified donors. As from April 2005, only donors willing to be identified could donate. In the lead-up period to the change in legislation, a number of U.K. clinics reported a considerable shortage of sperm donors (34).

With the lead up to and the removal of anonymity in a number of countries, there has been a plethora of studies discussing the impact of these changes on the number of sperm donors, suggesting alternative/complementary methods to recruit semen donors. The evidence is not easy to interpret but suffice it to say that removal of anonymity did initially reduce the number of donors (35). However, it is clear that what is required is a more comprehensive understanding of the needs of the donors and thus, subsequently, tailoring the recruitment and selection strategy (Table 4) (33). If this is performed, the precipitous decline in the number of donors can be halted (35) As such, reassuringly, any decline in sperm donor numbers following removal of anonymity appears to be temporary (see Table 5 and Fig. 2). In Sweden (the first country to change legislation), there was a temporary decline in numbers, followed by an increase in sperm donors reaching a level higher than that prior to legislation (36). The most recent data in the United Kingdom show a 6% increase in men registering as sperm donors (32). However, despite this, there are still considerable difficulties in obtaining donated sperm in many U.K. clinics. One probable reason is that the number of donors available is not sufficient to meet the demand; that is, we have our calculations wrong.

As part of a national strategy, it is essential to determine the number of donors required. CECOS have been doing this for years. For example, in 1989, 600 donors were required for 3600 patients (11). As more than 740 donors were recruited in

Table 4 Sperm Donor Recruitment

Potential sperm donor contacts the donor center

Record details
- Name
- Address
- Date of birth

Ask whether have previously donated sperm

Not suitable as sperm donor
- Age 46 or older or younger than 18 years
- Previously donated sperm and exceeded the limit of 10 families

Advise not suitable as sperm donor

Suitable for further assessment as sperm donor
- Age between 18 and 45 years
- Either not previously donated sperm, or if donated not reached the limit of 10 families

Information pack posted
- Medical questionnaire (current health, past medical history, fertility history, family/genetic history, sexual history)
- Information on consent to disclosure of information
- What you need to know about donating sperm, eggs, or embryos (HFEA leaflet)
- Donor Information
- Donor center information sheets including information for sperm donors, counselling information, and blood-borne virus screening

Donor contacts unit

Yes → **Arrange a clinic appointment**

No → **No further action**

Semen analysis arranged

Donor attends clinic appointment
- Assess result of the semen sample
- Assess medical history, using completed questionnaires and any relevant further questioning
- Perform general and genital examination

(*Continued*)

Table 4 Sperm Donor Recruitment *(Continued)*

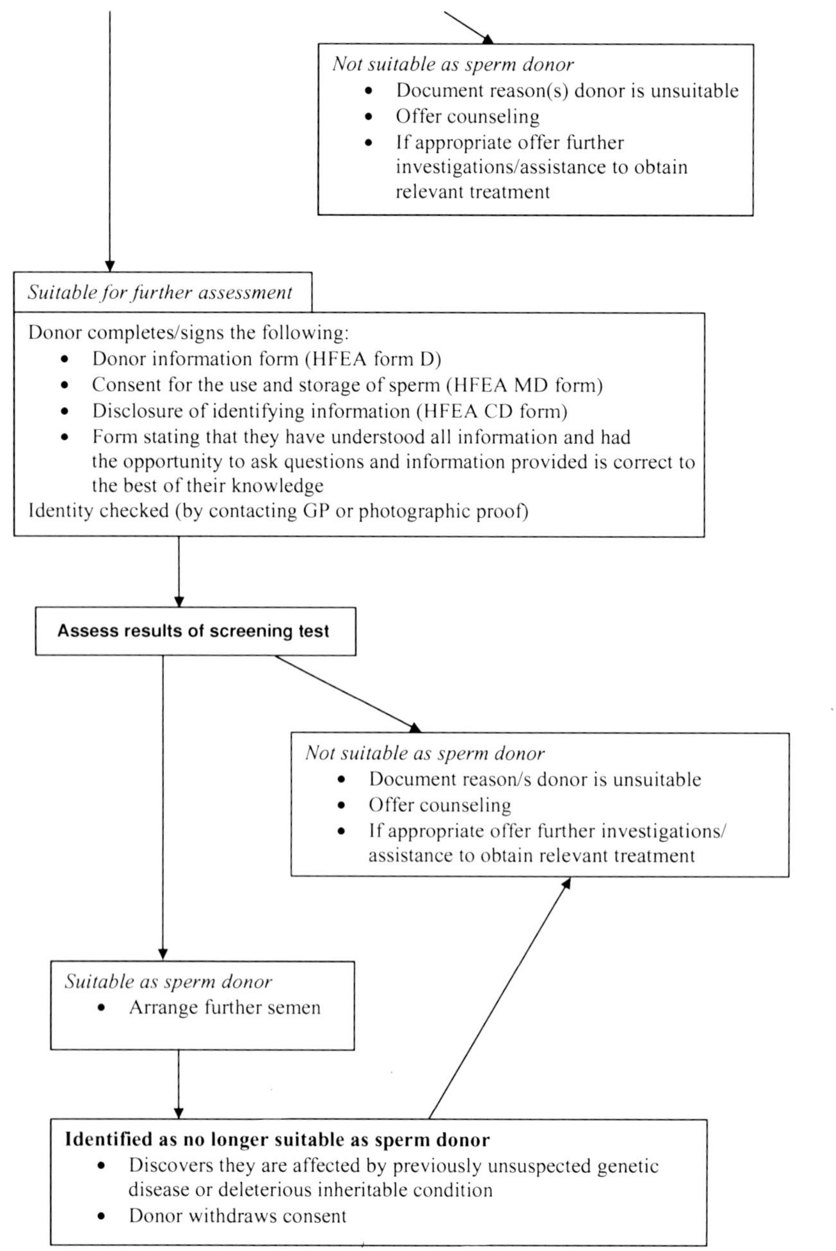

that year, this was sufficient. It is difficult to generate accurate calculations about the numbers, but if we use U.K. data and assume that ICSI was widely available in 1997, then we would assume that the number of patients requiring DI is approximately 5200 (Table 2). From this, it is possible to calculate (estimate) the number of donors that are required to serve this demand. If we assume that 2000 births are likely to be required (>40% of patients should get a birth), and only a maximum number of 10 livebirths per donor are allowed, then accounting for different ethnicity, some flexibility in matching characteristics, etc., we would need 1200 donors (200 if we allow no choice). There were only 356 new registered donors in 1997 in the United Kingdom—a considerable shortfall (Table 5, Fig. 2). Thus, we conclude that a shortage of donors is exacerbating the decline in the availability of treatment. Therefore, the starting point in any national strategy should be to determine how

Table 5 Number of Registered Donors with the HFEA (as on December 4, 2007)

Year	Number of registered donors
1992	369
1993	431
1994	422
1995	418
1996	421
1997	356
1998	265
1999	308
2000	325
2001	328
2002	278
2003	255
2004	247
2005	259
2006	307

Abbreviations: HFEA, Human Fertilisation and Embryology Authority.

many patients we expect to treat and thus, how many donors will we need.

One important factor that has been shown to strongly influence the recruitment of sperm donors is the use of financial incentives. Regulations vary across different countries, with an increasing number of countries restricting the financial incentives. In the United Kingdom, a nationwide report [the SEED review 2005 (32)] concluded that in addition to expenses, donors could be compensated for loss of earnings up to £55.19 per day (maximum £250 for each course of sperm donation although "course" was not rigorously defined). The SEED review concluded that financial reasons should not be the primary motivation for donation and thus, financial benefits are restricted. Not surprisingly, there have been fears among health care providers that this will result in a reduction in men being prepared to provide sperm. To date it is unclear what will happen in Europe with the implementation of the new EU regulations (37), but it is likely that financial incentives for gamete donors will be restricted.

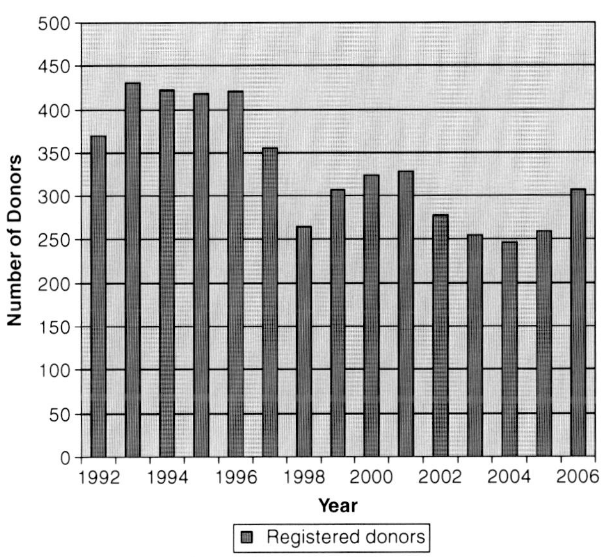

Figure 2 Number of registered donors with the HFEA.

With the change in financial compensation for semen donors, the characteristics of sperm donors may change. For example, older men are more prepared to donate sperm when there is no financial incentive than younger men (30). Interestingly, there is evidence that men who are prepared to donate sperms without financial incentives are more willing to be identified to offspring (38). Data from the Human Fertilisation and Embryology Authority (32) demonstrate changes in characteristics of sperm donors in the United Kingdom over the last 10 years: sperm donors are more likely to be family men (41.5% vs. 21% had children) and older (69% vs. 32.2% older than 30 years). In addition, there appears to be more homosexual men seeking to become sperm donors, with two out of eight men in our unit being homosexual in 2007. This may reflect more openness regarding homosexuality and also a desire of homosexual men to further their gene line. However, there are concerns regarding homosexual men being more likely to be infected with blood-borne viruses, including HIV. This resulted in the FDA making the controversial decision to ban homosexual sperm donors in America in 1995. However, sexual orientation does not reflect individual sexual behavior, and therefore, any criteria for rejection should be based on promiscuous sexual behavior.

There is limited evidence about the views of recipients over homosexual sperm donors. The sexual preference of oocyte donors was considered essential information for 60% of recipients (39). Conversely, some recipients may prefer a homosexual donor; for example, a group of lesbian and bisexual women in America have recommended that they have access specifically to gay sperm donors (40). Sexual orientation should not be used to discriminate when selecting semen donors; however, recipients should not be denied information regarding their donor.

All the above changes in sperm donor characteristics require individual clinics to modify their recruitment practices to attract these new groups of sperm donors. There is now strong evidence that improved counseling, support, and information are mandatory for the development of an effective recruitment program (33).

Screening of Semen Donors

Since 1985, there has been guidance that semen donors need to be screened for HIV. Currently, this involves retesting the donor for HIV antibodies in the serum, following a quarantine period of six months. This long-term quarantine creates a number of problems, for example, (1) requirement for considerable storage capacity and (2) difficulties with donors agreeing to rescreening. If we could have a more rapid screening method, for example, HIV RNA of the semen, then perhaps we could screen each sample, thus reducing the need for such a long quarantine period. Rapid screening methods for HIV RNA do exist (41), and it will be interesting to see whether they can be adapted for screening semen donors. If this could be done, then the process of recruiting and screening semen donors would be significantly shortened and, importantly, made easier.

CHANGES IN INDICATION FOR DONOR INSEMINATION

There are numerous indications for DI treatment. In a 12-year retrospective review of more than 1800 cycles by Zuzuarregui et al. (42), the commonest was azoospermia (46.8%), followed by oligozoospermia (40.2%). Other indications for DI included HIV seropositive male (0.9%), genetic disease (1.9%), ICSI failure (2.5%), and women without a male partner (7.5%). Since the successful introduction of ICSI, there are changes in the clinical indications for DI. Most men with oligozoospermia now opt for ICSI rather than DI although for personal or financial reasons a significant proportion (33%) will still prefer DI (43). Hence, the proportion of men with oligozoospermia having DI has and will decrease. This should result in improved DI success rates as the female partners of men with oligozoospermia have reduced fertility, with cumulative pregnancy rates over six cycles of 64% in azoospermic patients versus 32% in severe male factor patients (42). With the development and establishment of a number of other new techniques, including sperm washing for HIV discordant couples and preimplantation genetic diagnosis of genetic disease, further changes in the indications for DI are expected.

One specific area that is likely to significantly increase is the number of women without a male partner seeking treatment (44). This may reflect a widespread acceptance by society of single parents and gay couples. Evidence shows that offspring from single mothers and same-sex couples are not disadvantaged (45,46). However, there remains contention in many countries over whether women without a male partner should have the same rights to treatment as do couples. In the United Kingdom, there has recently been a change in the regulation that no longer requires taking into account the need for a father when considering the welfare of the child. However, concerns about being accused of discrimination by not treating women without a male partner remains to be rigorously tested.

FUTURE OPPORTUNITIES

DI provides an excellent tool for research, for example, examining the role of female factors on success. Specific questions such as the timing of inseminations (and site of insemination) can be rigorously addressed. However, what is surprising is that it is relatively poorly used (47) and perhaps what is required is a national/regional network to direct such studies.

With alterations in regulation (particularly, regarding anonymity and financial compensation), the characteristics of semen donors and recipients are dramatically changing and presumably will continue to change. This provides an excellent tool to study the developments in society's attitudes to reproductive choices, essential if we are to maintain public confidence regarding any advances in treatment and research. In addition, to optimize the recruitment of high quality semen donors, it is important to further our understanding of the characteristics and motivation of current donors.

CONCLUSION

With the decline in DI, there have been changes in the clinical indications for use. Unfortunately, ongoing pregnancy rates remain low, with poor quality semen and reduced female fertility being the main contributory factors. There is inconsistent data regarding optimal timing and methods of insemination. With changes in regulations, the characteristics of sperm donors and recipients are altering, with more donors who are family men and older, and an increasing number of recipients being women without male partners. Such changes have implications for future recruitment and clinical practices.

RECOMMENDATIONS

1. DI is a relatively simple effective treatment but is being used less frequently than before (A, 1b).
2. DI is often performed under suboptimal conditions (A, 2a). We have shown that success rates can be improved.
3. A number of key factors affect success; these include female infertility, for example, age, and practical aspects such as timing of inseminations and semen quality. Simple steps can be taken to control for these and also to improve the number and quality of the semen donors (A, 1b).

Grade of guideline recommendations (uppercase alphabets) and levels of evidence (lowercase alphabets with numerals) are given in parentheses.

REFERENCES

1. Bunge RG, Keettel WC, Sherman JK. Clinical use of frozen semen: Report of four cases. Fertil Steril 1954; 5:520–529.
2. Stewart GJ, Tyler JP, Cunningham AL, et al. Transmission of human T-cell lymphotropic virus type III (HTLV-III) by artificial insemination by donor. Lancet 1985; 14:581–585.
3. National Perinatal Statistics, 2007. http://www.npsu.unsw.edu.au/.
4. Nyboe Andersen A, Carlsen E, Loft A. Trends in the use of intracytoplasmatic sperm injection marked variability between countries. Hum Reprod Update 2008; 14:593–604.
5. David G, Czyglik F, Mayaux MJ, et al. Artificial insemination with frozen sperm: Protocol, method of analysis and results for 1188 women. Br J Obstet Gynaecol 1980; 87:1022–1028.
6. Barratt CLR, Cooke ID, eds. Donor Insemination. Cambridge, United Kingdom: Cambridge University Press, 1993:231.

7. Chauhan M, Barratt CL, Cooke S, et al. A protocol for the recruitment and screening of semen donors for an artificial insemination by donor programme. Hum Reprod 1988; 3:873–876.
8. Keel BA, Webster BW. Semen cryopreservation methodology and results. In: Barratt CLR, Cooke ID, eds. Donor Insemination. Cambridge, United Kingdom: Cambridge University Press, 1993:71–96.
9. Mortimer D. Current and future concepts and practices in human sperm cryobanking. Reprod Biomed Online 2004; 9: 134–151.
10. Lenton EA Ovulation timing. In: Barratt CLR, Cooke ID, eds. Donor Insemination. Cambridge, United Kingdom: Cambridge University Press, 1993:97–110.
11. Le Lannou D, Lansac J; Federation CECOS. Artificial procreation with frozen donor semen: The French experience of CECOS. In: Barratt CLR, Cooke ID, eds. Donor Insemination. Cambridge, United Kingdom: Cambridge University Press, 1993:152–169.
12. Wolf DP, Patton PE, Burry KA, et al. Intrauterine insemination-ready versus conventional semen cryopreservation for donor insemination: A comparison of retrospective results and a prospective, randomized trial. Fertil Steril 2001; 76:181–185.
13. Marshburn PB, McIntire D, Carr BR, et al. Spermatozoal characteristics from fresh and frozen donor semen and their correlation with fertility outcome after intrauterine insemination. Fertil Steril 1992; 58:179–186.
14. http://www.statistics.gov.uk.
15. Ferrara I, Balet R, Grudzinskas JG. Intrauterine insemination with frozen donor sperm. Pregnancy outcome in relation to age and ovarian stimulation regime. Hum Reprod 2002; 17:2320–2324.
16. http://www.iotf.org.
17. Wang JX, Davies M, Norman RJ. Body mass and probability of pregnancy during assisted reproduction treatment: Retrospective study. BMJ 2000; 321:1320–1321.
18. Van der Steeg JW, Steures P, Eijkemans MJC, et al. Obesity affects spontaneous pregnancy chances in subfertile, ovulatory women. Hum Reprod 2008; 23(2):324–328.
19. Zaadstra BM, Seidell JC, Van Noord PA, et al. Fat and female fecundity: Prospective study of effect of body fat distribution on conception rates. BMJ 1993; 306:484–487.
20. PHLS, Department of Health, Social Services, and Public Safety Northern Ireland, Scottish ISD(D) 5 Collaborative Group. Sexually transmitted infections in the UK: New episodes seen at genitourinary medicine clinics, 1995 to 2000. London, United Kingdom: Public Health Laboratory Service, 2001.
21. Paavonen J, Eggert-Kruse W. *Chlamydia trachomatis:* Impact on human reproduction. Hum Reprod Update 1999; 5:433–447.
22. Bradshaw KD, Guzick DS, Grun B, et al. Cumulative pregnancy rates for donor insemination according to ovulatory function and tubal status. Fertil Steril 1987; 48:1051–1054.
23. Stovall DW, Christman GM, Hammond MG, et al. Abnormal findings on hysterosalpingography: Effects on fecundity in a donor insemination program using frozen semen. Obstet Gynecol 1992; 80:249–252.
24. Balasch B. Investigation of the infertile couple in the era of assisted reproductive technology: A time for reappraisal. Hum Reprod 2000; 15:2251–2257.
25. Emperaire JC, Gauzere Soumireu E, Audebert AJ. Female fertility and donor insemination. Fertil Steril 1982; 37: 90–93.
26. National Institute for Health and Clinical Excellence. NICE Guidelines. Fertility: Assessment and treatment for people with fertility problems, Clinical Guideline 11, February 2004.
27. Tanahatoe S, Hompes PGA, Lambalk CB. Accuracy of diagnostic laparoscopy in the infertility work-up before intrauterine insemination. Fertil Steril 2003; 79:361–366.
28. Lalos A, Daniels K, Gottlieb C, et al. Recruitment and motivation of semen providers in Sweden. Hum Reprod 2003; 18:212–216.
29. De Jonge C, Barratt CL Gamete donation: A question of anonymity. Fertil Steril 2006; 85:500–501.
30. Cook R, Golombok S. A survey of semen donation: Phase 2—The view of the donors. Hum Reprod 1995; 10;951–959.
31. Lui SC, Weaver SM. Attitudes and motives of semen donors and non-donors. Human Reprod 1996; 11:2061–2066.
32. http://www.hfea.gov.uk.
33. Frith L, Blyth E, Farrand A. UK gamete donors' reflections on the removal of anonymity: Implications for recruitment. Hum Reprod 2007; 22:1675–1680.
34. Paul S, Harbottle S, Stewart JA. Recruitment of sperm donors: The Newcastle-upon-Tyne experience 1994–2003. Hum Reprod 2006; 21:150–158.
35. Janssens PM, Simons AH, van Kooij RJ, et al. A new Dutch Law regulating provision of identifying information of donors to offspring: Background, content and impact. Hum Reprod 2006; 21:852–856.
36. Daniels K, Lalos O. The Swedish insemination act and the availability of donors. Human Reprod 1995; 10:1871–1874.
37. EU Tissue and Cells Directive, 2004.
38. Daniels K, Feyles V, Nisker J, et al. Sperm donation: Implications of Canada's Assisted Human Reproduction Act 2004 for Recipients, Donors, Health Professionals, and Intuitions. J Obstet Gynaecol Can 2006; 608–615.
39. Voll S, Hamacher P, Toner J. Pertinent oocyte donor characteristics—What oocyte recipients wish to know about oocyte donors. Fertil Steril 1996; 66(suppl i):S25.
40. Ross LE, Steele L, Epstein R. Lesbian and bisexual women's recommendations for improving the provision of assisted reproductive technology services. Fertil Steril 2006; 86:735–738.

41. Schumacher W, Frick E, Kauselmann M, et al. Fully automated quantification of human immunodeficiency virus (HIV) type 1 RNA in human plasma by the COBAS AmpliPrep/COBAS TaqMan system. J Clin Virol 2007; 38;304–312.
42. Zuzuarregui JL, Meseguer M, Garrido N, et al. Parameters affecting the results in a program of artificial insemination with donor sperm. A 12-year retrospective review of more than 1800 cycles. J Assist Reprod Genet 2004; 21, 4:109–118.
43. Vernaeve V, Festre V, Baetens P, et al. Reproductive decisions by couples undergoing artificial insemination with donor sperm for severe male infertility: Implications for medical counselling. Int J Androl 2005; 28:22–26.
44. http://www.bancodesemeninternacional.net.
45. Murray C, Golombok S. Solo mothers and their donor insemination infants: Follow-up at age 2 years. Hum Reprod 2005; 20:1655–1660.
46. Gartrell N, Deck A, Rodas C, et al. The national lesbian family study: 4. Interviews with the 10-year-old children. Am J Orthopsychiatry 2005; 75:518–524.
47. Barratt CL, Chauhan M, Cooke ID. Donor insemination—A look to the future. Fertil Steril 1990; 54:375–387.

18 Male contraception

Ahmed Mahmoud and Guy T'Sjoen

INTRODUCTION

The impact of the development of a reliable hormonal contraception for males will likely be far less than the development of the contraceptive pill for the female. However, several studies indicate that such a contraceptive is desired by males as well as their female partners (1,2). The challenge to develop a male hormonal contraceptive that is convenient, reversible, and environmentally friendly (3) with few or no side effects is ongoing despite many recent advances in the field (4).

In order to logically explain the working mechanisms of hormonal contraception for males, it is appropriate to summarize the physiology of sperm production.

SPERM PRODUCTION

Spermatogenesis can be subdivided into four major steps (5), namely, *mitosis*, which is the multiplication of spermatogonia; *meiosis* (reduction division), which reduces the chromosome number from diploid to haploid (The cells, now called "primary spermatocytes," divide to form secondary spermatocytes, and then divide again to form round spermatids.); *spermiogenesis*, which is the transformation of the round spermatid into the complex structure of the spermatozoon; and *spermiation*, during which the spermatozoa are released into the lumen of the seminiferous tubule.

Sperm Transport, Storage, and Maturation

After spermatozoa have been released into the lumen of the seminiferous tubules, they are transported to the rete testis and pass through the epididymis. During this passage, spermatozoa undergo multiple changes in their membrane composition and in their metabolic activity, resulting in activation of motility. Spermatozoa are stored in the epididymis and in the ampulla of the vas deferens. During the first fraction of ejaculation, these spermatozoa are expelled together with the secretions of the prostate, and the second fraction of the ejaculate contains mostly the secretory products of the seminal vesicles. The ejaculation process is controlled by the sympathic nervous system, and the activity of the accessory sex glands is androgen dependent (6).

HORMONAL CONTROL OF SPERMATOGENESIS

In addition to sperm production, the testes produce steroid hormones. Spermatogenesis and steroidogenesis take place in two compartments that are morphologically and functionally well distinguished from each other: the tubular compartment, consisting of the seminiferous tubules, and the interstitial compartment between the seminiferous tubules. Although anatomically divided, both compartments are functionally connected to each other, and their integrity is necessary for quantitatively and qualitatively normal spermatogenesis (review: 7).

The function of the testis and thereby also the function of its compartments are primarily influenced by the hypothalamus and the pituitary gland, whereas at the testicular level, various local regulators (paracrine and autocrine factors) modulate the endocrine hormone actions in somatic and gamete cells directly.

Pulsatile secretion of gonadotropin-releasing hormone (GnRH) from the hypothalamus stimulates the production and release of the gonadotropins, luteinizing hormone (LH), and follicle-stimulating hormone (FSH) by the pituitary. LH stimulates Leydig cells to produce high levels of intratesticular testosterone (T). Intratesticular levels of T are several folds greater than in the systemic circulation (8). T in blood exerts a negative feedback on the hypothalamus, where it is aromatized to estradiol.

Sertoli cells play a pivotal role in the initiation and maintenance of spermatogenesis (9). Their function is stimulated mainly by FSH (reviews: 9,10). In response to FSH, Sertoli cells secrete, among many other substances, inhibin B, which, in turn, is part of the negative feedback loop regulating FSH secretion. The integrity of the spermatogenic process appears to be a second fundamental component in the regulation of inhibin B secretion from the testis.

A much-debated subject is the relative importance of FSH and LH/intratesticular T for the initiation and maintenance of human spermatogenesis. Studies indicate that either hormone can solely initiate or maintain spermatogenesis to some extent. Both hormones, however, are needed for the initiation and maintenance of a quantitatively and qualitatively normal spermatogenesis compatible with normal fertility (11,12).

HORMONAL CONTRACEPTION

Because spermatogenesis is under tight hormonal control, the hormonal approach via the suppression of pituitary gonadotrophins, and as a result suppression of LH/intratesticular T and FSH production, has been used to develop clinically applicable contraceptives for men (13). Studies from the World Health Organization (WHO) indicate that a sperm concentration below 3 million/mL is acceptable since the pregnancy rate is 1.4/100 years, which is similar to that obtained from the female contraceptive pill (14,15).

Androgens Alone

Several forms of T have been tested as a male contraceptive including intramuscular injections of T, both short-acting preparations such as T enanthate (weekly injections) as well as long-acting preparations (T buciclate, T undecanoate) and subcutaneous T and 7α-methyl-19-nortestosterone implants (reviews: 6,13,16). Several studies indicate that high normal or supraphysiological levels of androgens are needed to achieve acceptable suppression of spermatogenesis (6,13). Moreover, trials by the WHO revealed that azoospermia could be achieved in more than 90% of Asian men, but in only approximately 60% of Caucasian men (review: 16). The remaining men maintain a low rate of spermatogenesis. These high levels of circulating T result in unacceptably frequent side effects, including weight gain, gynecomastia, lowering of high-density lipoprotein (HDL) cholesterol concentration and potentially increased risk of atherogenesis, and adverse effects on the prostate (6,13).

Combined Therapy

In this approach, nonandrogenic agents were used to suppress pituitary gonadotrophins including progestins, progestin in combination with antiandrogen, oestrogens, and GnRH analogues (both agonists and antagonists) (reviews: 6,13). To counteract the side effects of the resultant systemic hypoandrogenism, exogenous T supplementation is added. This aims at achieving adequate physiological levels of T in peripheral circulation to maintain essential extragonadal androgenic actions including secondary sex characteristics, sexual function, bone, muscle, and hematopoiesis. Of these combinations, the androgen–progestin treatment regimens are the most extensively studied and the most promising.

Recently, the International Hormonal Male Contraception Summit Group reviewed its combined data to demonstrate that androgen–progestin contraceptive regimens (1) can be widely applied in men of differing ages, ethnicity, and other baseline characteristics; (2) are superior to androgens administered alone and compare favorably with vasectomy in terms of time of onset of contraceptive action; and (3) allow spermatogenesis to fully recover to levels consistent with normal male fertility in all men after cessation of androgen with and without progestin treatments (review: 4) (level of evidence: 1b).

Similarly, a recent double-blind, multicenter study assessed spermatogenesis suppression and safety of a new combination of etonogestrel subcutaneous implants combined with T undecanoate injections for male contraception using six different dose regimens. The study is the first large placebo-controlled study for male hormonal contraception (17). From six European countries, 354 healthy men were randomized to receive either a low- or high-release etonogestrel implant, SC, combined with intramuscular T undecanoate injections (750 mg every 10 or 12 weeks or 1000 mg every 12 weeks) or placebo implant and injections. Treatment duration was 42 or 44 weeks and posttreatment follow-up at least 24 weeks. Overall, spermatogenesis was suppressed to 1 million/mL or less at week 16 in 89% of men. Suppression was maintained up to the end of the treatment period in 91% of men. For all men who completed the treatment period, 3% never achieved a sperm concentration of 1 million/mL or less. Median recovery time to a sperm concentration of greater than 20 million/mL was 15 weeks. Although therapy was well tolerated, more men in the active treatment groups reported adverse events such as weight gain, mood changes, acne, sweating, or libido change. For both spermatogenesis suppression and safety, differences were small between the six active treatment groups (17) (level of evidence 1b). Despite this impressive progress, the authors indicate that this method of male hormonal contraception needs further refinement.

Factors Affecting the Recovery of Spermatogenesis

Although the reversibility of male hormonal contraception is well established, few data are available on factors affecting the speed of recovery of spermatogenesis. A multivariate analysis of the literature showed higher rates of recovery of spermatogenesis after cessation of hormonal contraception with older age, Asian origin, shorter treatment duration, shorter-acting T preparations, higher sperm concentrations at baseline, faster suppression of spermatogenesis, and lower blood concentrations of LH at baseline (18) (level of evidence 1b).

The Nonsuppressibles

Several studies explored the possible reasons for the polymorphism of spermatogenic suppression in response to exogenous T between Asian and European men.

Intratesticular androgenic bioactivity was found to be three times higher than that of intratesticular T during contraception treatment with T enanthate and levonorgestrel, suggesting that other androgens may be prevalent in the low intratesticular T environment (8). One possible compensation may be an increase in 5-α-reductase activity within the testes, resulting in relatively higher intratesticular levels of the more potent androgen dihydro T despite severe gonadotropin suppression (19), providing a possible explanation as to why spermatogenesis in some men could not be suppressed (8). Others have shown that after T enanthate administration there is a selective increase in 5-α-reductase in those men who remain oligozoospermic but not in those who become azoospermic (20).

Elevated end-of-treatment serum insulinlike growth factor 3, a marker of Leydig cell function, has been reported to be associated with failure to completely suppress spermatogenesis in men receiving male hormonal contraception (21).

Partial suppression of spermatogenesis (induced by 500 mg T undecaneoate monthly injections) was reported to be weakly influenced by hormonal and clinical features but not by polymorphism in androgen or FSH receptor genes (22). Differences in the pharmacokinetics or pharmacodynamics of T or in the sensitivity of the hypothalamic–pituitary–testicular axis to sex steroid inhibition are unlikely the cause of this discrepancy (23).

MECHANICAL CONTRACEPTION

Vasectomy

A review of the literature indicated that vasectomy is a simple and highly effective contraceptive method with a low morbidity rate and an extremely low mortality rate. Pregnancy rates associated with vasectomy are reported in the range of 0% to 2%, with most reporting <1% (24). Currently, the two most common surgical techniques for approaching the vas during vasectomy are the incisional method and the no-scalpel technique. A recent Cochrane review indicated that the no-scalpel approach to the vas resulted in less complications as well as a shorter operation time than the traditional incision technique. There was no difference in effectiveness between the two approaches (25).

Early complications, including hematoma, infection, sperm granulomas, epididymitis–orchitis, and congestive epididymitis, occur in 1% to 6% of men undergoing vasectomy. The weight of the evidence regarding prostate and testicular cancer suggests that men with vasectomy are not at increased risk of these cancers (24,26). Although the pathogenesis of postvasectomy pain syndrome is unknown, vasectomy reversal may provide effective relief in carefully selected individuals.

Frequency of Control Semen Analysis

The presence of spermatozoa in the ejaculate or in urine during the first few months and up to one year after vasectomy is common and does not necessarily indicate vasectomy failure. Spermatozoa remaining within the male reproductive tract rapidly become immotile, often within a few days of the vasectomy operation and usually by three weeks (review: 27). The patient has to be informed about the possibility of causing a pregnancy during this period and other contraceptive methods should be used if necessary.

Recommendations regarding the timing and number of semen analyses after vasectomy vary widely. For example, the British Andrology Society guidelines recommend that initial assessment is undertaken 16 weeks postvasectomy and after the patient has produced at least 24 ejaculates. If no sperms are seen, they recommend examining the centrifugate for the presence of motile and nonmotile spermatozoa. They recommend that the clinician should give the "all clear" after the production of two consecutive sperm-free ejaculates (review: 27). A special clearance is given when semen contains less than 100,000 nonmotile spermatozoa in the ejaculate (27). The presence of motile spermatozoa or a substantial number of nonmotile spermatozoa is considered as failure.

On the other hand, the Dutch Urology Association recommends clearing patients with less than 100,000 immotile sperms per milliliter in a single semen sample 12 weeks after vasectomy (28).

Although examination of semen centrifugate is usually recommended in cases with azoospermia following vasectomy, microscopic examination of uncentrifuged specimens was found to be a reliable method for identifying semen samples after vasectomy with more than 100,000 sperm per milliliter (29).

Recently, a home immunodiagnostic test kit (SpermCheck® Vasectomy) has been shown to be a simple test that can provide evidence of vasectomy success or failure with a sensitivity and specificity of 93% and 97%, respectively, offering an alternative to postvasectomy monitoring by semen analysis (30).

Fertility Preservation and Restoration

With increasing divorce rates and the establishment of second relationships, the demand for fertility by vasectomy patients is increasing. Sperm cryopreservation may be offered to patients before undergoing vasectomy.

The Practice Committee of the American Society for Reproductive Medicine has recently recommended that before vasectomy reversal is performed to restore fertility, an evaluation of the female partner's reproductive potential should take place (31).

The choice between vasectomy reversal and assisted reproductive techniques (ART) also should consider whether the couple plans to have one or more children as well as the comparative costs of the two strategies (31). Vasectomy reversal appears more cost-effective than percutaneous testicular sperm extraction (TESE) and microepididymal sperm aspiration (MESA) for the treatment of obstructive azoospermia when the impact of indirect costs is considered (32).

The choice of whether to perform vasovasostomy or epididymovasostomy depends on the gross characteristics of vasal fluid and careful examination of the epididymis during surgery (31).

There is now consensus that with microsurgery the results of vasovasostomy are superior to those of other methods using less magnification, with patency rates of approximately 90% (review: 33). Despite these high patency rates, spontaneous pregnancy rates may be lower than in normal couples because of testicular and epididymal changes (34) and the development of antisperm antibodies. Careful monitoring of semen quality after surgery is mandatory to promptly identify patients who are likely to develop reobstruction (31). Alternatively, testicular or epididymal spermatozoa can be used in ICSI, although studies show microsurgical vasectomy reversal to be more cost-effective. On the other hand, pregnancy can usually be achieved sooner after ICSI than after reanastomosis (33). Boyle (35) has reported that sperm retrieval with cryopreservation at the time of vasectomy reversal is not a cost-effective management strategy.

Other Mechanical Methods

Abstinence during the fertile period and coitus interruptus (withdrawal before ejaculation) have unacceptably high failure rates. Male condom remains the most commonly used method of male contraception. Although male condom use is generally associated with unacceptably high failure rates of approximately 19% in inexperienced users, it is a fairly effective method of contraception among stable, experienced condom users with a failure rate of 0.8% to 4% (36,37). The use of male condom has the advantage of protecting against sexually transmitted diseases including HIV/AIDS, reducing the risk of HIV transmission by roughly 80% (38,39). The additional use of a water-based external lubricant may significantly reduce male condom failure rates among experienced condom users (37).

CONCLUSIONS AND PERSPECTIVES

For the time being, condoms and vasectomy remain the only widely available methods for male contraception. Despite a considerable progress in male hormonal contraception, further improvements on different levels are still needed. The most promising hormonal regimen to achieve this goal seems to be a combination of T and a progestin. Because of the recent advances in molecular biology and genetics, several target genes and proteins influencing sperm production and possible vaccines have been identified as a potential male contraceptive, such as indenopyridines, selective androgen receptor modulators, sperm-specific Na^+/H^+ exchanger, and antibodies against eppin (40,41).

REFERENCES

1. Glasier AF, Anakwe R, Everington D, et al. Would women trust their partners to use a male pill? Hum Reprod 2000; 15:646–649.
2. Martin CW, Anderson RA, Cheng L, et al. Potential impact of hormonal male contraception: Cross-cultural implications for development of novel preparations. Hum Reprod 2000; 15:637–645.
3. Ehiri JE, Birley M. Environmental impact of contraceptive use: An overview of available evidence. Environ Manag Health 2009; 13:55–65
4. Liu PY, McLachlan RI. Male hormonal contraception: So near and yet so far. J Clin Endocrinol Metab 2008; 93:2474–2476.
5. de Kretser DM, Loveland KL, Meinhardt A, et al. Spermatogenesis. Hum Reprod 1998; 13(suppl 1):1–8.
6. Comhaire FH. Male contraception: Hormonal, mechanical and other. Hum Reprod 1994; 9(suppl 2):22–27.
7. Weinbauer GF, Wessels J. "Paracrine" control of spermatogenesis. Andrologia 1999; 31:249–262.
8. Coviello AD, Bremner WJ, Matsumoto AM, et al. Intratesticular testosterone concentrations comparable with serum levels are not sufficient to maintain normal sperm production in men receiving a hormonal contraceptive regimen. J Androl 2004; 25:931–938.
9. Morales C, Clermont Y. Structural changes of the Sertoli cell during the cycle of the seminiferous epithelium. In: Russel LD, Griswold MD, eds. The Sertoli Cell. Clearwater, FL: Cache River Press, 1993:305–330.
10. Parvinen M. Cyclic function of Sertoli cells. In: Russel LD, Griswold MD, eds. The Sertoli Cell. Clearwater, FL: Cache River Press, 1993:331–347.
11. McLachlan RI. The endocrine control of spermatogenesis. Baillieres Clin Endocrinol Metab 2000; 14:345–362.
12. Nieschlag E, Simoni M, Gromoll J, et al. Role of FSH in the regulation of spermatogenesis: Clinical aspects. Clin Endocrinol (Oxf) 1999; 51:139–146.
13. Oxynos C, Wu FC. Male hormonal contraception. Baillieres Best Pract Res Clin Endocrinol Metab 2000; 14:473–487.
14. WHO. Rates of testosterone-induced suppression to severe oligozoospermia or azoospermia in two multinational clinical studies. World Health Organization Task force on Methods for The Regulations of Male Fertility. Int J Androl 1995; 18:157–165.
15. Griffin D. Research on the regulation of male fertility—The WHO programme. In: Rajalakshmi M, Griffin PD, eds. Male contraception: Present and future. New Delhi, India: New Age International, 1999: 27–39.
16. Handelsman DJ, Waites GM. Hormonal male contraception. In: Schill WB, Comhaire F, Hargreave T, eds. Andrology for the Clinician. Berlin, Germany: Springer-Verlag, 2006:520–524.
17. Mommers E, Kersemaekers WM, Elliesen J, et al. Male hormonal contraception: A double-blind, placebo-controlled study. J Clin Endocrinol Metab 2008; 93:2572–2580.
18. Liu PY, Swerdloff RS, Christenson PD, et al. Rate, extent, and modifiers of spermatogenic recovery after hormonal male contraception: An integrated analysis. Lancet 2006; 367:1412–1420.
19. McLachlan RI, O'Donnell L, Stanton PG, et al. Effects of testosterone plus medroxyprogesterone acetate on semen quality, reproductive hormones, and germ cell populations in normal young men. J Clin Endocrinol Metab 2002; 87:546–556.
20. Anderson RA, Wallace AM, Wu FC. Comparison between testosterone enanthate-induced azoospermia and oligozoospermia in a male contraceptive study. III. Higher 5 alpha-reductase activity in oligozoospermic men administered supraphysiological doses of testosterone. J Clin Endocrinol Metab 1996; 81:902–908.
21. Amory JK, Page ST, Anawalt BD, et al. Elevated end-of-treatment serum INSL3 is associated with failure to completely suppress spermatogenesis in men receiving male hormonal contraception. J Androl 2007; 28:548–554.
22. Li JW, Gu YQ. Predictors for partial suppression of spermatogenesis of hormonal male contraception. Asian J Androl 2008; 10:723–730.
23. Anderson RA, Wu FC. Comparison between testosterone enanthate-induced azoospermia and oligozoospermia in a male contraceptive study. II. Pharmacokinetics and pharmacodynamics of once weekly administration of testosterone enanthate. J Clin Endocrinol Metab 1996; 81:896–901.
24. Schwingl PJ, Guess HA. Safety and effectiveness of vasectomy. Fertil Steril 2000; 73:923–936.

25. Cook LA, Pun A, van Vliet H, et al. Scalpel versus no-scalpel incision for vasectomy. Cochrane Database Syst Rev 2007; CD004112 doi:10.1002/14651858.CD004112.pub3.
26. Holt SK, Salinas CA, Stanford JL. Vasectomy and the risk of prostate cancer. J Urol 2008; 180:2565–2567 doi:10.1016/j.juro.2008.08.042
27. Hancock P, McLaughlin E. British Andrology Society guidelines for the assessment of post vasectomy semen samples (2002). J Clin Pathol 2002; 55:812–816.
28. Dohle GR, Meuleman EJ, Hoekstra JW, et al. Revised guideline "Vasectomy" from the Dutch Urological Association. Ned Tijdschr Geneeskd 2005; 149:2728–2731.
29. Steward B, Hays M, Sokal D. Diagnostic accuracy of an initial azoospermic reading compared with results of post-centrifugation semen analysis after vasectomy. J Urol 2008; 180:2119–2123.
30. Klotz KL, Coppola MA, Labrecque M, et al. Clinical and consumer trial performance of a sensitive immunodiagnostic home test that qualitatively detects low concentrations of sperm following vasectomy. J Urol 2008; 180:2569–2576.
31. Practice Committee of the American Society for Reproductive Medicine.Vasectomy reversal. Fertil Steril 2008; 90:S78–S82.
32. Lee R, Li PS, Goldstein M, et al. A decision analysis of treatments for obstructive azoospermia. Hum Reprod 2008; 23:2043–2049.
33. Fox M. Failed vasectomy reversal: Is a further attempt using microsurgery worthwhile? BJU Int 2000; 86:474–478.
34. Thimon V, Calvo E, Koukoui O, et al. Effects of vasectomy on gene expression profiling along the human epididymis. Biol Reprod 2008; 79:262–273.
35. Boyle KE, Thomas AJ Jr, Marmar JL, et al. Sperm harvesting and cryopreservation during vasectomy reversal is not cost effective. Fertil Steril 2006; 85:961–964.
36. Handelsman DJ, Waites GM. Problem: Male contraception. Traditional methods. In: Schill WB, Comhaire F, Hargreave T, eds. Andrology for the Clinician. Berlin, Germany: Springer-Verlag, 2006:122–124.
37. Gabbay MB, Thomas J, Gibbs A, et al. A randomized crossover trial of the impact of additional spermicide on condom failure rates. Sex Transm Dis 2008; 35:862–868.
38. Heikinheimo O, Lahteenmaki P. Contraception and HIV infection in women. Hum Reprod Update 2009; 15:165–176.
39. Weller S, Davis K. Condom effectiveness in reducing heterosexual HIV transmission. Cochrane Database Syst Rev 2002; CD003255.
40. Mruk DD. New perspectives in non-hormonal male contraception. Trends Endocrinol Metab 2008; 19:57–64 doi:10.1016/j.tem.2007.11.002
41. Page ST, Amory JK, Bremner WJ. Advances in male contraception. Endocr Rev 2008; 29:465–493.

19 Prevention of male infertility: Environmental and systemic disease effects on male fertility

Jens Peter Bonde and Jorma Toppari

INTRODUCTION

It is reasonable to assume that the apparent secular trends and regional differences in male reproductive health have causes that are greatly fluctuating in prevalence over time and across boundaries. Our environment, working conditions, and way of living have changed dramatically over the past century and it is likely that the key to an understanding of the changing occurrence of male reproductive disorders is found in social and environmental factors. Identification of one or more necessary links of the causal chain leading to disease is needed for rational prevention but examples are plenty that a complete understanding of causes and pathogenic processes are not necessary for successful prevention of diseases. In this chapter, current knowledge on impact of environmental factors (including life style and occupation) and systemic disease on male reproductive health is reviewed. This knowledge is the basis for counseling the infertile man in the clinical setting.

TOBACCO SMOKING

The habit of smoking tobacco was brought to Europe after the discovery of America in 1492. When introduced, smoking was recommended for medical purposes and it was not until the second half of the 19th century that evidence was mounting that pipe smoking caused cancer of the lip and tongue (1). With the growing habit of smoking cigarettes among doctors and all social classes of society, the sense that tobacco smoking could be a threat to health was ignored for many years. It was not until the 1950s that it became scientifically well documented that lung cancer and subsequently numerous diseases are related to tobacco smoking. Effects of smoking on male reproductive health are among outcomes that have been studied only very recently. During the 20th century, production and consumption of tobacco products increased worldwide until the 1960s, but by the 1980s, some countries in Europe and North America recorded a decline in smoking frequencies and in the total consumption of tobacco.

Figure 1 indicates prevalence and trends in tobacco smoking in selected European countries.

Smoking fume contains more than 3000 constituents including biologically active agents such as nicotine, polyaromatic hydrocarbons, nitrosamines, carbon monoxide, benzene, phenols, and several metals such as cadmium in small amounts.

In European studies of infertility, it was consistently shown that tobacco smoking in women is related to some 30% reduction in fecundability (probability of fertilization in one menstrual cycle) whereas smoking in men had no impact on couple fertility (2). These data indicate that the female reproductive system is more vulnerable to disrupting effects of tobacco smoking than is the male reproductive system. It has, however, become evident in the past few years that tobacco smokers have 15% to 20% reduction of sperm concentration and sperm counts in comparison with nonsmokers, while sperm motility and morphology seem to escape the effects of smoking (3–5). Although the fertility in terms of time taken to conceive is not affected in the average male smoker, there is increasing evidence that smoking is deleterious to spermatogenesis and that fertility may be impaired in susceptible men including men who are oligospermic for other reasons. Accordingly, it is well justified to advise cessation of smoking for both men and women in infertile couples. Nevertheless, it should be acknowledged that no studies are demonstrating that sperm counts increase after smoking cessation.

Involved mechanisms are unknown. There are indications that plasma concentrations of both androgens and luteinizing hormone are increased in male smokers, which is compatible with androgen insensitivity. It is, therefore, of interest that there is some experimental evidence indicating that constituents of tobacco smoke are inhibiting aromatase—the enzyme that converts androgens to estrogens (6).

Few recent studies indicate consistently that tobacco smoking during pregnancy is related to reduced sperm counts and semen volume among sons (7–11). Some of these studies demonstrate a dose related decline in sperm count that is more pronounced after prenatal exposure than after exposure during adulthood (Fig. 2). An early American follow-up study of a diethylstilbestrol cohort did not find indications of delayed effects of maternal tobacco smoking. An explanation of this apparent discrepancy with the more recent European studies may be the low prevalence of American women who smoked during pregnancy and that most female smokers are light smokers (12,13). The exact mechanisms are not known. Some studies show that benz(a)pyren, a constituent of tobacco smoke, in high doses given orally to pregnant mice causes dose-related atrophy of the seminiferous tubules (14). Tobacco smoking is estrogenic or antiandrogenic and could disrupt normal development of the male fetal gonads. So far the hormonal regulation in sons of smoking mothers has not been shown to be disrupted (15). In all circumstances, there seems now to be sufficient evidence to strongly advise pregnant mothers to abstain from smoking

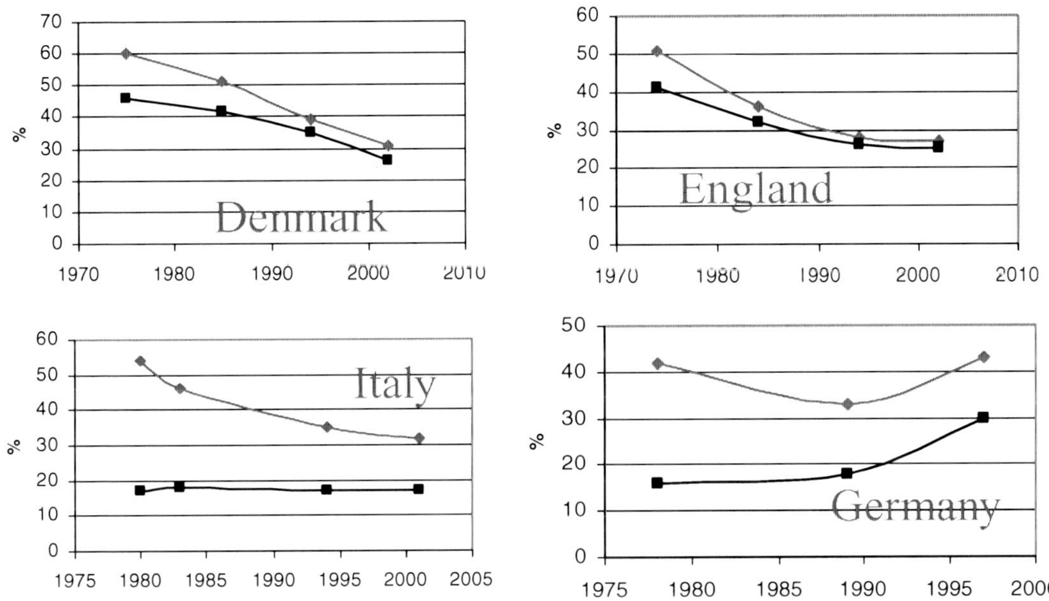

Figure 1 Trends in smoking prevalence in adult men (*upper lines*) and women (*lower lines*) in selected European countries. *Source:* Adapted from The Tobacco Atlas by The World Health Organization, 2002.

during pregnancy in order not to impair the fertility of the male offspring.

Effects of smoking on other male reproductive health endpoints are less obvious. In an Swedish ecological study, a striking correlation between trends in maternal smoking during pregnancy and incidence of testicular cancer was shown (16), but several case-control studies of testicular cancer have not convincingly demonstrated any relationship to smoking during pregnancy (17). New data indicate that maternal tobacco smoking may be related to cryptorchidism, but these data need to be corroborated (18). The picture is even more blurred with respect to hypospadias, where some studies indicate a protective effect of tobacco smoking (19). Although it might be possible to explain secular trends and geographical differences in male reproductive health by differences in smoking habits among pregnant women, it is far from obvious that smoking is a main contributor to testicular dysgenesis syndrome (20,21).

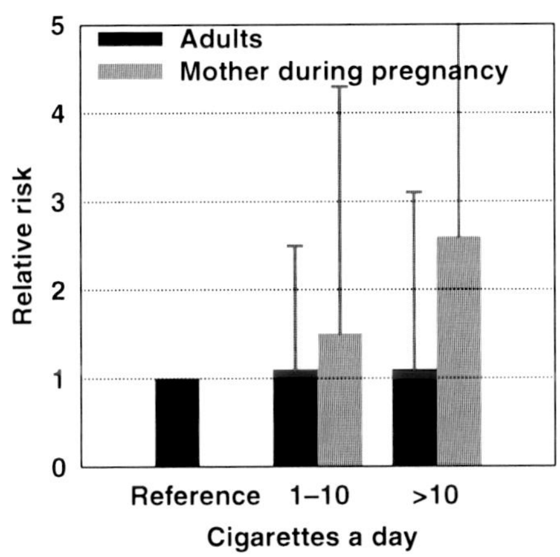

Figure 2 Risk for oligospermia according to smoking in adult men (3) and among mothers during pregnancy (11).

Few studies have demonstrated that male smokers have increased frequency of damage to the sperm genome in terms of aneuploidy (22–24) and in terms of damage to the DNA (25). Such findings are of importance when considering the possible risk for male-mediated developmental toxicity. There is a large body of evidence indicating that carcinogenic substances administered to pregnant rodents are related to an increased rate of fetal loss, congenital malformations, and impaired postnatal survival (26–29). There are also studies clearly demonstrating that the competition among sperms to fertilize the ovum does not protect against transmission of paternal chromosomal aberrations (30). Therefore, studies of effects such as congenital malformations and childhood cancer relative to paternal smoking are of importance. There is indeed limited evidence that paternal smoking is related to a moderately increased risk of cancer among children up to the age of five years (31,32). Similarly, there are some indications that paternal smoking is related to a moderately increased risk of congenital malformation in the offspring (33).

OVERWEIGHT AND ADIPOSITY

It is well established that overweight among women is related to subfertility but recent evidence demonstrates that overweight in

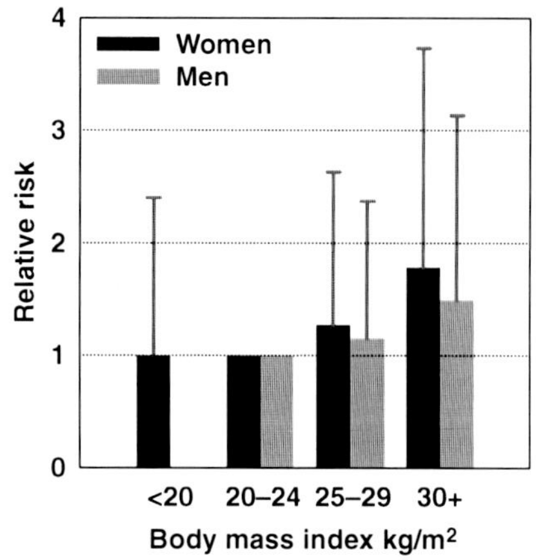

Figure 3 Relative risk of subfecundity according to body mass index in men and women (34).

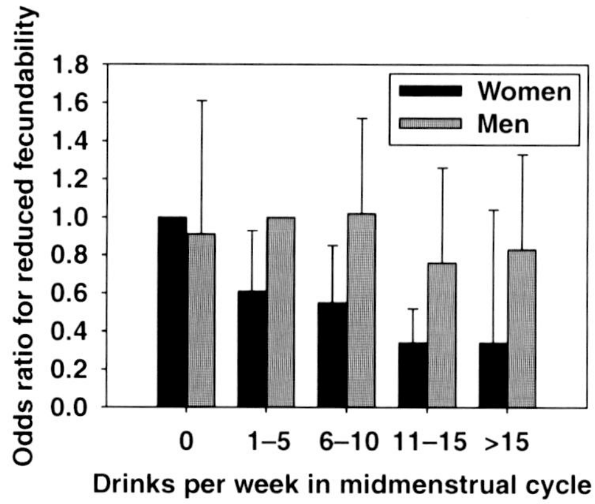

Figure 4 Fecundability odds ratios (95% confidence intervals) according to alcohol intake around time of ovulation (41).

the male is independently contributing to increased infertility of the same order of magnitude (34) (Fig. 3). Moreover, it seems that overweight in both partners in a couple has an additive effect on infertility and that infertility in overweight couples is not explained by altered sexual function (35). It is also well established that overweight is associated with disruption of normal hormonal homeostasis including sexual hormones, but so far the few studies in the field are not consistent with respect to associations with reduced sperm count (36,37). Hormonal imbalance toward higher oestrogen/androgen ratio has been suggested as a mechanism, but there is a lack of prospective studies to tell whether the hormonal disturbances related to infertility in overweight couples are primary or secondary. So far only one small-scale study indicates that the body mass index of the pregnant mother has bearings as to semen quality in the offspring (38).

ALCOHOLIC BEVERAGES

Intake of alcohol interferes with the endocrine system, and alcoholic liver damage disturbs the peripheral metabolism of hormones by interference with enzyme function, protein binding, and receptors. Experimental studies show that blood testosterone concentrations decline within hours after ingesting a sufficient amount of alcohol to produce hangover. In chronic alcoholism, levels of testosterone are low. Long-term effects of chronic alcoholism include reduced libido, erectile dysfunction, gynecomastia, testicular atrophy, and reduced sperm count and thus reduced fertility. Although several of these effects may be mediated by lowered serum testosterone level, findings of elevated luteinizing hormone level indicate that ethanol in high concentration may exert direct toxic actions on the testis (39,40).

Furthermore, serum concentrations of estrogens are increased in chronic alcoholism because of enhanced peripheral conversion of androgens to estrogens through increased activity of the enzyme aromatase in the liver and fat cells.

There are no indications that ingestion of alcoholic beverages in small amounts is associated with impaired male fertility. A prospective study of first pregnancy planners did not reveal effects of a weekly intake of alcohol in the range from 0 to more than 15 drinks a week on blood, concentration of sexual hormones, semen quality, or time taken to conceive (Fig. 4) (41). In counseling infertile couples it should, however, be acknowledged that acute high intake of alcohol is causing reduced testosterone levels in serum and possibly in the testis and hereby may cause reversible reduced fertility.

CAFFEINATED BEVERAGES

Caffeine (1,3,7-trimethyl xanthine) is a constituent of coffee, tea, soft drinks, and chocolate. The compound easily crosses biological membranes, is distributed throughout the body, and is also detectable in human semen. Biological effects of caffeine include stimulation of the central nervous system and increased activity of the sympathetic nervous system. The majority of studies addressing reproductive effects of caffeine focus on female-mediated infertility and possible teratogenic actions. Data in males are extremely limited. It is of interest, however, that a prospective study of first pregnancy planners found a dose-related decrease in fecundability in nonsmoking, but not among smoking, men (42). So far no studies have indicated effects of caffeine on semen quality, and possible mechanisms are obscure.

An effect of caffeine in nonsmokers only is biologically plausible because smoking interferes with the metabolism of caffeine and increases detoxification and elimination of caffeine metabolites.

SEDENTARY LIFESTYLE

Elevation of the testis temperature impairs and even inhibits spermatogenesis (43,45). Early experimental studies in humans show that external heating of the testis for a short period of time resolves in a dramatic but temporary decline in sperm count after six to eight weeks. It has also been known that elevation of the core temperature by fever or extreme sauna bathing reduces sperm count (45,46). Moreover, working in a hot occupational environment and exposure to radiant heat among welders, ceramic workers, bakery workers, and foundry workers may cause reduced sperm count (47–49). On this background, it is of concern whether sedentary work and lifestyle in affluent countries has an impact on testicular temperature regulation and subsequently on sperm count. Men sitting at a work for eight hours a day have an average 0.7°C increased temperature of scrotal skin during the day in comparison with employees spending less than eight hours in the sedentary body position. Although an increase in scrotal temperature of this order of magnitude might be sufficient to impair spermatogenesis, there are now several studies applying different designs that consistently indicate that office work is not related to decreased semen quality or fertility (50,51). It has also been speculated whether tight underwear could act as a testicular suspensorium, causing disruption of testicular temperature regulation and reduced sperm count. There is circumstantial evidence in support of this hypothesis (52).

In counseling the infertile couple, it seems justified to pay attention to extreme external heat exposures as in prolonged hot sauna bathing, particularly hot tubs and occupations with exposure to high levels of radiant heat and possibly among professional drivers, but office work and sedentary work positions in general are not related to male infertility.

PSYCHOLOGICAL STRESS

Interactions between the environment and the individual may result in stress that affects a large number of biological systems including the reproductive system. Since the work of Walter Cannon and Hans Selye more than 50 years ago, it has been established knowledge that the acute stress response involves activation of the sympathetic autonomic nerve system and of the hypothalamic–pituitary–adrenal (HPA) axis. Furthermore, severe long-term stress has a strong impact on several organ systems that may cause premature death in animals including monkeys (53,54). It is less obvious to which degree long-term psychological strain in ordinary work in daily life activate these systems. Ongoing fertility problems may have a strong impact on stress levels and emotions in both men and women. Whether psychological stress is causing dysfunction of the male reproductive system can, therefore, be examined only in prospective studies, where information on stressors is related to subsequent change in biological markers of fecundity. While there are many cross-sectional studies of infertility clients that document strong associations between fertility and high levels of mental stress, there are very few longitudinal studies. Limited experimental data in humans suggest that chronic or severe stress leads to decrease in sperm count, motility, and morphology (55). There is evidence that mild to severe emotional stress suppresses testosterone and perhaps interferes with spermatogenesis in humans. In a prospective study of pregnancy planners

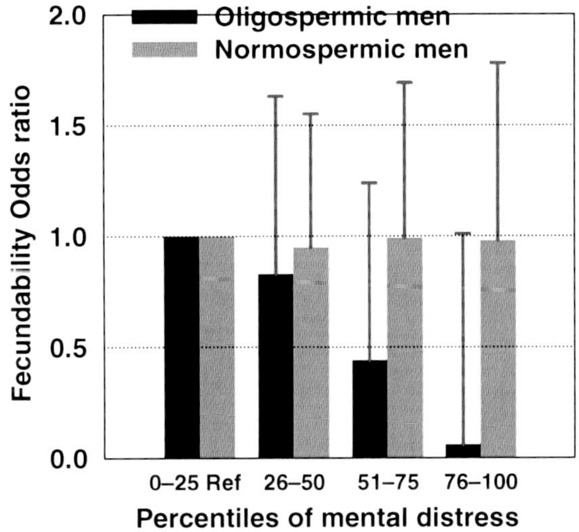

Figure 5 Adjusted odds ratio (OR) for pregnancy per menstrual cycle by male distress scores divided into quartiles. High values indicate high distress level. Analyses stratified by male sperm concentration (56).

where levels of emotional stress were recorded on a monthly basis, high levels of psychological distress predicted reduced fecundability, but only in men with reduced sperm count (Fig. 5) (56). If corroborated, this indicates that men who have reduced fecundity for one or more reasons are susceptible to effects of psychological distress. Considering the strong experimental data demonstrating effects of social stress on testosterone levels, sexual behavior, and testicular morphology, it seems reasonable to take mental stressors into account when counseling the infertile couples although the human evidence is limited.

FAMILY PLANNING

Easy access to effective contraceptive devices during the last century has strongly influenced the demographic transition and the balance between fertility rates and death rates (Fig. 6). Family planning may have an impact on the biological fertility in at least two different ways. First, women's participation in the workforce in affluent countries has resulted in delaying the age when the first child is born from less than 20 years, some 60 years ago, to more than 30 years at present. Since subfecundity is sharply increasing after 30 years of age in women, this development will result in increasing fertility problems even when population fecundity is not affected as such. Second, when families are restricting the number of children they have by use of family planning and effective contraception, the most fertile part of the population will have fewer children, while the lowest fertile part of the population will try to have the limited number of children they can, just as earlier. If genetic factors are important determinants of male fecundity, the result of family planning is expected to result in a genuine lower population

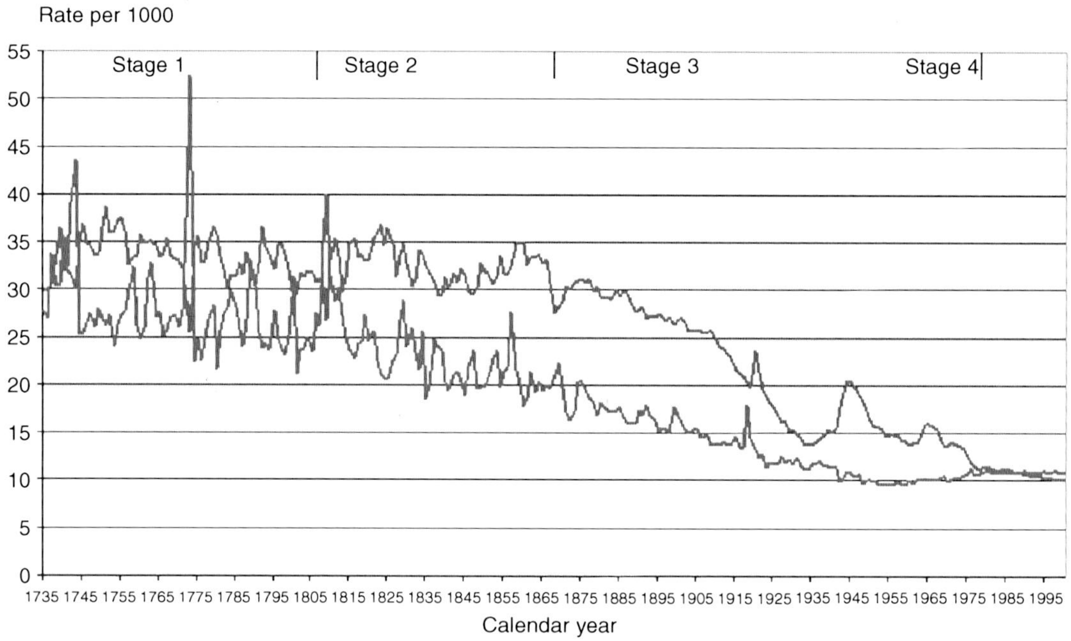

Figure 6 Demographic transition 1735 to 1995 in Sweden; lower line is death rate, upper line is birth rate. *Source:* Adapted from http://www.theoildrum. com/story/2005/12/18/1387/0641.

fecundity because of selection (57,58). There are data emerging from twin studies indicating that genetic factors, in fact, are major players in men's semen quality (59). This development is expected to accelerate further as a consequence of in vitro fertilization (IVF) techniques including intracytoplasmic sperm injection (ICSI). The magnitude that preferential selection of couples with lowest fertility, compared to earlier periods, have on average population fecundity is not known.

OCCUPATIONAL EXPOSURES

Workplace exposures are often considerably higher than environmental exposures experienced by the general population. Therefore, the individual risk can be high even if the exposure prevalence is low-- typically less than 1% to 5%. An overview of reported male reproductive hazards related to occupational exposures is given in Table 1.

The most well-established example of occupational effects on male reproduction is the adverse effects of the nematocide dibromochloropropane. It was discovered in 1977 that this pesticide causes severe reduction of sperm count among men involved in manufacture of dibromochloropropane (60). The problem was brought to light because spouses of male workers who manufactured the compound in a Californian company wondered why so many of them had difficulties in becoming pregnant. Subsequent semen analysis revealed azoospermia or oligospermia among the workers. Soon similar reports from agricultural workers in Israel confirmed that exposure to the compound is associated with severe impairment of spermatogenesis—even at low levels not causing clinical intoxication or reduced libido. In the majority of workers with oligospermia, the sperm count was recovered after discontinuation of exposure, but among workers with initial azoospermia some only recovered partly and others remained azoospermic through more than 10 years of follow-up (61). Testis biopsy shows a highly specific toxicity to the stem cells, which explains the ability of the compound to cause permanent azoospermia in cases where all stems cells have been destroyed. In some countries such as the United Kingdom, the compound was never manufactured because adverse effects on the testis were reported in several rodent species from 1960 onwards. In other countries such as the United States and Israel, the compound was banned after 1977.

Several other pesticides in current use are suspected for reproductive toxicity (Fig. 7). Other well-established occupational hazards to male reproductive function include ionizing radiation and radiant heat exposure. The testis is one of the most radiosensitive tissues of the body. A temporary reduction in sperm count occurs after a radiation dose of 0.15 Gy, while single exposures of approximately 2 Gy cause permanent azoospermia (62).

Working in hot occupational environments as in specialized welding operations, foundries, and bakeries may cause reversible reduction of sperm counts with recovery within weeks or months after discontinuation of exposure (44,47) (Fig. 8).

Exposure to hormonally active compounds such as chlordecone, some pesticides, carbon disulfide, several other organic

Table 1 Examples of Known and Suspected Occupational Hazards to Male Reproductive Function

Occupational exposure	Male reproductive effect
Anesthetic gas	Malformations in offspring?
Dinitrotoluene and toluene diamine	Reduced semen quality?
Metals	
Welding	Infertility, birth rate, semen quality, spontaneous abortion in spouse?
Chromium compounds	Testis toxicity?
Cadmium	Testis capillary bed
Lead	Reduced semen quality
Manganese	Reduced birth rate?
Mercury vapor (metallic)	Infertility?
Oral contraceptives and sexual hormones	Gynecomastia, reduced libido, impotence, reduced testicular function?
Organic solvents	
Carbon disulfide	Reduced libido and impotence
Chlorinated hydrocarbons	Poor semen quality?
Ethylene glycol ethers	Poor Semen quality
Halogenated hydrocarbons	Poor Semen quality?
Ethoxy ethanol	Poor Semen quality
Persistent organochlorine compounds	
Polychlorinated biphenyls (PCB)	Motility, sperm chromatin
p,p′-1, 1,1-bis-(4-chlorophenyl)-2, 2-dichloroethene (DDE) [a dichlordiphenyltrichlorethan (DDT) metabolite]	Reduced sperm count
Dioxin	Reduced sperm count
Pesticides	
Carbaryl	Abnormal sperm morphology?
Chloropren	Poor semen quality?
Dibromochloropropane	Sterility, infertility, oligospermia
Ethylene dibromide	Poor semen quality
Para-tertiary butyl acid	?
Chloroprene	?
Ionizing radiation, radium	Sterility, azoospermia oligospermia
Radar and microwaves	Poor semen quality?
Radiant heat	Reduced sperm count

solvents, boric acid, lead, and manganese has been reported to cause adverse reproductive effects including reduced semen quality (63). Inorganic lead is another example of a compound that interferes with reproductive function at exposure levels that are not associated with signs of clinical intoxication. Thus, reduced sperm count occurs at blood lead levels around 40 μg/dL of blood or higher, which is above levels occurring in the general population but below levels associated with clinical intoxication (64).

RISK ASSESSMENT AND COUNSELING

Suspicion of work-related male infertility is raised when a potential hazardous workplace exposure is present in a worker with reduced semen quality that is not explained by specific medical or andrological disease. In general, there are four criteria that must be fulfilled to establish that a case of infertility, most likely, is caused by a specified occupational exposure. First, the adverse reproductive effect—for instance, in terms of reduced libido, impotence, or reduced quantity and quality of semen—must fit with what is known about adverse effects of the suspected hazardous exposure (Box 1). Second, the exposure must be sufficient to cause the adverse effects. The occupational history is the main tool to obtain information on type, intensity, and duration of an exposure. Obviously, the mere presence of a toxic compound is not sufficient to cause damage. It is necessary to estimate the extent of exposure. Sometimes, occupational biological monitoring data on, for instance, blood lead values are available and enhance the validity of the exposure assessment. Moreover, data on occupational exposure standards in terms of threshold limit values or biological exposure indices are provided by national agencies such as The Health and Safety Executive in the United Kingdom. When considering

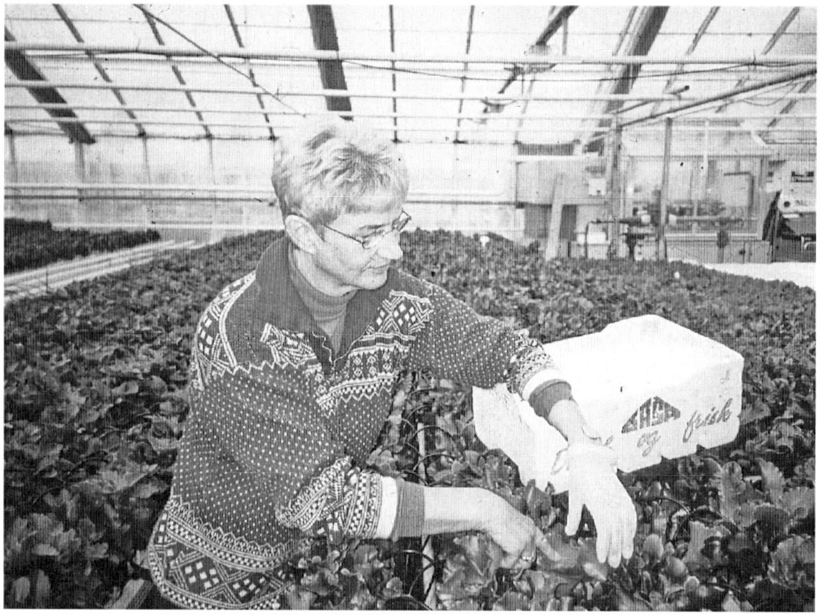

Figure 7 Manual handling of cultures may confer exposure to pesticides by skin contact. The fetal gonad may be vulnerable to trace amounts of chemicals and thereby early exposures may have bearings for fertility later in life.

hygienic standards, it should be kept in mind that the criteria for setting standards are seldom subclinical adverse effects on the reproductive tract. As the examples with dibromochloropropane, an inorganic lead, clearly demonstrates, severe effects impairing the fertility potential can occur at levels not associated with signs of intoxication and below threshold limit values. Third, the timing of exposure relative to the adverse effects must be relevant. Irreversible effects of earlier exposure are difficult to demonstrate. If, however, discontinuation of an ongoing exposure is associated with an increase in reproductive function during the subsequent weeks or months, it speaks in favor of causal associations. Chemical agents operating at the final stages of spermatogenesis such as some pesticides may have effects on sperm motility that may disappear in the weeks after cessation of exposure. On the contrary, chemical agents operating in the early stages of spermatogenesis may have effects lasting for several months after cessation of exposure because of the 72-day duration of human spermatogenesis. Fourth, other causes must

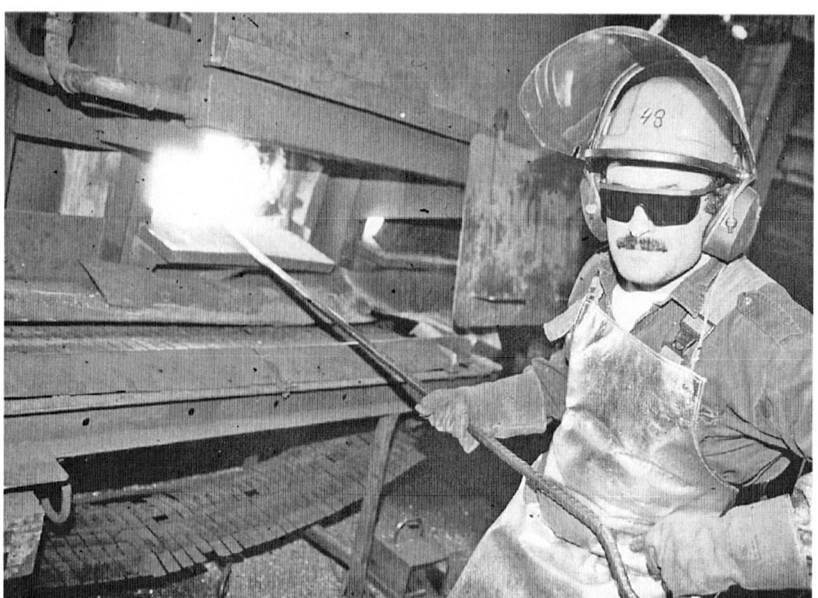

Figure 8 Radiant heat in the occupational environment as a foundry is an acknowledged risk factor for reduced sperm counts.

be excluded. The physician should consider alternative disorders that could explain the infertility. It is equally wrong to miss occupational disorders and hereby miss possibilities for prevention as inappropriately labeling a disease as occupational and thus missing an opportunity to provide the appropriate treatment.

Text Box 1 **On-line Information on Reproductive Toxicity of Industrial Chemicals**

General toxicological information is available at TOXNET (http://www.toxnet.mlm.nih.gov) and IPCS/INCHEM (http://www.inchem.org).

Material safety data sheets (http://www.hazards.com/msds and http://www.siri.org/msds) provide information about health hazards and recommended precautions to be taken by users of the product but no reproductive data are available.

Repro risk system of reproductive toxicity databases provides reviews of some 850 chemicals (http://www.micromidex.com/products/reprorisk).

Reprotox (http://www.reprotox.org) provides excellent brief reviews of reproductive toxicity based upon animal experiments as well as epidemiological and clinical studies.

PREVENTION AND WORKER'S COMPENSATION

Prevention of work-related reproductive disorders including male infertility relies on identification of potential hazards and appropriate regulation spanning the entire range of possible interventions from complete ban of a chemical to restricted use, encapsulation at the workplaces, exhaust ventilation, and use of personal protective devices and information. Infertility is not a prescribed occupational disorder in any country, and male infertility is not explicitly compensated by occupational health law acts. Nevertheless, identification of occupational reproductive disorders including male infertility is important for the individual worker who may be able to recover if the exposure is eliminated and to promote preventive measures at work places at large.

SYSTEMIC DISEASES AND IATROGENIC CAUSES OF INFERTILITY

Systemic diseases can affect reproductive maturation by delaying pubertal onset. Typical example of such disease is anorexia nervosa that is rare in boys but has similar effect as in girls; that is, hypothalamic ignition of pubertal development does not start normally. Systemic diseases can have both central (hypothalamic) and peripheral (direct gonadal) effects. Severe traumas, including large operations, burns, myocardial infarcts, and liver failures, are associated with declined serum testosterone levels while the LH levels do not change much and pulsatile LH secretion may diminish (65). Functional significance of diminished androgen levels in acute illness is not known, and randomized placebo-controlled studies with androgen substitution in this difficult patient group are missing.

Liver diseases, particularly liver cirrhosis, cause reproductive dysfunction irrespective of the reason for cirrhosis. Men with liver failure have impaired spermatogenesis, testicular atrophy, declined testosterone levels, alopecia abdomen, gynecomastia, and sexual dysfunction. Low testosterone level can be masked by elevated sex hormone binding globuline (SHBG), which maintains the total testosterone level relatively normal while the free testosterone level is subnormal. Estrogen and prolactin levels are typically elevated, whereas gonadotropin levels may remain unchanged. Severity of the liver disease determines how badly reproductive functions are compromised. Liver transplantation can normalize the reproductive functions (66).

Kidney diseases affect hypothalamic–pituitary–gonadal axis both centrally and peripherally. Uremia causes direct testicular effects that manifest as declined testosterone levels, impaired spermatogenesis, and infertility. Gonadotropin secretion does not respond as much as it should to compensate the compromised testicular function. Testicular atrophy, erectile dysfunction, and gynecomastia occur frequently in association with chronic renal failure (67). The only effective treatment of reproductive problems associated with end-stage kidney disease is renal transplantation.

Hemochromatosis may disturb several endocrine organs, including the testis, pituitary gland, and hypothalamus. Often, the pituitary gland is the most affected one of reproductive endocrine organs and gonadotropin induction can be used to restore fertility. Effective prevention by iron chelators and avoidance of excess iron load can postpone the hypogonadism and allow normal pubertal development, for example, in β-thalassemia patients (68). **Sickle cell anemia** can cause hypogonadism and fertility problems by thromboses and multiple infarcts, both in the hypothalamus and in the testes. The symptoms depend on location of main damage.

Cystic fibrosis is one of the most common hereditary metabolic diseases in Caucasian population. However, some populations, for example, Finns, have very low carrier frequency of the mutations in the cystic fibrosis transmembrane conductance regulator (*CFTR*) gene that are the cause of this condition. In European population, the most common mutation is deltaF508 deletion. Infertility is caused by the congenital bilateral absence of vas deference that causes obstructive azoospermia. Thus, the men can be effectively helped with artificial reproductive techniques because their spermatogenesis is usually normal. In Young syndrome, reproductive organs are structurally normal, but epididymis are clogged by viscous fluid. In both cystic fibrosis and Young syndrome, the respiratory symptoms are the main problems for patients.

Chronic **gastrointestinal diseases**, such as Crohn disease and ulcerative colitis, can be associated with impaired fertility. The underlying mechanisms include chronic inflammation and its mediators, fever, and medication. Salazosulfapyridine can disturb testicular function, whereas 5-aminosalinocylic acid does not (69). There are also reports of adverse effects of untreated celiac disease on male reproductive health (70), but in our population-based study we did not find any major influence (71). Gastric diseases are not associated with reproductive problems, but an old H_2- receptor blocker cimetidine is an androgen antagonist.

Some endocrine diseases affect fertility indirectly. **Thyroid disorders** can affect reproductive functions by alterations in SHBG levels that tend to increase in hyperthyroidism and decrease in hypothyroidism. Hyperprolactinemia can be induced secondarily by increased thyrotropin-releasing hormone (TRH) stimulation caused by primary hypothyroidism. **Hypercortisolism** suppresses LH secretion and may also affect testicular function directly.

Some neurological syndromes are associated with fertility problems. **Myotonic dystrophy** is caused by an expansion of tandem CTG repeats in the 3' untranslated region of the myotonin protein kinase gene. Patients have impaired spermatogenesis and secondary hypergonadotropism. Testosterone levels may remain normal. **Late-onset X-linked bulbospinal muscular atrophy (Kennedy disease)** is caused by an expansion of CAG repeats in androgen receptor gene impairing normal handling of gene product and gradual impairment of muscle function and testes. Several syndromes involve abnormal hypothalamic function and ensuing hypogonadotropic hypogonadism, for example, **Prader–Willi syndrome**.

Autoimmune diseases rarely affect fertility, but in autoimmune polyendocrinopathy–candidiasis–ectodermal dystrophy (APECED; autoimmune polyglandular syndrome 1, APS1), testicular autoantibodies can develop, leading to infertility. These may appear at any time during the disease (72), and cryopreservation of sperm can be recommended. The recessively inherited disease is caused by mutations in the autoimmune regulator (*AIRE*) gene. APECED is a rare disease, but it is enriched in Finnish disease heritage.

All infectious diseases can disturb testicular function in acute phase. Severe chronic infections, such as **AIDS**, can lead to testicular failure. **Tuberculosis** and **leprosy** can also directly affect testicular structures, causing impaired spermatogenesis and infertility. This is rarely seen in affluent countries but may occur in developing countries.

Cancer diseases can cause multiple organ failure and impairment of reproductive functions. However, other than malignancies of reproductive organs, these cancer diseases rarely affect fertility by themselves. It is rather their treatment that causes infertility (73) (see Chapter 30).

In addition to diseases themselves, treatment can affect hypothalamic–pituitary–gonadal axis. There are multiple mechanisms how these operate: cytotoxic effects (cancer chemotherapy and irradiation), receptor antagonism (antiandrogens, e.g., flutamide, bicalutamide, cyproterone acetate, spironolactone, cimetidine), inhibition of steroidogenic enzymes (e.g., aminoglutethimide, etomidate, ketoconazole), inhibition of GnRH and/or gonadotropin secretion (e.g., opiates, verapamil, phenothiazine, glucocorticoids), stimulation of androgen elimination (hepatic enzyme–inducing drugs, e.g., barbiturates, many anticonvulsants), and direct hormonal effects of estrogens, anabolic androgens, and GnRH analogues and antagonists. Many drugs function by influencing the autonomic nervous system and can, thereby, cause adverse effects in sexual functions. Typical examples are antihypertensives. Central nervous system drugs can also affect libido and sexual functions. For many drugs the mechanism of untoward actions is unknown.

Environmental Effects

Environmental influences on male fertility depend critically on the timing of exposure. As evidenced by many occupational exposures, men can often recover from damage caused by a temporary exposure during adulthood. In contrast, fetal or childhood exposure may cause permanent effects. Sperm production capacity depends on the number of Sertoli cells (74,75), which cease proliferating at the onset of spermatogenesis in puberty. Thus, at adulthood, sperm production capacity cannot be improved beyond the limits that Sertoli cells have set during development. If these limits are small, sperm numbers remain low. This is exactly what seems to have happened during the last two generations when sperm counts have been lower than those reported in our grandparents' youth. There are also regional differences in semen quality. The reasons for these changes are unknown, but many things point to the possibility that adverse environmental effects play a role. Impaired sperm production has been associated with other reproductive problems, such as cryptorchidism, hypospadias, and testicular cancer, all of which have their origin in abnormal fetal development (76). Potential environmental effectors are endocrine disrupting chemicals that have been shown to influence animal reproductive organs. These include anti-androgenic pesticides (e.g., DDE) and fungicides (e.g., vinclozoline, procymidone), certain phthalate esters (e.g., dibutyl phthalate and diethyl hexyl phthalate), some polybrominated diphenyl ethers, and an ever-increasing list of other commonly used chemicals. Some of these are very persistent (e.g., DDE) and therefore transfer from generation to generation even after phasing out of the compound. Exposure to individual chemicals remains usually below no adverse effect levels (NOAEL), but there is currently a great concern about the cumulative effects of mixtures of chemicals that we are exposed to in real life (77). In mixtures, endocrine-disrupting chemicals can indeed cause severe reproductive organ damage at doses that alone have no effects (78). Precautionary approach is, therefore, to protect fetuses and growing children from all unnecessary chemical exposures as long as we do not know enough of their potential endocrine and reproductive effects.

CONCLUSION

Knowledge about causes of male infertility related to environmental factors is sufficient to prevent part of the problem but the magnitude of the proportion of male infertility that is

Table 2 Recommendations for Counseling of the Infertile Male[a]

Recommendation	Level of evidence	Grade of evidence
Discontinue smoking, in particular among men with oligospermia	2a	B
Weight reduction if BMI > 30 kg/m^2	2b	C
Discontinue excessive intake of alcoholic beverages (>20–30/wk)	2b	C
Eliminate or reduce certain occupational exposures (ionizing radiation, radiant heat, PCB, DDT, some metals, some solvents, some pesticides)	2a	B

[a]The level and grade of evidence is classified according to criteria set up by the U.S. Department of Health and Human Services, Public Health Service, Agency for Health Care Policy and Research.
Abbreviations: BMI, body mass index; PCB, polychlorinated biphenyls; DDT.

preventable is unknown at present. It may be limited (<5%) or very large (>50%). Additional knowledge in the future is expected to provide a much better basis for rational prevention of conditions leading to male infertility. A list of recommendations of clinical relevance for counseling the infertile male is given in Table 2.

REFERENCES

1. Sömmering ST. De Morbis Vasorum Absorbentium Corporis Humani. Frankfurt, Germany: Varrentrapp & Wenner, 1795.
2. Bolumar F, Olsen J, Boldsen J. Smoking reduces fecundity: A European multicenter study on infertility and subfecundity. The European Study Group on Infertility and Subfecundity. Am J Epidemiol 1996; 143:578–587.
3. Ramlau-Hansen CH, Thulstrup AM, Aggerholm AS, et al. Is smoking a risk factor for decreased semen quality? A cross-sectional analysis. Hum Reprod 2007; 22: 186–196.
4. Vine MF, Margolin BH, Morrison HI, et al. Cigarette smoking and sperm density: A meta-analysis. Fertil Steril 1994; 61:35–43.
5. Vine MF. Smoking and male reproduction: A review. Int J Androl 1996; 19:323–337.
6. Osawa Y, Tochigi B, Tochigi M, et al. Aromatase inhibitors in cigarette smoke, tobacco leaves and other plants. J Enzyme Inhib 1990; 4:187–200.
7. Jensen TK, Henriksen TB, Hjollund NH, et al. Adult and prenatal exposures to tobacco smoke as risk indicators of fertility among 430 Danish couples. Am J Epidemiol 1998; 148:992–997.
8. Storgaard L, Bonde JP, Ernst E, et al. Does smoking during pregnancy affect sons' sperm counts?. Epidemiology 2003; 14:278–286.
9. Jensen TK, Jorgensen N, Punab M, et al. Association of in utero exposure to maternal smoking with reduced semen quality and testis size in adulthood: A cross-sectional study of 1770 young men from the general population in five European countries. Am J Epidemiol 2004; 159: 49–58.
10. Jensen MS, Mabeck LM, Toft G, et al. Lower sperm counts following prenatal tobacco exposure. Hum Reprod 2005; 20:2559–2566.
11. Ramlau-Hansen CH, Thulstrup AM, Storgaard L, et al. Is prenatal exposure to tobacco smoking a cause of poor semen quality? A follow-up study. Am J Epidemiol 2007; 165:1372–1379.
12. Ratcliffe JM, Gladen BC, Wilcox AJ, et al. Does early exposure to maternal smoking affect future fertility in adult males? Reprod Toxicol 1992; 6:297–307.
13. Baird DD, Wilcox AJ: Future fertility after prenatal exposure to cigarette smoke. Fertil Contracept 1986; 46:368–372.
14. MacKenzie KM, Angevine DM. Infertility in mice exposed in utero to benzo(a)pyrene. Biol Reprod 1981; 24: 183–191.
15. Ramlau-Hansen CH, Thulstrup AM, Olsen J, et al. Maternal smoking in pregnancy and reproductive hormones in adult sons. Int J Androl 2008; 31:565–572.
16. Pettersson A, Kaijser M, Richiardi L, et al. Women smoking and testicular cancer: One epidemic causing another? Int J Cancer 2004; 109:941–944.
17. Pettersson A, Akre O, Richiardi L, et al. Maternal smoking and the epidemic of testicular cancer—A nested case-control study. Int J Cancer 2007; 120:2044–2046.
18. Jensen MS, Toft G, Thulstrup AM, et al. Cryptorchidism according to maternal gestational smoking. Epidemiology 2007; 18:220–225.
19. Kallen K. Role of maternal smoking and maternal reproductive history in the etiology of hypospadias in the offspring. Teratology 2002; 66:185–191.
20. Skakkebaek NE. Testicular dysgenesis syndrome. Horm Res 2003; 60(suppl 3):49–49.
21. Sonne SB, Hoei-Hansen CE, Fisher JS, et al. Do environmental factors play a role in the aetiology of carcinoma in situ testis and the testicular dysgenesis syndrome? Verh Dtsch Ges Pathol 2004; 88:144–151.
22. Harkonen K, Viitanen T, Larsen SB, et al. Aneuploidy in sperm and exposure to fungicides and lifestyle factors. ASCLEPIOS. A European Concerted Action on Occupational Hazards to Male Reproductive Capability. Environ Mol Mutagen 1999; 34:39–46.
23. Robbins WA, Vine MF, Truong KY, et al. Use of fluorescence in situ hybridization (FISH) to assess effects of smoking, caffeine, and alcohol on aneuploidy load in sperm of healthy men. Environ Mol Mutagen 1997; 30:175–183.
24. Rubes J, Lowe X, Moore D, et al. Smoking cigarettes is associated with increased sperm disomy in teenage men. Fertil Steril 1998; 70:715–723.

25. Loft S, Kold-Jensen T, Hjollund NH, et al. Oxidative DNA damage in human sperm influences time to pregnancy. Hum Reprod 2003; 18:1265–1272.
26. Trasler JM, Hales BF, Robaire B. Paternal cyclophosphamide treatment of rats causes fetal loss and malformations without affecting male fertility. Nature 1985; 316:144–146.
27. Friedman JM. Implications of research in male-mediated developmental toxicity to clinical counsellors, regulators, and occupational safety officers. Adv Exp Med Biol 2003; 518:219–226.
28. Anderson D. Overview of male-mediated developmental toxicity. Adv Exp Med Biol 2003; 518:11–24.
29. Trasler JM. Translational research in male mediated developmental toxicity. Adv Exp Med Biol 2003; 518:279–284.
30. Marchetti F, Lowe X, Bishop J, et al. Absence of selection against aneuploid mouse sperm at fertilization. Biol Reprod 1999; 61:948–954.
31. Sorahan T, McKinney PA, Mann JR, et al. Childhood cancer and parental use of tobacco: Findings from the inter-regional epidemiological study of childhood cancer (IRESCC). Br J Cancer 2001; 84:141–146.
32. Ji BT, Shu XO, Linet MS, et al. Paternal cigarette smoking and the risk of childhood cancer among offspring of non-smoking mothers. J Natl Cancer Inst 1997; 89:238–244.
33. Zhang J, Savitz DA, Schwingl PJ, et al. A case-control study of paternal smoking and birth defects. Int J Epidemiol 1992; 21:273–278.
34. Ramlau-Hansen CH, Thulstrup AM, Nohr EA, et al. Subfecundity in overweight and obese couples. Hum Reprod 2007; 22:1634–1637.
35. Nguyen RH, Wilcox AJ, Skjaerven R, et al. Men's body mass index and infertility. Hum Reprod 2007; 22:2488–2493.
36. Jensen TK, Andersson AM, Jorgensen N, et al. Body mass index in relation to semen quality and reproductive hormones among 1558 Danish men. Fertil Steril 2004; 82:863–870.
37. Aggerholm AS, Thulstrup AM, Toft G, et al. Is overweight a risk factor for reduced semen quality and altered serum sex hormone profile? Fertil Steril 2008; 90:619–626.
38. Ramlau-Hansen CH, Nohr EA, Thulstrup AM, et al. Is maternal obesity related to semen quality in the male offspring? A pilot study. Hum Reprod 2007; 22:2758–2762.
39. Pajarinen JT, Karhunen PJ. Spermatogenic arrest and "Sertoli cell-only" syndrome–common alcohol-induced disorders of the human testis. Int J Androl 1994; 17(6):292–299.
40. Pajarinen J, Laippala P, Penttila A, Karhunen PJ. Incidence of disorders of spermatogenesis in middle aged Finnish men, 1981–91: Two necropsy series. BMJ 1997; 314(7073):13–18
41. Jensen TK, Hjollund NH, Henriksen TB, et al. Does moderate alcohol consumption affect fertility? Follow up study among couples planning first pregnancy. BMJ 1998; 317:505–510.
42. Jensen TK, Henriksen TB, Hjollund NH, et al. Caffeine intake and fecundability: A follow-up study among 430 Danish couples planning their first pregnancy. Reprod Toxicol 1998; 12:289–295.
43. Mieusset R, Bujan L. Testicular heating and its possible contributions to male infertility: A review. Int J Androl 1995; 18:169–184.
44. Thonneau P, Bujan L, Multigner L, et al. Occupational heat exposure and male fertility: A review. Hum Reprod 1998; 13:2122–2125.
45. Procope BJ. Effect of repeated increase of body temperature on human sperm cells. Int J Fertil 1965; 10:333–339.
46. Carlsen E, Andersson AM, Petersen JH, et al. History of febrile illness and variation in semen quality. Hum Reprod 2003; 18:2089–2092.
47. Bonde JP. Semen quality in welders exposed to radiant heat. Br J Ind Med 1992; 49:5–10.
48. Figa-Talamanca I, Cini C, Varricchio GC, et al. Effects of prolonged autovehicle driving on male reproduction function: A study among taxi drivers. Am J Ind Med 1996; 30:750–758.
49. Thonneau P, Ducot B, Bujan L, et al. Heat exposure as a hazard to male fertility. Lancet 1996; 347:204–205.
50. Hjollund NH, Bonde JP, Jensen TK, et al. Diurnal scrotal skin temperature and semen quality. The Danish First Pregnancy Planner Study Team. Int J Androl 2000; 23:309–318.
51. Stoy J, Hjollund NH, Mortensen JT, et al. Semen quality and sedentary work position. Int J Androl 2004; 27(1):5–11.
52. Jung A, Eberl M, Schill WB. Improvement of semen quality by nocturnal scrotal cooling and moderate behavioural change to reduce genital heat stress in men with oligoasthenoteratozoospermia. Reproduction 2001; 121:595–603.
53. Uno H, Tarara R, Else JG, et al. Hippocampal damage associated with prolonged and fatal stress in primates. J Neurosci 1989; 9:1705–1711.
54. Fuchs E, Flugge G, Ohl F, et al. Psychosocial stress, glucocorticoids, and structural alterations in the tree shrew hippocampus. Physiol Behav 2001; 73:285–291.
55. McGrady AV. Effects of psychological stress on male reproduction: A review. Arch Androl 1984; 13:1–7.
56. Hjollund NH, Bonde JP, Henriksen TB, et al. Reproductive effects of male psychologic stress. Epidemiology 2004; 15(1):21–27.
57. Hjollund H, Storgaard L, Bonde JP, et al. Can a negative time trend of sperm density be explained by changes in reproductive pattern? Epidemiology 2002; 13:746–748.
58. Czeizel AE, Rothman KJ. Does relaxed reproductive selection explain the decline in male reproductive health? A new hypothesis. Epidemiology 2002; 13:113–114.
59. Storgaard L, Bonde JP, Ernst E, et al. Genetic and environmental correlates of semen quality: A twin study. Epidemiology 2006; 17:674–681.
60. Whorton MD, Krauss RM, Marshall S, et al. Infertility in male pesticide workers. Lancet 1977; 2:1259–1261.

61. Whorton MD, Milby TH. Recovery of testicular function among DBCP workers. J Occup Med 1980; 22:177–179.
62. Ogilvy-Stuart AL, Shalet SM. Effect of radiation on the human reproductive system. Environ Health Perspect 1993; 101(suppl 2):109–116.
63. Jensen TK, Bonde JP, Joffe M. The influence of occupational exposure on male reproductive function. Occup Med (Lond) 2006; 56:544–553.
64. Bonde JP, Joffe M, Apostoli P, et al. Sperm count and chromatin structure in men exposed to inorganic lead: Lowest adverse effect levels. Occup Environ Med 2002; 59: 234–242.
65. Woolf PD, Hamill RW, McDonald JV, et al. Transient hypogonadotropic hypogonadism caused by critical illness. J Clin Endocrinol Metab 1985; 60(3):444–450.
66. Handelsman DJ, Strasser S, McDonald JA, et al. Hypothalamic-pituitary-testicular function in end-stage non-alcoholic liver disease before and after liver transplantation. Clin Endocrinol (Oxf) 1995; 43(3):331–337.
67. Handelsman DJ. Hypothalamic-pituitary gonadal dysfunction in renal failure, dialysis and renal transplantation. Endocr Rev 1985; 6(2):151–182.
68. Wang C, Tso SC, Todd D. Hypogonadotropic hypogonadism in severe beta-thalassemia: Effect of chelation and pulsatile gonadotropin-releasing hormone therapy. J Clin Endocrinol Metab 1989; 68(3):511–516.
69. Zelissen PM, van Hattum J, Poen H, et al. Influence of salazosulphapyridine and 5-aminosalicylic acid on seminal qualities and male sex hormones. Scand J Gastroenterol 1988; 23(9):1100–1104.
70. Farthing MJ, Dawson AM. Impaired semen quality in Crohn's disease—Drugs, ill health, or undernutrition?. Scand J Gastroenterol 1983; 18(1):57–60.
71. Lohi S, Lohi O, Vierula M, et al. Coeliac disease autoantibodies in seminal plasma from cases with screen-detected coeliac disease. Scand J Gastroenterol 2009; 44(4):509–511.
72. Perheentupa J. Autoimmune polyendocrinopathy-candidiasis-ectodermal dystrophy. J Clin Endocrinol Metab 2006; 91(8):2843–2850.
73. Viviani S, Santoro A, Ragni G, et al. Gonadal toxicity after combination chemotherapy for Hodgkin's disease. Comparative results of MOPP vs. ABVD. Eur J Cancer Clin Oncol 1985; 21(5):601–605.
74. Johnson L, Zane RS, Petty CS, Neaves WB. Quantification of the human Sertoli cell population: Its distribution, relation to germ cell numbers, and age-related decline. Biol Reprod 1984; 31(4):785–795.
75. Sharpe RM, Skakkebaek NE. Testicular dysgenesis syndrome: Mechanistic insights and potential new downstream effects. Fertil Steril 2008; 89(suppl 2):e33–e38.
76. Skakkebaek NE, Rajpert-De Meyts E, Main KM. Testicular dysgenesis syndrome: An increasingly common developmental disorder with environmental aspects. Hum Reprod 2001; 16(5):972–978.
77. Kortenkamp A. Low dose mixture effects of endocrine disrupters: Implications for risk assessment and epidemiology. Int J Androl 2008; 31(2):233–240.
78. Rider CV, Furr J, Wilson VS, Gray LE Jr. A mixture of seven antiandrogens induces reproductive malformations in rats. Int J Androl 2008; 31(2):249–262.

20 Infertility and testis cancer

Patrick de Geeter and Peter Albers

- At the time of diagnosis, an abnormal semen analysis report is a frequent finding in patients with testicular cancer. Approximately 50% of the men with initial oligozoospermia or azoospermia will recover normal sperm quality within 4 to 19 months after orchiectomy and before any additional treatment.
- Advances in surgical techniques have allowed for the preservation of ejaculatory function and significantly reduced the risk for infertility associated with retroperitoneal lymph node dissection (RPLND).
- In general, approximately 25% of the patients after four cycles of (cis)platin–vinblastin–bleomycin (PVB) chemotherapy can be expected to be azoospermic. Two cycles of (cis)platin–etoposide–bleomycin (PEB) chemotherapy have only a small transient impact upon fertility when initial sperm counts are within a normal range. Higher cisplatin doses are definitely more harmful with regard to fertility.
- Men receiving adjuvant infradiaphragmatic radiotherapy for seminoma may experience a transient decrease in sperm counts but can anticipate a recovery of spermatogenesis within three years.
- There is no increased risk for congenital malformations after chemotherapy.
- The ability to preserve fertility through assisted reproductive technologies is an option for men who have persistent azoospermia or anejaculation after treatment of testicular cancer, and cryopreservation should always be recommended to enhance the potential for paternity.

INTRODUCTION

Testicular cancer (TC) represents the most common solid organ tumor in men between 25 and 35 years of age, with an incidence of 3 to 6 new cases occurring per 100,000 males /yr in Western society and up to 9 to 10 new cases per 100,000 males/yr in Germany and Scandinavian countries (1). Fortunately, TC is also one of the most curable malignancies, with an excellent survival rate due to a standardized multimodality treatment. After the introduction of cisplatin-based chemotherapy into the treatment of TC in the 1970s, the cancer-specific five-year survival rates for these patients approach 95% in the Western world (2). Consequently, the objective of contemporary TC treatment is not only cure but also the prevention of therapy-induced late toxicity, which has been observed in approximately 20% of TC survivors.

One of the major concerns is infertility (3). Infertility in TC survivors is related to both the malignancy itself and/or the treatment (4). It is very important to determine how TC and infertility are interrelated and to what extent TC might be exacerbated by different treatment modalities to preserve natural fertility by the best means possible.

INFERTILITY IN PATIENTS WITH TC AT DIAGNOSIS

At the time of diagnosis, an abnormal semen analysis report is a frequent finding in patients with TC: among them, 54% to 57% presented with oligozoospermia and 11% to 13% with azoospermia before orchidectomy. It is, therefore, not surprising that 30% of these patients will have an elevated follicle-stimulating hormone (FSH) level (5,6); in addition, up to 20% of the patients might show elevated luteinizing hormone (LH) levels although testosterone level is generally in the normal range indicating a normal Leydig cell function. From the literature, even more data are available on postorchiectomy parameters in patients presenting with TC, and one can derive from those data that an impaired spermatogenesis is initially present in approximately 50% to 70% of these patients before any cytotoxic therapy (7).

As an example, in a study from the University of Indiana, there was a 77% incidence of oligozoospermia at the time of diagnosis, including 17% azoospermia (8). The most frequent findings include low sperm concentration, poor motility, or low semen volume. Some studies verified the marked decline in sperm quality among patients with TC in comparison with healthy volunteers (9). Other investigations revealed that impaired spermatogenesis was neither related to the stage of the disease nor was correlated with the duration and severity of symptoms attributed to the TC (5,7). However, there might be a difference in sperm production between seminoma and nonseminomatous germ cell tumors (NSGCT) patients, although this issue is rather controversial. Some reports found a superior sperm quality in seminoma patients (9), whereas others found no differences between both entities (7) and even lower sperm counts in seminoma patients (10). It is possible that the more advanced age of most seminoma patients and not the type of disease was the main reason for a lower sperm count. Other studies confirmed histologically that the semen quality in patients with pure seminoma was higher than that in patients with a pure embryonal tumor and these differences persisted after stratification for patients' age and tumor size and stage (9,11). Although both tumors exhibited equally poor spermatogenesis in the proximate regions, men with embryonal carcinomas had significantly lower scores than those with seminomas in regions remote from the tumor. A continuum in the malignant transformation of the germ cell might explain these differences. There is some evidence that the first state of malignant transformation is in the direction of a seminoma tumor, which bears a greater resemblance to the normal germ cells than do more aggressive tumors. In a further transformation, these cells lose any resemblance to the functioning germ cells and gain more aggressive characteristics, through embryonal carcinoma, the primitive embryonal tissues (teratoma), and extraembryonic tissue (yolk sac carcinoma and choriocarcinoma). This may explain why spermatogenesis is more severely affected in NSGCT compared with seminoma tumors.

In conclusion, impaired spermatogenesis is a very frequent finding in the presence of TC, either seminoma or NSGCT. At the same time, it is important to note that this effect might be reversible under certain conditions as some investigators report that approximately 50% of the men with initial oligospermia or azoospermia will recover normal sperm quality within 4 to 19 months after orchiectomy and before any additional treatment. Further evidence is available from men successfully followed on surveillance who can expect a stable or improved semen quality postorchiectomy (12,13). In general, however, impaired spermatogenesis will be further exacerbated by additional anticancer treatments postorchiectomy. Nevertheless, the exact etiology for initially impaired spermatogenesis in patients with TC is still unknown and there is much evidence that the causes might be multifactorial. Many possible etiologies have to be considered, that is, abnormal testicular development, systemic cancer effects, local tumor effects, and endocrine factors.

Abnormal Testicular Development

Abnormalities in testicular maturation, such as cryptorchidism, are often associated with infertility and TC. However, this condition should not be confounded with retractile or ectopic testes. Fertility is often reduced in men with undescended and therefore unpalpable testis, even after orchiopexy in infancy. In case of unilateral cryptorchidism, the incidence of infertility is only slightly elevated with a reported rate of approximately 10% (compared with approximately 6% for the general population of adult men) but is more pronounced after orchiopexy for bilateral cryptorchidism with a rate of approximately 38%, which is six times higher than that of the general population. Although the elevated intra-abdominal temperature is at least one major contributing factor for impaired spermatogenesis in cryptorchid testes, further research in the last decades suggest that this issue might be more complex and that intrinsic anomalies of the undescended testis and additional factors such as a high rate of anomalies of the epididymis could be even more important. Especially those factors that cause the lack of descent of the testis are believed to impair the development of spermatogenic tissue as well. One of the strongest arguments for early orchiopexy is prevention of TC, as the reported relative risk for TC in patients who have cryptorchidism is 3 to 14 times higher than the expected incidence (14,15). Until recently, it was controversial whether early orchiopexy actually reduces the chance of developing TC, although it was recognized that orchiopexy would at least make cancer more easily recognizable at an earlier stage. In a large recently published retrospective study from Sweden, early orchiopexy was clearly associated with a decreased risk of developing TC. In that study, the relative risk for TC was 2.23 if orchiopexy was performed before the age of 13 years and increased to 5.4 when orchiectomy took place after that age (16). These results were confirmed by a meta-analysis of four studies, placing the cutoff point for early orchiopexy at 10 years of age; orchiectomy after the age of 10 was associated with a relative risk of 5.8 for TC (17). Therefore, recent evidence indicates that early orchiopexy reduces the risk of developing TC. As with infertility, the causes of cancer associated with cryptorchidism are not very well known. Again, most evidence suggests that cancer risk is due to an inherent abnormality of the undescended testis. Impaired spermatogenesis, cryptorchidism, and germ cell tumors represent a spectrum of abnormal testicular development and are often interrelated. Andersson and Skakkebaek and colleagues propose that this spectrum of testicular maldevelopment should be classified as testicular dysgenesis syndrome (18). Their hypothesis advocates a common cause, either genetic or environmental, for cryptorchidism, hypospadias, impaired spermatogenesis, and testis cancer (19). Further support for this hypothesis was given by Hoei-Hansen et al. from a study where ultimately 25.2% of patients who had germ cell tumors had evidence of testicular dysgenesis and 8.7% had carcinoma in situ in the contralateral testis (20).

Together with other findings concerning the incidence of TC in cohorts of patients with infertility, this raises the question regarding the nature of the relationship between abnormal spermatogenesis and TC: Is this association a "chicken" or "egg" phenomenon? Does TC and its precursor lesions induce infertility or does abnormal spermatogenesis generate critical cells that ultimately produce germ cell malignancies? Indeed, some studies are available documenting an increased risk for TC in patients presenting with infertility. This connection is clearly documented in a large population-based study in Denmark including 32,442 men who underwent semen analysis from 1963 to 1995, where men who had abnormal semen analysis results had an increased risk for developing TC compared with the general Danish population (21). The authors of a more recent evaluation of 3800 men presenting with infertility and abnormal semen analysis results in the United States concluded that infertile patients have a risk of testicular tumor development that is 20 times higher than that in the normal population (22). All these arguments indicate a close interrelationship between infertility and TC, which seems to depend to a major extent upon developmental anomalies.

Systemic Cancer Effects

Despite the possibility of a common developmental origin, the association between germ cell tumors and infertility may also result from malignancy itself, which can have a wide range of effects on the body, including metabolic derangements, hormonal imbalances, and thermoregulatory changes. Investigations in young men with TC or Hodgkin disease revealed a substantial number of patients with abnormal semen analysis results before the initiation of treatment. The risk for impaired spermatogenesis increased with elevated levels of acute-phase reactants and advanced stage. Some changes may result from the tumor itself or from the body's response by means of cytokines, interleukins, or tumor necrosis factors (23).

Local Tumor Effects

TC not only disrupts the architecture of the testis but also its functionality, being more pronounced in more advanced tumors, which are generally associated with worse semen quality than are tumors of lower stage. This seems to be related in part to a disturbance of the blood–testis barrier, which normally prevents the formation of antisperm antibodies, which could affect spermatogenesis. Although normal fertile men have a 5% to 8% incidence of antisperm antibodies, studies have reported men who have TC to have an 18%, 21%, and 73% incidence, suggesting that germ cell tumors disturb the blood–testis barrier to some extent (24). This is also evident from histopathologic studies comparing orchiectomy specimens of benign versus malignant tumors, where benign tumors revealed significantly fewer abnormalities in spermatogenesis (25). As already mentioned, many reports describe an improvement in semen quality after orchiectomy in patients with TC, adding more evidence to the role of local tumor effects on spermatogenesis (12,13).

Endocrine Factors

Germ cell tumors, especially NSGCT, can produce β-human chorionic gonadotropin (β-HCG) and α-fetoprotein (AFP). Some investigators found a quantifiable correlation between increased β-HCG levels and decreased spermatogenesis in the contralateral testis (26). An endocrine mechanism has been postulated in which β-HCG stimulation of intratesticular estradiol impairs spermatogenesis. The exact influence of AFP on spermatogenesis is rather unclear, although there is some evidence that elevated AFP levels were associated with decreased sperm counts in NSGCTs. In up to 30% of patients with TC, serum FSH levels are elevated (5), serving as an indicator for impaired spermatogenesis. Men who have TC and elevated FSH levels before treatment generally have more posttreatment fertility disturbances compared with patients with normal FSH levels, irrespective of the kind of anticancer treatment. On the other hand, malignancy itself seems to be able to disturb the hypothalamic–pituitary axis, and FSH and LH levels are often abnormal in patients with a malignant disease. As an example, men with untreated Hodgkin disease were found to have significantly decreased FSH and testosterone levels compared with healthy controls; in addition, low testosterone level was not compensated by high LH levels suggestive for some dysfunction of the hypothalamic–pituitary axis (27).

Other Factors

The mere fact that after orchiectomy one should expect a 50% reduction in the germinal epithelium might, in itself, explain the reduced capacity for sperm production. Ferreira et al. examined men with one testis and found that regardless of the etiology, 50% had a sperm concentration of less than 20×10^6/mL (28), and similar findings have been reported recently by Lin et al. who evaluated semen quality after unilateral testicular injury (29).

TC TREATMENT AND INFERTILITY

The association between the development of testicular germ cell cancer and infertility is well known although the causative factors are still being investigated. Also documented is the potential for improved fertility after the primary tumor is removed at radical orchiectomy. Cancer treatment, therefore, has the potential to reverse impaired spermatogenesis associated with testicular neoplasia, although the treatment of testicular neoplasm is a complex paradigm involving histology, stage, and patient selection. After radical orchiectomy, four treatment options are currently available: surveillance, retroperitoneal lymph node dissection (RPLND), chemotherapy, and radiation therapy. Unfortunately, these treatments can have further impact on reproductive function and have distinct implications for post-treatment fertility (4).

Surveillance

Postorchiectomy surveillance is a realistic treatment option for men with low-risk criteria and stage I disease, provided patients strictly adhere to the surveillance protocol. Through surveillance, potential post-RPLND ejaculatory disturbances and gonadotoxic therapies can be avoided in the majority of these patients, although approximately 20% of men eventually relapse and will then require additional treatment. Advocates of primary RPLND will argue that men who relapse on surveillance protocols and require gonadotoxic treatments may be at greater risk for infertility than men initially treated with nerve-sparing RPLND (30).

In men successfully followed with a surveillance policy without relapse, semen analysis parameters, including sperm concentrations, may remain stable or actually improve after orchiectomy. Carroll et al. described that approximately 50% of the men with initial oligospermia or azoospermia will recover normal sperm quality within 4 to 19 months after orchiectomy. Jacobsen et al. confirm this by finding a significant increase in sperm concentration at one year postorchiectomy (12,13). In general, men successfully followed on surveillance can expect a stable or improved semen quality postorchiectomy.

Retroperitoneal Lymph Node Dissection

RPLND can influence fertility due to the risk of postoperative ejaculatory disorders, whether performed with primary intention or as residual tumor resection (RTR) after previous cytotoxic therapy. Removal of the retroperitoneal lymph nodes may compromise the postganglionic sympathetic nerve fibers, which arise from both sides of the aorta and join in the midline to form the hypogastric plexus in the pelvis. These delicate nerves innervate the seminal vesicles, the ampullary part of the vas deferens, internal sphincter and periurethral musculature, and glands. An intraoperative lesion of these nerves can result in retrograde ejaculation or even anejaculation depending on the severity of the nerve injury. Until 1980 this occurred rather systematically after a routine staging lymphadenectomy in which all lymphatic tissue around the great vessels was removed (standard radical bilateral lymphadenectomy) from the renal hilum down to the aortic bifurcation. Since the early 80s, the risk for this complication diminished substantially—at least for staging lymphadenectomies—with the introduction of technical modifications based on topographic anatomical studies. These techniques allow nerve preservation by adhering to so-called dissection templates or even nerve sparing due to intraoperative identification of the nerves. By using a dissection template in staging lymphadenectomy, antegrade ejaculation could be preserved in roughly 75% of the patients, whereas this percentage increased to 98% with the nerve sparing technique, introduced by Donohue (31). In an updated study, the same group documented 76% of men after nerve-sparing RPLND for stage 1 NSGCT being successful after their attempts to conceive (32). Although equally good results are hardly possible in cases of RTR, introduction of identical technical modifications could diminish the incidence of retrograde ejaculation in these cases. However, anejaculation, diminished ejaculatory volume, and retrograde ejaculation will be present in at least 50% of patients after RTR. In those cases, ejaculatory problems often aggravate pre-existing fertility disturbances, which necessitate specific treatment (33). In case of retrograde ejaculation after RPLND, sympathomimetics may temporarily restore antegrade ejaculation. In a small series, Jonas et al. describe the efficacy of an intravenous injection of 30 mg midodrin in 7 out of 10 patients. Later reports on the use of oral midodrin were less successful (34). In some patients with anejaculation, electroejaculation (in general anesthesia) by means of a rectal probe could deliver viable sperm for subsequent in vitro fertilization (IVF). In summary, advances in surgical techniques have allowed for the preservation of ejaculatory function and significantly reduced the risk for infertility associated with RPLND.

Chemotherapy

Current cisplatin-based chemotherapy regimens have significantly increased the survival of patients with TC and therefore, potential side effects might gain more importance. Gonadal dysfunction is one of the most common side effects of chemotherapy (35). Both the endocrine and exocrine compartments of the testis are affected by chemotherapy. The serum FSH levels rise immediately after initiation of chemotherapy, indicating a dysfunction of the germinal epithelium (8,36–39). Although the Leydig cells of the testes are more resistant to cytotoxic damage than is the germinal epithelium, the increased LH levels in men suggest an endocrine dysfunction (38–40). This probably represents a compensatory mechanism resulting from reduced negative feedback by testosterone at the hypothalamic–pituitary level. Testicular exocrine function, however, is more affected by systemic chemotherapy, which targets rapidly dividing cells, explaining the vulnerability of germinal cells. Especially, the differentiating spermatogonia with a pronounced mitotic and meiotic activity, such as spermatogonia Ap (pale) and spermatogonia B, are very vulnerable cells, whereas spermatogonia Ad (dark) seem to be less sensitive and represent some kind of cellular reserve (37). The duration and severity of the spermatogenic depression depends upon the dose and duration of chemotherapy and baseline testis function prior to therapy, where initial FSH levels serve as a good indicator (41). Alkylating agents especially, such as cisplatin, are the most toxic drugs with regard to spermatogenesis. Damage to both spermatogenesis and testicular endocrine function will be temporary, provided that the cumulative cisplatin dose does not exceed 400 mg/m^2. Combination with ifosfamide (42 g/m^2) seems to increase toxicity (42). In an already mentioned study from Indiana University, changes in fertility at diagnosis and with subsequent follow-up evaluations at 6, 12, and 24 months following four cycles of PVB chemotherapy (20 mg/m^2 cisplatin from day 1 to 5 in each cycle) were documented (8).

In that study, there was a 77% incidence of oligospermia at the time of diagnosis, including 17% incidence of azoospermia. At six months following chemotherapy, all patients were azoospermic. At two years, oligospermia was still present in 75%, including 25% who were azoospermic. Other studies that have investigated sperm concentrations following chemotherapy with PVB have shown similar results, emphasizing that severe disturbances in spermatogenesis, observed one to three years after chemotherapy in patients with NSGCT, are likely to be the expression of a highly impaired pretreatment sperm cell production and only to a lesser degree dependent on the influence of chemotherapy on exocrine testicular function (6). In 1987, Nijman et al. (43) reported their results with 54 patients treated with four cycles of PVB chemotherapy. They found a 48% incidence of oligospermia and a 28% incidence of azoospermia after two years. A 1990 report by Hansen et al. (38) described a similar two-year incidence of azoospermia (27%), following PVB chemotherapy at a median follow-up time of 64 months. They did not state the exact incidence of oligospermia but indicated that more than half of the patients had persistent oligospermia. In general, however, around 25% of the patients after four cycles of PVB chemotherapy can be expected to be azoospermic. This is a very important finding, whereas oligospermia might have less severe consequences. Indeed, some studies were able to show that many patients who fathered children after chemotherapy were indeed oligospermic with sperm concentrations below 5×10^6/mL. This indicates that a low sperm concentration does not in itself preclude fatherhood (38).

Higher doses of chemotherapy certainly have an even more pronounced effect on fertility. Petersen and colleagues compared semen analyses and hormonal profiles from 33 men treated with conventional-dose PEB to data obtained from 21 men treated with high-dose PEB and found azoospermia in 19% and 47% of men treated with conventional-dose PEB and high-dose PEB, respectively (44). In addition, FSH levels were significantly higher in men who received high-dose PEB. No difference in testosterone or LH level was noted between the groups. These abnormalities in semen analyses and hormone levels are not necessarily permanent, and the potential for normalization of endocrine and spermatogenic function exists. On the other hand, lower cisplatin doses administered as two cycles of adjuvant chemotherapy (cumulative cisplatin dose of <240 mg/m^2) in patients with (high-risk) stage I NSGCT seem to produce only minor fertility disturbances although a slight risk of long-term impairment of spermatogenesis (azoospermia) could not be excluded (45). In the meantime, two cycles of adjuvant, cisplatin-based combined chemotherapy for patients with high-risk, stage I nonseminomatous germ cell tumor result in excellent long-term disease control. It needs to be emphazised that this therapy is associated with only mild short-term and minimal long-term toxicity, particularly with regard to fertility and sexual activity. Therefore, two cycles of modified PEB adjuvant chemotherapy can provide a valuable treatment option, particularly for patients with a possibly compromised follow-up. Recovery of spermatogenesis depends on the level of spermatogonial stem cells killed and the rate at which the surviving stem cells can repopulate the seminiferous tubule and resume differentiation. Despite an early depression in spermatogenesis, a reasonable number of patients show recovery within one to two years after treatment with variable sperm counts in their ejaculates (39,43,46). Although some reports indicate that abnormal sperm counts two years after treatment will no longer improve with time (38), more recent findings tend to give a more optimistic view, as indicated by a study from the Royal Marsden Hospital (United Kingdom). In their summary, further improvement and even normalization of semen parameters can be expected even five years after therapy (47). A review of semen analyses from patients who had germ cell neoplasms treated with cisplatin-based chemotherapy at the Royal Marsden Hospital demonstrated that improved sperm counts were present in 48% and 80% of patients at two and five years postchemotherapy, respectively. Even more encouraging, the probability of achieving normal sperm counts was 22% and 58% at two and five years, respectively. High pretreatment sperm counts and the use of carboplatin versus cisplatin were associated with an increased probability of improved fertility postchemotherapy. In summary, systemic chemotherapy for germ cell malignancies affects both Sertoli cell and Leydig cell function and has the potential to permanently impair spermatogenesis. Recovery of spermatogenesis is possible, but men who have elevated FSH level, high-dose cisplatin therapy, and low pretreatment sperm counts are at increased risk for long-term infertility. Interestingly, the only significant difference between patients who received chemotherapy and those who did not was the sperm concentration, while no significant differences were found in morphology or motility of the spermatozoa. At this point it remains uncertain whether classical semen analysis gives the right information about the status of semen from men with testis carcinoma. Indeed, some studies indicate that sperm DNA integrity in general remained poor compared with that in healthy controls after chemotherapy. It is still unknown whether these changes in sperm integrity represent a lack of apoptosis of abnormal cells during chemotherapy (abortive apoptosis) or whether the postchemotherapy matured sperms present (persisting?) intrinsic genomic damage. Therefore, it might be prudent to evaluate semen from cancer patients, not only by routine analysis but also by genomic integrity analysis, as external characteristics of spermatozoa do not necessarily correlate with their DNA integrity (48).

Radiotherapy

The testis is a very radiosensitive organ. Gonadotoxicity depends upon several variables such as direct or diffused irradiation, total applied dose, and especially, the number and duration of fraction. This is different from other organ systems, where fractionation of radiation generally reduces cellular damage. Men diagnosed with clinical stage (CS) 1, 2A, and 2B seminoma often receive adjuvant infradiaphragmatic radiation therapy. Patients with CS 1 disease receive 20 Gy directed upon the paracaval and paraaortic region. In patients with CS 2A and 2B disease, the dose is higher, 30 and 36 Gy, respectively, and the primary field is further extended (so called dog leg) to cover the ipsilateral iliac region. Although gonadal shielding minimizes irradiation of the testis, it is rather unpractical and far from perfect, and unintended gonadal exposure doses occur, especially with increasing doses and when the boundaries of the primary field get closer (49).

During abdominopelvic radiotherapy, the scattered testicular dose may vary between 1% and 2% of the total dose applied to the tumor, that is, somewhere between 10 to 100 cGy and even up to 300 cGy according to some authors. Centola et al. documented a mean testicular radiation dose of 44 cGy with a range from 28 cGy to 90 cGy in men receiving infradiaphragmatic radiation treatment of seminoma with gonadal shielding (50). Once again, the spermatogonia are the most vulnerable cells and radiation doses between 15 and 35 cGy will cause oligospermia. Azoospermia occurs with doses between 35 and 50 cGy, whereas this effect remains reversible for doses below 200 cGy. At higher doses, permanent damage is more and more likely. Centola et al. found that no recovery of spermatogenesis was observed after radiation doses of 1.4 to 2.6 Gy, which represents a threshold for permanent testicular damage (50). The effect of the radiation on spermatogenesis is usually visible after a delay of some months, with a nadir around four to six months after the end of treatment. Time to recovery depends on the dose but usually starts around 1 year after the end of the radiation therapy and up to 10 to 18 months might be required for complete recovery (50). This is demonstrated in a retrospective study from Hahn et al. in patients receiving infradiafragmatic radiotherapy with ipsilateral iliac field at a dosage of 32 Gy, in which the scattered dose to the remaining and shielded testis was approximately 78 cGy. The majority of this (small) group of 14 patients was azoospermic 2.5 to 7.5 months after the irradiation and had a recovery of their previous sperm counts within 7.5 to 20 months (49). In another study where irradiation was limited to a lumbar para-aortic field with 20 to 24 Gy, as recommended for CS I seminomas by the national Medical Research Council (MRC, United Kingdom), gonadotoxicity was significantly reduced and no azoospermia was seen. The sperm counts after 18 months were significantly higher in this group compared with those in another group of patients that received additional ipsilateral irradiation. In addition, FSH levels were almost unchanged in the group receiving limited radiation therapy, whereas those levels increased significantly in the case of associated iliac irradiation and normalized within three years (51). LH levels generally remain unchanged after adjuvant infradiaphragmatic irradiation for seminoma (41). This is different in the case of direct testicular irradiation, where Leydig cells are damaged by radiation doses over 15 Gy; with doses greater than 20 Gy, damage might be irreversible (52). After exploring patients undergoing testicular radiation with different doses (16, 18, 20 Gy) because of testicular intraepithelial neoplasia (TIN) lesions, testosterone level was found to be reduced for more than five years in all patients, even at lower doses and the need for androgen substitution was similar at all dose levels (53). With respect to spermatogenesis, direct testicular radiation with doses greater than 16 Gy results in a Sertoli-cell–only (SCO) syndrome (54).

In conclusion, however, men receiving adjuvant infradiaphragmatic radiotherapy for seminoma may experience a transient decrease in sperm counts but can anticipate a recovery of spermatogenesis. Compared with standard chemotherapy regimens, especially carboplatin based, differences in favor of chemotherapy may exist with respect to pregnancy rates as demonstrated in a large French multicenter trial. In this study, cumulative conception rates for patients who were treated with radiotherapy were significantly lower compared with the rates for patients who were treated with chemotherapy, confirming the more deleterious effect of radiotherapy compared with chemotherapy (55).

PRESERVATION AND RESTORATION OF FERTILITY

Protection of Spermatogenesis

In animal models it has been possible to prevent gonadotoxicity during irradiation or chemotherapy by means of gonadotropin-releasing hormone (GNRH) analogues, FSH, and steroids with partially encouraging results (56).

Testicular hypothermia was proven to be rather successful in rats under the same conditions. Some clinical trials with the intention to protect spermatogenesis in men with TC were performed using GNRH analogues or medroxyprogesterone, unfortunately without any relevant protective effect on gonadal function (57,58). From a practical standpoint, the pretreatment period with GnRH analogues in men has been much shorter (one week) compared with that in animal trials, where longer pretreatment periods (six weeks) were possible and it might explain the completely different outcomes. Besides this, there have been no reports on the successful use of testicular cooling in the same setting in humans.

Sperm Cryopreservation and Assisted Reproductive Techniques

Currently, men who have TC have many options available to preserve fertility and potential paternity. The availability of sperm cryopreservation, advances in assisted reproductive techniques (ART), and testicular sperm extraction (TESE) provide the potential for fatherhood for men unable to conceive as a result of TC treatments (4).

It should be noted that men who had chemotherapy for TC have decreased fertilization rates per IVF or intracytoplasmic sperm injection (ICSI) cycle and a decreased pregnancy rate compared with men who have TC treated without chemotherapy (59).

Sperm cryopreservation has been available for more than 20 years for the preservation of fertility in patients with cancer. Freezing occurs at $-196°C$ in liquid nitrogen and freeze damage is limited by the use of an appropriate cryoprotective solution. French investigators from the Cochin hospital advocate sperm sampling for cryopreservation even before orchiectomy, which might be rather unpractical in most cases; alternatively, cryopreservation should then be performed as early as possible after orchiectomy. These recommendations have been confirmed by other groups (60,61). Sperm cryopreservation remains the best preventive strategy to cope with potential infertility problems after TC treatment, even when the individual risk for infertility might seem to be minimal. Too frequently, the possibility of sperm banking remains unknown to the patient and in some recently published series only 24% of the younger patients with cancer used the possibility of pretherapeutic sperm banking (62,63).

In some counties, however, as in France, informed consent on this specific issue is regulated by law (64). At the same time, there is some evidence that ultimately cryopreserved sperm might not be used in many cases, but even then a positive psychological effect is guaranteed (65). The success of cryopreservation depends upon the sperm quality after reviving the sample, as some sperm cells die in the process and those surviving are in general less functional with reduced motility. The quality of the sperm after thawing depends to a great extent upon the initial quality, which is generally reduced in patients with TC. This has been verified in a large comparitive French study, where the initial sperm quality from patients with TC was definitely lower compared to that from sperm donors. At the same time, sperms of patients with TC were significantly more vulnerable after the freeze–thawing process (66). To be of use in intrauterine insemination (IUI), the sample should after thawing have more than 5 million motile sperm cells/mL with a good grade of motility. If the grade of motility is poor, 10 million motile cells/mL is required. For IVF, lower sperm concentrations are needed, but at least 100,000 sperms/mL. With even lower sperm counts, ICSI can be used for fertilization.

In addition, the issue of teratogenicity is not completely solved, but it seems that at least in the setting of IVF there is no increase in genetic malformations or other developmental anomalies in the offspring conceived from cryopreserved sperm; however, in the setting of ICSI, some doubts persist why no prospective data are available. In a study evaluating the ultimate outcomes with cryopreserved sperms obtained from men before antineoplastic treatment revealed an overall 18.3% pregnancy rate and 7%, 23%, and 37% pregnancy rates with IUI, IVF, and ICSI, respectively (67). Roughly 50% of men who cryopreserved sperm seem to use this possibility afterwards. Records of 67 couples referred for ART for male factor infertility following treatment of malignancies, including TC and lymphoma, were reviewed to determine the options used and the success of various treatment modalities. Eighty-two percent of men cryopreserved sperm before treatment and 58% of men used cryopreserved sperm for ART. A total of 151 cycles of ART were completed, including 55 IUI, 82 ICSI, and 14 ICSI-frozen embryo replacements, with a corresponding delivery rate of 11.1%, 30.5%, and 21% (68). In men who have true anejaculation or azoospermia or in men where prior cryopreservation was omitted or had failed, TESE can provide viable sperms for ICSI. In very special cases, TESE can even be performed upon orchiectomized tissue (69,70).

An evaluation of 12 men who had azoospermia status post chemotherapy documented motile spermatozoa in 41.6% of men after TESE (71).

In 17 azoospermic men postchemotherapy, testicular biopsies performed at the time of TESE revealed Sertoli-cell–only syndrome in 76% of patients and hypospermatogenesis in 24% if patients. Of these patients, 45% had successful sperm extraction that resulted in livebirths in 22% of couples (72). Comparable results were published in a previous study from the UCSF and Boston University (73). The ability to preserve fertility through ART is an option for men who have persistent azoospermia or anejaculation after treatment of TC, and cryopreservation should always be recommended to enhance the potential for paternity.

Teratogenicity

TC treatment has a very high cure rate and current reproductive technologies allow many TC survivors to become new fathers. Keeping in mind the possibility of an underlying testicular dysgenesis together with the gonadotoxic potential of the anticancer treatment, concerns regarding the potential risk for congenital anomalies may arise. To get further information concerning this issue, basically two main tests can be performed on a sperm sample: an aneuploidy test to see whether there are any chromosomal abnormalities in the sperm [detected with fluorescent in situ hybridization (FISH)] and a sperm chromatin structure assay (SCSA), which looks at DNA fragmentation and stainability. In humans, assessment of sperm DNA integrity before and after treatment of germ cell neoplasms did not reveal a higher DNA fragmentation index after diagnosis of germ cell tumors in comparison with controls but did reveal a higher DNA fragmentation index up to two years after radiotherapy. This increased DNA fragmentation index was not noted after chemotherapy (74), although recent studies may change the chemotherapy issue (48). FISH analysis of semen specimens from five men after PEB treatment revealed a significantly increased frequency of diploidy and disomy 16, 18, and XY in comparison with healthy controls at 6 to 17 months after treatment (75).

However, another study using FISH to assess the risk for disomy for chromosomes 1, 12, X, Y, and XY in men treated with PEB found no increased risk for numerical chromosomal abnormalities (76).

Many retrospective studies involving patient-reported pregnancy outcomes have investigated the risk for early pregnancy loss and perinatal morbidity and mortality in children fathered by men who had TC and found no increased risk for pregnancy loss or congenital anomalies (77).

Spermon and colleagues sent questionnaires to 305 men who had germ cell tumors from 1982 to 1999, 226 of whom responded, to evaluate fertility before and after treatment (78).

They documented a 66% and 43% conception rate in patients attempting to conceive within one year before the diagnosis of TC and after treatment, respectively. The rate of congenital anomalies was approximately 4% before and after treatment of germ cell neoplasms. This data regarding the potential for genetic abnormalities in the posttreatment period provide additional arguments for sperm cryopreservation before the initiation of gonadotoxic treatment. In addition, in all men with TC, effective contraceptive methods should be employed from the very beginning and patients should be counseled to postpone conception for approximately 12 to 18 months after treatment to minimize the risk for potential fetal anomalies (61,79).

REFERENCES

1. Huyghe E, Matsuda T, Thonneau P. Increasing incidence of testicular cancer worldwide: A review. J Urol 2003; 170: 5–11.
2. Coleman MP, Gatta G, Verdecchia A, et al. EUROCARE-3 summary: Cancer survival in Europe at the end of the 20th century. Ann Oncol 2003; 14(suppl 5):128–149.
3. Kollmannsberger C, Kuzcyk M, Mayer F, et al. Late toxicity following curative treatment of testicular cancer. Semin Surg Oncol 1999; 17(4):275–281.
4. Lambert SM, Fisch H. Infertility and testis cancer. Urol Clin North Am 2007; 34:269–277.
5. Hansen PV, Glavind K, Panduro J, et al. Paternity in patients with testicular germ cell cancer: Pretreatment and post-treatment findings. Eur J Cancer 1991; 27:1385–1389.

6. Siener R, Albers P, Kliesch S, et al; German Testicular Cancer Study Group. Fertility in patients with stage I nonseminomatous germ-cell tumors (NSGCT). Analysis of the German prospective multicenter trial. J Clin Oncol, ASCO Annual Meeting Proceedings 2002; 21. Abstract 752.
7. Fossa SD, Aabyholm T, Aakvaag A. Spermatogenesis and hormonal status after orchiectomy for cancer and before supplementary treatment. Eur Urol 1984; 10:173–177.
8. Drasga RE, Einhorn LH, Williams SD. Fertility after chemotherapy for testicular cancer. J Clin Oncol 1983; 1:179–183.
9. Botchan A, Hauser R, Yogev L, et al. Testicular cancer and spermatogenesis. Hum Reprod 1997; 12 (4):755–758.
10. Hansen PV, Trykker H, Andersen J, et al. Germ cell function and hormonal status in patients with testicular cancer. Cancer 1989; 64:956–961.
11. Agarwal A, Tolentino MV Jr, Sidhu RS. Effect of cryopreservation on semen quality in patients with testicular cancer. Urology 1995; 46:382–389.
12. Carroll PR, Morse MJ, Whitmore WF Jr. Fertility status of patients with clinical stage I testis tumors on a surveillance protocol. J Urol 1987; 138(1):70–72.
13. Jacobsen KD, Theodorsen L, Fossa SD. Spermatogenesis after unilateral orchiectomy for testicular cancer in patients following surveillance policy. J Urol 2001; 165(1): 93–96.
14. Henderson BE, Benton B, Jing J. Risk factors for cancer of the testis in young men. Int J Cancer 1979; 23(5):598–602.
15. Farrer JH, Walker AH, Rajfer J. Management of the postpubertal cryptorchid testis: A statistical review. J Urol 1985; 134:1071–1076.
16. Pettersson A, Richiardi L, Nordenskjold A, et al. Age at surgery for undescended testis and risk of testicular cancer. N Engl J Med 2007; 356(18):1835–1841.
17. Walsh TJ, Dall'Era MA, Croughan MS, et al. Prepubertal orchiopexy for cryptorchidism may be associated with lower risk of testicular cancer. J Urol 2007; 178(4, pt 1): 1440–1446.
18. Bay K, Asklund C, Skakkebaek NE. Testicular dysgenesis syndrome: Possible role of endocrine disruptors. Best Pract Res Clin Endocrinol Metab 2006; 20(1):77–90.
19. Skakkebaek NE. Rajpert-De Meyts E. Jørgensen N. et al. Germ cell cancer and disorders of spermatogenesis: An environmental connection? APMIS 1998; 106(1):3–11.
20. Hoei-Hansen CE, Holm M, Rajpert-De Meyts E. Histological evidence of testicular dysgenesis in contra lateral biopsies from 218 patients with testicular germ cell cancer. J Pathol 2003; 200(3): 70–74.
21. Jacobsen R, Bostofte E, Engholm G. Risk of testicular cancer in men with abnormal semen characteristics: Cohort study. BMJ 2000; 321:789–792.
22. Raman JD, Nobert CF, Goldstein M. Increased incidence of testicular cancer in men presenting with infertility and abnormal semen analysis. J Urol 2005; 174(5):1819–1822.
23. Rueffer U, Breuer K, Josting A. Male gonadal dysfunction in patients with Hodgkin's disease prior to treatment. Ann Oncol 2001; 12(9):1307–1311.
24. Guazzieri S, Lembo A, Ferro G. Sperm antibodies an infertility in patients with testicular cancer. Urology 1985; 26(2):139–142.
25. Ho GT, Gardner H, Mostofi K. The effect of testicular nongerm cell tumors on local spermatogenesis. Fertil Steril 1994; 62(1):162–166.
26. Hayashi T, Arai G, Hyochi N. Suppression of spermatogenesis in ipsilateral and contra lateral testicular tissues in patients with seminoma by human chorionic gonadotropin beta subunit. Urology 2001; 58(2): 251–257.
27. Vigersky RA, Chapman RM, Berenberg J. Testicular dysfunction in untreated Hodgkin's disease. Am J Med 1982; 73(4):482–486.
28. Ferreira U, Netto NR Jr, Esteves SC. Comparative study of the fertility potential of men with only one testis. Scand J Urol Nephrol 1991; 25:255.
29. Lin WW, Kim ED, Quesada ET. Unilateral testicular injury from external trauma: Evaluation of semen quality and endocrine parameters. J Urol 1998; 159:841.
30. Herr HW, Bar-Chama N, O'Sullivan M. Paternity in men with stage I testis tumors on surveillance. J Clin Oncol 1998; 16(2):733–734.
31. Donohue JP, Foster RS, Rowland RG, et al. Nerve-sparing retroperitoneal lymphadenectomy with preservation of ejaculation. J Urol 1990; 144:287–291.
32. Foster RS, McNulty A, Rubin LR. The fertility of patients with clinical stage 1 testis cancer managed by nerve sparing retroperitoneal lymph node dissection. J Urol 1994; 152(4):1150–1151.
33. Turek PJ, Lowther DN, Carroll PR. Fertility issues and their management in men with testis cancer. Urol Clin North Am 1998; 25:517–532.
34. Jonas D, Linzbach P, Weber W. The use of midodrin in the treatment of ejaculations disorders following retroperitoneal lymphadenectomy. Eur Urol 1979; 5:184–187.
35. DeSantis M, Albrecht W, Holtl W, et al. Impact of cytotoxic treatment on long-term fertility in patients with germ-cell cancer. Int J Cancer 1999; 83:864–865.
36. Hendry WF, Stedronska J, Jones CR, et al. Semen analysis in testicular cancer and Hodgkin's disease: Pre- and post-treatment findings and implications for cryopreservation. Br J Urol 1983; 55:69–773.
37. Meistrich ML. Relationship between spermatogonial stem cell survival and testis function after cytotoxic therapy. Br J Cancer Suppl 1986; 7:89–101.
38. Hansen SW, Berthelsen JG, von der Maase H. Long-term fertility and Leydig cell function in patients treated for germ cell cancer with cisplatin, vinblastine, and bleomycin versus surveillance. J Clin Oncol 1990; 8:1695–1698.

39. Howell SJ, Radford JA, Ryder WD, et al. Testicular function after cytotoxic chemotherapy: Evidence of Leydig cell insufficiency. J Clin Oncol 1999; 17:1493–1498.
40. Brennemann W, Stoffel-Wagner B, Helmers A, et al. Gonadal function of patients treated with cisplatin based chemotherapy for germ cell cancer. J Urol 1997; 158: 844–850.
41. Brennemann W, Stoffel-Wagner B, Wichers M, et al. Pretreatment follicle-stimulating hormone: A prognostic serum marker of spermatogenesis in patients treated for germ cell cancer. J Urol 1998; 159:1942–1946.
42. Pont J, Albrecht W. Fertility after chemotherapy for testicular germ cell cancer. Fertil Steril 1997; 68:1.
43. Nijman JM, Schraffordt Koops H, Kremer J, et al. Gonadal function after surgery and chemotherapy in men with stage II and III nonseminomatous testicular tumors. J Clin Oncol 1987; 5:651–656.
44. Petersen PM, Hansen SW, Giwercman A. Dose-dependent impairment of testicular function in patients treated with cisplatin-based chemotherapy for germ cell cancer. Ann Oncol 1994; 5(4):355–358.
45. Böhlen D, Burkhard FC, Mills R, et al. Fertility and sexual function following orchiectomy and 2 cycles of chemotherapy for stage I high risk nonseminomatous germ cell cancer. J Urol 2001; 165:441–444.
46. Costabile RA. The effects of cancer and cancer therapy on male reproductive function. J Urol 1993; 149:1327–1330.
47. Lampe H, Horwich A, Norman A. Fertility after chemotherapy for testicular germ cell cancers. J Clin Oncol 1997; 15(1):239–245.
48. Spermon JR, Ramos L, Wetzels AMM, et al. Sperm integrity pre- and post-chemotherapy in men with testicular germ cell cancer. Hum Reprod 2006; 21(7):1781–1786.
49. Hahn EW, Feingold SM, Simpson L. Recovery from aspermia induced by low-dose radiation in seminoma patients. Cancer 1982; 50(2):337–340.
50. Centola GM, Keller JW, Henzler M, et al. Effect of low-dose testicular irradiation on sperm count and fertility in patients with testicular seminoma. J Androl 1994; 15:608–613.
51. Fossa SD, Horwich A, Russel JM, et al. Optimal planing target volume for stage I testicular seminoma: A Medical Research Council randomized trial. J Clin Oncol 1999; 17:1146–1154.
52. Meistrich ML, Vassilopoulou-Sellin R, Lipshultz L. Adverse effects of treatment: Gonadal dysfunction. In: DeVita VT, Hellman S, Rosenberg SA, eds. Cancer: Principles and Practice of Oncology, 7th ed. Philadelphia: Lippincott Williams & Wilkins, 2005:2560–2574.
53. Petersen PM, Giwercman A, Daugaard G, et al. Effect of graded testicular doses of radiotherapy in patients treated for carcinoma-in-situ in the testis. J Clin Oncol 2002; 15:1537–1543.
54. Classen J, Dieckmann K, Bamberg M. German Testicular Cancer Study Group. Radiotherapy with 16 Gy may fail to eradicate testicular intraepithelial neoplasia: Preliminary communication of a dose-reduction trial of the German Testicular Cancer Study Group. Br J Cancer 2003; 88:828–831.
55. Huyghe E, Matsuda T, Daudin M, et al. Fertility after Testicular Cancer Treatments. Results of a Large Multicenter Study. Cancer 2004; 100 (4):732–737.
56. Velez De La Calle JF, Ben Hassel M, Jegou B. Protection gonadique contre les effets iatrogènes des traitements anticancéreux: Données expérimentales. Andrologie 1995; 5:498–503.
57. Blumenfeld Z, Haim N. Prevention of gonadal damage during cytotoxic therapy. Ann Med 1997; 29:199–206.
58. Fossa SD, Klepp O, Norman N. Lack of gonadal protection by medroxyprogesterone acetate-induced transient medical castration during chemotherapy for testicular cancer. Br J Urol 1988; 62:449–453.
59. Hakim LS, Lobel SM, Oates RD. The achievement of pregnancies using assisted reproductive technologies for male factor infertility after retroperitoneal lymph node dissection for testicular carcinoma. Fertil Steril 1995; 64(6):1141–1146.
60. Petersen PM, Skakkebaek NE, Rorth M, et al. Semen quality and reproductive hormones before and after orchiectomy in men with testicular cancer. J Urol 1999; 161:822–826.
61. Krege S, et al. European Consensus Conference on Diagnosis and Treatment of Germ Cell Cancer: A Report of the Second Meeting of the European Germ Cell Cancer Consensus group (EGCCCG)-Part I. Eur Urol 2008; 53:478–96. doi:10.1016/j.eururo.2007.12.024.
62. Schover LR, Brey K, Lichtin A. Knowledge and experience regarding cancer, infertility, and sperm banking in younger male survivors. J Clin Oncol 2002; 20:1880–1889.
63. Edge B, Holmes D, Makin G. Sperm banking in adolescent cancer patients. Arch Dis Child 2006; 91: 149–152.
64. Arrêté du 12 janvier 1999 relatif aux règles de bonnes pratiques cliniques et biologiques en assistance médicale à la procréation. Journal Officiel de la République Française (28 février) 1999:3061–3069.
65. Saito K, Suzuki K, Iwasaki A, et al. Sperm cryopreservation before cancer chemotherapy helps in the emotional battle against cancer. Cancer 2005; 104:521–524.
66. Thepot F, Mayaux MJ, Czyglick F, et al. Incidence of birth defects after artificial insemination with frozen donor spermatozoa: A collaborative study of the French CECOS federation on 11,535 pregnancies. Hum Reprod 1996; 11:2319–2323.
67. Agarwal A, Ranganathan P, Kattal N. Fertility after cancer: A prospective review of assisted reproductive outcomes with banked semen specimens. Fertil Steril 2004; 81(2):342–348.

68. Schmidt KL, Larsen E, Bangsboll S. Assisted reproduction in male cancer survivors: Fertility treatment and outcome in 67 couples. Hum Reprod 2004; 19(12):2806–2810.
69. Binsaleh S, Sircar K, Chan PT. Feasibility of simultaneous testicular microdissection for sperm retrieval and ipsilateral testicular tumor resection in azoospermic men. J Androl 2004; 25:867–871.
70. Baniel J, Sella A. Sperm extraction at orchiectomy for testis cancer. Fertil Steril 2001; 75:260–262.
71. Mesequer M, Garride N, Remohi J, et al. Testicular sperm extraction (TESE) and ICSI in patients with permanent azoospermia after chemotherapy. Hum Reprod 2003; 18(6):1281–1285.
72. Chan PT, Palermo GD, Veeck LL. Testicular sperm extraction combined with intracytoplasmic sperm injection in the treatment of men with persistent azoospermia postchemotherapy. Cancer 2001; 92(6):1632–1637.
73. Damani MN, Master V, Meng MV, et al. Postchemotherapy ejaculatory azoospermia: Fatherhood with sperm from testis tissue with intracytoplasmic sperm injection. J Clin Oncol 2002; 20:930–936.
74. Stahl O, Eberhard J, Jepson K. The impact of testicular carcinoma and its treatment on sperm DNA integrity. Cancer 2004; 100(6):1137–1144.
75. De Mas P, Daudin M, Vincent MC. Increased aneuploidy in spermatozoa from testicular tumour patients after chemotherapy with cisplatin, etoposide and bleomycin. Hum Reprod 2006; 16(6):1204–1208.
76. Martin RH, Ernst S, Rademaker A. Chromosomal abnormalities in sperm from testicular cancer patients before and after chemotherapy. Hum Genet 1997; 99(2):214–218.
77. Hartmann JT, Albrecht C, Schmoll HJ, et al. Longterm effects on sexual function and fertility after treatment of testicular cancer. Br J Cancer 1999; 80(5–6):801–807.
78. Spermon JR, Kiemeney L, Meuleman E. Fertility in men with testicular germ cell tumors. Fertil Steril 2003; 79(3):1543–1549.
79. Wyrobek AJ, Schmid TE, Marchetti F. Relative susceptibilities of male germ cells to genetic defects induced by cancer chemotherapies. J Natl Cancer Inst Monogr 2005; 34:31–35.

21 Male aging and reproduction

Sabine Kliesch

Reproductive aging and increasing life expectancy play an increasingly important role in andrology. For Germany, the life expectancy for the total population is 79 years, and for males 76 years and females 82 years, respectively. This increase in life expectancy is accompanied by a slow but constant increase of female and male age when reproduction is desired. While in females the start of menopause clearly indicates the end of the reproductive phase and natural conception becomes impossible, no clear limits for reproduction are known in males. Birth statistics show that there are quite a number of children born to fathers older than 50 years in the general population, both in Western and Eastern countries (1). However, profound knowledge concerning male reproductive functions is necessary to correctly counsel patients starting their family planning with increasing age. Nowadays, the wish to father children gains practical relevance after setting up one's professional education and career.

While endocrine changes of testicular function with age have been extensively studied in recent years, research and the increase of knowledge concerning reproductive functions is still limited (2). Possible comorbidities and comedications as well as the process of aging itself influence the hypothalamic–pituitary–gonadal axis. Long-term studies on reproductive male aging do not exist.

This chapter will summarize the known age-related changes of reproductive functions in the male in respect to the clinically relevant changes of testicular morphology and sperm function and their possible genetic impact on reproduction.

AGE-RELATED MORPHOLOGIC CHANGES OF THE TESTIS

The number and functionality of Leydig cells decrease with advancing age, the basal membrane of the tubuli seminiferi thickens, and a constant reduction of androgen secretion is observed clinically as a result of reduced steroid synthesis (3–8). There is no clear cut off time point defined of when morphological changes can start. Moreover, arteriosclerotic lesions and reduced arterial perfusion of the testis are observed with increasing age. So far, no duplex sonographic studies could show a correlation between reduced perfusion and altered endocrine parameters. The increased thickness of the basal lamina of seminiferous tubules and the microscopical observation of reduced type A spermatogonia as well as the observation of increased numbers of megalospermatocytes in males older than 60 years are morphological changes of the tubuli seminiferi possibly due to aging (9). On account of missing access to testicular biopsies of aging healthy men, most results of testicular morphological analyses are based on testicular autopsy preparations that reveal reduced spermiogenesis and spermatid numbers. Reduced spermatogenic efficiency was documented (10). Another source for investigations of aging testes are testicles from prostate cancer patients that were orchiectomized for hormonal ablation. In up to one-third of cases, no significant differences to young males can be observed. No general decrease in testicular volume can be observed (11).

INTERPRETATION OF SEMEN PARAMETERS AND FUNCTION IN AGING MALES

Studies on semen parameters so far were inconsistent: No changes of semen volumes were observed between men younger then 37 years and those older than 60 years (12), while Ng et al. (13) revealed significantly different seminal volumes between young and old men (Table 1). Because of reduced semen volumes, the sperm concentrations were increased in older men, while total sperm numbers were reduced. Moreover, significantly increased follicle stimulating hormone serum levels could be observed in older men, reflecting to some extent testicular spermatogenic function (14). Inhibin B as a possible marker for spermatogenesis shows a moderate but significant decrease reflecting the aging process that possibly affects spermatogenesis (15). Concerning sperm motility, a significant decrease is observed with increasing age as well as decreased normal sperm morphology (Fig. 1) (16–18). For sperm morphology, an increasing decline of normally formed spermatozoa can be observed with a percentage of 0.2% to 0.9% per year (16,19). In old men with normozoospermia, a reduction of the percentage of progressively motile sperm was observed (20). Decreased sperm motility may be a result of increased abstinence time with aging because of reduced frequency of cohabitation or masturbation (21). However, Eskenazi et al. (22) showed in a sample of healthy men that semen volume and sperm motility decrease continuously between 22 and 80 years of age with no evidence of a threshold. Recently, Hellstrom et al. (23) demonstrated in a screening population of 1174 men aged 45 to 80 (mean 52.9 years), showing up for participation in a study for erectile dysfunction treatment that the normal WHO criteria for semen analysis were met only by 46% of the study population (24). Moreover, they demonstrated a significant decline of the median semen volume, sperm motility, and morphology (Fig. 2) (23).

While sperm concentration, motility, and morphology are mainly descriptive parameters, sperm function in respect to

Table 1 Sperm Concentration Vs. Total Number of Spermatozoa According to Ng et al. (13)

	Young men	Old men	
Sperm concentration (10^6/mL)	73	64	NS
Sperm volume (mL)	3.2	1.8	$P < 0.05$
Total number of spermatozoa (10^6/mL)	206	74	$P < 0.05$

fertilization capacity could help to give more insight in age effects. Zenzes et al. (25) investigated the heterologous oocyte penetration tests in younger (24–37 years) and older (60–88 years) males without significant differences between the two groups. The main effect could possibly be attributed to the prolonged duration of sperm storage in the genital tract after maturation with an effect on sperm function. Similar results were found for acrosome reactions and chromatin condensation tests in younger (< 35 years) and older (> 45 years) men not showing significant differences between the two groups (17). However, missing differences in these tests do not necessarily truly reflect the influence of aging on fertilization and pregnancy induction.

COUNSELLING OF COUPLES FOR FATHERHOOD IN ADVANCED AGE

The mean age of fathers has increased in most Western countries, and by now a significantly large percentage of men father a child in their 50s (16,26). While this trend is mainly attributed to the fact that the woman decides to delay the first child, which is clearly associated with a decline in female fertility, it still remains unclear whether the above-mentioned mild changes in semen quality might become clinically important. Although changes in the endocrine profile with a constant decline in testosterone serum levels after the age of 50 years are well documented (3)

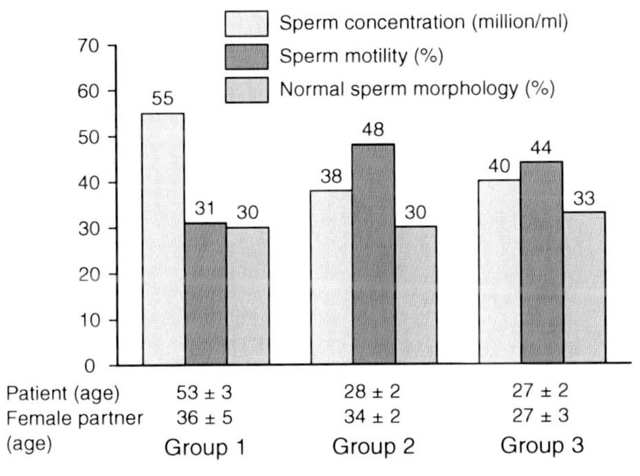

Figure 1 Comparison of semen parameters between older and younger men of infertile couples. *Source:* From Ref. 44.

and some changes of the seminal composition are observed, these data do not prove a decline in overall male fertility.

There is some recent evidence that parental age decreases offspring sex ratio (27). Altogether 3049 deliveries from five community-based hospitals in Osaka, Japan were prospectively evaluated. The male-to-female birth ratio was significantly decreased in the paternal age group >40 years to 0.75 compared to 1.17 in males aged between 30 and 34 years. The same was found in the maternal age group between 35 and 39 years with a decreased male-to-female birth ratio of 0.87 compared to 1.12 in females aged between 30 and 34 years. The authors concluded that the paternal ages synergistically decrease the male-to-female birth ratio (27).

There are some important studies clearly indicating the effect of male age on the time to conception and an increased risk for abortions.

Rolf et al. (18) investigated the pregnancy rates of three groups of couples (Table 2). With 30% and 23.3%, the cumulative pregnancy rates between group II and III showed no significant differences, respectively. However, with 60.7% the pregnancy rate in group I was significantly higher. The authors concluded that maternal age significantly influences pregnancy rates, while paternal age plays a limited role (Fig. 3).

The time to pregnancy was shown to be increased up to three times in men older than 40 years in comparison to 25-year-old men in a study investigating 638 pregnant females (Fig. 4) (28). A population study showed a negative effect of paternal age on time to conception, after adjustment for nine variables including the age of the women being independently related to the time to conception (29). Ford et al. (29) showed that the odds ratio for conception within 12 months decreases by 3% per year of the man's age. This study compared the chance of conception within 12 months for women whose partners were at least five years older with women whose partners were the same age or younger as the female. The resulting odds ratio was 0.73 (29).

In assisted reproduction, the fertilization of spermatozoa from older men can be investigated (at least in countries with the option of heterologous oocyte donation); the increased age of men do not change the results of fertilization or implantation. However, the rate of abortions increase with males older than 50 years (30,31). Pregnancies from fathers older than 50 years have a doubled risk for abortion (32). Pregnancies of females older than 30 years and males with increased age also have an increased risk for abortion (33,34).

CHROMOSOMAL AND GENETIC IMPACT ON SPERM FUNCTION IN AGING MALES

By means of assisted reproduction more insight can be gained into sperm function and embryo development after using sperm from the elderly, possibly with an important impact on genetic and chromosomal aspects especially in respect to the offspring.

A nondisjunction of homologous chromosomes during meiotic division results in abnormal numbers of chromosomes and

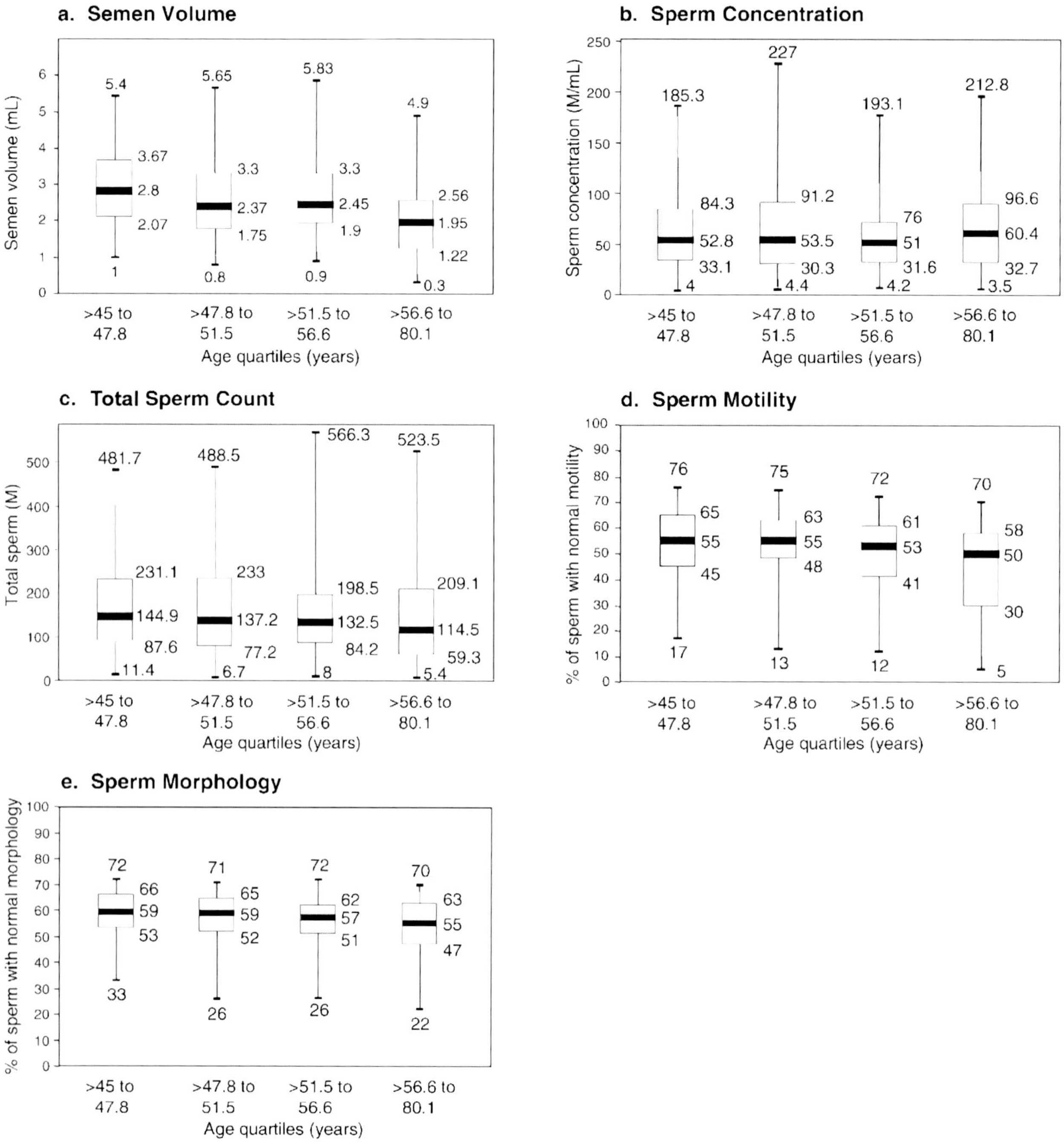

Figure 2 Reference ranges by age quartile for (A) semen volume (mL), (B) sperm concentration (M/mL), (C) total sperm count (M), (D) sperm motility (percentage of normal sperm motility), and (E) sperm morphology (percentage of sperm with normal morphological features). Each box represents the distribution of data between the 25th and 75th percentile. The median is indicated by a band across each box. Whiskers on each box represent the 95% reference range for the data set. There were 247 to 294 subjects per age quartile. *Source:* From Ref. 23.

Table 2 Pregnancy Rates of Three Groups of Couples According to Rolf et al. (18)

Group	Age males (years) (mean ± SEM)	Age females (years) (mean ± SEM)	Cumulative pregnancy rate
I $n = 39$	< 30 (27.4 ± 1.6)	< 30 (26.6 ± 2.7)	62.2% (17/28)
II $n = 39$	< 30 (27.5 ± 1.5)	> 33 (33.9 ± 2.4)	30.3% (9/30)
III $n = 39$	> 50 (53.5 ± 7.8)	> 33 (35.7 ± 5.1)	23.3% (6/26)

can be observed in 4.7% of spermatozoa of healthy men (35). In infertile men with oligozoospermia, the number of chromosomal changes is increased. An age-related increase of numeral changes could be observed only for the sex chromosomes, not for the autosomes (34). With increasing paternal age, increased chromosomal aberrations in spermatozoa are observed more with structural than numeral changes (14, 36–38) (Table 3).

The genetic quality of sperm produced by older men may be reduced for several reasons, among which age-related increases in germ cell mutations, impairment of DNA repair mechanisms, and apoptotic processes are the most likely. The incidence of several autosomal dominant diseases, such as achondroplasia, polyposis coli, Marfan syndrome, Apert syndrome, or basal cell nevus is associated with advanced paternal age, whereas there is no clear evidence for a paternal effect on structural or numeral chromosomal anomalies (38). The increased number of structural chromosomal aberrations shows a correlation with age and increases from 2.8% in males aged between 20 and 24 years up to 13.6% in males older than 45 years. The reasons are not well understood; possibly this is due to the long exposing time to potentially mutagenic substances. With increasing paternal age, the risk for birth defects—such as heart defects, chondrodystrophia, or visceral inversion—increases (39). However, when investigating aneuploidy rates in younger and older men, no significant differences in disomy rates (0.1–2.3% vs. 0.1–1.8%, respectively) and aneuploidy rates for both sex chromosomes and chromosomes 9 and 18 could be detected (14). Thus, men of advanced age (> 60 years) do not have significantly increased risks of procreating offspring with chromosomal abnormalities compared with younger males (< 30 years), at least in regard to the investigated chromosomes (Table 3).

IS GENETIC TESTING INDICATED IN OLDER MEN?

Although the genetic understanding of reproduction is slowly growing, no clear evidence can be given concerning the genetic risk of the elderly. According to our present knowledge, men of advanced age do not have significantly increased risks of procreating offspring with chromosomal abnormalities compared with younger males. The frequency of chromosomal anomalies and disomies increases with male age, but paternal age is not associated with numerical or de novo structural abnormalities in newborns (possibly excepting trisomy 21) (36,40). The types of genetic abnormalities that occur in spermatozoa are more likely to cause early abortion rather than result in the birth of abnormal children.

Nevertheless there do exist chromosomal anomalies that are, to a high proportion, of paternal origin: de novo structural rearrangements (80%), the XYY karyotype (100%), and 45,X Turner's syndrome (80%) as well as Klinefelter's syndrome (50%). However, a relationship between paternal aging and an increase of the proportion of chromosomal anomalies in the offspring has not been proven. It remains difficult to establish a clear relationship, because most of the chromosomal abnormalities do not produce a recognizable phenotype and remain possibly underdiagnosed. In addition, the increase is not as marked as in some anomalies of maternal origin. To our present knowledge, the increased paternal age is not an indication for prenatal diagnosis.

Thus, no systematic genetic testing of aging men can be recommended. If assisted reproductive techniques (ART) will be offered, genetic counselling should follow the same rules for the elderly as for the younger males, including karyotyping and

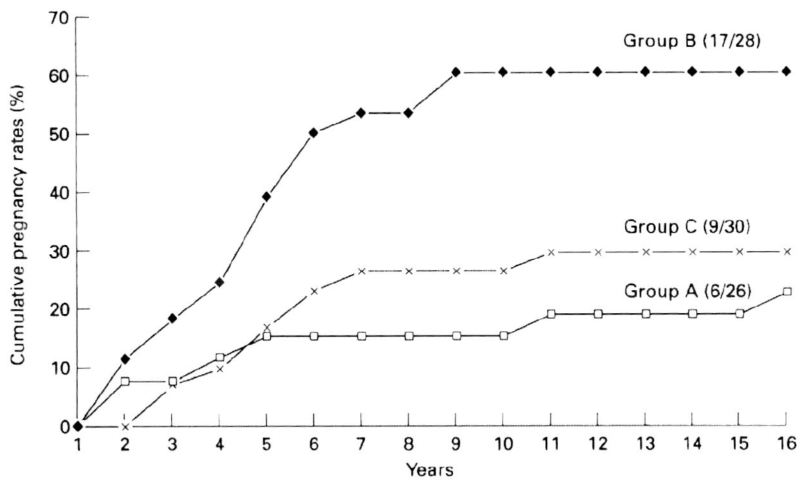

Figure 3 Cumulative percentage pregnancy rates in groups A, B, and C from the beginning of infertility. *Source:* From Ref. 18.

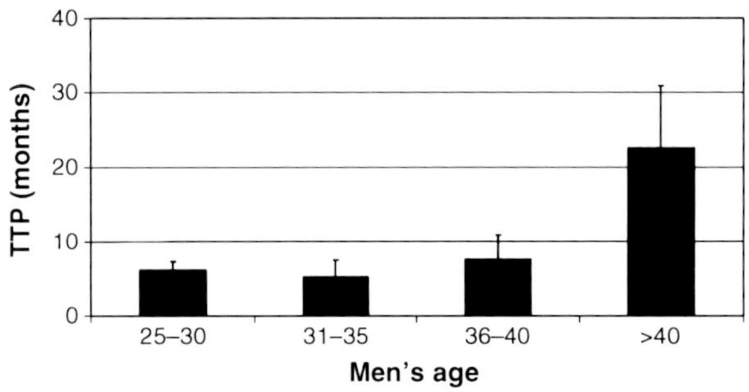

Figure 4 Time-to-pregnancy (TTP) in women younger than 25 years ($n = 638$) in relation to partner's age. *Source:* From Ref. 44.

screening, for example, Y-chromosomal microdeletions if indicated by clinical findings of infertility or phenotype. Genetic counselling should be offered to the couple irrespective of their age when ART is applied.

CRYOPRESERVATION OF SEMEN IN OLDER MEN

For aging males the same indications for cryopreservation of semen may be applied as for younger males (41). Cryopreservation of semen can be applied to males who wish to preserve their fertility potential prior to planned vasectomy, prior to ART, or to prevent fertility damage due to potentially gonadotoxic treatment either because of benign (arthritis, transplantation, chronic bowel disease) or malignant diseases. In general, the storage of semen for fertility preservation can be offered irrespective of the male patient's age. However, this depends on the type of oncological diseases and the prognosis for survival that may substantially differ between younger and older men. While young patients with testis cancer have an excellent prognosis and good chances for long-term survival, the prognosis for example of prostate, renal, or bladder cancer is different and depends on the age at the time of diagnosis, the initial clinical stage, and treatment options of the disease. Thus, one has to keep in mind that cryopreservation of semen offers the chance for paternity in severely ill men. There are ethical questions being raised that are neither thoroughly discussed nor clearly regulated in different countries. In Germany, it is contractually regulated to destroy the cryopreserved semen after the death of the patient. However, the use of cryopreserved spermatozoa of incurably ill males is not regulated and may confront the patient, his female partner, and the doctors with unresolved ethical conflicts.

Table 3 Chromosomal Anomalies in Advanced Paternal Age

Numerical anomalies in sperm
- No paternal age effect for chromosomes 6, 8, 12, 13, 14, 18
- Possible age effect for chromosomes 1, 9, 21
- Probable age effect for XY and linear effect for diploidy
- In newborns: probable effect for trisomy 21

Structural anomalies in sperm
- Increase in centromere/telomere deletions or duplications of chromosomes 1, 9, 3
- In newborns: no increase of de novo anomalies

Source: From Refs. 19 and 38.

Concerning cryopreservation of spermatozoa from semen donors for heterologous insemination, it is important to realize that it is because of the association between elevated paternal age and birth defects that the age of semen donors is limited to 40 years in certain countries (42,43).

ASSISTED REPRODUCTION IN THE TREATMENT OF OLDER MEN

From studies concerning ART we were able to learn that not the implantation rate but obviously the early abortions increase with male partners older than 50 years (30–34). Depending on the legal issues for ART in different countries, there are more or less limitations concerning female and male age in respect to refunding of the ART procedure by the insurance companies.

These restrictions, however, do not necessarily reflect the clinical and ethical impact on ART in the elderly. Most publications consider the maternal age to be important in respect to ART. There are considerations of egg or embryo freezing to give women more options to delay childbearing. Even among fertility experts, the discussion is mainly regarding the female role in reproduction. For the male part, it seems to be accepted to have semen storage for later use in ART. However, there are more questions being raised than answers being prepared concerning the social implications of delayed parenthood, either maternal or paternal or both: What about the future of the children born to elderly patients? What about the impact on the older parents? What is the demographic impact on the society as a whole? Will it contribute to a decline in fertility at the population level?

SUMMARY

The available data for testicular morphology, semen parameters, and fertility in aging males reflect a gradual functional deterioration with age. However, there is a broad individual variation spectrum to be considered. So far, we can summarize a moderate but obvious slow decline of semen parameters in aging males, while fertilization rates remain mainly unchanged. An increased incidence of abortions can be observed, while an increased risk for chromosomal anomalies in offspring is seldom observed. So far, the increased age of fathers at conception is no indication for an intensified prenatal diagnostic procedure (40,44). The most important parameter for pregnancy induction by an aging male is the young age of his female partner.

REFERENCES

1. Martin JA, Hamilton BE, Sutton PD, et al. Births: final data for 2002. Natl Vital Stat Rep 2003; 52:1–113.
2. Kaufman JM, Vermeulen A. The decline of androgen levels in elderly men and its clinical and therapeutic implications. Endocr Rev 2005; 26:833–876.

3. Gray A, Feldman HA, McKinlay JB, et al. Age, disease and changing sex hormone levels in middle aged men: results of the Massachusetts Male Ageing Study. J Clin Endocrinol Metab 1991; 73:1016–1025.
4. Feldman HA, Longcope C, Derby CA, et al. Age trends in the level of serum testosterone and other hormones in middle-aged men: longitudinal results from the Massachusetts male aging study. J Clin Endorinol Metab 2002; 87:587–598.
5. Neaves WB, Johnson L, Porter JC, et al. Leydig cell numbers, daily sperm production and serum gonadotropin levels in aging men. J Clin Endocr Metab 1984; 59:756–763.
6. Johnson L, Petty CS, Neaves WB. Influence of age on sperm production and testicular weights in men. J Reprod Fertil 1984; 70:211–218.
7. Takahashi J, Higashi Y, Lanasa JA, et al. Studies of the human testis. XVIII. Simultaneous measurement of nine intratesticular steroids, evidence for reduced mitochondrial function in testis of elderly men. J Clin Endocrinol Metab 1983; 56:1178–1187.
8. Zitzmann M. Testosterone and the brain. Aging Male 2006; 9:195–199.
9. Bergmann M, Kliesch S. Testicular biopsy and histology. In Nieschlag E, Behre HM, Nieschlag S, eds. Andrology – Male Reproductive Health and Dysfunction, 3rd ed. Heidelberg: Springer, 2009:151–163.
10. Johnson L, Grumbles JS, Bagheri A, et al. Increased germ cell degeneration during postprophase of meiosis is related to increased serum follicle-stimulating hormone concentrations and reduced daily sperm production in aged men. Biol Reprod 1990; 42:281–287.
11. Handelsman DJ, Staraj S. Testicular size: the effects of aging, malnutrition, and illness. J Androl 1985; 6:144–151.
12. Nieschlag E, Lammers R, Freischem CW, et al. Reproductive functions in young fathers and grandfathers. J Clin Endocrinol Metab 1982; 55:656–681.
13. Ng KK, Donat R, Chan L, et al. Sperm output of older men. Hum Reprod 2004; 19:1811–1815.
14. Luetjens CM, Rolf C, Gassner P, et al. Sperm aneuploidy rates in younger and older men. Hum Reprod 2002; 17:1826–1832.
15. Mahmoud AM, Goemaere S, El-Garem Y, et al. Testicular volume in relation to hormonal indices of gonadal function in community-dwelling elderly men. J Clin Endocrinol Metab 2003; 88:179–184.
16. Kidd SA, Eskenazi B, Wyrobek AJ. Effects of male age on semen quality and fertility: a review of the literature. Fertil Steril 2001; 75:237–248.
17. Haidl G, Jung A, Schill WB. Ageing and sperm function. Hum Reprod 1996; 11:558–560.
18. Rolf C, Behre HM, Nieschlag E. Reproductive parameters of older compared to younger men of infertile couples. Int J Androl 1996; 19:135–142.
19. Kühnert B, Nieschlag E. Reproductive functions of the ageing male. Hum Reprod Update 2004; 10:327–339.
20. Levitas E, Lunenfeld E, Weisz N, et al. Relationship between age and semen parameters in men with normal sperm concentration: analysis of 6022 semen samples. Andrologia 2007; 39:45–50.
21. Paulson RJ, Milligan RC, Sokol RZ. The lack of influence of age on male fertility. Am J Obstet Gynecol 2001; 184:818–822.
22. Eskenazi B, Wyrobek AJ, Slotzer E, et al. The association of age and semen quality in healthy men. Hum Reprod 2003; 18:447–454.
23. Hellstrom WJ, Overstreet JW, Sikka SC, et al. Semen and sperm reference ranges for men 45 years of age and older. J Androl 2006; 47:421–428.
24. World Health Organization. WHO laboratory manual for the examination of human semen and sperm-cervical mucus interaction, 4th ed. Cambridge, UK: Cambridge University Press, 1999.
25. Zenzes MT, Reed TE, Nieschlag E. Non-poisson distribution of sperm from grandfathers in zona-free hamster ova. J Androl 1991; 12:71–75.
26. Plas E, Berger P, Hermann M, et al. Effects of ageing on male fertility? Exp Gerontol 2000; 35:543–551.
27. Matsuo K, Ushioda N, Udoff LC. Parental aging synergistically decreases offspring sex ratio. J Obstet Gynaecol Res 2009; 35:164–168.
28. Hassan MA, Killick SR. Effect of male age on fertility: evidence for the decline in male fertility with increasing age. Fertil Steril 2003; 79(suppl 3):1520–1527.
29. Ford WC, North K, Taylor H, et al. Increasing paternal age is associated with delayed conception in a large population of fertile couples: evidence for declining fecundity in older men. The ALSPAC Study Team (Avon Longitudinal Study of Pregnancy and Childhood). Hum Reprod 2000; 15:1703–1708.
30. Gallardo E, Simon C, Levy M, et al. Effect of age on sperm fertility potential: oocyte donation as a model. Fertil Steril 1996; 66:260–264.
31. Fratarelli JL, Miller KA, Miller BT, et al. Male age negatively impacts embryo development and reproductive outcome in donor oocyte assisted reproductive technology cycles. Fertil Steril 2008; 90:97–103.
32. Nybo Andersen AM, Hansen KD, Andersen PK, et al. Advanced paternal age and risk of fetal death: a cohort study. Am J Epidemiol 2004; 160:1214–1222.
33. La Rochebrochard E, Thonneau P. Paternal age and maternal age are risk factors for miscarriage; results of a multicentre European study. Hum Reprod 2002; 17:1649–1656.
34. Sartorius G, Nieschlag E. Paternal age and reproduction. Hum Reprod Update; 16:65–79 [Advance Access published August 20, 2009].

35. Bordson BL, Leonardo VS. The appropriate upper age limit for several semen donors: a review of the genetic effects of paternal age. Fertil Steril 1991; 56:397–401.
36. Martin RH, Rademaker AW. The effect of age on the frequency of sperm chromosomal abnormalities in normal men. Am J Hum Genet 1987; 41:484–492.
37. Murray MJ, Meacham RB. The effect of age on male reproductive function. World J Urol 1993; 11:137–140.
38. Rolf C, Nieschlag E. Reproductive functions, fertility and genetic risks of ageing men. Exp Clin Endocrinol Diabetes 2001; 109:68–74.
39. Lian ZH, Zack MM, Erickson JD. Paternal age and the occurrence of birth defects. Am J Hum Genet 1976; 39:648–660.
40. ESHRE Capri Workshop Group. Fertility and ageing. Hum Reprod Update 2005; 11:261–276.
41. Kliesch S, Kamischke A, Cooper TG, et al. Cryopreservation of human spermatozoa. In: Nieschlag E, Behre HM, Nieschlag S, eds. Andrology – Male Reproductive Health and Dysfunction, 3rd ed. Heidelberg: Springer, 2009:499–514.
42. American Society for Reproductive Medicine. Guidelines for therapeutic donor insemination: sperm. Fertil Steril 1998; 70(suppl 3):1S–3S.
43. British Andrology Society. British Andrology Society guidelines for the screening of semen donors for donor insemination. Hum Reprod 1999; 14:1823–1826.
44. Rolf C, Zitzmann M, Nieschlag E. The aging male and late-onset hypogonadism. In Nieschlag E, Behre HM, Nieschlag S, eds. Andrology – Male Reproductive Health and Dysfunction, 3rd ed. Heidelberg: Springer, 2009:235–257.

22 Sex steroids in men: Biosynthesis, transport, metabolism, interaction with receptors, and cellular (Genomic and Nongenomic) and biological actions

Jemima Gaytant, Katrien Venken, and Dirk Vanderschueren

INTRODUCTION

Androgens and estrogens are known as sex steroids. Estrogens are C-18 steroid hormones originating from aromatization of androgens. Androgens are C-19 steroids secreted from the testes and from the adrenals. Biological effects of sex steroids in men ultimately depend on a complex process involving not only regulation of biosynthesis but also transport, metabolism, and genomic and/or nongenomic actions. In the following chapter, these different steps will be discussed in chronological order.

BIOSYNTHESIS

More than 95% of the major circulating androgen, testosterone (T) is synthesized and secreted by the Leydig cells in the testes (1). In addition to testicular T production, other androgens such as dehydroepiandrosterone (DHEA), its sulphate (DHEAS), and androstenedione are produced in the adrenal cortex (2,3). By further peripheral conversion, these adrenal androgens also contribute to the T production in men.

Cholesterol is the precursor of androgen production. Cholesterol can either be synthesized de novo within the cell or derived from the plasma pool by endocytosis of low-density lipoprotein into the cell. As shown in Figure 1, five enzymatic processes are involved in this conversion of cholesterol to T (1,4–6).

1. *Cholesterol side-chain cleavage* with formation of pregnenolone. This reaction is catalyzed within the mitochondria by the P450 side-chain cleavage enzyme, which is encoded by the CYP11A gene. The delivery of cholesterol to this enzyme, located in the inner mitochondrial membrane, requires the steroidogenic acute regulatory protein (StAR). The conversion of cholesterol to pregnenolone is also the rate-limiting reaction in T synthesis. This conversion rate is, however, not determined by the activity of the P450 side-chain cleavage enzyme. Instead, StAR determines the rate of delivery of cholesterol to the enzyme in the inner mitochondrial membrane and thereby the conversion rate. This process is also the main site of action of luteinizing hormone (LH) (7,8). All further reactions take place in the endoplasmic reticulum.
2. *3β-hydroxysteroid dehydrogenase-$\Delta^{4,5}$-isomerase complex (3β-HSD).* Pregnenolone can be further converted to T by two alternative routes: the Δ^4 pathway or the Δ^5 pathway, which are the dominant routes in the adrenals and the testis, respectively. In the Δ^4 pathway, pregnenolone is first metabolized to progesterone. This step is initialized by 3β-HSD. In the Δ^5 pathway formation of T goes via 17-hydroxypregnenolone.
3. *17α-hydroxylase.* 17α-hydroxylase catalyzes the synthesis of 17-hydroxypregnenolone from pregnenolone and 17-hydroxyprogesterone from progesterone. Both 17α-hydroxylase and 17,20-lyase reside in a single cytochrome P450 enzyme (P450c17) that is encoded by the CYP17 gene.
4. *17,20-lyase.* The Δ^4 pathway mediates the formation of androstenedione. In the Δ^5 pathway 17,20-lyase catalyzes the conversion of 17-hydroxypregnenolone to DHEA.
5. *17β-hydroxysteroid dehydrogenase (17β-HSD)* catalyzes the formation of T from androstenedione. It is also involved in the transformation of DHEA to androstenediol. The latter is converted to T by 3β-HSD.

Besides production in the gonads and adrenal glands, sex steroids are also synthesized and/or converted locally in peripheral tissues, for example, T can be converted to the more potent 5α-dihydrotestosterone (DHT) or is aromatized into 17β-estradiol (E_2) (see transport and metabolism) (3).

Regulation of Sex Steroid Secretion

Testes

Testosterone is secreted in a pulsatile fashion under the control of LH. Hormonal regulation of the gonadotropin LH involves interactions between the hypothalamus, anterior pituitary gland, and the testes, a relationship known as the hypothalamic–pituitary–testicular axis (see chapter 23 "Gonadotropins and Their Receptors" for more details). Secretion of LH from the anterior pituitary is controlled by the hypothalamic gonadotropin-releasing hormone (GnRH). GnRH is secreted into the hypophyseal portal system in a pulsatile fashion. It elicits pulsatile secretion of LH by binding to receptors on pituitary gonadotropes. LH in turn binds to LH receptors on the Leydig cells, activating a cAMP-mediated signalling cascade that stimulates the expression of steroidogenic enzymes (see earlier) involved in T biosynthesis (1,4). An increase of serum T will inhibit LH secretion by acting both at the pituitary and hypothalamic level. This negative feedback is partially mediated by aromatization of T into E_2 (9).

Adrenal Glands

In contrast with LH, adrenocorticotropin (ACTH) is the major determinant of the production of androgens in the adrenal

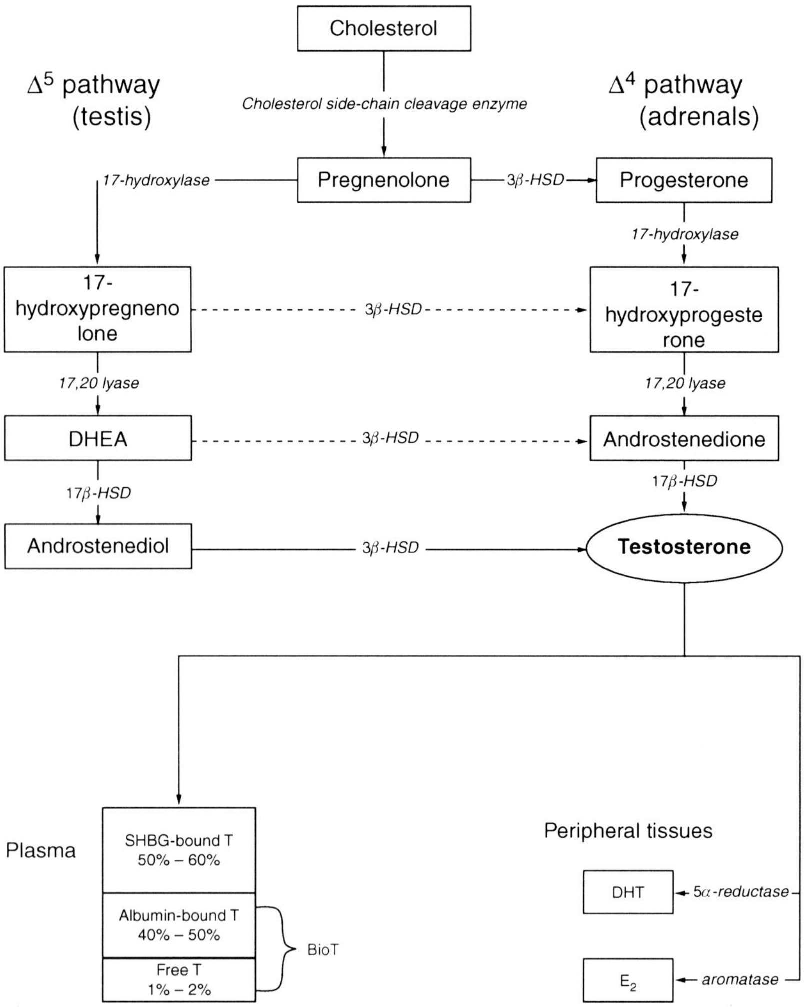

Figure 1 Pathways of testosterone (T) synthesis in humans and the destiny of T in plasma and peripheral tissues. T synthesis: there are two pathways of T synthesis; the Δ^4 pathway and the Δ^5 pathway, which are respectively the dominant routes in the adrenals and the testis. In plasma the majority of T is bound to sex hormone binding globulin (SHBG) (50–60%), about 40% to 50% of T binds to albumin. Only 1% remains free. The albumin-bound T and free T are also referred to as bioavailable T (BioT). In peripheral tissues T is converted into the more potent dihydrotestosterone (DHT) or T is aromatized into estradiol (E_2). 3β-hydroxysteroid dehydrogenase-$\Delta^{4,5}$-isomerase complex (3β-HSD), 17β-hydroxysteroid dehydrogenase (17β-HSD), dehydroepiandrosterone (DHEA).

gland. ACTH indeed stimulates not only synthesis and release of glucocorticoids, but also of androgens via cAMP-dependent mechanisms. The immediate actions of ACTH on steroid synthesis are to increase cholesterol esterase, as well as transport cholesterol to and across the mitochondrial membrane and cholesterol binding to P450 side-chain cleavage enzyme thereby enhancing pregnenolone production (10).

TRANSPORT AND METABOLISM

In plasma the majority (50–60%) of T is bound to sex hormone binding globulin (SHBG) with high affinity (Fig. 1). SHBG is synthesized in the liver and its concentration may be affected by a number of clinical conditions, which are listed in Table 1. SHBG also binds between 20% and 40% of circulating E_2. About 40% to 50% of the circulating T is bound to albumin with low affinity. Only 1% to 2% of T remains free. The free T and the albumin-bound T represent the fractions available for biological action and are therefore referred to as the bioavailable T (BioT) (Fig. 1). Unbound T diffuses passively through the cell membranes into the target cell, where it binds to the specific androgen receptor (AR) (11) (Fig. 2). The albumin-bound T dissociates during tissue transit and thereby comes bioavailable. Binding of T to SHBG on the other hand prevents the bound hormone from diffusing out of the bloodstream, thereby preventing hormone binding to the intracellular androgen and estrogen receptors. Binding to SHBG also decreases the metabolic clearance rate of T (12).

In healthy adult males, serum T shows circadian variations with amplitude between 20% and 40%, indicating highest concentrations in the morning and lowest concentrations in the late afternoon (13,14). Morning levels of serum T typically vary between around 10.4 and 35 nmol/L (300 and 1000 ng/dL). The reason for this large interindividual variation is still poorly understood. However, there is evidence for the involvement of a genetic component in the determination of T blood concentrations. Indeed, the CAG repeat polymorphism of the AR affects

Table 1 Different Clinical Conditions That May Be Associated With an Increase or a Decrease of SHBG Concentration.

Conditions with abnormal SHBG concentrations	
[SHBG] increase	Aging Androgen deficiency Growth hormone deficiency Thyrotoxicosis Estrogen treatment Alcoholic cirrhosis Hepatitis
[SHBG] decrease	Androgen treatment Hypothyroidism Obesity Hyperinsulinemia Hypercortisolemia Acromegaly Nephrotic syndrome Familial

SHBG, sex hormone binding globulin; [SHBG], concentration of sex hormone binding globulin.

not only androgen action, but may also contribute to the variability of serum T level through modulation of the negative feedback control of the hypothalamic–pituitary–testicular axis. Longer CAG repeats are associated with diminished androgen feedback and relative elevation of circulating T. These findings have potential implications for interpretation of epidemiological studies, diagnosis of hypogonadism in borderline situations, and possibly individualization of androgen therapies in men (15).

Other androgens in the systemic circulation include: DHT, androstenedione, DHEA, and DHEAS. The serum concentration of DHT is much lower than T and varies between 0.7 and 3 nmol/L (20–80 ng/dL). The most abundant androgen in serum is DHEAS: its mean concentration in young males is about 6 μmol/L (220 μg/dL), and its secretion decreases rapidly with age. Due to its slow metabolism, serum DHEAS concentrations do not show circadian variations (3). Serum concentrations of sex steroids, however, do not accurately reflect their biological action. A large proportion of androgens and estrogens in men are indeed synthesized locally in peripheral target tissues from adrenal DHEA and DHEAS. The synthesis

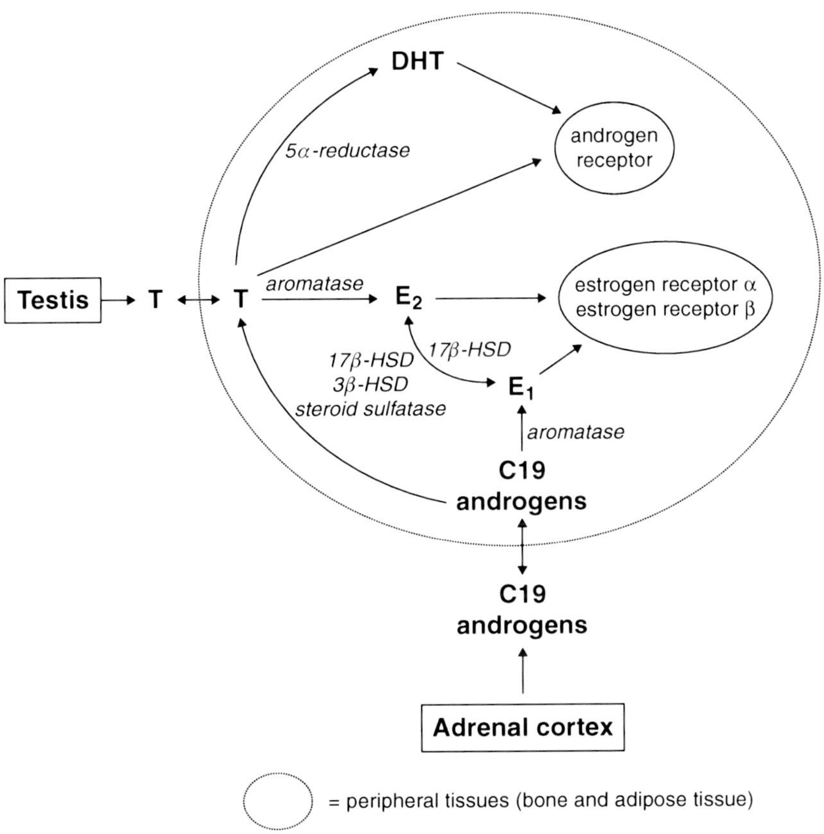

Figure 2 Overview of the metabolism and action of sex steroids in men. HSD, hydroxysteroid dehydrogenase.

of the active steroids therefore takes place in the target cells where the steroid action is exerted without release of the active hormones in the extracellular space or in the general circulation. This process is called intracrinology. Serum DHEAS levels in adult men are 100 to 500 times higher than those of testosterone, thus providing a large reservoir of substrate for conversion into androgens and/or estrogens in peripheral intracrine tissues. Intracrinology provides autonomous control to target tissues, which are able to adjust the formation and metabolism of sex steroids according to local requirements (16,17). Transformation of DHEAS and DHEA into androgens and/or estrogens in peripheral target tissues depends to a large extent upon the level of expression of the various steroidogenic and metabolizing enzymes in each of these tissues (18). DHEA and DHEAS can be metabolized to estrone (E_1) by the aromatase enzyme or to T by steroid sulfatase, 17β-HSD, and/or 3β-HSD (Fig. 2).

In peripheral tissues expressing 5α-reductase, T can also be irreversibly converted to the more potent DHT. There are two 5α-reductase isoenzymes (19). Type 1 is expressed in the liver and nongenital skin, whereas type 2 is expressed in the male urogenital tract, genital skin, and in the liver.

Most T entering prostate tissue is transformed into DHT, and in most tissues, with the important exception of muscle tissue, DHT is the principal active androgen, which acts mainly locally, only a small fraction escaping into the general circulation. In addition, T has the unique feature that it can be converted into 17β-estradiol (E_2) by the P450 aromatase enzyme, and subsequently exerts its effects through estrogen receptor α (ERα) or β (ERβ) (Fig. 2). Only 20% of E_2 is directly secreted by the testes; the remaining 80% of E_2 in men is solely derived from the aromatization of T and androstenedione in peripheral tissues, mainly in adipose tissue and striated muscles, although, aromatase activity is also present in many other tissues including bone and the brain. Hence, action of T is the resultant of tissue availability and locally achieved T concentrations, of local T metabolism, of expression of AR and/or ERs, as well as the expression of a number of coactivators and repressors of these receptors. These determining factors of T action can be differentially regulated in the tissues, thus offering a large potential for differential regulation of sex steroid action in the different tissues (3).

Depending on the relative activity of P450 aromatase, 5α-reductase, 17β-HSD, 3β-HSD and steroid sulfatase, T, and C-19 androgens may either predominantly activate the AR or the ERs.

A large part of the catabolism of sex steroids takes place in the liver. The degradation of T involves 5α/5β reduction of the double bond between carbons 4 and 5, 3α/3β reduction in ring A, and 17β hydroxyl oxidation. DHEA is first converted to androstenedione and the subsequent metabolism is identical to that of T. The end metabolites of endogenous androgens, i.e., androsterone, etiocholanolone, and 5α/5β androstane-3α, 17β diol are excreted by the kidneys (3).

Serum sex steroid levels fall progressively with age in healthy men from the fourth decade onwards (20, 21). Total T concentrations decrease only marginally (between 0.4% and 1.5% each year), whereas total E_2 concentrations remain constant. However, SHBG increases (+ 120%) markedly in aging men resulting in reduction of the bioavailable T and E_2 (22). SHBG concentration increases at an earlier age than the decrease in T levels. The mechanisms responsible for the age-associated increase of serum SHBG remains to be established (12,23,24). Although the androgen decline may to some extent be related with age-related clinical changes, such as decreased libido, impotence, reduced cognitive function, increased obesity, and a decrease in muscle mass, muscle strength, and bone mineral density, a causal relationship of such clinical manifestations and declining hormones also remains to be established (3,25).

RECEPTORS, GENOMIC, AND NONGENOMIC ACTIONS

Cellular actions of (sex) steroids are exerted in several ways. The genomic pathway involves hormone binding to classic receptors and subsequent modulation of gene expression followed by protein synthesis. Alternatively, the cellular effects of the sex steroids may also be mediated via nongenomic pathways.

Sex Steroid Receptors

The AR, ERα, and ERβ are all sex steroid receptors that belong to the same nuclear receptor family, i.e., a family of ligand-activated transcription factors (26). They are composed of three independent but interacting functional domains: the NH_2-terminal, the DNA-binding domain (DBD), and the COOH-terminal or ligand-binding domain (Fig. 3) (27–29). The sequence homology in the DBD is high among the sex steroid receptors. The N-terminal domain of these receptors encodes a ligand-independent activation function (AF-1), a region of the receptor involved in protein–protein interactions, and transcriptional activation of target gene expression. The ligand-binding domain (LBD), mediates ligand binding, heat shock protein interaction, receptor dimerization, nuclear translocation, and transcription of target gene expression (Fig. 4) (30). The LBD also consists of a ligand-inducible activation function (AF-2) (28,31).

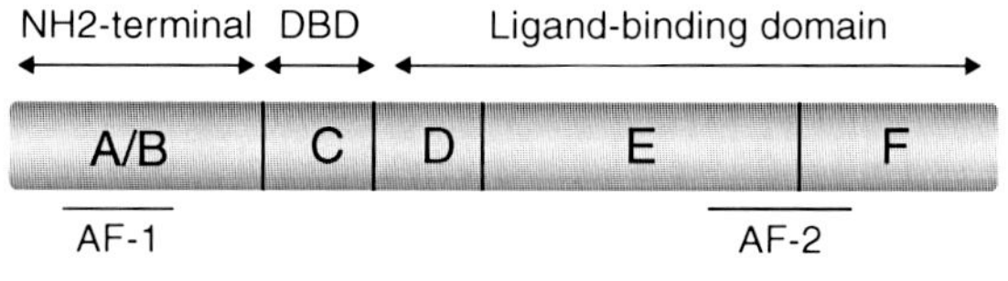

Figure 3 Representation of the domain structure of nuclear receptors. The A/B domain at the NH_2 terminus contains the AF-1 site where other transcription factors interact. The C or DNA-binding domain (DBD) and the D/E/F or ligand-binding domain, which also contain the AF-2 domain that directly contacts coactivator peptides.

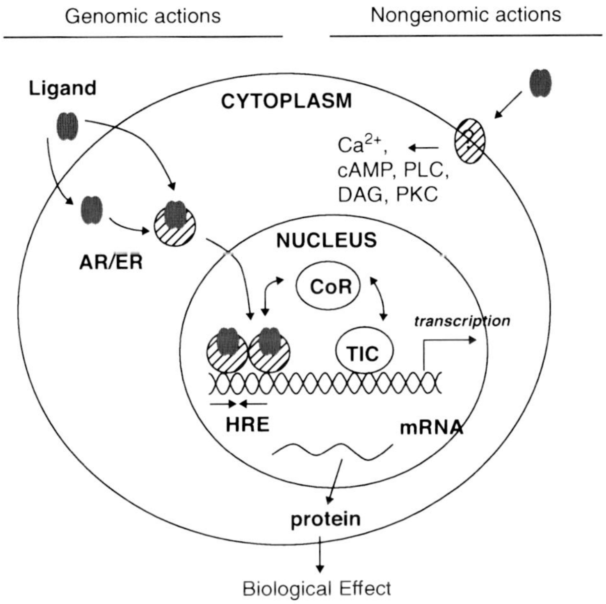

Figure 4 Genomic and nongenomic gonadal steroid signaling. Genomic action: The ligand binds to its specific receptor, which induces a conformational change. The receptor translocates to the nucleus and undergoes dimerization. The receptor dimer binds to specific DNA sequences, so called hormone response elements. The DNA-bound receptor contacts the general transcription initiation complex (TIC) either directly or indirectly through coregulatory proteins (CoR). Nongenomic action: The ligand binds a, yet undefined, plasma membrane receptor, which results in the activation of second messenger signal transduction pathways including Ca^{2+}, (PLC), cyclic AMP (cAMP), phospholipase C, diacylglycerol (DAG), protein kinase C (PKC). ER, estrogen receptor, AR, androgen receptor, HRE, hormone response element.

The AR receptor gene is located on the long arm (Xq11–12) of the X chromosome. Exon 1 of the gene consists of two polymorphic repeats (CAG and GGN) (32). The CAG repeat length and AR transactivation potential are inversely correlated (33), and the CAG repeat length is associated with a series of androgen-related clinical effects (an involvement of prostate tissue, spermatogenesis, bone density, hair growth, cardiovascular risk factors, and psychological factors have been demonstrated) (15,34–36). As mentioned earlier, longer CAG repeats are also associated with diminished androgen feedback and relative elevation of circulating T (15).

Genomic Sex Steroid Action

In the absence of hormone, the receptor is kept in an inactive state and it forms a multiprotein complex with chaperone molecules such as heat shock proteins (Hsp), Hsp70 and Hsp 90. Hormone binding induces an activating conformational change within the receptor, resulting in dissociation of the chaperone proteins, translocation of the receptor to the nucleus, and increased phosphorylation (Fig. 4). Then, the hormone-bound receptor dimerizes with another hormone-bound receptor and this dimer binds with high affinity to specific DNA sequences, i.e., estrogen or androgen responsive elements (ERE or ARE), respectively, located within the regulatory region of the target gene (37). To regulate transcription, the DNA-bound receptor must contact the general transcription machinery. This may be achieved either by direct contact between the receptor and the general transcription apparatus or indirectly via coregulatory proteins that act coordinated in order to influence the transcription of the target gene. These coregulatory proteins may include either factors enhancing transactivation (coactivators) or factors reducing transactivation (corepressors). The length of time between hormone entry and the accumulation of significant amounts of newly formed proteins is in the order of hours. The genomic pathway is also characterized by a sensitivity towards inhibitors of transcription and translation, e.g., actinomycin D and cycloheximidine (31,38).

The above-mentioned mechanism provides an explanation for the regulation of genes with a functional responsive element sequence within the promoter region. Reports of hormone-bound receptor activation of genes without a responsive element sequence led to the discovery that sex steroid receptors can also modulate gene expression at alternative regulatory DNA sequences such as activating protein-1 (AP-1) (39–41) and specificity protein-1 (SP-1) (42). In this context, the sex steroid receptor is recruited to the specific promoter complex where it interacts with other DNA-bound transcription factors such as c-Jun, c-Fos, and other coactivator proteins.

Nongenomic Sex Steroid Action

Some physiological effects of sex steroids are not mediated by nuclear action as shown by their insensitivity toward appropriate inhibitors and/or their ability to respond to sex steroids within seconds or minutes. Such rapid sex steroid effects are likely to be mediated by receptors with properties distinct from those of the classic nuclear steroid receptors. However, these nuclear receptors may also be involved in nongenomic steroid action. Sex steroids may indeed elicit nongenomic effects, possibly through cell-surface receptors linked to intracellular signal transduction proteins (43,44). Binding sites for estrogens and androgens have been identified on plasma membranes. Nongenomic cellular actions of sex steroids may result in regulation of G protein-coupled receptors, transmembrane ion fluxes, and activation of conventional second messenger transduction cascades, including activation of protein kinase A (PKA), protein kinase C (PKC), tyrosine kinases, mitogen-activated protein kinases (MAPKs), phosphoinositide-3 kinase (PI3K), and Akt- and Src/Shc/ERK signalling (Fig. 4) (45,46).

BIOLOGICAL ACTIONS

Androgens play a crucial role in a number of physiological events. In the first place they induce male sexual differentia-

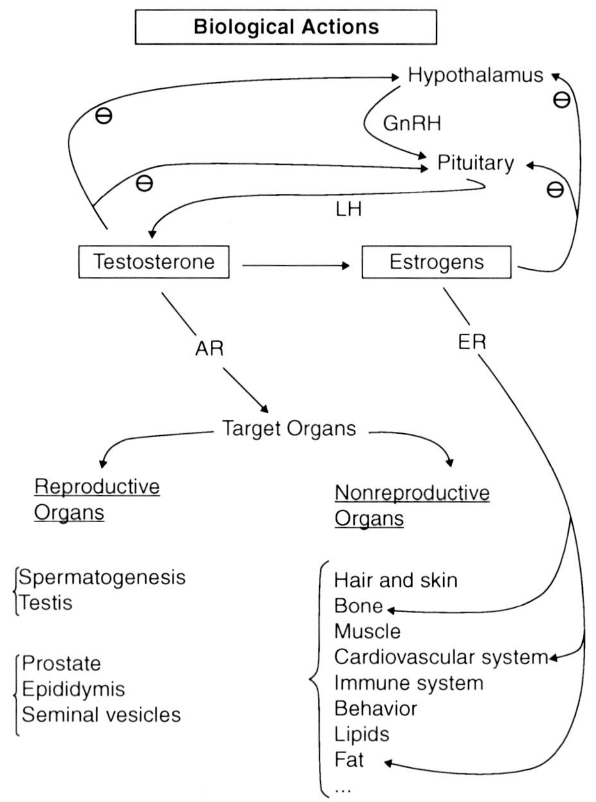

Figure 5 Schematic overview of the biological actions of T. GnRH, gonadotropin-releasing hormone; LH, luteinizing hormone; AR, androgen receptor; ER, estrogen receptor.

tion before birth. Interestingly, neonatal males also have high T concentrations (median concentrations are 200–300 ng/dL), which may be involved in the imprinting of the typical male pattern of growth hormone secretion (47). Second, androgens induce sexual maturation during puberty. Finally, as shown in Figure 5, T may also have a number of important actions in adult men. It is well established that T is necessary to maintain spermatogenesis and therefore reproduction. T is also responsible for the maintenance of the full integrity of other male reproductive organs including prostate, seminal vesicles, and epididymis. Testosterone even has an important impact on a number of other nonreproductive organs, including hair and skin (48), bone (49), muscle (50), as well as the cardiovascular system (51,52).

Part of the beneficial actions of androgens may be related to the aromatization of T into estrogens and stimulation of the ER (53,54). For instance, it is well established that the stimulation of longitudinal growth of the male skeleton and epiphyseal bone are solely dependent on the aromatization of androgens. Also, aromatization of androgens is involved in the reduction of fat mass in men. On the other hand, other aspects of androgen action such as androgen action on skin, muscle tissue, or reproductive organs appear to be mainly AR dependent. Finally, T is involved in the regulation of its own synthesis by a negative feedback on the hypothalamus and the pituitary. Again, part of this important feedback mechanism appears to be estrogen dependent. Estrogen also has dual sites of negative feedback, acting both on the hypothalamus and the pituitary (55,56).

CASE REPORTS

The following patients were referred by their family doctor to a clinical andrologist for androgen replacement therapy.

Case 1

A 45-year-old man consulted his family doctor because of persistent fatigue. An evening blood sample was drawn to assess his T concentration. Compared to the references of the laboratory (10.4–35 nmol/L), T concentration was below normal (9 nmol/L).

Should this man receive androgen replacement therapy?

Answer

Further chemical analysis revealed that the LH concentration (3.4 IU/L) of the patient was within normal references (1.7–8.6 IU/L). Moreover, T concentration was determined in a control serum sample drawn before 10 a.m. T was significantly higher (12 nmol/L) in this morning sample and therefore within normal reference range. The earlier lower (−30%) evening T was entirely explained by diurnal variation. Therefore, androgen replacement therapy is probably not necessary in this patient.

Case 2

A 63-year-old, obese man with low libido as well as low T concentration (9 nmol/)L was referred to a clinical andrologist. Clinical genital examination was completely normal. Should this patient receive androgen replacement therapy?

Answer

Additional investigation revealed that the LH concentration of this patient was normal (5.3 IU/L), but his SHBG concentration was low (0.56 μg/dL) (reference range SHBG [0.70–1.60 μg/dL]). Bioavailable and free T were in the low normal range. It is well established that obesity is associated with low SHBG concentration as well as low total T concentration. Although a trial T therapy is a potential option, its efficacy is very uncertain in this case.

Case 3

A 25-year-old man consulted his family doctor because of his relative lack of facial and body hair. Measurement of T (19.4 nmol/L), LH (4.9 IU/L), and FSH (6.3 IU/L) were within normal references of the laboratory ([10.4–35 nmol/L], [1.7–8.6 IU/L], and [1.2–7.7 IU/L] for T, LH, and FSH, respectively). Is androgen therapy an option?

Answer

The typical characteristics of virilization are not only determined by serum T concentrations but also interindividual differences of T metabolism and action. These mostly genetically determined differences in androgen action and metabolism will not be influenced by androgen therapy, which is therefore not indicated in this case.

REFERENCES

1. Griffin HG, Wilson JD. Disorders of the testes and male reproductive tract. In: Wilson JD, Foster DW, eds. Textbook of Endocrinology. Philadelphia, PA: Saunders, 1994:799–852.
2. Endoh A, Kristiansen SB, Casson PR, et al. The zona reticularis is the site of biosynthesis of dehydroepiandrosterone and dehydroepiandrosterone sulfate in the adult human adrenal cortex resulting from its low expression of 3 beta-hydroxysteroid dehydrogenase. J Clin Endocrinol Metab 1996; 81(10):3558–3565.
3. Kaufman JM, Vermeulen A. The decline of androgen levels in elderly men and its clinical and therapeutic implications. Endocr Rev 2005; 26(6):833–876.
4. Payne AH, Youngblood GL. Regulation of expression of steroidogenic enzymes in Leydig cells. Biol Reprod 1995; 52(2):217–225.
5. Payne AH, Hales DB. Overview of steroidogenic enzymes in the pathway from cholesterol to active steroid hormones. Endocr Rev 2004; 25(6):947–970.
6. Winters SJ, Clark BJ. Testosterone synthesis, transport and metabolism. In: Bremner WJ, Bagatell CJ, eds. Androgens in Health and Disease. Humana Press Inc., Totowa, New Jersey 2003:3–22.
7. Stocco DM, Clark BJ. The role of the steroidogenic acute regulatory protein in steroidogenesis. Steroids 1997; 62(1):29–36.
8. Stocco DM. StAR protein and the regulation of steroid hormone biosynthesis. Annu Rev Physiol 2001; 63:193–213.
9. Hayes FJ, Decruz S, Seminara SB, et al. Differential regulation of gonadotropin secretion by testosterone in the human male: absence of a negative feedback effect of testosterone on follicle-stimulating hormone secretion. J Clin Endocrinol Metab 2001; 86(1):53–58.
10. Nussey S, Whitehead A. The adrenal gland. In: Andrea Bosher, ed. Endocrinology: An Integrated Approach. Taylor & Francis. BIOS Scientific Publishers Lt 2001; 115–168.
11. Giorgi EP, Stein WD. The transport of steroids into animal cells in culture. Endocrinology 1981; 108(2):688–697.
12. de Ronde W, van der Schouw YT, Muller M, et al. Associations of sex-hormone-binding globulin (SHBG) with non-SHBG-bound levels of testosterone and estradiol in independently living men. J Clin Endocrinol Metab 2005; 90(1):157–162.
13. Bremner WJ, Vitiello MV, Prinz PN. Loss of circadian rhythmicity in blood testosterone levels with aging in normal men. J Clin Endocrinol Metab 1983; 56(6):1278–1281.
14. Resko JA, Eik-nes KB. Diurnal testosterone levels in peripheral plasma of human male subjects. J Clin Endocrinol Metab 1966; 26(5):573–576.
15. Crabbe P, Bogaert V, De Bacquer D, et al. Part of the interindividual variation in serum testosterone levels in healthy men reflects differences in androgen sensitivity and feedback set point: contribution of the androgen receptor polyglutamine tract polymorphism. J Clin Endocrinol Metab 2007; 92(9):3604–3610.
16. Labrie F, Luu-The V, Lin SX, et al. Intracrinology: role of the family of 17 beta-hydroxysteroid dehydrogenases in human physiology and disease. J Mol Endocrinol 2000; 25(1):1–16.
17. Labrie F, Belanger A, Cusan L, et al. Physiological changes in dehydroepiandrosterone are not reflected by serum levels of active androgens and estrogens but of their metabolites: intracrinology. J Clin Endocrinol Metab 1997; 82(8):2403–2409.
18. Labrie F, Luu-The V, Labrie C, et al. DHEA and its transformation into androgens and estrogens in peripheral target tissues: intracrinology. Front Neuroendocrinol 2001; 22(3):185–212.
19. Russell DW, Wilson JD. Steroid 5 alpha-reductase: two genes/two enzymes. Annu Rev Biochem 1994; 63:25–61.
20. Behre HM, Kliesch S, Leifke E, et al. Long-term effect of testosterone therapy on bone mineral density in hypogonadal men. J Clin Endocrinol Metab 1997; 82:2386–2390.
21. Feldman HA, Longcope C, Derby CA, et al. Age trends in the level of serum testosterone and other hormones in middle-aged men: longitudinal results from the Massachusetts male aging study. J Clin Endocrinol Metab 2002; 87(2):589–598.
22. Khosla S, Melton LJ 3rd, Atkinson EJ, et al. Relationship of serum sex steroid levels and bone turnover markers with bone mineral density in men and women: a key role for bioavailable estrogen. J Clin Endocrinol Metab 1998; 83(7):2266–2274.
23. Vermeulen A, Kaufman JM, Giagulli VA. Influence of some biological indexes on sex hormone-binding globulin and androgen levels in aging or obese males. J Clin Endocrinol Metab 1996; 81(5):1821–1826.
24. Kahn SM, Hryb DJ, Nakhla AM, et al. Sex hormone-binding globulin is synthesized in target cells. J Endocrinol 2002; 175(1):113–120.
25. Orwoll E, Lambert LC, Marshall LM, et al. Testosterone and estradiol among older men. J Clin Endocrinol Metab 2006; 91(4):1336–1344.
26. Mangelsdorf DJ, Thummel C, Beato M, et al. The nuclear receptor superfamily: the second decade. Cell 1995; 83(6):835–839.

27. Wierman ME. Sex steroid effects at target tissues: mechanisms of action. Adv Physiol Educ 2007; 31(1):26–33.
28. Nilsson S, Makela S, Treuter E, et al. Mechanisms of estrogen action. Physiol Rev 2001; 81(4):1535–1565.
29. Quigley CA, De Bellis A, Marschke KB, et al. Androgen receptor defects: historical, clinical, and molecular perspectives. Endocr Rev 1995; 16(3):271–321.
30. Williams GR, Franklyn JA. Physiology of the steroid-thyroid hormone nuclear receptor superfamily. Baillieres Clin Endocrinol Metab 1994; 8(2):241–266.
31. Beato M, Klug J. Steroid hormone receptors: an update. Hum Reprod Update 2000; 6(3):225–236.
32. Rajender S, Singh L, Thangaraj K. Phenotypic heterogeneity of mutations in androgen receptor gene. Asian J Androl 2007; 9(2):147–179.
33. Chamberlain NL, Driver ED, Miesfeld RL. The length and location of CAG trinucleotide repeats in the androgen receptor N-terminal domain affect transactivation function. Nucleic Acids Res 1994; 22(15):3181–3186.
34. Lapauw B, Goemaere S, Crabbe P, et al. Is the effect of testosterone on body composition modulated by the androgen receptor gene CAG repeat polymorphism in elderly men? Eur J Endocrinol 2007; 156(3):395–401.
35. Davis-Dao CA, Tuazon ED, Sokol RZ, et al. Male infertility and variation in CAG repeat length in the androgen receptor gene: a meta-analysis. J Clin Endocrinol Metab 2007; 92(11):4319–4326.
36. Zitzmann M, Nieschlag E. The CAG repeat polymorphism within the androgen receptor gene and maleness. Int J Androl 2003; 26(2):76–83.
37. Tsai MJ, O'Malley BW. Molecular mechanisms of action of steroid/thyroid receptor superfamily members. Annu Rev Biochem 1994; 63:451–486.
38. McKenna NJ, Lanz RB, O'Malley BW. Nuclear receptor coregulators: cellular and molecular biology. Endocr Rev 1999; 20(3):321–344.
39. Kushner PJ, Agard DA, Greene GL, et al. Estrogen receptor pathways to AP-1. J Steroid Biochem Mol Biol 2000; 74(5):311–317.
40. Whitmarsh AJ, Davis RJ. Transcription factor AP-1 regulation by mitogen-activated protein kinase signal transduction pathways. J Mol Med 1996; 74(10):589–607.
41. Wiren KM, Toombs AR, Zhang XW. Androgen inhibition of MAP kinase pathway and Elk-1 activation in proliferating osteoblasts. J Mol Endocrinol 2004; 32(1):209–226.
42. Safe S. Transcriptional activation of genes by 17 beta-estradiol through estrogen receptor-Sp1 interactions. Vitam Horm 2001; 62:231–252.
43. Losel RM, Falkenstein E, Feuring M, et al. Nongenomic steroid action: controversies, questions, and answers. Physiol Rev 2003; 83(3):965–1016.
44. Falkenstein E, Tillmann HC, Christ M, et al. Multiple actions of steroid hormones–a focus on rapid, nongenomic effects. Pharmacol Rev 2000; 52(4):513–556.
45. Hammes SR., Levin ER. Extranuclear Steroid Receptors: Nature and Actions. Endocr Rev 2007;28(7):726–741.
46. Kousteni S, Bellido T, Plotkin LI, et al. Nongenotropic, sex-nonspecific signaling through the estrogen or androgen receptors: dissociation from transcriptional activity. Cell 2001; 104(5):719–730.
47. Knickmeyer RC, Baron-Cohen S. Fetal testosterone and sex differences. Early Hum Dev 2006; 82(12):755–760.
48. Zouboulis CC, Degitz K. Androgen action on human skin – from basic research to clinical significance. Exp Dermatol 2004; 13(suppl 4):5–10.
49. Vanderschueren D, Vandenput L, Boonen S, et al. Androgens and bone. Endocr Rev 2004; 25(3):389–425.
50. Brodsky IG, Balagopal P, Nair K.S. Effects of testosterone replacement on muscle mass and muscle protein synthesis in hypogonadal men–a clinical research center study. J Clin Endocrinol Metab 1996; 81(10):3469–3475.
51. Wu FC, von Eckardstein A. Androgens and coronary artery disease. Endocr Rev 2003; 24(2):183–217.
52. Liu PY, Death AK, Handelsman DJ. Androgens and Cardiovascular Disease. Endocr Rev 2003; 24(3):313–340.
53. de Ronde W, Pols HA, van Leeuwen JP, et al. The importance of oestrogens in males. Clin Endocrinol (Oxf) 2003; 58(5):529–542.
54. Lombardi G, Zarrilli S, Colao A, et al. Estrogens and health in males. Mol Cell Endocrinol 2001; 178(1–2):51–55.
55. Hayes FJ, Seminara SB, DeCruz S, et al. Aromatase inhibition in the human male reveals a hypothalamic site of estrogen feedback. J Clin Endocrinol Metab 2000; 85(9):3027–3035.
56. Vanderschueren D., Bouillon R. Estrogen deficiency in men is a challenge for both the hypothalamus and pituitary. J Clin Endocrinol Metab 2000; 85(9):3024–3026.

23 Gonadotropins and gonadotropin receptors

Ilpo Huhtaniemi and Maria Alevizaki

INTRODUCTION

Gonadotropin function is the master switch in the regulation of all testicular functions. Missing gonadotropin action has differential phenotypic effects depending on the age it occurs. Congenital absence of gonadotropins or their receptors interferes with masculinization of the male fetus. At puberty it blocks the normal sexual maturation, and if it occurs in adult age, the consequences are hypogonadism and infertility. The purpose of this chapter is to review the basic information about the structure, regulation, normal functions, and pathologies of the key molecules involved in gonadotropin action, that is, the gonadotrophic hormones and their cognate receptors.

THE STRUCTURE OF GONADOTROPINS AND THEIR RECEPTORS

Gonadotropins

The pituitary gonadotropins, luteinizing hormone (LH) and follicle-stimulating hormone (FSH), and the placental LH analogue human chorionic gonadotropin (hCG) belong together with thyroid-stimulating hormone (TSH) to the family of glycoprotein hormones (1). They all are large dimeric glycoproteins with molecular mass of 30 to 40 kDa, consisting of a common α-subunit (Cα) bound noncovalently to the hormone-specific β-subunit (LHβ, hCGβ, FSHβ, and TSHβ, respectively). Only the α/β dimers of the glycoprotein hormones are biologically active. The mature Cα protein consists of 92 amino acid residues and is encoded by a single gene comprising four exons, localized on chromosome 6q12.21 (Fig. 1). There are 10 cysteines in the Cα protein, which participate in the formation of intra-subunit cystine bridges, and there are two N-linked glycosylation sites in the protein. The structures of carbohydrate side chains are heterogenous between individual molecules, for which reason gonadotropins appear in the circulation as multiple "isoforms" with differing intrinsic bioactivities (2). All β-subunit genes are located on different chromosomes. There is a cluster of one *LH*β and six *hCG*β genes and pseudogenes on chromosome 19q13.32 (3). Most of the steady-state *hCG*β mRNA is transcribed from genes 3, 5, and 8 (4); hCG, and mostly its free β-subunit, is also produced in men in testicular germ cell tumors and biliary and pancreatic cancer, and therefore, it is a sensitive marker for these malignancies (4,5). The single genes of *FSH*β and *TSH*β are located on chromosomes 11p13 and 1p13, respectively (3).

The mature β-subunit proteins range in length from 110 to 145 amino acids (Fig. 1), and they contain 12 cysteine pairs forming six intra-subunit disulphide bridges. The main difference between LHβ and hCGβ is the 24-amino acid C-terminal peptide (CTP) extension in the latter. There is one N linked glycosylation site in LHβ, two in FSHβ, and hCGβ has two N-linked and four O-linked glycosylation sites in its CTP. The differential degrees of glycosylation determine the differential circulatory half-lives of the hormones (LH, 20 minutes; hCG, 24 hours, FSH, 3–4 hours). Although the β-subunits confer the functional specificity of the hormones, they have considerable amino acid identity, ranging from 32% for the LH–TSH pair to 83% for the LH–hCG pair (excluding the CTP of hCGβ). The *hCG*β subunit is thought to have evolved most recently from *LH*β through a frameshift mutation with addition of the CTP. Attachment of the CTP to a recombinant form of FSH is now being exploited clinically in the form of a long-acting FSH preparation (6).

As expected, the crystal structures of deglycosylated hCG and FSH are very similar (7,8) and reveal that both subunits contain so-called "cystine knot structures" that are similar to some remotely related growth factor–type signaling molecules. Each subunit has elongated shape, with two β-hairpin loops on one side of the central cystine knot and a single long loop on the other side. The noncovalent interaction between the two subunits is stabilized by a segment of the β-subunit that extends like a "seatbelt" around the α-subunit and is locked by a disulphide bridge (7,8).

Gonadotropin Receptors

Similar to their ligands, the LH receptor (R) and FSHR (as well as TSHR) are structurally related, belonging to class A rhodopsin-like G protein–coupled receptors (GPCRs) (Fig. 2) (9). The molecular size of these receptors is approximately 80 kDa, and they are also glycosylated. They each have a serpentine transmembrane domain that traverses the plasma membrane as seven α-helices that are connected by three extracellular and three intracellular loops (Figs. 3 and 4). The transmembrane region is the integral part in signal transduction of LH/hCG and FSH across the plasma membrane. Approximately half of the size of the receptor molecule is composed of the long extracellular tail, whose distinctive part is formed by a stretch of leucine-rich repeats forming a kind of elongated concave structure that functions as the primary site of hormone–receptor interaction (9). In this sense, the receptors resemble other molecules with a known role in protein–protein interaction. The extracellular and transmembrane domains are connected by a short hinge region, which apparently partly determines the receptor's ligand specificity, as shown with a human *LHR* mutation lacking

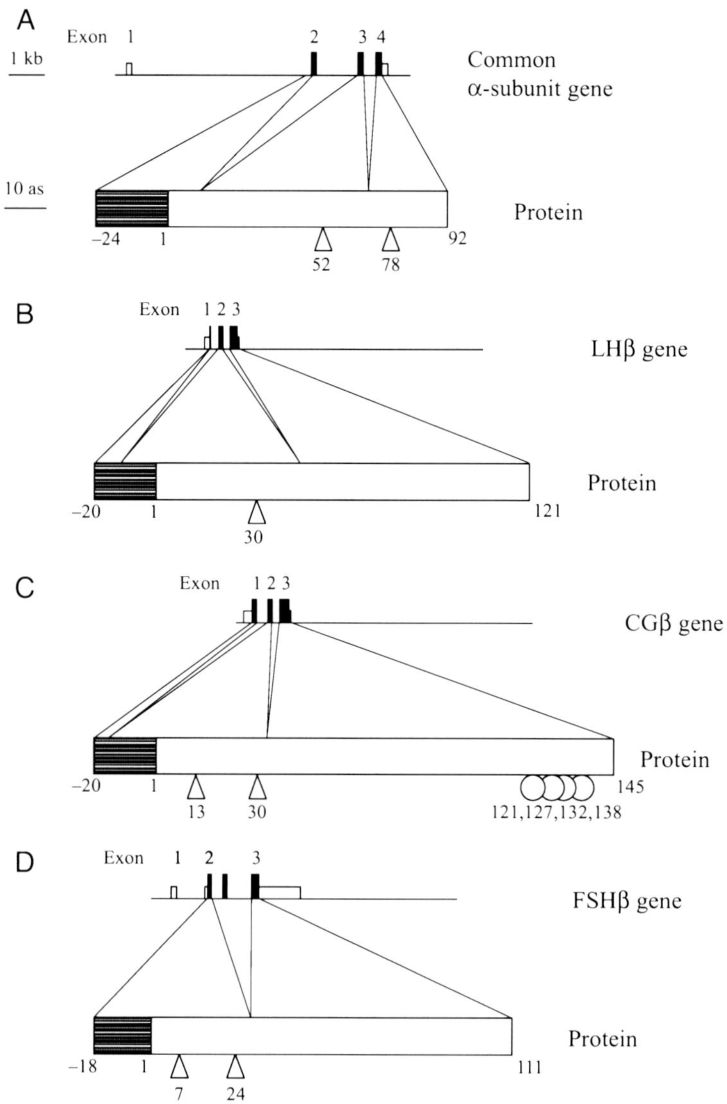

Figure 1 Schematic presentation of the human gonadotropin subunit genes and proteins. The *top part* of each scheme depicts the gene. The open bars indicate non–protein-coding exon sequences. The closed bars indicate the sequences that comprise the protein-coding open reading frame. The horizontal line depicts intronic sequence. The genes are drawn to scale. In the *bottom part* of each scheme the protein structure is shown. The signal peptide is indicated by the shaded bar, and the mature protein is depicted by the open bar. The numbers below the protein signify the start and end of the signal peptide and the length of the mature protein product, taking the first amino acid of the mature protein as 1. Below the protein the positions (and number of amino acid) of the N-linked glycosylation sites are indicated by inverted triangles and in the case of CGβ, the O-linked glycosylation sites (*circles*). The connecting lines between the coding exons in the top part of the scheme and the protein structure in the bottom part serve to indicate the sections of the protein encoded by the respective exon. Note that the β-genes consist of three exons and that the common α-subunit gene is much longer mainly because of addition of the first, noncoding exon and long intron 1. In contrast to the other β-genes, the first exon of *FSHβ* is noncoding and exon 3 encodes a long 39-untranslated region (*open bar*). *Source*: From Ref. 1, with permission.

this region, and consequently being able to bind only hCG but not LH (10). The fourth functional domain of the gonadotropin receptors is the intracellular tail, which participates in the desensitization and internalization of the receptor following hormone binding and signal transduction (please refer to the following section).

While FSHR binds only FSH, LHR binds both LH and hCG, hence the latter can be considered functionally an LH agonist. Both gonadotropin receptors are located next to each other on chromosome 2p, and especially, their transmembrane domains are structurally very similar. The clearest structural difference between the gonadotropin receptor genes is that *LHR* has 11 and *FSHR* 10 exons; however, in both molecules the longest last exon encodes the entire transmembrane and intracellular domains. The liganded extracellular domains of FSHR have been crystallized (9), and the hormone appears to bind in a handclasp fashion to an elongated, curved receptor.

REGULATION OF GONADOTROPIN SYNTHESIS AND SECRETION

Stimulation of Gonadotropin Gene Expression, Synthesis, and Secretion

Gonadotropins are produced by the gonadotroph cells of the anterior pituitary gland. The proximal regulator of gonadotropin synthesis and secretion is the hypothalamic gonadotropin-releasing hormone (GnRH) produced by nuclei of the anterior hypothalamus (11). GnRH neurons send axons to the median eminence of the hypophysial stalk, from where GnRH is released into the hypophysial portal circulation to

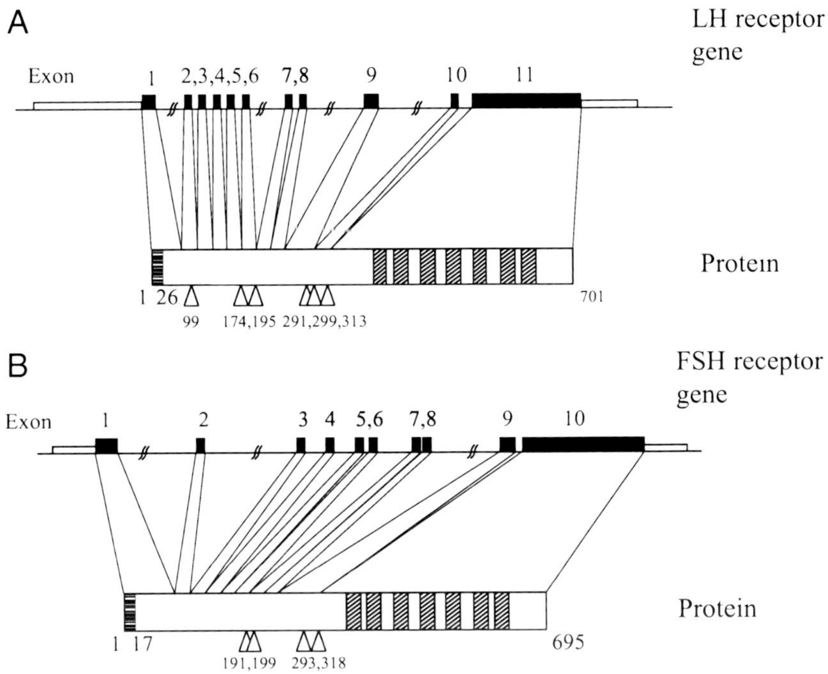

Figure 2 Schematic presentation of the human gonadotropin receptor genes and proteins. The structure of the genes is depicted in the *top part of the drawings*. The open bars indicate non–protein-coding exon sequences. The closed bars indicate the sequences that comprise the protein-coding open reading frame. The horizontal line depicts intronic sequences. Although the genes are not drawn to scale, exons that are grouped in the gene are also drawn grouped. The total length of *LHR* is approximately 69 kb and that of FSHR approximately 192 kb. The relation between the intron/exon structure of the gene and the domains of the protein are indicated by the broken lines. The horizontally hatched part of the protein indicates the signal peptide, and the cross-hatched bars signify the seven segments of the transmembrane domain. The numbers below the proteins indicate the start and end of the signal peptide and the length of the total protein product including the signal peptide. The numbered inverted triangles below the protein indicate the positions of N-linked glycosylation sites. Note that the receptor genes are very similar in structure with the exception of an additional exon 11 in the *LHR*. Exon 1 encodes the signal peptide and a small part of the extracellular domain; the following eight or nine exons encode the rest of the extracellular domain, including the leucine-rich repeat motifs. In both the receptor genes, the final exon is the largest and contains the information for the transmembrane signal transduction domain. *Source:* From Ref. 1, with permission.

reach the anterior pituitary gland, and to interact, subsequently, with its cognate receptors on the plasma membrane of gonadotroph cells. GnRH secretion is under direct and indirect upstream regulation of multiple neurotransmitters, including glutamate, GABA, neuropeptide Y, opiates, dopamine, noradrenaline, kisspeptin, and nitric oxide (Fig. 5) (12).

A novel regulatory mechanism, the kisspeptin/GPR54 system, has received particular attention recently, and it is now considered the master switch in turning on the hypothalamic–pituitary–gonadal axis at puberty (13). For the stimulation of gonadotropin synthesis, it is vital that GnRH is secreted in short bursts every 60 to 90 minutes. If GnRH secretion is tonic, as occurs during GnRH agonist treatments, the effect is opposite, that is, desensitization and cessation of gonadotropin synthesis.

Approximately 6% to 10% of the anterior pituitary cells are gonadotrophs, and most of them secrete both LH and FSH (14). The action of GnRH is mediated by its cognate receptor, GnRHR, also a GPCR (15), with the unique structural feature that it lacks the intracellular tail, which makes it more resistant to desensitization than other GPCRs. The rapid signaling of GnRHR involves activation of phospholipase C (PL-C), followed by hydrolysis of membrane phosphoinositides and increase in intracellular inositol phosphates, followed by rapid mobilization of calcium from intracellular stores and through voltage-gated channels. In the long term, GnRH stimulation involves the activation of the protein kinase C/MAP kinase/ERK/JNK cascade. Pulsatile GnRH can maintain GnRHR expression, but continuous exposure, or prolonged GnRH deficiency, leads to receptor decline and suppressed gonadotropin subunit gene expression.

The basal and GnRH-stimulated expression of gonadotropin subunit genes are regulated by an array of transcription factors

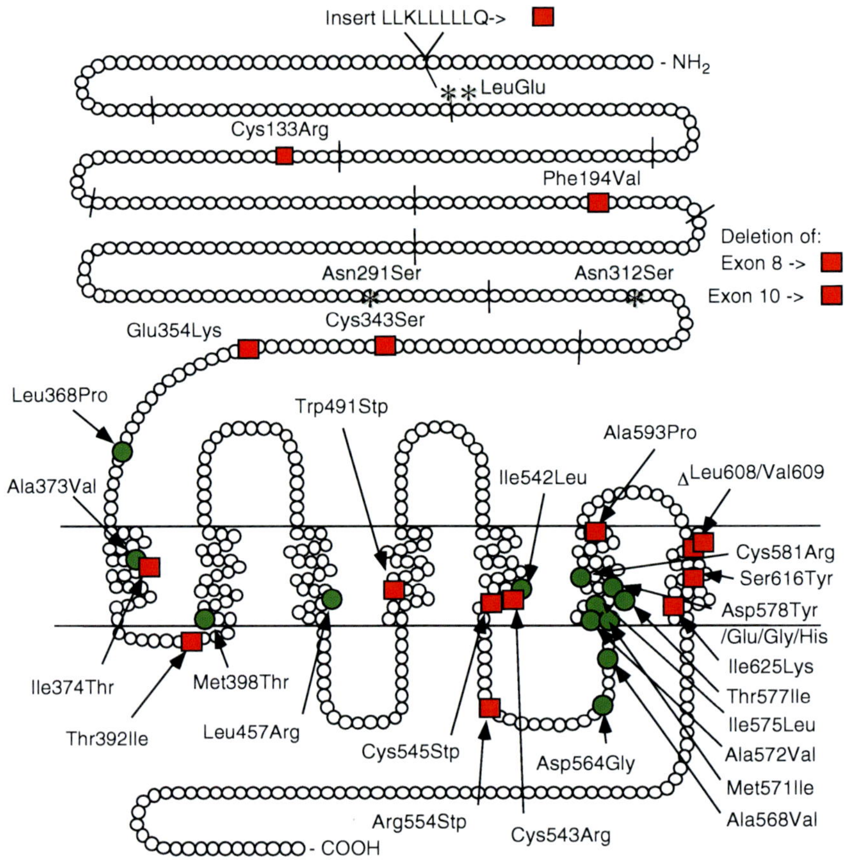

Figure 3 Currently known mutations in the human LHR gene. Schematic structures of the receptor proteins in association with plasma membrane (extracellular side above) are presented. Open squares indicate inactivating and closed circles activating mutations, and asterisks depict nonsynonymous polymorphisms. The short lines across the amino acid chain separate the 11 exons encoding the receptor protein. For further details, please refer to the text.

binding to the promoter regions of the gonadotropin subunit genes (16). A limited number of transcription factors are active in basal conditions, and when GnRH signaling is activated, additional transcription factors are bound with consequently stimulated gene expression. *C*α expression is basally relatively high, and GnRH stimulation upregulates more clearly that of the β-subunits. Cα is always produced in excess of the β-subunits, for which reason free Cα is readily measurable in circulation also during inhibitory treatment with GnRH analogues (17).

Feedback Regulation of Gonadotropins

The negative feedback regulation of gonadotropins is under the influence of the gonadal steroids and peptides, acting partly directly on the pituitary gonadotrophs and partly indirectly through hypothalamus to suppress the GnRH secretion (Fig. 5). In the absence of the gonadal input, as in primary hypogonadism or after gonadectomy, gonadotropin levels rise. The main steroid hormone mediating the testicular feedback is testosterone (T), and its conversion to oestradiol in the brain is essential for this action (18). Animal experiments emphasize the importance of GnRH secretion as the target of steroid negative feedback (19), but experiments in men have shown that the oestrogen effect consists of two components—decreased GnRH pulse frequency and decreased pituitary responsiveness to GnRH (20). Conspicuously, the GnRH neurons lack oestrogen and androgen receptors, and it has recently been established that these effects appear to go through inhibition of kisspeptin neurons (13).

There are similarities and differences in the feedback regulation of LH and FSH (Fig. 5). LH secretion is mainly under the negative feedback regulation of T and its metabolite oestradiol. Besides gonadal steroids, two pituitary paracrine factors, follistatin and activin, and one testicular peptide hormone, inhibin-B, selectively regulate FSH secretion at the pituitary level. Activin and inhibin belong to the TGF-β family of peptides, and follistatin is an activin-binding protein (17). Therefore, although the same GnRH pulses stimulate both LH and FSH secretion, there is some discordance between them. The testicular feedback on

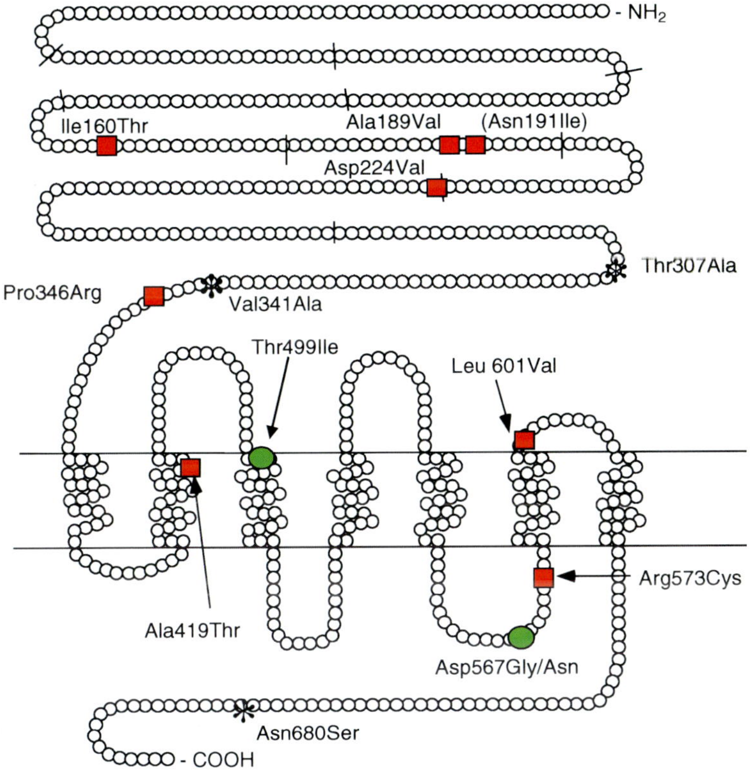

Figure 4 Currently known mutations in the human FSHR gene. Schematic structures of the receptor proteins in association with plasma membrane (extracellular side above) are presented. Open squares indicate inactivating and closed circles activating mutations, and asterisks depict nonsynonymous polymorphisms. The short lines across the amino acid chain separate the 10 exons encoding the receptor protein. For further details, please refer to the text.

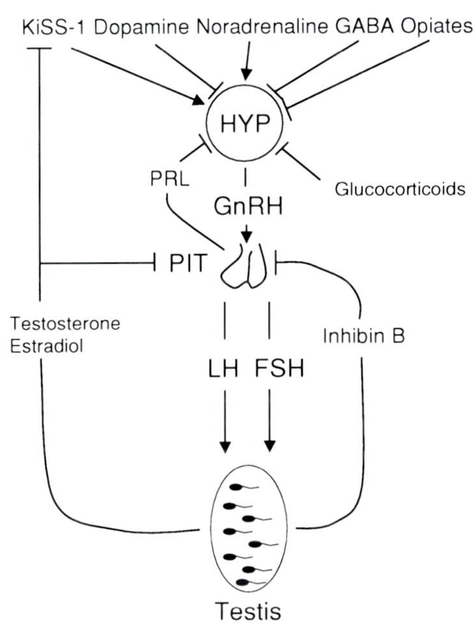

Figure 5 A simplified scheme for the stimulation, actions, and feedback control of gonadotropins. *Abbreviations:* HYP, hypothalamus; PIT, pituitary gland; –>, stimulatory effect; –I, inhibitory effect.

FSH secretion is mainly mediated by inhibin-B, predominately produced by Sertoli cells, and to some extent by Leydig cells (21). Inhibins are heterodimers of two peptide chains, the α-subunit and either βA or βB. Only α and βB chains are produced by the testis, hence the testicular inhibin is of the B type. Testicular inhibin-B also functions as an intratesticular paracrine regulator, but its inhibitory effect on FSH secretion at the pituitary level is better characterized.

FSH is the main stimulator of testicular inhibin secretion by upregulating *α-subunit* expression, whereas the factors regulating *βB subunit* remain unclear. The regulator(s) apparently originate from germ cells because cancer chemotherapy destroying spermatogenesis suppresses plasma levels of inhibin-B but not those of α-subunit (22). Circulating inhibin-B levels reflect closely the number and function of Sertoli cells, and although this peptide has a negative feedback effect on pituitary FSH secretion, the reciprocity is less strict than between LH and T.

The other component in the role of inhibin peptides on gonadotropin secretion takes place in the pituitary gland, where activin and its binding protein follistatin participate in paracrine regulation of FSH synthesis (23). Activin is composed of two inhibin β chains (βA and βB) and the βB/βB form predominates in the pituitary gland. It stimulates FSHβ mRNA synthesis and prolongs its half-life (24). Activin action is antagonized by follistatin that binds to it and neutralizes its bioactivity, as does inhibin by competing with activin by binding and blocking its receptors (23); inhibin can, thus, be considered an activin antagonist.

MOLECULAR ASPECTS OF GONADOTROPIN ACTION

The molecular events mediating the actions of LH and FSH on Leydig and Sertoli cells, respectively, are, in principle, similar (25–27). There are differences in details of these actions, and all aspects have not been explored to the same extent with both hormones. Moreover, the molecular mechanisms of gonadotropin action in the human testis have not been studied in great detail, and much of the information is based on animal experiments and in vitro studies on immortalized cell lines. We present in the following a simplified view of these actions, recognizing that all details on LH and FSH action in the human testis are not yet known.

The first step after binding of LH/hCG or FSH to their cognate receptor is a conformational change in their transmembrane receptor domain, which catalyses the activation of a specific stimulatory guanosine triphosphate (GTP) binding protein, Gs (Fig. 6). It is a heterotrimer ($\alpha/\beta/\gamma$) whose α-subunit binds in the inactive state guanosine diphosphate (GDP). Upon ligand-induced activation of the receptor, GDP is replaced by GTP and the α-subunit (Gs_{α}) dissociates from $G_{\beta//\gamma}$. The former activates cell membrane–associated adenylyl cyclase, catalyzing the conversion of ATP to cyclic adenosine-3':5'-monophosphate (cAMP), which functions as the intracellular second messenger of the LH/LHR and FSH/FSHR signaling cascades; cAMP binds to the regulatory subunit of protein kinase A (PK-A), which in inactive form is a tetramer of two regulatory and two catalytic subunits. The active catalytic subunit of PK-A then catalyses the phosphorylation of an array of target proteins, thereby stimulating or inhibiting their activities, and also leading to changes in gene expression. One of the target proteins is a transcription factor, cAMP response element binding (CREB) protein, which binds to a specific cAMP response element (CRE) sequence of gonadotropin responsive genes. Such genes are, for example, *CREB* itself, the *inducible cAMP early repressor of cAMP-mediated gene transcription* (*ICER*) and other genes responding directly to LH or FSH stimulation.

Also other signaling pathways mediate gonadotropin actions. With respect to LH, they concern Leydig cell proliferation and differentiation and involve the PL-C–activated inositol phosphate pathway and Ca^{2+} fluxes (28). Which G protein, Gs, Gi_2, or Gq/11 is participating in this signalling is not fully explored; furthermore, the $G_{\beta/\gamma}$ dimer may function as the activator of PL-C. The activation of PL-C is apparently dependent on LHR density, and it is only observed at a high concentration of the receptor. This leaves the physiological function of PL-C activation open, and it may prevail only in specific physiological or pathophysiological situations, for example, in connection with specific LHR mutations (please refer to the following section).

In the case of FSH, the cAMP response has been shown to activate several other signaling pathways (29,30). One of them is the MAP kinase, ERK, and p38 pathway, which probably play a role in the promotion of Sertoli cell proliferation. Another one is FSH-stimulated influx of intracellular free Ca^{2+} through plasma membrane ion channels and from intracellular stores, again through a cAMP-mediated mechanism. Calcium binds to calmodulin (CaM), and then activates CaM-dependent kinases, stimulates Sertoli–Sertoli cell junctional dynamics, and activates cytoskeletal structures and gene expression. Another cAMP-initiated signaling cascade is the phosphatidylinositol-3-kinase (PI3-K) pathway, which generates specific inositol phospholipids that activate protein kinase B encoded by the *akt* gene. It is important for Sertoli cell metabolism, including glucose uptake, amino acid transport, and maintenance of activity of lactate dehydrogenase. Finally, the activation of phospholipase A_2 leads to the release of arachidonic acid and its subsequent metabolism to prostaglandin E_2 and other eicosanoids—all functioning as intracellular messengers.

The cessation of LHR and FSHR action is in principle similar through desensitization of signaling and downregulation of receptors (Fig. 6). In this process, the intracellular loops of the receptors become phosphorylated by specific G protein–coupled receptor kinases (GRKs), which facilitate the binding of arrestin to the receptor. Finally, by interacting with clathrin the receptors concentrate in clathrin-coated pits, which become endocytosed and either transported to lysosomes for protein degradation or recycled to the cell membrane. A concomitant event is the postsignaling activation of phosphodiesterase, which converts cAMP to inactive AMP, thereby reverting PK-A back to its inactive tetramer state and terminating the intracellular responses to gonadotrophic stimulation.

GONADOTROPIN SECRETION AND ACTIONS THROUGHOUT THE MALE LIFE SPAN

Fetal pituitary gonadotropin synthesis starts between weeks 12 to 13 of gestation (31), reaches its intrauterine peak around the middle of pregnancy, and declines thereafter towards the end of gestation, apparently as a result of placental and fetal testicular negative feedback regulation (32) (Fig. 7). The levels are lower in male fetuses because of active fetal testicular androgen production; significant ovarian steroidogenesis does not start until puberty. Fetal testes express LHR and FSHR mRNA and protein in the turn of the first and second trimesters of pregnancy, but the ovaries only after birth (33–35). It is uncertain whether the fetal pituitary gonadotropins are functionally important because hCG is present in higher concentrations in fetal circulation and apparently provides the trophic stimulus for the fetal testes to produce T necessary for male fetal masculinization. The role of hCG is emphasized by the findings that males with inactivating *LH*β mutation are normally masculinized at birth, whereas those with *LHR* inactivation fail to masculinize (1). What exactly FSH does in fetal life is not known, and animal experiments suggest that the first function FSH assumes in males is to stimulate Sertoli cells' proliferation at puberty (36).

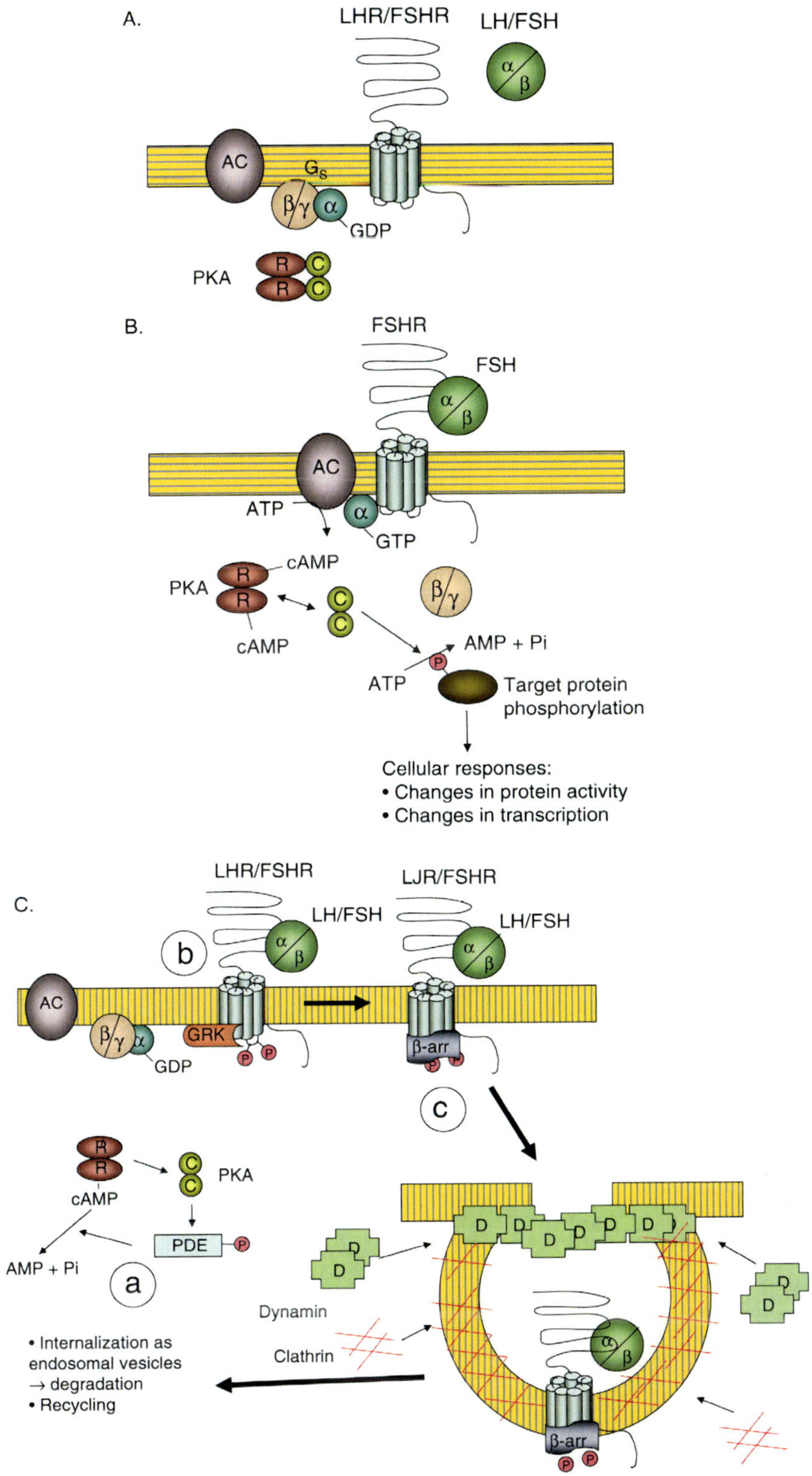

Figure 6 Molecular events in the stimulation, desensitization, and downregulation of gonadotropin receptor function. *Panel A* presents the resting stage, *panel B* presents events upon acute signal transduction, and *panel C* presents events upon attenuation of the signal after the stimulatory phase. (A) In resting stage, with no hormone–receptor interaction, the Gs protein remains as an inactive α/β/γ trimer and the α-subunit binds guanosine diphosphate (GDP). Protein kinase A (PK-A) is an inactive tetramer in which each catalytic subunit (C) is associated with one regulatory subunit (R). (B) Upon ligand binding, the α-subunit of Gs protein dissociates from β/γ, binds guanosine triphosphate (GTP), and activates adenylyl cyclase (AC), which catalyses the conversion of adenosine triphosphate (ATP) to the second messenger, cyclic adenosine monophosphate (cAMP); cAMP binds to the regulatory subunits of PKA, activating the dissociated catalytic subunits, which thereafter catalyze phosphorylation of target proteins, altering their activities and bringing about the cellar responses to hormonal stimulation. (C,a) Levels of the second messenger, cAMP, are decreased through activation of phosphodiesterase (PDE) through PKA-stimulated phosphorylation. (C,b) G protein–coupled receptor kinase (GRK) phosphorylates serine and threonine residues in intracellular loops of the receptors, which blocks coupling of Gs protein with the receptor, hence attenuating signaling pathway. (C,c) The phosphorylated receptor binds β-arrestin (β-ARR), which provides an additional hindrance to receptor–Gs coupling. The receptor–β-arrestin complex then binds to the clathrin–dynamin (D) endocytotic machinery and becomes internalized in endosomal vesicles. Consequently, the number of receptors on plasma membrane decreases, that is, becomes downregulated. The intracellular fate of the endocytosed receptor is either to become degraded or to enter the rapid recycling pathway.

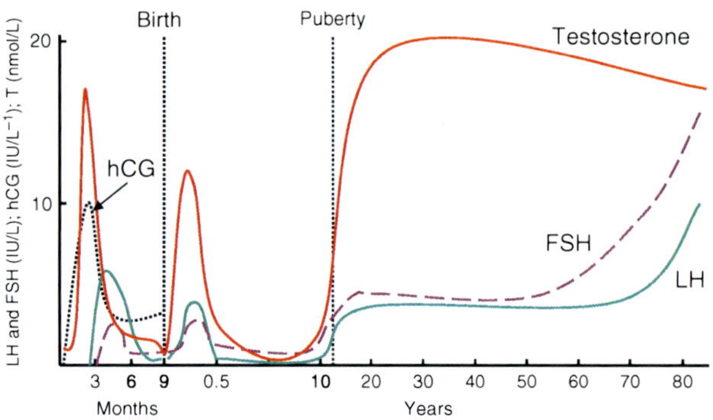

Figure 7 Circulating gonadotropin and testosterone levels in a male from fetal life until old age. The red line depicts testosterone, the green line LH, the purple dashed line FSH, and the black dashed line hCG. Please note the different scale of the hCG level (IU/L × 10–1).

After birth, there is a transient increase in gonadotropin secretion up to approximately six months of life (37) with a concomitant increase in T secretion ("mini-puberty") (Fig. 7). No function has been assigned to this temporary activation of the pituitary–gonadal axis, and it is possible that it represents merely an adaptational period following the elimination of the high intrauterine levels of placental steroids and their strong negative feedback effects. The prepubertal period of male development is typified by very low gonadotropin secretion and testicular endocrine activity. However, gonadotropin levels are not totally absent, and sensitive assays are able to detect low gonadotropin secretory activity especially at nighttime (38). Prepubertal testes also express gonadotropin receptors, as shown indirectly by their response to stimulation with hCG and FSH (39).

Puberty represents the period of reawakening of gonadotropin secretion (Fig. 7), and it is now known to occur because of activation of the kisspeptin/GPR54 system, which then turns on GnRH secretion (13). At this time, both LH and FSH reach their adult levels and pulsatile secretion patterns. LH activates the proliferation, growth, and steroidogenic activity of Leydig cells, and FSH stimulates Sertoli cell proliferation and the multitude of their metabolic functions needed for the paracrine maintenance of spermatogenesis. Whether FSH action is mandatory for the pubertal initiation of spermatogenesis is somewhat controversial because the phenotypes of the different clinical situations and experimental models with inactivation of FSH action do not agree (please refer to the following section). In any case, it is clear that FSH action is necessary for the maintenance of qualitatively and quantitatively normal spermatogenesis (40).

Testicular androgen production and gametogenesis decline gradually with age, and recent studies have clarified that they occur mainly due to aging-related changes at the testicular level (41). Initially, increased gonadotropin levels can maintain normal testicular function, and the situation appears as "compensated" hypogonadism, with T levels in the normal range, while LH is high normal or increased. When this condition progresses, it gradually develops into genuine primary hypogonadism with subnormal T and elevated gonadotropin levels. When obesity, metabolic syndrome, and/or serious comorbidities are associated with aging, the type of hypogonadism is secondary, with suppressed gonadotropin and androgen levels. However, it should be emphasized that the decrease of T because of aging per se is minimal, only about 1% per year.

GENETIC DISTURBANCES IN GONADOTROPIN SECRETION AND ACTION

A descriptive term hypogonadotrophic hypogonadism (HH) is used for a part of these conditions, when the pathogenesis includes aberrations in the upstream control of GnRH synthesis, the synthesis and action of GnRH, as well as the synthesis of gonadotropins. In contrast, the inactivation of gonadotropin receptors brings about gonadotropin resistance with hypergonadotrophic hypogonadism, and the reverse is observed with activating *LHR* and *FSHR* mutations when gonadotropin signaling is constitutively activated. Many of these cases remain idiopathic, and in the following we have reviewed the known mutations causing these conditions with known molecular pathogenesis. The phenotypes of those affecting the genes of GnRH, gonadotropins, and their receptors are summarized in Table 1.

Mutations Affecting the Hypothalamic Control of Gonadotropin Synthesis and Secretion

Two factors regulating the function of GnRH neurons have received attention recently, that is, kisspeptin and leptin, both upstream regulators of GnRH neurons. Although kisspeptin mutations are not yet known, several HH patients with inactivating missense, nonsense, and nonstop mutation in *GPR54*, that is, its receptor in GnRH neurons, have been identified (42,43). Both congenital deficiency of leptin and leptin receptor have been found to cause severe early-onset obesity and HH. These cases are rare and only approximately 10 of each are currently known (44,45). The mechanism of leptin action in regulating gonadotropin secretion is possibly due to its role in the release of neurotransmitters, such as neuropeptide Y, which then regulate GnRH secretion (46).

Kallmann Syndrome

The commonest form of HH affecting GnRH neuronal function is Kallmann syndrome (KS), with a prevalence of 1:8000 in boys and five to seven times less in girls (47). KS patients have HH combined with the lack of sense of smell, caused by a developmental disturbance of the olfactory placode. Besides disturbed olfaction, the migration of GnRH neurons in embryonic life from the nasal cavity to the hypothalamus is blocked. Consequently, the GnRH neurons do not reach the location from which they can secrete GnRH into the hypophysial portal circulation, to reach the adenohypophysis

Table 1 The Types of Mutations Detected in Men in *GnRH*, *Common α-Subunit*, *LHβ*, *FSHβ*, and the Receptors (R) of the Cognate Hormones (*LHR and FSHR*)[a]

Gene	Type of mutation	Phenotype
GnRH	• Inactivating	Hypogonadotrophic hypogonadism, no anosmia
GnRHR	• Inactivating	Hypogonadotrophic hypogonadism, no anosmia
Common α-subunit	• No mutations detected	
LHβ	• Inactivating	Hypergonadotrophic hypogonadism, normal masculinization at birth, no spontaneous puberty
LHR	• Activating	Gonadotropin-independent precocious puberty
	• Inactivating	Pseudohermaphroditism (no masculinization in utero)
FSHβ	• Activating	Azoospermia
FSHR	• Inactivating	Spermatogenesis in the absence of gonadotropins (posthypophysectomy)
	• Inactivating	Variable impairment of spermatogenesis

[a]For references, see the text.

and to stimulate gonadotroph cells (48,49). Most cases of KS are sporadic and usually diagnosed in adolescence, when the absence of spontaneous puberty and deficient olfaction are observed. Without androgen replacement, the KS patients do not develop male secondary sex characteristics at the normal age of puberty. They remain azoospermic unless treated with GnRH or gonadotropins—androgen therapy does not initiate spermatogenesis.

KS is genetically heterogeneous, with X-linked, autosomal dominant and autosomal recessive forms of inheritance (50). Two KS-related loci are known today. *KAL1*, encoding anosmin-1, is responsible for a small proportion of X-linked form of KS, and *KAL2,* encoding the fibroblast growth factor receptor 1 (FGFR1), is mutated in some cases of autosomal dominant KS. Anosmin-1 has several functions including a role as an axonal guidance factor, probably directing the normal migration of GnRH neurons. It is an extracellular glycoprotein interacting with plasminogen activator and FGFR1. The genetic background of the majority of KS cases still remains obscure, but candidate genes include the DNA-binding protein *CHD7* (51), guidance molecule for olfactory axonal outgrowth *NELF* (52,53), and prokinetin receptor *PKR2* (54). Finally, very recent reports add *fibroblast growth factor (FGF)* 8 (55) and *neurokinin B* (56) to the growing list of genes whose mutations can cause HH.

Mutations Affecting the Function of GnRH

Although the *GnRH* gene is a natural candidate for mutations causing HH, the first mutations in this gene, disrupting GnRH synthesis, were only very recently reported (57,58). Instead, a total of approximately 20 inactivating mutations of the *GnRHR* gene have been reported (see Text Box 1 for a case report). These mutations are found in complete or incomplete HH without anosmia. The phenotype in males includes delayed puberty, decreased libido, poor masculinization, and reduced testis size with asthenoteratozoospermia (59). Basal gonadotropin levels are low or normal, with normal frequency but low amplitude of peaks and variable response to GnRH stimulation. Mutations occur in all parts of the *GnRHR* gene with no specific hot spot, and they display either dramatically reduced ligand binding and/or reduced signaling.

Text Box 1 **Case Report: A Typical Case of Inactivating *GnRHR* Mutation**

This was the first published report on a male patient with inactivating mutation in *GnRHR*. The propositus was a 22-year-old man referred because of hypogonadism. He had puberty at the age of 16, his height was 180 cm, weight 84 kg, and arm span 186 cm. He reported impaired libido, but it remained unclear whether he ever had sexual intercourse. Physical examination revealed the absence of facial hair, sparse pubic hair (Tanner stage 3), a penis of 6 cm, and scrotal testes (volume 8/8 mL) and no gynecomastia. He had a normal sense of smell, no mirror movements of the upper limbs, no abnormal eye movements, no color blindness, and no renal or craniofacial abnormalities. Audiometry and magnetic resonance imaging of the head were normal. The karyotype was 46,XY. His serum testosterone concentration was 2.8 nmol/L (normal range 9–24 nmol/L). The basal levels of serum LH and FSH were 4.0 and 5.9 IU/L, respectively (normal range 1.0–5.0 and 0.9–5.7, respectively), and they responded normally to GnRH challenge. Evaluation of pulsatile LH secretion revealed a mean LH concentration of 3.7 IU/L, a normal number of 4.5 pulses in 8 hours, but a decreased amplitude of 0.8 IU/L (normal 3.9). Results of other pituitary hormones were normal. Semen volume was 0.1 mL, with a sperm density of 39 million/mL, 5% motility, and 43% normal morphology.

The patient's older sister (37 years) had a history of primary amenorrhea and infertility. His 62-year-old mother and his younger sister (34 years old) had normal pubertal development and regular menstrual cycles. The 64-year-old father of the propositus was normally virilized, and his serum gonadotropin and testosterone concentrations were normal. There was no indication of parental consanguinity.

Source: Abbreviated from Ref. 60.

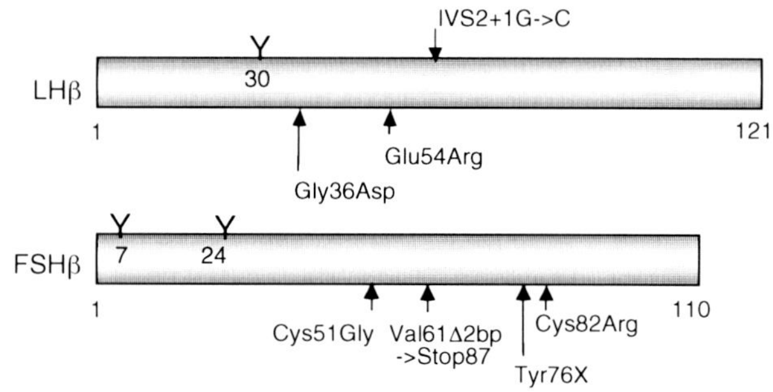

Figure 8 The currently known inactivating mutations in the LHβ abd *FSHβ* genes. The numbers indicate order in amino acids in the subunit proteins. Y indicates the position of carbohydrate side chain. IVS2 + 1G->C indicates the approximate location of a point mutation in position +1 of intron 2, which destroys a 5' splice-donor site (60). No inactivating mutations have been detected in the *common-α* and *hCGβ* genes. For further details, please refer to the text.

Mutations of Gonadotropin Subunit Genes

There is apparently effective selection against mutations in gonadotropin subunits because they directly impair reproduction and are thus likely to be quickly eliminated from the genetic pool. Hence, quite understandably, these mutations are extremely rare. However, a few homozygous cases of such mutations have been described (Fig. 8) (61).

The Cα subunit is shared by all gonadotropins and TSH, and thus inactivating mutations of this gene would have widespread consequences in the form of hypogonadism, hypothyroidism, and male pseudohermaphroditism. Moreover, pregnancy would probably be impossible in the absence of hCG and apparently for this reason no germ-line mutations of *Cα* have been detected.

Three men with inactivating *LHβ* mutation have been described (62–64). They are normally masculinized at birth but totally lack sexual maturation at puberty (see Text Box 2 for a case report). The reason for their normal intrauterine masculinization is that placental hCG is able to stimulate fetal testicular T production in the absence of pituitary LH, but when hCG is eliminated after birth, no trophic stimulus is available for postnatal Leydig cells. In contrast, when there is an inactivating mutation in *LHR*, also the fetal testis lacks the LH/hCG stimulus, which prevents the normal intrauterine masculinization driven by fetal testicular T.

Text Box 2 **A Typical Case of Inactivating LHβ Mutation**

The patient presented at the age of 17 years because of delayed puberty. He was normally masculinized at birth. He was treated for two years with testosterone, but there was no evidence for onset of spontaneous puberty after withdrawal of the treatment. His serum immunoreactive LH was found twice to be normal (but it was subsequently found to be biologically inactive), and his serum FSH was normal. In contrast, his serum testosterone was low. His karyotype was 46,XY. A testicular biopsy revealed an arrest of spermatogenesis, and no mature Leydig cells could be identified. Long-term treatment with hCG resulted in testicular enlargement, normal virilization, and a sperm count of 11 million/mL, with 50% motility. He subsequently was unable to father children despite treatments with hCG and testosterone. There was a history of consanguinity from both maternal and paternal side, and three of maternal uncles had a history of infertility, without apparent delay of puberty or hypogonadism.

Source: Modified from Ref. 63.

Three men with *FSHβ* mutations have been described in the literature (65–67). They all were normally masculinized but azoospermic. Two of them were detected upon screening of azoospermic men, the third was a brother of a woman with *FSHβ* mutation. This phenotype differs from that described in connection with an inactivating *FSHR* mutation (68), where variable spermatogenesis was detected in all subjects (please refer to the following section). Neither are knockout mice for *FSHβ* or *FSHR* azoospermic; their testis size is somewhat reduced but they have roughly normal fertility (69–71). As discussed in more detail elsewhere (1), two of the three men with *FSHβ* mutation may have another pathology contributing to their azoospermia. Additional cases must be identified before the male phenotype of totally missing FSH action can be conclusively defined.

Mutations of Gonadotropin Receptor Genes

LHR

Activating *LHR* mutation was the first one detected in the genes of gonadotropins and their receptors, apparently because of its striking phenotype (1,72,73). These patients present with early-onset familial male-limited precocious puberty, also termed 'testotoxicosis' (see Text Box 3 for a case report). Affected boys develop signs of puberty as early as at two to three years of age; conspicuously, girls with the same mutations have no phenotype. The mutations are located in the transmembrane region of the *LHR* or in its vicinity, with a hot spot in transmembrane region 6 (Fig. 3). The mutated receptors show clear constitutive activity in the absence of hormone, which explains why Leydig cell T production is activated in affected boys well before the normal pubertal onset of LH secretion. The early puberty causes short stature in adult age, but apart from the apparent psychological symptoms of the early puberty, the affected men are normal. Normal fertility of the affected men explains why this mutation is the commonest of those affecting gonadotropin action. The other reason is that also heterozygotes have the phenotype of these gain-of-function mutations.

Text Box 3 **A Typical Case of Activating LHR *Mutation***

The patient showed early signs of precocious puberty. He started to grow rapidly and showed signs of puberty at the age of 3 years. When he was first seen by a physician at the age of 4.5 years, he was 128 cm tall (+5.8 SD for chronological age) and had a muscular build, deep voice, and facial acne. He was classified as Tanner stage G3 (increased testicular size and penile enlargement) and PH2 (pubic hair). His bone age was 10.5 years. His basal level of serum testosterone was midpubertal (6.0 nmol/L), whereas serum LH and FSH levels remained prepubertal, that is, were undetectable (<0.5 IU/L). Gonadotropin levels did not respond to GnRH challenge. Testicular biopsy revealed active spermatogenesis and aggregates of steroidogenically active Leydig cells.

Source: Modified from Refs. 74 and 75.

With respect to loss-of-function mutations, both alleles must be inactivated to provide a phenotype, which is possible through homozygous or compound heterozygous mutations. After unraveling of the structure of *LHR*, the first inactivating mutation of this gene was soon discovered—an A593P missense mutation near the extracellular side of the plasma membrane (Fig. 3) (76). It was found in a 46,XY pseudohermaphrodite adult subject, born from consanguineous parents, who presented with female external genitalia, primary amenorrhoea, and lack of breast development at the age of puberty. As expected, the parents were nonsymptomatic heterozygous carriers for the same mutation. Cryptorchid testicular tissue of the subject showed hyalinized seminiferous tubules with total lack of spermatogenesis and immature-type Leydig cells in the interstitial space. When expressed in vitro, the mutated receptor displayed low level of ligand binding and total lack of cAMP production in response to hCG.

Currently, more than 20 loss-of-function mutations of *LHR* have been identified, ranging from partial to complete inactivation of the receptor function (Fig. 3). In the complete form all LHR activity is lost, and in partial mutations some receptor activation remains. The hallmark of the complete form is Leydig cell hypoplasia and male pseudohermaphroditism with complete lack of secondary sex characteristics with absent breast development. The latter symptom differentiates this condition from complete androgen insensitivity syndrome (CAIS; testicular feminization) due to inactivating mutation of the *androgen receptor*, where female breast development occurs because of peripheral aromatization of T produced by the testes. Individuals with complete LHR inactivation have female external genitals, low T and high LH levels, normal FSH levels, a total lack of response to LH/hCG stimulation, and no development of secondary male or female sex characteristics at puberty. In incomplete forms of *LHR* inactivation (1,77), some testicular androgen production remains, and consequently, some masculinization is induced, ranging from cryptorchidism and micropenis (78) to severe perineoscrotal hypospadias (79). In these cases, the differential diagnosis must be made between partial androgen insensitivity syndrome (PAIS) caused by incomplete androgen receptor inactivation.

FSHR

The only apparently activating mutation of *FSHR* has been detected in a male who was previously hypophysectomized due to a pituitary tumor, but still maintained normal spermatogenesis in spite of undetectable gonadotropins (80). Surprisingly, no other activating *FSHR* mutations have been detected since the first case over 10 years ago. Attempts to find such mutations in candidate diseases, including premature ovarian failure, ovarian tumors, megalotestes, precocious puberty, and twin pregnancies have been unsuccessful (81–86). It remains, therefore, a possibility that activating *FSHR* mutations in otherwise normal individuals have no phenotype or that it totally differs from our educated guesses. Another explanation is that the phenotype appears only in extreme situations, such as after hypophysectomy (80).

Only few loss-of-function mutations of the *FSHR* have been described so far (Fig. 4), probably because their phenotypes are less clear and/or clinically less striking. Because of the known role of FSH in spermatogenesis, inactivating *FSHR* mutations could be expected in connection with high serum FSH, small testicles, and impaired spermatogenesis in normally androgenized males. In line with this hypothesis, *FSHR* mutations have been searched in men with candidate phenotypes including absent, low, or aberrant sperm production with high FSH levels (87) and in idiopathic infertility (88). However, all searches based on candidate phenotypes have been unsuccessful in detecting *FSHR* mutations.

The only loss-of-function mutations of *FSHR* in men have been found in brothers of women, harboring the Finnish-type *FSHR* mutation, that is, A189V in exon 7 (68). All five men identified to be homozygous were normally masculinized, indicating normal Leydig cell function. Their T levels were normal, LH normal or slightly elevated, FSH moderately elevated, inhibin-B low, and their testis volumes were slightly to severely reduced. A semen sample was obtained from each man, and the sperm counts ranged from normal to severe oligozoospermia, with low volume and teratozoospermia in one man, but notably, none of the men was azoospermic. Two of the men had two children each. It was concluded that FSH contributes to the quality and quantity of spermatogenesis but is not mandatory for this process per se. The normal androgen production alone in the mutant men is evidently sufficient to maintain their spermatogenesis and fertility, although at a reduced level. Unlike previously suggested, normal FSH action is not compulsory for the pubertal onset of spermatogenesis. These findings also indicate that attempts to reduce spermatogenesis for contraceptive purposes by inhibiting FSH secretion or action do not offer a viable alternative.

NONGENETIC DISTURBANCES IN GONADOTROPIN SECRETION OR ACTION

Also many acquired disturbances of the hypothalamic–pituitary function can cause gonadotropin deficiency with subsequent hypogonadism and/or infertility. Such conditions include pituitary infarctions, primary or metastatic tumors, granulomatous processes, and radiation injury, which usually cause panhypopituitarism and secondary testicular failure. Isolated functional impairment of hypothalamic GnRH secretion (analogous to hypothalamic amenorrhoea in women) can occur in connection with fasting or critical illness (89,90).

Secondary gonadotropin deficiency through inhibition of GnRH secretion can be caused by cortisol in Cushing syndrome (91) and by prolactin in hyperprolactinemia (92). Hemochromatosis can cause iron deposits in the pituitary gland and testes with subsequent HH (91). Finally, HH can also be idiopathic, with altered GnRH pulse frequency for unknown reasons (as reviewed in Ref. 93).

Considerable attention has recently been received by the hypogonadism occurring in aging men (41,94). The frequency of serum T levels in the low normal/mildly suppressed range increases with age, and it can be associated with increased, normal, or suppressed LH levels. The former situation, that is, normal or somewhat suppressed T and increased LH level, indicating primary hypogonadism, is a typical finding specifically associated with aging. Secondary hypogonadism, with suppressed T, but low gonadotropins because of lack of the hypothalamic–pituitary compensation, also appears during aging but is not caused by the increased age per se. In particular, obesity decreases both T and gonadotropin levels, but a similar response is observed in association with comorbidities (e.g., atherosclerosis, diabetes mellitus, metabolic syndrome). Often, however, the status of the pituitary–testicular function of aging men represents combined effects of aging and comorbidities.

Finally, certain medications can affect gonadotropin secretion and induce various symptoms of hypogonadism and/or sub/infertility. Most typically, androgen treatment suppresses gonadotropin secretion due to enhanced negative feedback regulation. Hence, although androgen can restore and increase peripheral androgen action, the simultaneous suppression of gonadotropins causes androgen deficiency within the testis tissue, with consequent impairment of spermatogenesis. Therefore, androgen therapy is not suitable for the treatment of hypogonadism, if restoring of fertility is desired. This principle is even being tested for male contraception (95). For the same reason, decreased testis size and oligo/azoospermia are common findings amongst abusers of androgenic/anabolic steroids. Finally, the hyperprolactinemia associated with neuroleptic drugs may disturb gonadotropin secretion, which is a poorly recognized side effect of psychiatric treatments (96).

REFERENCES

1. Themmen APN, Huhtaniemi IT. Mutations of gonadotropins and gonadotropin receptors: Elucidating the physiology and pathophysiology of pituitary-gonadal function. Endocr Rev 2000; 21(5):551–583.
2. Stanton PG, Burgon PG, Hearn MT, et al. Structural and functional characterisation of hFSH and hLH isoforms. Mol Cell Endocrinol 1996; 125(1–2):133–141.
3. Bousfield G, Perry W, Ward D. Gonadotropins. Chemistry and biosynthesis. In: Knobil E, Neill JD, eds. The Physiology of Reproduction, 2nd ed. New York: Raven Press, 1994:1749–1792.
4. Bo M, Boime I. Identification of the transcriptionally active genes of the chorionic gonadotropin beta gene cluster in vivo. J Biol Chem 1992; 267(5):3179–3184.
5. Stenman UH, Alfthan H, Hotakainen K. Human chorionic gonadotropin in cancer. Clin Biochem 2004; 37(7):549–561.
6. Klein J, Lobel L, Pollak S, et al. Pharmacokinetics and pharmacodynamics of single-chain recombinant human follicle-stimulating hormone containing the human chorionic gonadotropin carboxyterminal peptide in the rhesus monkey. Fertil Steril 2002; 77(6):1248–1255.
7. Fox KM, Dias JA, Van Roey P. Three-dimensional structure of human follicle-stimulating hormone. Mol Endocrinol 2001; 15(3):378–389.
8. Lapthorn AJ, Harris DC, Littlejohn A, et al. Crystal structure of human chorionic gonadotropin. Nature 1994; 369(6480):455–461.
9. Fan QR, Hendrickson WA. Structure of human follicle-stimulating hormone in complex with its receptor. Nature 2005; 433(7023):269–277.
10. Gromoll J, Eiholzer U, Nieschlag E, et al. Male hypogonadism caused by homozygous deletion of exon 10 of the luteinizing hormone (LH) receptor: Differential action of human chorionic gonadotropin and LH. J Clin Endocrinol Metab 2000; 85(6):2281–2286.
11. Song T, Nikolics K, Seeburg PH, et al. GnRH-prohormone-containing neurons in the primate brain: Immunostaining for the GnRH-associated peptide. Peptides 1987; 8(2):335–346.
12. Urbanski HF, Kohama SG, Garyfallou VT. Mechanisms mediating the response of GnRH neurones to excitatory amino acids. Rev Reprod 1996; 1(3):173–181.
13. Popa SM, Clifton DK, Steiner RA. The role of kisspeptins and GPR54 in the neuroendocrine regulation of reproduction. Annu Rev Physiol 2008; 8:213–238.
14. Childs GV. Division of labor among gonadotropes. Vitam Horm 1995; 50:215–286.
15. Millar RP, Lu ZL, Pawson AJ, et al. Gonadotropin-releasing hormone receptors. Endocr Rev 2004; 25(2):235–275.

16. Brown P, McNeilly AS. Transcriptional regulation of pituitary gonadotrophin subunit genes. Rev Reprod 1999; 4(2):117–124.
17. Lemay A, Lourdusamy M. Gonadotrophin releasing hormone agonist suppressive treatment of ovarian function decreases serum LH-beta and bioactive LH but maintains elevated levels of LH-alpha. Clin Endocrinol (Oxf) 1991; 34(3):191–196.
18. Finkelstein JS, Whitcomb RW, O'Dea LS, et al. Sex steroid control of gonadotropin secretion in the human male. I. Effects of testosterone administration in normal and gonadotropin-releasing hormone-deficient men. J Clin Endocrinol Metab 1991; 73(3):609–620.
19. Tilbrook AJ, Clarke IJ. Negative feedback regulation of the secretion and actions of gonadotropin-releasing hormone in males. Biol Reprod 2001; 64(3):735–742.
20. Hayes FJ, Seminara SB, Decruz S, et al. Aromatase inhibition in the human male reveals a hypothalamic site of estrogen feedback. J Clinical Endocrinol Metab 2000; 85(9):3027–3035.
21. Burger HG, Robertson DM. Editorial: Inhibin in the male–progress at last. Endocrinology 1997; 138(4):1361–1362.
22. Wallace EM, Groome NP, Riley SC, et al. Effects of chemotherapy-induced testicular damage on inhibin, gonadotropin, and testosterone secretion: A prospective longitudinal study. J Clin Endocrinol Metab 1997; 82(9):3111–3115.
23. Bilezikjian LM, Blount AL, Donaldson CJ, et al. Pituitary actions of ligands of the TGF-beta family: Activins and inhibins. Reproduction 2006; 132(2):207–215.
24. Pangas SA, Woodruff TK. Activin signal transduction pathways. Trends Endocrinol Metab 2000; 11(8):309–314.
25. Dias JA, Van Roey P. Structural biology of human follitropin and its receptor. Arch Med Res 2001; 32(6):510–519.
26. Simoni M, Gromoll J, Nieschlag E. The follicle-stimulating hormone receptor: Biochemistry, molecular biology, physiology, and pathophysiology. Endocr Rev 1997; 18(6):739–773.
27. Ascoli M, Fanelli F, Segaloff DL. The lutropin/choriogonadotropin receptor, a 2002 perspective. Endocr Rev 2002; 23(2):141–174.
28. Ascoli M. Potential Leydig cell mitogenic signals generated by the wild-type and constitutively active mutants of the lutropin/choriogonadotropin receptor (LHR). Mol Cell Endocrinol 2007; 260–262:244–248.
29. Burger LL, Haisenleder DJ, Aylor KW, et al. Regulation of luteinizing hormone-beta and follicle-stimulating hormone (FSH)-beta gene transcription by androgens: Testosterone directly stimulates FSH-beta transcription independent from its role on follistatin gene expression. Endocrinology 2004; 145(1):71–78.
30. Walker WH, Cheng J. FSH and testosterone signaling in Sertoli cells. Reproduction 2005; 130(1):15–28.
31. Asa SL, Kovacs K, Singer W. Human fetal adenohypophysis: Morphologic and functional analysis in vitro. Neuroendocrinology 1991; 53(6):562–572.
32. Kaplan SL, Grumbach MM, Aubert ML. The ontogenesis of pituitary hormones and hypothalamic factors in the human fetus: Maturation of central nervous system regulation of anterior pituitary function. Recent Prog Horm Res 1976; 32:161–243.
33. Huhtaniemi IT, Korenbrot CC, Jaffe RB. hCG binding and stimulation of testosterone biosynthesis in the human fetal testis. J Clin Endocrinol Metab 1977; 44(5):963–967.
34. Huhtaniemi IT, Yamamoto M, Ranta T, et al. Follicle-stimulating hormone receptors appear earlier in the primate fetal testis than in the ovary. J Clin Endocrinol Metab 1987; 65(6):1210–1214.
35. O'Shaughnessy PJ, Baker PJ, Monteiro A, et al. Developmental changes in human fetal testicular cell numbers and mRNA levels during the second trimester. J Clin Endocrinol Metab 2007; 92(12):4792–4801.
36. Orth JM. The role of follicle-stimulating hormone in controlling Sertoli cell proliferation in testes of fetal rats. Endocrinology 1984; 115(4):1248–1255.
37. Forest MG, De Peretti E, Bertrand J. Hypothalamic-pituitary-gonadal relationships in man from birth to puberty. Clin Endocrinol (Oxf) 1976; 5(5):551–569.
38. Wu FC, Butler GE, Kelnar CJ, et al. Patterns of pulsatile luteinizing hormone and follicle-stimulating hormone secretion in prepubertal (midchildhood) boys and girls and patients with idiopathic hypogonadotropic hypogonadism (Kallmann's syndrome): A study using an ultrasensitive time-resolved immunofluorometric assay. J Clin Endocrinol Metab 1991; 72(6):1229–1237.
39. Raivio T, Toppari J, Perheentupa A, et al. Treatment of prepubertal gonadotrophin-deficient boys with recombinant human follicle-stimulating hormone. Lancet 1997; 350(9073):263–264.
40. Plant TM, Marshall GR. The functional significance of FSH in spermatogenesis and the control of its secretion in male primates. Endocr Rev 2001; 22(6):764–786.
41. Wu F, Tajar A, Pye S, et al. Hypothalamic-pituitary-testicular axis disruptions in older men are differentially linked to age and modifiable risk factors—Baseline results from the European Male Aging Study (EMAS). J Clin Endocrinol Metab 2008; 93(7):1374–1385.
42. Seminara SB. Mechanisms of disease: The first kiss—A crucial role for kisspeptin-1 and its receptor, G-protein-coupled receptor 54, in puberty and reproduction. Nat Clin Pract Endocrinol Metab 2006; 2(6):328–334.
43. de Roux N. GnRH receptor and GPR54 inactivation in isolated gonadotropic deficiency. Best Pract Res Clin Endocrinol Metab 2006; 20(4):515–528.
44. Farooqi IS, Wangensteen T, Collins S, et al. Clinical and molecular genetic spectrum of congenital deficiency of the leptin receptor. N Engl J Med 2007; 356(3):237–247.

45. O'Rahilly S, Farooqi IS. Genetics of obesity. Philos Trans R Soc Lond B Biol Sci 2006; 361(1471):1095–1105.
46. Gamba M, Pralong FP. Control of GnRH neuronal activity by metabolic factors: The role of leptin and insulin. Mol Cell Endocrinol 2006; 254–255:133–139.
47. Cadman SM, Kim SH, Hu Y, et al. Molecular pathogenesis of Kallmann's syndrome. Horm Res 2007; 67(5):231–242.
48. Schwanzel-Fukuda M, Pfaff DW. Origin of luteinizing hormone-releasing hormone neurons. Nature 1989; 338(6211):161–164.
49. Wray S, Grant P, Gainer H. Evidence that cells expressing luteinizing hormone-releasing hormone mRNA in the mouse are derived from progenitor cells in the olfactory placode. Proc Natl Acad Sci U S A 1989; 86(20):8132–136.
50. Oliveira LM, Seminara SB, Beranova M, et al. The importance of autosomal genes in Kallmann syndrome: Genotype-phenotype correlations and neuroendocrine characteristics. J Clin Endocrinol Metab 2001; 86(4):1532–1538.
51. Pinto G, Abadie V, Mesnage R, et al. CHARGE syndrome includes hypogonadotropic hypogonadism and abnormal olfactory bulb development. J Clin Endocrinol Metab 2005; 90(10):5621–5626.
52. Miura K, Acierno JS Jr, Seminara SB. Characterization of the human nasal embryonic LHRH factor gene, NELF, and a mutation screening among 65 patients with idiopathic hypogonadotropic hypogonadism (IHH). J Hum Genet 2004; 49(5):265–268.
53. Pitteloud N, Quinton R, Pearce S, et al. Digenic mutations account for variable phenotypes in idiopathic hypogonadotropic hypogonadism. J Clin Invest 2007; 117(2): 457–63.
54. Dode C, Teixeira L, Levilliers J, et al. Kallmann syndrome: Mutations in the genes encoding prokineticin-2 and prokineticin receptor-2. PLoS Genet 2006; 2(10):e175.
55. Raivio T, Cole LW, Hayes FJ, et al. FGF8 is a key ligand for FGFR1 in GnRH ontogeny: Evidence for a human disease model. Endocrine Society, Annual Meeting; 2007:P4–354.
56. Topaloglu AK, Reimann F, Guclu M, et al. TAC3 and TAC3R mutations in familial hypogonadotropic hypogonadism reveal a key role for Neurokinin B in the central control of reproduction. Nat Genet 2009; 41(3):354–358.
57. Bouligand J, Ghervan C, Tello JA, et al. Isolated familial hypogonadoropic hypogonadism and GNRH1 mutation. N Engl J Med 2009; 360(26):2742–2748.
58. Chan YM, de Guillebon A, Lang-Muritano M, et al. GNRH1 mutations in patients with idiopathic hypogonadotropic hypogonadism and GnRH1 mutation. Proc Natl Acad Sci USA 2009; 106(28):11703–11708.
59. Bedecarrats GY, Kaiser UB. Mutations in the human gonadotropin-releasing hormone receptor: Insights into receptor biology and function. Semin Reprod Med 2007; 25(5):368–378.
60. de Roux N, Young J, Misrahi M, et al. A family with hypogonadotropic hypogonadism and mutations in the gonadotropin-releasing hormone receptor. N Engl J Med 1997; 337(22):1597–1602.
61. Lofrano-Porto A, Barra GB, Giacomini LA, et al. Luteinizing hormone beta mutation and hypogonadism in men and women. N Engl J Med 2007; 357(9):897–904.
62. Daly AF, Salvi R, Menage J-J, et al. Identification of a family harboring a novel LHbeta subunit mutation associated with hypogonadism. The Endocrine Society, 88th Annual Meeting; 2006: OR52–5.
63. Valdes-Socin H, Salvi R, Daly AF, et al. Hypogonadism in a patient with a mutation in the luteinizing hormone beta-subunit gene. N Engl J Med 2004; 351(25):2619–2625.
64. Weiss J, Axelrod L, Whitcomb RW, et al. Hypogonadism caused by a single amino acid substitution in the beta subunit of luteinizing hormone. N Engl J Med 1992; 326(3):179–183.
65. Layman LC, Porto AL, Xie J, et al. FSH beta gene mutations in a female with partial breast development and a male sibling with normal puberty and azoospermia. J Clin Endocrinol Metab 2002; 87(8):3702–3707.
66. Lindstedt G, Nystrom E, Matthews C, et al. Follitropin (FSH) deficiency in an infertile male due to FSHbeta gene mutation. A syndrome of normal puberty and virilization but underdeveloped testicles with azoospermia, low FSH but high lutropin and normal serum testosterone concentrations. Clin Chem Lab Med 1998; 36(8):663–665.
67. Phillip M, Arbelle JE, Segev Y, et al. Male hypogonadism due to a mutation in the gene for the beta-subunit of follicle-stimulating hormone. N Engl J Med 1998; 338(24):1729–1732.
68. Tapanainen JS, Aittomaki K, Min J, et al. Men homozygous for an inactivating mutation of the follicle-stimulating hormone (FSH) receptor gene present variable suppression of spermatogenesis and fertility. Nat Genet 1997; 15(2):205–206.
69. Dierich A, Sairam MR, Monaco L, et al. Impairing follicle-stimulating hormone (FSH) signaling in vivo: Targeted disruption of the FSH receptor leads to aberrant gametogenesis and hormonal imbalance. Proc Natl Acad Sci U S A 1998; 95(23):13612–13617.
70. Abel MH, Wootton AN, Wilkins V, et al. The effect of a null mutation in the follicle-stimulating hormone receptor gene on mouse reproduction. Endocrinology 2000; 141(5):1795–1803.
71. Kumar TR, Wang Y, Lu N, et al. Follicle stimulating hormone is required for ovarian follicle maturation but not male fertility. Nat Genet 1997; 15(2):201–204.
72. Kremer H, Mariman E, Otten BJ, et al. Cosegregation of missense mutations of the luteinizing hormone receptor gene with familial male-limited precocious puberty. Hum Mol Genet 1993; 2(11):1779–1783.

73. Shenker A, Laue L, Kosugi S, et al. A constitutively activating mutation of the luteinizing hormone receptor in familial male precocious puberty. Nature 1993; 365(6447):652–654.
74. Yano K, Hidaka A, Saji M, et al. A sporadic case of male-limited precocious puberty has the same constitutively activating point mutation in luteinizing hormone/choriogonadotropin receptor gene as familial cases. J Clin Endocrinol Metab 1994; 79(6):1818–1823.
75. Yano K, Saji M, Hidaka A, et al. A new constitutively activating point mutation in the luteinizing hormone/choriogonadotropin receptor gene in cases of male-limited precocious puberty. J Clin Endocrinol Metab 1995; 80(4):1162–1168.
76. Kremer H, Kraaij R, Toledo SP, et al. Male pseudohermaphroditism due to a homozygous missense mutation of the luteinizing hormone receptor gene. Nat Genet 1995; 9(2):160–164.
77. Huhtaniemi IT, Themmen AP. Mutations in human gonadotropin and gonadotropin-receptor genes. Endocrine 2005; 26(3):207–217.
78. Toledo SP, Arnhold IJ, Luthold W, et al. Leydig cell hypoplasia determining familial hypergonadotropic hypogonadism. Prog Clin Biol Res 1985; 200:311–314.
79. Latronico AC, Anasti J, Arnhold IJ, et al. Brief report: Testicular and ovarian resistance to luteinizing hormone caused by inactivating mutations of the luteinizing hormone-receptor gene. N Engl J Med 1996; 334(8):507–512.
80. Gromoll J, Simoni M, Nieschlag E. An activating mutation of the follicle-stimulating hormone receptor autonomously sustains spermatogenesis in a hypophysectomized man. J Clin Endocrinol Metab 1996; 81(4):1367–1370.
81. Sundblad V, Chiauzzi VA, Escobar ME, et al. Screening of FSH receptor gene in Argentine women with premature ovarian failure (POF). Mol Cell Endocrinol 2004; 222 (1–2):53–59.
82. Giacaglia LR, Kohek MB da F, Carvalho FM, et al. No evidence of somatic activating mutations on gonadotropin receptor genes in sex cord stromal tumors. Fertil Steril 2000; 74(5):992–995.
83. de la Chesnaye E, Canto P, Ulloa-Aguirre A, et al. No evidence of mutations in the follicle-stimulating hormone receptor gene in Mexican women with 46,XX pure gonadal dysgenesis. Am J Med Genet 2001; 98(2):125–128.
84. Montgomery GW, Duffy DL, Hall J, et al. Dizygotic twinning is not linked to variation at the alpha-inhibin locus on human chromosome 2. J Clin Endocrinol Metab 2000; 85(9):3391–3395.
85. Tong Y, Liao WX, Roy AC, et al. Absence of mutations in the coding regions of follicle-stimulating hormone receptor gene in Singapore Chinese women with premature ovarian failure and polycystic ovary syndrome. Horm Metab Res 2001; 33(4):221–226.
86. Takakura K, Takebayashi K, Wang HQ, et al. Follicle-stimulating hormone receptor gene mutations are rare in Japanese women with premature ovarian failure and polycystic ovary syndrome. Fertil Steril 2001; 75(1):207–209.
87. Tuerlings JH, Ligtenberg MJ, Kremer JA, et al. Screening male intracytoplasmic sperm injection candidates for mutations of the follicle stimulating hormone receptor gene. Hum Reprod 1998; 13(8):2098–2101.
88. Simoni M, Gromoll J, Hoppner W, et al. Mutational analysis of the follicle-stimulating hormone (FSH) receptor in normal and infertile men: Identification and characterization of two discrete FSH receptor isoforms. J Clin Endocrinol Metab 1999; 84(2):751–755.
89. Aloi JA, Bergendahl M, Iranmanesh A, et al. Pulsatile intravenous gonadotropin-releasing hormone administration averts fasting-induced hypogonadotropism and hypoandrogenemia in healthy, normal weight men. J Clinical Endocrinol Metab 1997; 82(5):1543–1548.
90. Takahashi J, Higashi Y, LaNasa JA, et al. Studies of the human testis. XVIII. Simultaneous measurement of nine intratesticular steroids: Evidence for reduced mitochondrial function in testis of elderly men. J Clin Endocrinol Metab 1983; 56(6):1178–1187.
91. Baker HW. Reproductive effects of nontesticular illness. Endocrinol Metab Clin North Am 1998; 27(4):831–850.
92. Davis JL. Lowering prolactin level in a hyperprolactinemic man: Responses of luteinizing hormone, follicle-stimulating hormone, and testosterone. Arch Intern Med 1982; 142(1):146–148.
93. Griffin J, Wilson J. Disorders of the testis and the male reproductive tract. In: Williams' Textbook of Endocrinology, 2006: 709–769.
94. Kaufman JM, Vermeulen A. The decline of androgen levels in elderly men and its clinical and therapeutic implications. Endocr Rev 2005; 26(6):833–876.
95. Anderson RA, Baird DT. Male contraception. Endocr Rev 2002; 23(6):735–762.
96. Haddad PM, Wieck A. Antipsychotic-induced hyperprolactinaemia: Mechanisms, clinical features and management. Drugs 2004; 64(20):2291–2314.

24 Androgen effects in reproductive and nonreproductive organs

Michael Zitzmann

INTRODUCTION

In men, testosterone (T) is essential for the development and maintenance of various specific tissues with reproductive and nonreproductive tasks. In general, T exerts a widespread pattern of effects on metabolism, psyche, and body composition. This is most obviously seen in the difference between men and women. T-deficiency is associated with a magnitude of pathophysiological symptoms, clinically known as hypogonadism. Physicians define this condition by adverse traits in physical appearance, disturbed mental and cognitive traits, shifts in body composition, namely increased body fat content and reduced muscle mass. Physical abilities in androgen-deficient men are further attenuated by lower oxygen supply due to decreased hemoglobin concentrations and by poor glucose utilization. Also bone tissue is subject to strong regulation by T and its aromatization product, estradiol.

PHYSIOGENOMIC BACKGROUND

T and its metabolite dihydro-T exert their effects on gene expression and thus affect maleness via the androgen receptor (AR). A wide range of clinical conditions starting with complete androgen insensitivity are related to mutations in the AR. Subtle modulations of the transcriptional activity induced by the AR have also been described and can be assigned to a polyglutamine stretch of variable length within the N-terminal domain of the receptor. This stretch is encoded by CAG-triplets in exon 1 of the AR gene, which is located on the X-chromosome. Longer triplet residues mitigate binding of androgen receptor coactivators and, hence, facilitate decreased androgenicity. A marked relation to androgenic traits can not only be seen in men with an elongation of more than 37 CAG repeats, but also in those with CAG repeats within the normal range (1,2).

REPRODUCTIVE TISSUES

Introduction

T is able and necessary to qualitatively initiate, maintain and reinitiate spermatogenesis and formation of spermatozoa. T acts synergistically to follicle stimulating hormone (FSH), which is also a prerequisite for spermatogenesis. Under physiological circumstances, only the combination of T and FSH yields quantitatively and qualitatively normal spermatozoa. T acts indirectly via somatic testicular cells on spermatogenesis. These are most likely Sertoli cells. The testicular effects of T are thus paracrine. These effects are partly mediated by its metabolization products, estradiol and dihydrotestosterone. T and FSH cooperate during regulation of spermatogenesis but act via different pathways (3).

Basic Features of Intratesticular Testosterone

T production and spermatogenesis are the two primary functions of the testis in man. Normal testicular function is dependent on the intratesticular activity of the pituitary gonadotropins, luteinizing hormone (LH) and FSH. LH stimulates Leydig cells to produce T within the testis. Intratesticular T (ITT) is an absolute prerequisite for normal spermatogenesis. FSH is also vital for normal testicular function and is necessary for quantitatively normal spermatogenesis in man. Specifically, FSH is thought to play an important role early in spermatogenesis during spermatogonial maturation as well as late in the process during spermiation. The relative roles of intratesticular androgens and FSH are not fully understood in man (3).

Control of the intratesticular hormonal environment is in a large part regulated through negative feedback of T at the level of the hypothalamus and the pituitary. Exogenous T has been shown to dramatically suppress gonadotropin release when administered as supraphysiological as well as physiological doses. Administration of T alone has been shown to reduce sperm production in the majority of men. Gonadotropin withdrawal has also been shown to dramatically reduce ITT, which, in turn, decreases sperm production. However, suppression of spermatogenesis is not uniform, and why some men are nonresponders is not clear. Possibilities include incomplete gonadotropin suppression, particularly with regard to FSH as well as inconsistencies in ITT suppression (4).

The Clinical-Human Model of Hypogonadotropic Hypogonadism for Understanding the Effects of Androgens on Testicular Development and Architecture

In male hypogonadotropic hypogonadism, T therapy is sufficient for maturation and maintenance of secondary sex characteristics. For stimulation of spermatogenesis, administration of gonadotropins is necessary. If pulsatile gonadotropin-releasing hormone (GnRH) is not indicated or desired, human chorionic gonadotropin (hCG) is used as the source of (LH) activity to stimulate T secretion by Leydig cells, whereas human menopausal gonadotropin (hMG) is used as the source of FSH. More recently, recombinant gonadotropins have also been used clinically. Several animal studies have investigated the relative contributions of both gonadotropins for induction and maintenance of spermatogenesis. Therefore FSH and LH/T in combination are required to maintain spermatogenesis to full extent (5,6).

Thus, idiopathic hypogonadotropic hypogonadism (IHH) is an important disease model in the human male. Men suffering from this disorder classically display a number of clinical symptoms including absent pubertal development, lack of secondary sexual characteristics, and infertility. Microadenomas with functional significance (producing hormone or leading to hypopituitarism) exclude the diagnosis of IHH. However, radiologic anomalies of the pituitary gland without functional significance is occasionally seen in IHH as well as in a small proportion of normal healthy adults, which is confirmed by a nearly uniform response to physiological regimens of exogenous GnRH-replacement therapy (6).

A small subset of patients with this disorder presents with a partial form of GnRH deficiency as assessed by some degree of testicular growth despite hypogonadal T levels. In contrast to most other causes of male infertility, IHH is typically curable in many patients. Indeed, long-term GnRH therapy or gonadotropins successfully induce spermatogenesis in the majority of these patients. However, 20% to 30% of IHH with the most severe form of GnRH deficiency remain azoospermic. This latter observation has attracted the attention of many clinicians and researchers to focus their attention on the management of IHH and the role of T (6).

Many of the IHH patients have a testis that resembles the prepubertal testis. Precocious puberty can be induced in immature monkeys following various hormonal regimens, and in these experiments it was demonstrated that there was an increased proliferation of Sertoli cells accompanied by germ cell proliferation, a process regulated by both FSH and LH, thus T (for review see 7).

Testicular Histology in Relation to Testosterone Action

While testicular biopsy was accepted as a diagnostic tool for the assessment of infertility in the 1970s, the evolution of assisted reproduction techniques (i.e., IVF and ICSI), has popularized the usage of testicular biopsies during the course of treatment of infertile men. Additionally, testicular biopsies have been used in previous studies to rule out äSertoli cell-only syndrome prior to starting therapy in IHH men as well as to monitor the efficacy in inducing spermatogenesis. These histological studies revealed that most IHH men had prepubertal testes. However, these studies included few subjects and focused mostly on seminiferous tubule diameter, basement membrane thickness, and the ratio of germ cells to Sertoli cells.

While a great deal is known about the histology of the normal adult testes, less is known about prepubertal testes, and there is an even greater paucity of information regarding the histology of IHH testes. The normal adult human testis is composed of seminiferous tubules resting on a tunica propria containing a number of myoid cell layers separated from the seminiferous epithelium by a zone of connective tissue and a basement membrane. The seminiferous epithelium contains the nonproliferating fully mature Sertoli cells and the proliferating and differentiating generations of germ cells, from spermatogonia to fully mature spermatozoa (8). The interstitium has clusters of Leydig cells in the angular intervals between the seminiferous tubules. In the prepubertal testis, only immature Sertoli cells and type A spermatogonia are present. The prevailing view is that among the type A spermatogonia resides a stem cell population and that these stem cells must be stimulated directly or indirectly via Sertoli cells, in order for spermatogenesis to be initiated. Normal spermatogenic activity in healthy men is due to the interaction of Sertoli cell-produced growth factors and germ cells with the support of T produced by the Leydig cells (9).

Sertoli Cells and Androgens

The role of androgens in the proliferation and maturation of Sertoli cells (SC) and the development of their capacity to support spermatogenesis is not fully understood. Such functions can be compared in complete androgen receptor knockout (ARKO) and SC-selective androgen receptor knockout (SCARKO) mice. Compared with controls, ARKO mice exhibit a progressive reduction in SC number/testis, while SCARKO mice have only minor changes, suggesting that androgen effects on SC number are not mediated via direct action on SCs. Immunoexpression of anti-Mullerian hormone (AMH) which changes according to SC maturational status, occurs normally in ARKO and SCARKO mice. Functional capacity of SCs to support spermatogonia is obviously similar in SCARKOs and controls, whereas ARKOs showed reduced capacity with age. SC capacity to support total germ cells reveals, however, major deficits in ARKO and SCARKO adults, particularly with respect to postmeiotic germ cells. In ARKO as well as SCARKO mice, expression of fatty acid binding protein, platelet-derived growth factor-A, and transferrin are markedly reduced, whereas FSH receptor and AMH are uniformly increased, highlighting these as potentially androgen-regulated SC genes that merit further study. In conclusion, androgen action is not required for maturation-dependent changes of the SCs but is essential for expression of other SC genes, the attainment of normal SC number, and the support of meiotic and postmeiotic germ cell development (10). Latest evidence suggests that FSH and androgens act synergistically to stimulate and maintain spermatogenesis. FSH acts directly on SCs to stimulate germ cell number. Discrimination between direct effects of FSH on spermatogenesis and effects mediated indirectly through androgen action shows that FSH acts to stimulate spermatogenesis through an increase in spermatogonial number and subsequent entry of these cells into meiosis, but has no direct effect on the completion of meiosis, although FSH effects on Leydig cell number (thus LH-mediated androgen production) are mediated through interstitial ARs (11).

The Prostate

Testosterone is the major growth and functional regulator of the prostate, an organ being composed functionally into stem cell units, transit amplifying cells, intermediate cells, and secretory luminal cells. Androgens are able to stimulate the proliferation of transit amplifying cells and their survival. Prostate cancer cells usually derive from such cells, undergoing molecular changes inducing a conversion from a paracrine to an autocrine pathway, allowing the androgen receptor to directly stimulate proliferation of malignant cells (12). For several decades it has been assumed that higher T concentrations lead to greater growth of benign and malign prostate tissue, but this view has come under greater scrutiny over the last several years. Although there are as yet no large-scale, long-term controlled studies of T therapy to provide a definitive assessment of risk, numerous smaller clinical trials as well as population-based longitudinal studies consistently fail to support the historical idea that T therapy poses an increased risk of prostate cancer or exacerbation of symptoms due to benign prostatic hyperplasia. This lack of prostate risk despite increased serum T appears to be explained by data showing that exogenous T does not raise intraprostatic concentrations of T or dihydrotestosterone, suggesting a saturation model (13,14).

NONREPRODUCTIVE TISSUES

Figure 1 summarizes the effects of testosterone both on the above-mentioned effects on reproductive organs as well as nonreproductive tissues, which are elucidated below.

Erythropoiesis

T administration for anemia in patients with renal failure has been common medication before synthetic erythropoietin was available (15). T acts directly on bone marrow at the level of polychromatophilic erythroblasts and enhances the synthesis of ribosomal RNA or its precursors and stimulates a nuclear ribonuclease. It is postulated that erythropoietin and T act synergistically to maintain and foster the biochemical machinery for hemoglobin synthesis (16). In agreement, hypogonadal men often present with anemia. Elevation of T levels, irrespective of the used preparation, will increase hemoglobin levels in these patients (17–20). Substitution effects will reach a plateau after approximately 6 to 9 months (21). The above-mentioned studies demonstrate a marked variability in responsiveness of the hematopoietic system to T and strengthen the necessity for surveillance of substitution therapy: in some men, unacceptably high levels of hemoglobin concentration and hematocrit can develop, so that the dose has to be adjusted in order to prevent adverse vascular events (20). Age plays a pivotal role in modulating the T effects on erythropoiesis: older men seem to be much more susceptible than younger men (22). In addition, it has been demonstrated that pharmacogenetic effects of the CAG repeat polymorphism are visible during T replacement therapy and have to be considered for evaluating erythropoiesis and hematocrit (2).

Androgens and Hair

Androgens are the main regulator of human hair growth, having paradoxical effects on hair follicles depending on their body site. They can stimulate the formation of large hairs, e.g., beard and axilla but inhibit follicles of the scalp. All such effects are gradual and genetically modified, requiring the expression of the androgen receptor in hair follicles. A major component is the 5α-reductase metabolite of T, DHT, which acts via the cells of the dermal papilla, altering production of regulatory paracrine factors acting on keratinocytes, melanocytes, or endothelial cells (23)

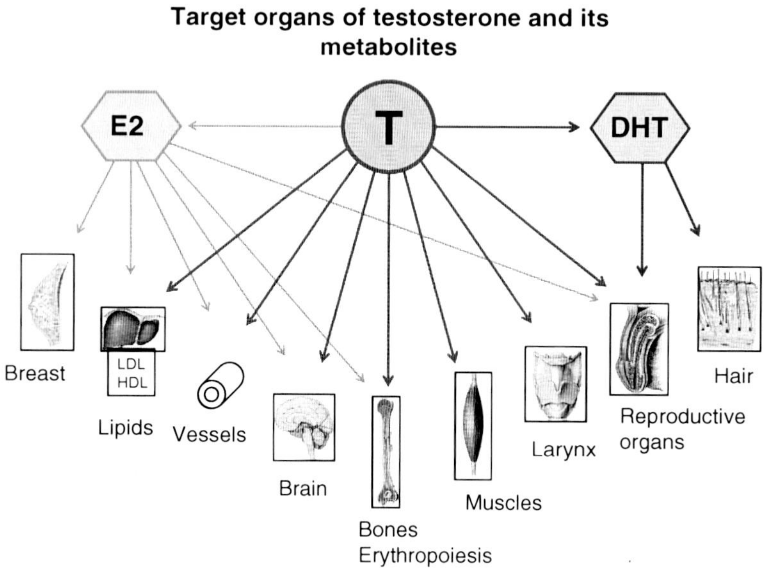

Figure 1 Graphical summary of androgens and their target tissues.

Body Composition

Bone Tissue

In conditions of T deficiency, bone mineral density is decreased and markers of bone turnover are usually elevated (24–27). Especially in hypogonadal men, whose trabecular bone density is decreased, T substitution is effective in regard to significant increase in bone density, particularly in those patients with a marked baseline deficit (28–32). The type of hormone substitution as well as the disease causing low androgen levels do not influence the effectiveness of T substitution on bone density. Nevertheless, there is a tendency of higher T substitution levels to contribute to higher bone density, albeit marginally, since androgen influence on bone tissue seems to be nonlinear: the effect is much stronger in alterations within the low range than in the high range and is influenced by the CAG repeat polymorphism (33).

The underlying mechanisms depend on both T and estradiol, as they contribute to higher bone density. These effects are probably exerted via different pathways: T inhibits osteoclastic activity, while estradiol seems to activate osteoblasts (34,35). Since an interactive, paracrine positive feedback exists between both types of cells (36), both hormones take effect on both types of cells. The mediators of these effects are still unclear. Indications are that androgens act mainly via inhibition of secretion of the cytokine interleukin-6, thus down-regulating osteoclastic activity (37,38), but also via the insulin-like growth factor system of osteoblasts (39). External T administration leads to reduction of markers of bone turnover (38). It is possible that increased muscle strength during T substitution contributes to the gain of bone tissue by enhancing traction forces, a positive stimulus for osteoblasts (40). Overall, bone fracture rates in older men have been related to lower T concentrations in a large epidemiological approach (41).

Muscle Tissue

In addition to the effects of T deficiency on body fat content, a loss of fat-free mass and decrease in muscle protein synthesis is observed in hypogonadal men (42). In agreement, when androgens are substituted in such patients, fat-free mass increases significantly, which can be attributed to muscle growth (43,44). The growth of muscle tissue seems to follow a linear dose–response relationship over a wide range of T levels, as was demonstrated in healthy young men receiving androgen ablation by a GnRH agonist and subsequent T administration in various doses to achieve low-to-supraphysiological levels. As fat-free mass increased with the increasing T dose, so did volumes of thigh muscles (45). Muscle biopsies in these men demonstrated a homogenous increase in cross-sectional areas of both type I and II muscle fibers, which maintained their proportion. Because muscle fiber hypertrophy involves the addition of newly formed myonuclei via the fusion of myogenic cells, the myonuclear number increased in direct relation to the increase in muscle fiber diameter. Muscle cell hyperplasia did not play a significant role (46).

Body Fat

Cross-sectional investigations in healthy, eugonadal men have demonstrated a negative relationship between body fat content and levels of total T (47,48). This applies in particular to abdominal fat tissue (49,50). In healthy obese men, the issue is complicated by simultaneously decreasing levels of sex hormone binding globuline (SHBG), thus levels of free or bioavailable T are often maintained (51).

In hypogonadal men, an increased total body mass index (BMI) is regularly observed as well as a reduced lean BMI (measured with DEXA or bioimpedance), both in comparison to age-matched healthy controls. This suggests higher body weight due to increased fat mass in the presence of lower muscle mass (52,53). T treatment can significantly reduce body fat content in hypogonadal men, and vice versa it can increase lean body mass, an observation which is not only due to shifts in proportions but also to growth of muscle tissue (as mentioned later) (19,20,43,54–58).

This is exerted via a redistribution of body fat during which mainly visceral and intermuscular fat depots are affected, but subcutaneous tissue seems to be spared (59); it is likely that fat cell size itself is modulated by androgens (60). The process seems to follow a linear dose–response relationship to T (59), but the exact mechanism by which fat cells are subject to androgen influence is not known. It can be speculated that this is mediated via increased insulin sensitivity and improved glucose utilization, resulting in lower insulin levels and, thus, a less amount of lipid storage.

Visceral fat tissue plays a central role within the metabolic syndrome, which is mentioned in detail later, acting as a source of inflammatory, anti-insulinergic, and atherogenically relevant cytokines such as TNF-α and IL-6 (61,62). Fat tissue also functions as an endocrine organ: its product, adiponectin plays an important role in metabolism and is related to cardiovascular risk factors. It is produced by fat cells in large quantities, yet its levels are inversely associated with total body fat mass, which is most likely caused by auto-/paracrine down-regulation via inflammatory cytokines. Improvement of insulin sensitivity and inhibition of various atherogenic processes within the vessel wall are direct effects of adiponectin (63). Leptin is another hormone secreted by fat cells. Hypophagia to reduce fat mass is supported by leptin signals, but adipose tissue fosters further food intake by facilitating leptin resistance at the hypothalamic level via afferent nerve signals (64). A vicious circle is thus induced as leptin resistance increases further adipocyte-related production of this hormone. There are indications that high levels of leptin can mitigate T secretion (65,66).

T seems to have various effects on fat cells and insulin resistance. A study in mouse pluripotent stem cells indicates that T regulates body composition by promoting the commitment of these mesenchymal cells into the myogenic lineage and inhibiting their differentiation into the adipogenic lineage. This provides a unifying explanation for the reciprocal effects of androgens on muscle and fat mass in men (59). A inhibiting effect of T has also been described concerning the differentiation of pre-adipocytes in 3T3-L1 cells that differentiate to form fat cells in adipogenic medium. T inhibits adipocyte differentiation in vitro through an androgen receptor–mediated nuclear translocation of β-catenin and activation of downstream Wnt signaling (such Wnt signals direct distinct fates of differentiation in precursor cell types) (67). In addition, T increases lipolysis and the number of adrenoreceptors in male rat adipocytes (68).

T may facilitate insulin sensitivity both in fat and muscle cells by up-regulating the expression of insulin-induced downstream protein expression. Respective dose-dependent effects of T on insulin receptor substrate-1 and glucose transporter 4 expression were seen in cell models (69). Recent models of insulin resistance also suggest a pivotal role of mitochondrial function with the decreased transcription of oxidative phosphorylation genes in skeletal muscle of insulin-resistant subjects. This leads to decreased oxidative phosphorylation, decreased lipid oxidation, intracellular accumulation of triglycerides in skeletal muscle, and ultimately insulin resistance (70). A study in 60 men demonstrated T levels to correlate positively with mitochondrial capacity assessed by measuring maximal aerobic capacity and also expression of oxidative phosphorylation genes (71).

As discussed above, leptin resistance and consequently up-regulated adipocyte leptin secretion play a pivotal role in obesity. T substitution in hypogonadal men is able to reduce leptin secretion of fat cells, probably by an androgen receptor–mediated pathway (72), thus breaking the described vicious circle of leptin resistance and obesity (28,56,73,74).

Mental Issues

Physical performance is strongly influenced by the mental status. Especially mood changes in terms of depression and aggression are likely to modulate physical abilities. Both parameters are subject to androgen influence and an interdependence of physical performance with both hormone levels and mood is likely to exist (75).

Depressiveness

A relation of T levels to depressive mood disorders has been demonstrated by investigations in patients treated for a major depression (76,77). Viewing the aspect from the angle of hypogonadism, clinical consensus exists that this condition in men is related to depressive symptoms. Low T levels seem to be associated with depressive symptoms and late life dysthymia (78). When T level and depressive symptoms were collected in a large sample of elderly men ($n = 856$, mean age $= 70.2 \pm 9.2$ years), Beck Depression Inventory scores and free T levels were inversely correlated with high significance (79).

In a large sample of healthy older men, T levels and modulation of androgen activity by the CAG repeat polymorphism of the androgen receptor gene are associated with depressed mood (80). Therefore, it is no surprise that hypogonadal men profit largely from T substitution in regard of mood improvement, an effect that seems to be independent from substitution modalities (20,81,82).

Aggression

Indications are strong that there is an interdependent feedback mechanism between T and aggression, which is modified by experiences of victory and defeat, as well as by educational, cultural, and socioeconomic background (83). The immense variety of individual response patterns to androgens is demonstrated by a controlled trial in which exceptionally high doses of 600 mg testosterone-cypionate per week were administered: aggressive effects were reported in 16% of the men. The psychological behavior of the others remained unremarkable (84). The effects of external administration of T on aggressive behavior in eugonadal men are seen controversially (85–87).

In hypogonadal men, several subparameters associated with aggression such as tension, anger, and fatigue can be reduced by T substitution and, simultaneously, vigor can increase. There is obviously a level of negative effect experienced by hypogonadal men, which can be reduced by elevation of androgen levels (88).

Metabolic Aspects and Glucose Metabolism

Within the last century, life circumstances have changed in developed countries as physical activity has become less frequent and, simultaneously, an oversupply of food is present. This results in an increasing prevalence of overweight and obesity, particularly over the past two decades. As a consequence, a complex disorder consisting of visceral obesity, dyslipidemia, insulin resistance, and hypertension emerges with increasing incidence: the so-called metabolic syndrome contributes to a symptomatology, which progressively leads to the manifestation of diabetes type 2 and cardiovascular disease. While the pathogenesis of the metabolic syndrome and each of its components is complex and not well understood, central obesity and insulin resistance are acknowledged as important causative factors (89–92). Persons affected are twice as likely to die from and three times as likely to suffer a heart attack or stroke compared to those free of the metabolic syndrome (93). They also have a fivefold greater risk of developing type 2 diabetes mellitus, if not already present (94).

The International Diabetes Federation has recently updated the criteria for diagnosis of the metabolic syndrome (Table 1). In men, obesity as the central component of the metabolic

Table 1 Key Messages

- Intratesticular testosterone action, as being stimulated by gonadotropins, is pivotal for the development of spermatogenesis and normal function of reproductive organs (evidence level 1b).
- Testosterone supplementation can restore these functions at least partially in androgen-deficient men (evidence level 1b).
- Testosterone exerts fundamental and, for male physiology, essential effects on various components of body composition, erythropoiesis, metabolism, and psychological aspects (evidence level 1a).

syndrome is associated with low T concentrations (Table 2) (e.g., 49,50,72,95).

In men, T deficiency may contribute to the development of the metabolic syndrome. In turn, states of hyperinsulinemia and obesity lead to a reduction in testicular testosterone production. T has reciprocal effects on the generation of muscle and visceral adipose tissue by influencing the commitment of pluripotent stem cells and by inhibiting the development of preadipocytes. Insulin sensitivity of muscle cells is increased by augmenting mitochondrial capacity and fostering expression of oxidative phosphorylation genes. T has a protective effect on pancreatic β cells, which is possibly exerted by androgen receptor–mediated mechanisms and have an influence on inflammatory cytokines. As some, but not all, epidemiological and interventional studies indicate, T substitution might be helpful in preventing or attenuating the metabolic syndrome in aging men with late-onset hypogonadism and in hypogonadal patients with type 2 diabetes mellitus, but larger controlled trials are needed to confirm such hypotheses (97).

Metabolic Perspectives for Men

Among hypogonadal men, especially the group of Klinefelter patients exhibit an increased prevalence of the metabolic syndrome (98). Special efforts to detect this under-diagnosed chromosome disorder and mitigate the increased mortality of these men due to complications of diabetes mellitus and cardiovascular events (98) are necessary. Although approaches examining the effects of T on sub-parameters of the metabolic syndrome have been made (as mentioned earlier), prospective studies investigating its incidence in hypogonadal men receiving T substitution therapy are needed. Such studies should take the modulatory effect of the androgen receptor into account to fully elucidate the putative potential of T to attenuate or prevent the metabolic syndrome in men.

Table 2 The International Diabetes Federation: Updated Criteria for the Diagnosis of the Metabolic Syndrome

Central obesity, defined as waist circumference (> 102 cm for North American Men, > 94 cm for European men, and 90 cm for Asian men), along with any two of the following four factors:

- concentration of fasting triglycerides >150 mg/dL (1.7 mmol/L), or specific treatment for this lipid abnormality
- concentration of HDL cholesterol <40 mg/dL (1.0 mmol/L) in males, or specific treatment for this lipid abnormality
- systolic blood pressure >130 or diastolic blood pressure >85 mm Hg, or treatment of previously diagnosed hypertension
- concentration of fasting plasma glucose >100 mg/dL (5.6 mmol/L), or previously diagnosed diabetes mellitus type 2

Source: From Ref. 96.

REFERENCES

1. Canale D, Caglieresi C, Moschini C, et al. Androgen receptor polymorphism (CAG repeats) and androgenicity. Clin Endocrinol (Oxf) 2005; 63:356–361.
2. Zitzmann M. Mechanisms of disease: pharmacogenetics of testosterone therapy in hypogonadal men. Nat Clin Pract Urol 2007; 4:161–166.
3. Weinbauer GF, Niehaus M, Nieschlag E. The role of testosterone in spermatogenesis. In: Nieschlag E, Behre HM, editors. Testosterone: Action, Deficiency, Substitution. 3rd edn. Cambridge, UK: Cambridge University Press, 2004: 173–206.
4. McLachlan RI, O'Donnell L, Meachem SJ, et al. Identification of specific sites of hormonal regulation in spermatogenesis in rats, monkeys, and man. Recent Prog Horm Res 2002; 57:149–179.
5. Pitteloud N, Dwyer AA, DeCruz S, et al. The relative role of gonadal sex steroids and gonadotropin-releasing hormone pulse frequency in the regulation of follicle-stimulating hormone secretion in men. J Clin Endocrinol Metab 2008; 93(7):2686–2692.
6. Pitteloud N, Hayes FJ, Dwyer A, et al. Predictors of outcome of long-term GnRH therapy in men with idiopathic hypogonadotropic hypogonadism. J Clin Endocrinol Metab 2002; 87(9):4128–4136.
7. Raivio T, Falardeau J, Dwyer A, et al. Reversal of idiopathic hypogonadotropic hypogonadism. N Engl J Med 2007; 357(9):863–873.
8. Denolet E, De Gendt K, Allemeersch J, et al. The effect of a sertoli cell-selective knockout of the androgen receptor on testicular gene expression in prepubertal mice. Mol Endocrinol 2006; 20(2):321–334.
9. Chemes HE, Rey RA, Nistal M, et al. Physiologic androgen insensitivity of the fetal, neonatal, and early infantile testis is explained by the ontogeny of the androgen receptor expression in sertoli cells [published online ahead of print August 19, 2008]. J Clin Endocrinol Metab 2008; 93:4408–4412.
10. Tan KA, De Gendt K, Atanassova N, et al. The role of androgens in sertoli cell proliferation and functional maturation: studies in mice with total or Sertoli cell-selective

ablation of the androgen receptor. Endocrinology 2005; 146:2674–2683.

11. O'Shaughnessy PJ, Morris ID, Huhtaniemi I, et al. Role of androgen and gonadotrophins in the development and function of the Sertoli cells and Leydig cells: data from mutant and genetically modified mice. Mol Cell Endocrinol 2009; 10:2–8.
12. Isaacs JT. Role of androgens in prostatic cancer. Vitam Horm 1994; 49:433–502.
13. Isbarn H, Pinthus JH, Marks LS, et al. Testosterone and prostate cancer: revisiting old paradigms [published online ahead of print April 8, 2009]. Eur Urol 2009; 56:48–56.
14. Marks LS, Mazer NA, Mostaghel E, et al. Effect of testosterone replacement therapy on prostate tissue in men with late-onset hypogonadism: a randomized controlled trial. JAMA 2006; 296:2351–2361.
15. Von Hartitzsch B, Kerr DN, Morley G, et al. Androgens in the anaemia of chronic renal failure. Nephron 1977; 18(1):13–20.
16. Perretta M, Valladares L, Romero C, et al. Hormone action on the cell nucleus: effect of erythropoietin and testosterone on bone marrow. Arch Biol Med Exp 1976; 10(1–3):35–40.
17. Liu PY, Wishart SM, Handelsman DJ. A double-blind, placebo-controlled, randomized clinical trial of recombinant human chorionic gonadotropin on muscle strength and physical function and activity in older men with partial age-related androgen deficiency. J Clin Endocrinol Metab 2002; 87(7):3125–3135.
18. Ly LP, Jimenez M, Zhuang TN, et al. A double-blind, placebo-controlled, randomized clinical trial of transdermal dihydrotestosterone gel on muscular strength, mobility, and quality of life in older men with partial androgen deficiency. J Clin Endocrinol Metab 2001; 86(9):4078–4088.
19. Sih R, Morley JE, Kaiser FE, et al. Testosterone replacement in older hypogonadal men: a 12-month randomized controlled trial. J Clin Endocrinol Metab 1997; 82(6):1661–1667.
20. Wang C, Swedloff RS, Iranmanesh A, et al. Transdermal testosterone gel improves sexual function, mood, muscle strength, and body composition parameters in hypogonadal men. Testosterone Gel Study Group. J Clin Endocrinol Metab 2000; 85(8):2839–2853.
21. Von Eckardstein S, Nieschlag E. Treatment of male hypogonadism with testosterone undecanoate injected at extended intervals of 12 weeks: a phase II study. J Androl 2002; 23(3):419–425.
22. Coviello AD, Kaplan B, Lakshman KM, et al. Effects of graded doses of testosterone on erythropoiesis in healthy young and older men. J Clin Endocrinol Metab 2008; 93(3):914–919.
23. Randall VA. Androgens and hair: a biological paradox. In: Nieschlag E, Behre HM, eds. Testosterone – Action, Deficiency, Substitution, 3rd ed. United Kingdom: Cambridge University Press, 2004:207–232.
24. Erben RG, Eberle J, Stahr K, et al. Androgen deficiency induces high turnover osteopenia in aged male rats: a sequential histomorphometric study. J Bone Miner Res 2000; 15:1085–1098.
25. Fukuda S, Iida H. Effects of orchidectomy on bone metabolism in beagle dogs. J Vet Med Sci 2000; 62:69–73.
26. Scopacasa F, Horowitz M, Wishart JM, et al. The relation between bone density, free androgen index, and estradiol in men 60 to 70 years old. Bone 2000; 27:145–149.
27. Stepan JJ, Lachman M, Zverina J, et al. Castrated men exhibit bone loss: effect of calcitonin treatment on biochemical indices of bone remodeling. J Clin Endocrinol Metab 1989; 69:523–527.
28. Behre HM, Kliesch S, Leifke E, et al. Long-term effect of testosterone therapy on bone mineral density in hypogonadal men. J Clin Endocrinol Metab 1997; 82:2386–2390.
29. Kenny AM, Prestwood KM, Gruman CA, et al. Effects of transdermal T on bone and muscle in older men with low bioavailable T levels. J Gerontol A Biol Sci Med Sci 2001; 56:M266–M272.
30. Leifke E, Korner HC, Link TM, et al. Effects of testosterone replacement therapy on cortical and trabecular bone mineral density, vertebral body area and paraspinal muscle area in hypogonadal men. Eur J Endocrinol 1998; 138: 51–58.
31. Snyder PJ, Peachey H, Hannoush P, et al. Effect of testosterone treatment on bone mineral density in men over 65 years of age. J Clin Endocrinol Metab 1999; 84:1966–1972.
32. Wang C, Swerdloff RS, Iranmanesh A. Effects of transdermal T gel on bone turnover markers and bone mineral density in hypogonadal men. Clin Endocrinol (Oxf) 2001; 54:739–750.
33. Zitzmann M, Brune M, Vieth V, et al. Monitoring bone density in hypogonadal men with phalangeal ultrasound. Bone 2002; 31:422–429.
34. Damien E, Price JS, Lanyon LE. Mechanical strain stimulates osteoblast proliferation through the estrogen receptor in males as well as females. J Bone Miner Res 2000; 15:2169–2177.
35. Fohr B, Schulz A, Battmann A. Sex steroids and bone metabolism: comparison of in vitro effects of 17beta-estradiol and testosterone on human osteosarcoma cell lines of various gender and differentiation. Exp Clin Endocrinol Diabetes 2000; 108:414–423.
36. Ziegler R. Der Knochen und seine Erkrankungen, Teil II. Dtsch Med Wochenschr 1995; 120:571–572.
37. Bellido T, Jilka RL, Boyce BF, et al. Regulation of interleukin-6, osteoclastogenesis, and bone mass by

androgens. The role of the androgen receptor. J Clin Invest 1995; 95:2886–2895.

38. Zitzmann M, Nieschlag E. Testosterone and bone metabolism. In: Nieschlag E, Behre HM, editors. Testosterone: Action, Deficiency, Substitution. 3rd edn. Cambridge, UK: Cambridge University Press, 2004: 233–254.
39. Gori F, Hofbauer LC, Conover CA. et al. Effects of androgens on the insulin like growth factor system in an androgen-responsive human osteoblastic cell line. Endocrinology 1999; 140:5579–5586.
40. Aparicio LF, Jurkovic M, DeLullo J. Decreased bone density in ambulatory patients with duchenne muscular dystrophy. J Pediatr Orthop 2002; 22(2):179–181.
41. Amin S, Zhang Y, Felson DT, et al. Estradiol, testosterone, and the risk for hip fractures in elderly men from the Framingham Study. Am J Med 2006; 119(5):426–433.
42. Mauras N, Hayes V, Welch S, et al. Testosterone deficiency in young men: marked alterations in whole body protein kinetics, strength, and adiposity. J Clin Endocrinol Metab 1998; 83:1886–1892.
43. Bhasin S, Storer TW, Berman N, et al. A replacement dose of testosterone increases fat-free mass and muscle size in hypogonadal men. J Clin Endocrinol Metab 1997; 82:407–413.
44. Brodsky IG, Balagopal P, Nair KS. Effects of testosterone replacement on muscle mass and muscle protein synthesis in hypogonadal men—a clinical research center study. J Clin Endocrinol Metab 1996; 81:3469–3475.
45. Bhasin S, Woodhouse L, Casaburi R, et al. Testosterone dose-response relationships in healthy young men. Am J Physiol Endocrinol Metab 2001; 281(6):E1172–E1181
46. Sinha-Hikim I, Artaza J, Woodhouse L, et al. Testosterone-induced increase in muscle size in healthy young men is associated with muscle fiber hypertrophy. Am J Physiol Endocrinol Metab 2002; 283(1):E154–E164
47. Simon D, Charles MA, Nahoul K, et al. Association between plasma total testosterone and cardiovascular risk factors in healthy adult men: The Telecom Study. J Clin Endocrinol Metab 1997; 82:682–685.
48. Vermeulen A, Goemaere S, Kaufman JM. Testosterone, body composition and aging. J Endocrinol Invest 1999; 22(suppl 5):110–116.
49. Khaw KT, Barrett-Connor E. Lower endogenous androgens predict central adiposity in men. Ann Epidemiol 1992; 2:675–682.
50. Marin P, Arver S. Androgens and abdominal obesity. Baillieres Clin Endocrinol Metab 1998; 12:441–451.
51. Vermeulen A, Kaufman JM, Giagulli VA. Influence of some biological indexes on sex hormone-binding globulin and androgen levels in aging or obese males. J Clin Endocrinol Metab 1996; 81(5): 1821–1826.
52. Katznelson L, Finkelstein JS, Schoenfeld DA, et al. Increase in bone density and lean body mass during testosterone administration in men with acquired hypogonadism. J Clin Endocrinol Metab 1996; 81:4358–4365.
53. Marin P. Testosterone and regional fat distribution. Obes Res 1995; 3(suppl 4):609–612.
54. Behre HM, von Eckardstein S, Kliesch S, et al. Long-term substitution therapy of hypogonadal men with transscrotal testosterone over 7–10 years. Clin Endocrinol 1999; 50:629–635.
55. Marin P, Holmang S, Jonsson L, et al. The effects of testosterone treatment on body composition and metabolism in middle-aged obese men. Int J Obes Relat Metab Disord 1992; 16:991–997.
56. Rolf C, von Eckardstein S, Koken U, et al. Testosterone substitution of hypogonadal men prevents the age-dependent increases in body mass index, body fat and leptin seen in healthy ageing men: results of a cross-sectional study. Eur J Endocrinol 2002; 146:505–511.
57. Snyder PJ, Peachey H, Berlin JA, et al. Effects of testosterone replacement in hypogonadal men. J Clin Endocrinol Metab 2000; 85(8):2670–2677.
58. Allan CA, Strauss BJ, McLachlan RI. Body composition, metabolic syndrome and testosterone in ageing men. Int J Impot Res 2007; 19:448–457.
59. Woodhouse LJ, Gupta N, Bhasin M, et al. Dose-dependent effects of testosterone on regional adipose tissue distribution in healthy young men. J Clin Endocrinol Metab 2004; 89:718–726.
60. Garaulet M, Perex-Llamas F, Fuente T, et al. Anthropometric, computed tomography and fat cell data in an obese population: relationship with insulin, leptin, tumor necrosis factor-alpha, sex hormone-binding globulin and sex hormones. Eur J Endocrinol 2000; 143(5):657–666.
61. Grimble RF. Inflammatory status and insulin resistance. Curr Opin Clin Nutr Metab Care 2002; 5:551–559.
62. Guerre-Millo M. Adipose tissue hormones. J Endocrinol Invest 2002; 25:855–861.
63. Diez JJ, Iglesias P. The role of the novel adipocyte-derived hormone adiponectin in human disease. Eur J Endocrinol 2003; 148:293–300.
64. Yamada T, Katagiri H, Ishigaki Y, et al. Signals from intra-abdominal fat modulate insulin and leptin sensitivity through different mechanisms: neuronal involvement in food-intake regulation. Cell Metab 2006; 3:223–229.
65. Isidori AM, Caprio M, Strollo F, et al. Leptin and androgens in male obesity: evidence for leptin contribution to reduced androgen levels. J Clin Endocrinol Metab. 1999; 84:3673–3680.
66. Isidori, AM, Strollo F, Morè M, et al. Leptin and aging: correlation with endocrine changes in male and female healthy adult populations of different body weights. J Clin Endocrinol Metab 2000; 85:1954–1962.

67. Singh R, Artaza JN, Taylor WE, et al. Testosterone inhibits adipogenic differentiation in 3T3-L1 cells: nuclear translocation of androgen receptor complex with beta-catenin and T-cell factor 4 may bypass canonical Wnt signaling to down-regulate adipogenic transcription factors. Endocrinology 2006; 147:141–154.
68. Xu XF, De Pergola G, Björntorp P. Testosterone increases lipolysis and the number of beta-adrenoreceptors in male rat adipocytes. Endocrinology 1991; 128:379–382.
69. Chen X, Li X, Huang HY, et al. Effects of testosterone on insulin receptor substrate-1 and glucose transporter 4 expression in cells sensitive to insulin. Zhonghua Yi Xue Za Zhi 2006; 86:1474–1477.
70. Mootha VK, Lindgren CM, Eriksson KF, et al. PGC-1alpha-responsive genes involved in oxidative phosphorylation are coordinately downregulated in human diabetes. Nat Genet 2003; 34:267–273.
71. Pitteloud N, Mootha VK, Dwyer AA, et al. Relationship between testosterone levels, insulin sensitivity, and mitochondrial function in men. Diabetes Care 2005; 28:1636–1642.
72. Zitzmann M, Gromoll J, von Eckardstein A, et al. The CAG repeat polymorphism in the androgen receptor gene modulates body fat mass and serum concentrations of leptin and insulin in men. Diabetologia 2003; 46: 31–39.
73. Jockenhövel F, Blum WF, Vogel E, et al. Testosterone substitution normalizes elevated serum leptin levels in hypogonadal men. J Clin Endocrinol Metab 1997; 82:2510–2513.
74. Mayes JS, Watson GH. Direct effects of sex steroid hormones on adipose tissues and obesity. Obes Rev 2004; 5:197–216.
75. Filaire E, Bernain X, Sagnol M, et al. Preliminary results on mood state, salivary testosterone:cortisol ratio and team performance in a professional soccer team. Eur J Appl Physiol 2001; 86(2):179–184.
76. Schweiger U, Deuschle M, Weber B, et al. Testosterone gonadotropin and cortisol secretion in male patients with major depression. Psychosom Med 1999; 61:292–296.
77. Unden F, Ljunggren JG, Beck-Friis J, et al. Hypothalamic-pituitary-gonadal axis in major depressive disorders. Acta Psychiatr Scand 1988; 78:138–146.
78. Seidman SN, Araujo AB, Roose SP, et al. Low testosterone levels in elderly men with dysthymic disorder. Am J Psychiatry 2002; 159(3):456–459.
79. Barrett-Connor E, Von Mühlen DG, Kritz-Silverstein D. Bioavailable testosterone and depressed mood in older men: the Rancho Bernardo Study. J Clin Endocrinol Metab 1999; 84(2):573–577.
80. Seidman SN, Araujo AB, Roose SP, et al. Testosterone level, androgen receptor polymorphism, and depressive symptoms in middle-aged men. Biol Psychiatry 2001; 50:371–376.
81. Burris AS, Banks SM, Carter CS, et al. A long-term prospective study of the physiologic and behavioural effects of hormone replacement in untreated hypogonadal men. J Androl 1992; 13:297–304.
82. Rabkin JG, Wagner GJ, Rabkin R. A double-blind, placebo-controlled trial of testosterone therapy for HIV-positive men with hypogonadal symptoms. Arch Gen Psychiatry 2000; 57(2):141–147.
83. Zitzmann M, Nieschlag E. Testosterone levels in healthy men and the relation to behavioural and physical characteristics: facts and constructs. Eur J Endocrinol 2001; 144(3):183–197.
84. Pope HG Jr, Kouri EM, Hudson JI. Effects of supraphysiologic doses of testosterone on mood and aggression in normal men: a randomized controlled trial. Arch Gen Psychiatry 2000; 57:133–140.
85. Christiansen K. Behavioural correlates of testosterone. In: Nieschlag E, Behre HM, eds. Testosterone: Action Deficiency Substitution, 2nd ed. Berlin: Springer, 1998:107–142.
86. Kouri EM, Lukas SE, Pope HG Jr, et al. Increased aggressive responding in male volunteers following the administration of gradually increasing doses of testosterone cypionate. Drug Alcohol Depend 1995; 40:73–79.
87. Tricker R, Casaburi R, Storer TW, et al. The effects of supraphysiological doses of testosterone on angry behaviour in healthy eugonadal men–a clinical research center study. J Clin Endocrinol Metab 1996; 81:3754–3758.
88. O'Connor DB, Archer J, Hair WM, et al. Exogenous testosterone, aggression, and mood in eugonadal and hypogonadal men. Physiol Behav 2002; 75(4):557–566.
89. Anderson PJ, Critchley JA, Chan JC, et al. Factor analysis of the metabolic syndrome: obesity vs insulin resistance as the central abnormality. Int J Obesity 2001; 25:1782–1788.
90. Carr DB, Utzschneider KM, Hull RL. Intra-abdominal fat is a major determinant of the National Cholesterol Education Program Adult Treatment Panel III criteria for the metabolic syndrome. Diabetes 2004; 53:2087–2094.
91. Cassells HB, Haffner SM. The metabolic syndrome: risk factors and management. J Cardiovasc Nurs 2006; 21:306–313.
92. Eisenmann JC. Secular trends in variables associated with the metabolic syndrome of North American children and adolescents: a review and synthesis. Am J Hum Biol 2003; 15:786–794.
93. Isomaa B, Almgren P, Tuomi T. Cardiovascular morbidity and mortality associated with the metabolic syndrome. Diabetes Care 2001; 24:683–689.
94. Stern M, Williams K, Gonzalez-Villalpando C. Does the metabolic syndrome improve identification of individuals at risk of type 2 diabetes and/or cardiovascular disease? Diabetes Care 2004; 27:2676–2681.

95. Van Den Beld AW, de Jong FH, Grobbee DE, et al. Measures of bioavailable serum testosterone and estradiol and their relationships with muscle strength, bone density, and body composition in elderly men. J Clin Endocrinol Metab 2000; 85:3276–3282.
96. http://www.idf.org/webdata/docs/MetSyndrome_FINAL.pdf.
97. Zitzmann M. Testosterone deficiency, insulin resistance and the metabolic syndrome [published online ahead of print October 27, 2009]. Nat Rev Endocrinol 2009; 5:673–681.
98. Bojesen A, Kristensen K, Birkebaek NH, et al. The metabolic syndrome is frequent in Klinefelter's syndrome and is associated with abdominal obesity and hypogonadism. Diabetes Care 2006a; 29:1591–1598.

25 Clinical aspects of male sex differentiation

Johan Svensson and Yvonne Lundberg Giwercman

SYNOPSIS

Disorders of sex determination are devastating conditions for parents of a newborn. Correct management and rational sex assignment is, therefore, of crucial importance. Clinical diagnosis is, however, often complex and knowledge of normal sexual differentiation is necessary for understanding these disorders. In the following, the principles of sexual development as well as disorders related to different steps during sex differentiation are described. For the clinician who is confronted with a child with a disorder of sex determination, it is of outmost importance not to guess the gender but to initiate a proper diagnostic procedure. Diagnosis generally requires a thorough clinical examination of the child and careful family history taking. The further diagnostic procedure includes cytogenetic, hormonal, and mutational analyses. Advances in molecular techniques are continuously providing tools for detection of genetic defects and primary diagnosis. These methods may also be applied for prenatal diagnosis and carrier identification. Some helpful keys in the diagnosis of children with disorders of sex determination are, therefore, provided.

INTRODUCTION

During the first six weeks of normal human fetal development, male and female embryos have the same phenotype although the chromosomal content differs; 46,XY and 46,XX, respectively. The embryo at that stage develops two bipotential gonads and two double ductal systems, the Wolffian ducts, and the Müllerian ducts. Thereafter, the gonads will develop to either testes or ovaries because of different genetic events. Classic animal studies by Alfred Jost in 1947 founded the research on mammalian sex determination (1). Jost surgically removed the gonadal ridges, from which both testes and ovaries are derived, from developing rabbit fetuses and then allowed the castrated animals develop to term. The experiment showed that embryonic castration of male rabbits before a critical stage of development resulted in female differentiation of the internal as well as external genitalia, whereas unilateral castration resulted in female genitals unilaterally. Jost suggested that locally acting hormones from the fetal testis were crucial for normal male development.

The testicular hormones that are essential for male development are testosterone secreted from the testicular Leydig cells and anti-Müllerian hormone (AMH), also recognized as Müllerian-inhibiting hormone or Müllerian-inhibiting substance, produced by the Sertoli cells. Testosterone acts on the Wolffian ducts by stimulating the male internal genital development resulting in vas deferens, epididymis, and the seminal vesicles. AMH acts on the cells of the Müllerian ducts, resulting in regression of these ducts and also preventing a formation of uterus and fallopian tubes. In the same manner, the external genital organs in males and females are identical until gestational week 6 (Fig. 1). Under the influence of high androgen levels locally in males, the genital tubercle grows and differentiates to a penis, the urethral plate gradually closes to a urethra that opens on the tip of the glans, a scrotum is formed by fusion in the midline, and the testes migrate from the initial abdominal position to the scrotum.

Because of this developmental cascade of events, disorders of the sex development in the male occur as different degrees of undermasculinization. In mild forms, boys present with hypospadias, with a urethral meatus located near the glans. In the most severe forms, the meatus is located in the perineum, often associated with a small and curved penis. Other associated malformations are cryptorchidism and micropenis. In females, virilization causes different degrees of enlargement of clitoris or midline closure to a urogenital sinus and scrotum. The most common cause of these conditions in females is congenital adrenal hyperplasia (CAH).

Ambiguous genitalia in the newborn may also occur as a result of chromosome abnormalities. The most common chromosome abnormality is 45,X/46,XX mosaicism associated with mixed gonadal dysgenesis. The phenotype encompasses a wide spectrum, ranging from hypospadias with normal penile size to severe undermasculinization and micropenis. However, more than 90% of children with a prenatally 45X/46,XY diagnosis have normal male genitalia (2). The gonadal morphology in children with ambiguous genitalia is usually a testis on one side and a streak gonad on the other. The streak gonad should be removed because of risk of malignancy (3). In childhood, stigmata like those in Turner syndrome may develop.

In children with a 46,XX/47,XXY karyotype, the phenotype varies depending on the nature of the gonads. Ovotestis (true hermaphroditism) is a histological diagnosis based on the presence of both ovarian and testicular tissue in the individual. Internal and external phenotype varies, but the most frequent karyotype is 46,XX.

Also, other disorders have been of importance to define the process of sexual differentiation, thereby identifying key genes (Table 1). Mutations in any of these genes lead to different disorders of sexual differentiation (see Case Story).

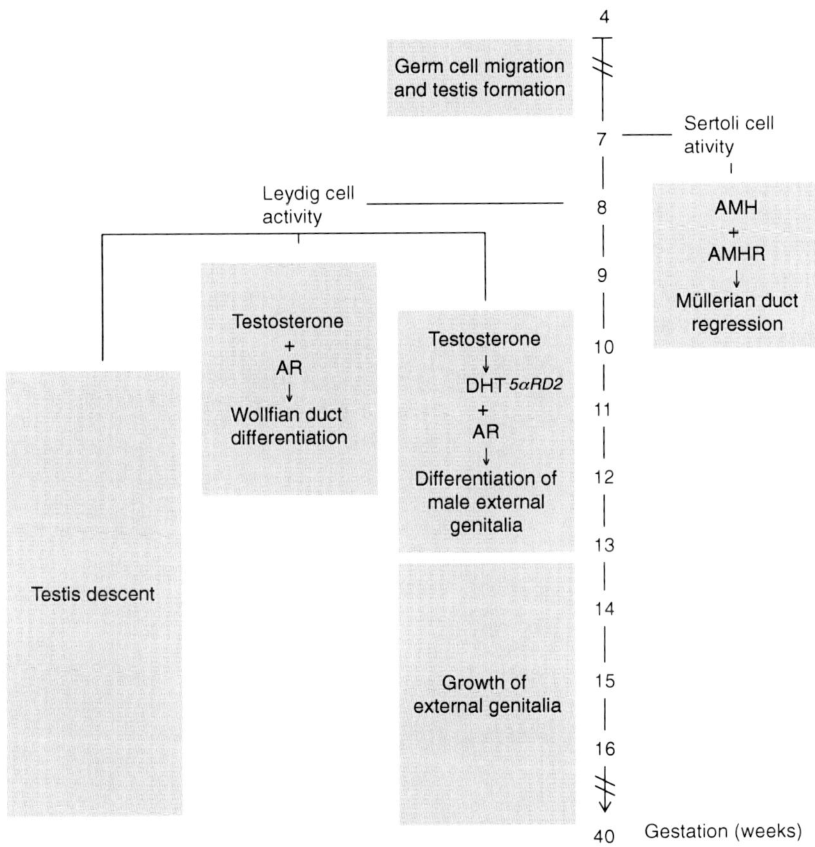

Figure 1 Schematic events in the embryology of male sex development.

NORMAL SEX DETERMINATION AND DIFFERENTIATION

Male sexual differentiation can be defined as three different developmental stages:

1. Fetal period
2. Neonatal period and infancy
3. Puberty and adulthood

Fetal Period

The events in fetal male sex development, related to gestational age, are shown in Fig. 1.

Sex determination and differentiation comprise a cascade of events in the developing embryo, beginning with the establishment of chromosomal sex, which is defined by the inheritance of an X or a Y chromosome from the father. Human embryos with either 46,XX or 46,XY karyotype develop identically for the first six weeks of gestation, both being endowed with bipotential primordial gonadal tissue, two sets of internal genital ducts (Wolffian and Müllerian), and undifferentiated external genitalia.

In the presence of a Y chromosome, male gonadal sex is established. After formation of the testes, male sex differentiation proceeds under the control of hormones produced by the fetal testis.

Neonatal Period and Infancy

In newborn boys, there is a significant activation of the hypothalamic–pituitary–testicular axis. At the age of two to three months, the serum levels of gonadotropins, testosterone, and inhibin B are approaching pubertal levels, but fall to non-measurable concentrations after a few months and remain at this low level until the initiation of puberty. The physiological background for such endocrine activity in neonatal boys is still unclear. However, a significant increase in the number of Sertoli cells was found to occur in the human testis during the first three months of life.

Puberty and Adulthood

Puberty is characterized by an increase in growth rate and the appearance of striking somatic sex differences. The first sign of male puberty is growth of the testes above the infantile size of 2 to 4 mL, increasing gradually to the normal adult size of 15 to 30 mL each. This testicular growth is primarily due to Sertoli cell proliferation and subsequent initiation of spermatogenesis. The period of pubertal development is characterized by significant

Table 1 Suggested Classification of Disorders of Sex Development (Ref. 34)

Sex chromosome DSD	46,XY DSD	46,XX DSD
A. 45,X (Turner syndrome and variants)	A. Disorders of gonadal (testicular) development • Complete or partial gonadal dysgenesis (SRY, SOX9, SF1, WT1 DAX1 dupl, WNT4 dupl) • Gonadal/testis regression • Ovotesticular DSD	A. Disorders of gonadal (ovarian) development • Gonadal dysgenesis • Testicular DSD (SRY, SOX9 dupl, RSP01) • Ovotesticular DSD
B. 47,XXY (Klinefelter syndrome and variants)	B. Disorders of androgen synthesis and action 1. *Disorders of androgen synthesis* • Leydig cell hypoplasia, aplasia (LHCGR defects) • Congenital lipoid adrenal hyperplasia (StAR) • Cholesterol side-chain cleavage enzyme deficiency (CYP 11A1) • 17α-hydroxylase/17,20-lyase deficiency (CYP17A1) • 3β-hydroxysteroid dehydrogenase 2 (HSD3B2) • 17β-hydroxysteroid dehydrogenase deficiency (HSD17B3) • 5α-reductase 2 deficiency (SRD5A2) • P450 oxireductase deficiency (POR) • Smith–Lemi–Opitz syndrome (DHCR7) 2. *Disorders of androgen action* • Androgen insensitivity syndrome (AR receptor mutation) • Drugs and environmental modulators	B. Androgen excess 1. *Fetal* • 21-hydroxylase deficiency (CYP21A2) • 3β-hydroxysteroid dehydrogenase 2 (HSD3B2) • 11β-hydroxylase deficiency (CYP11B1) • P450 oxidoreductase deficiency (POR) 2. *Fetoplacental* • Aromatase deficiency (CYP19) • Oxidoreductase deficiency (POR) 3. Maternal • Maternal virilizing tumors • Androgenic drugs
C. 45,X/46,XY (mixed gonadal dysgenesis, ovotesticular DSD)	C. Other • Persistent Müllerian duct syndrome (AMH and AMHR) • Vanishing testis syndrome • Congenital hypogonadotropic hypogonadism (DAX1) • Cryptorchidism (INSL3, LGR8) • Isolated hypospadias (CX0rf6) • Syndromic associations of male genital development (e.g., cloacal anomalies, Robinow, Aarskog, hand–foot–genital, popliteal pterygium)	C. Other • Müllerian agenesis/hypoplasia (e.g., MURCS) • Vaginal atresia (McKusick–Kaufman syndrome) • Uterine abnormalities (e.g., MODY 5) • Labial adhesions • Syndromic associations (e.g., cloacal anomalies)
D. 46,XX/46,XY (Chimeric, ovotesticular DSD)		

Abbreviations: DSD, disorders of sex development; SRY, sex-determining region of the Y chromosome; SOX9, SRY-related *HMG-BOX* gene 9; SF1, steroidogenic factor 1; WT1, Wilms tumor 1; DAX1, DSS–AHC critical region on the X chromosome, gene 1; Wnt4, wingless-type integration site family member 4; MMTV, mouse mammary tumor virus; StAR, steroidogenic acute regulatory protein; SRD, steroid reductase; AR, androgen receptor; AMH, anti-Müllerian hormone; AMHR, anti-Müllerian hormone receptor; INSL3; LGR8, luceine-rich repeat-containing G protein-coupled receptor 8; dupl, duplicated; RSPO1, roof plate–specific spondin family, member 1; LHCGR, luteinizing hormone/choriogonadotropin receptor; DHCR7, delta-7-sterol reductase; MURCS, Müllerian duct aplasia, unilateral renal aplasia, and cervicothoracic somite dysplasia; CXOrf6, chromosome X opening reading frame 6; MODY5, maturity-onset diabetes of the young, type 5.

increase in serum levels of gonadotropins, inhibin B, and testosterone. Initially, this increase may be difficult to detect since it is not constant, but rather manifests as short peaks, mainly during the sleeping period. It is still unclear which factors are triggering the pubertal development that in normal boys is initiated between the age of 10 and 14 years. Testosterone, which increases more than 20-fold (normal adult range of 10–30 nM), plays a crucial role for the development of secondary sex characteristics, stimulating growth of muscles, bone, and penis as well as facial, body, and pubic hair. In hypogonadal individuals, all sex characteristics—with the only exception of testicular growth—can be evoked by use of testosterone only. However, increase in gonadal size requires a concerted action of androgens and gonadotropins.

DISORDERS OF MALE SEX DETERMINATION AND DIFFERENTIATION

As discussed in the previous section, embryonic sex determination and differentiation results from a cascade of events involving proteins that are encoded by autosomal as well as sex chromosomal genes. Mutations in any of these genes can result in aberrant sex differentiation, as discussed in the following section. An outline of the genes expressed in male sex development is given in Fig. 2.

Defects in Testis Determination

SRY

SRY (*s*ex-determining *r*egion of the *Y* chromosome) is the initial factor that starts the cascade of events that differentiates the bipotential gonad to testis leading to a normal male genital differentiation. The gene is located on the short arm of the Y chromosome and functions as a transcription factor. A lack of normal SRY function always leads to a complete gonadal dysgenesis with streak gonads. Recent studies have revealed that mutations or deletions of the *SRY* gene occur in two of three patients with the complete form of XY gonadal dysgenesis, which is a much higher incidence than previously thought (5). This condition is associated with a substantial risk of gonadal tumors. However, all other stigmata are lacking. In addition, approximately 80% to 90% of all XX males have an *SRY* gene translocation, usually to the X chromosome. Surprisingly, some XY female cases have inherited the *SRY* mutation from their healthy father. The mechanism is unknown but is thought to arise because of gonadal mosaicism. To add even more to the complexity of genital development, a few cases were reported with a XX male phenotype, but lacking the *SRY* gene, indicating that other sex reversal genes may stimulate normal male development even without *SRY*.

SF1

SF1 (steroidogenic factor 1), also known as adrenal 4-binding protein (Ad4BP), is an orphan receptor and a member of the nuclear receptor superfamily, which like other members of this family regulates transcription of target genes. SF1 plays a direct role in regulating genes involved in sexual differentiation, reproduction, and steroidogenesis by regulating the expression of steroidogenic enzymes involved in the production of testosterone. In males, SF1 participates in sexual development by regulating expression of AMH. In 1999, the first patient was described with a mutation in the *SF1* gene (6). As predicted from the mouse model, this patient presented with adrenal crisis and female phenotype despite 46,XY karyotype. The phenotype was due to absence of gonads and adrenals. Since then, mutations have been reported in karyotypic males with a spectrum of phenotypes ranging from adrenal and gonadal failure at the most severe end of the spectrum to mild gonadal dysgenesis and impaired virilization with normal adrenal function at the other end. Very recently it was also reported that the same mutation could cause discordant phenotypes in siblings

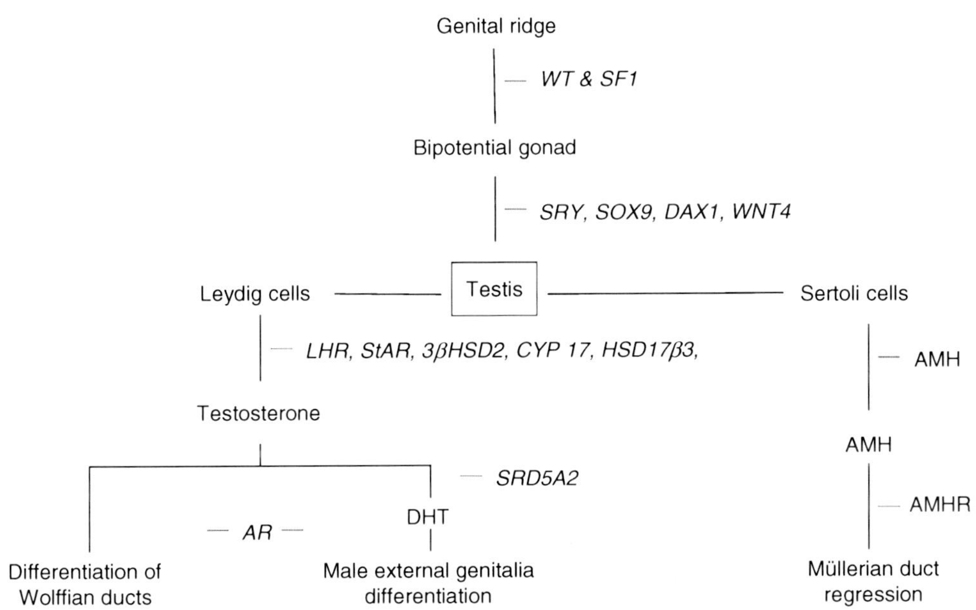

Figure 2 Outline of male sex determination and differentiation with key genes, where clinical investigation may lead to mutation analysis. Gene abbreviations are defined in the text.

(7) as well as in dizygotic twins (8). With respect to the twins, one of the boys presented with bilateral anorchia and micropenis, whereas the twin had progressed through puberty. Adrenal function was normal in both brothers. The authors suggest that epigenetic variability, modifying factors, or environmental influences could account for the differences in phenotype seen.

WT1

WT1 (the Wilms tumor 1) gene was initially identified because of its role in Wilms tumor or nephroblastoma, a pediatric kidney tumor (9). Wilms tumor is one of the most common solid tumors of childhood, occurring in 1 in 10,000 children and accounting for 8% of childhood cancers. The gene is located in the chromosomal region 11p13, and loss of this chromosomal region is seen in children with Wilms tumor, aniridia, genitourinary anomalies, and mental retardation (WAGR) syndrome—a multigene disorder with aniridia, genital malformations, mental retardation, and Wilms tumor (10). Because of the very specific expression pattern, both in a spatially and timely manner in the early genital ridge, gonads, and kidneys, this gene was identified to cause Denys–Drash syndrome (11). This unusual syndrome consists of early renal insufficiency due to mesangial sclerosis, gonadal dysgenesis, and Wilms tumor. In boys the syndrome is more easily recognised because of the male pseudohermaphroditism caused by the gonadal deficiency. In girls on the other hand, a very high grade of suspicion only will reveal the diagnosis before the Wilms tumor has already given symptoms. Therefore, this syndrome must always be suspected in small girls with renal insufficiency in order to diagnose tumors early. It has also been proposed that some of the patients reported as cases of Denys–Drash syndrome, in fact, had a different disorder for which the designation Frasier syndrome was suggested. In several patients, the diagnosis was established only after successful kidney transplantation during evaluation for primary amenorrhea. It was later shown that the molecular difference between Frasier syndrome and Denys–Drash syndrome was caused by a mutation in the donor splice site of intron 9 of the *WT1* gene, resulting in an altered ratio of the 2 splice isoforms of the protein. In the Denys–Drash syndrome, the tumor risk is much greater than in Frasier syndrome.

SOX9

SOX9 (SRY-related *HMG-BOX* gene 9) is an autosomal gene situated on chromosome band 17q24. One of the earliest effects of SRY expression is to induce upregulation of *SOX9* gene expression in the developing gonad. Before sexual differentiation, SOX9 protein is initially found in the cytoplasm of undifferentiated gonads from both sexes, but at the time of testis differentiation, it becomes localized to the nuclear compartment in males, whereas it is downregulated in females. Inactivating heterozygote mutations of this gene cause a skeletal dysplasia, so called campomelic dysplasia, with characteristically bent limbs, in combination with a total or a partial gonadal dysgenesis in 75% of all XY females (12). Type II collagen, the major cartilage matrix protein, is directly regulated by SOX9 during chondrocyte differentiation and implicated in abnormal regulation of chondrogenesis as a cause of the skeletal abnormalities associated with campomelic dysplasia.

DSS

Dosage-sensitive sex reversal (DSS) refers to a region on the X chromosome (p21–22), containing the *DAX1* gene, which has been duplicated in some 46,XY females. The existence of an X-specific gene involved in human sex determination was first identified when present in duplicate, resulted in male-to-female sex reversal (13). This region is normally thought to be X-inactivated since 47,XXY and 48,XXXY individuals are phenotypic males, whereas in DSS subjects, who have two active copies of the region, the function of SRY is overridden and testes development fails. Recently, in a 21-year-old 46,XY female, a deletion with a distal breakpoint upstream of the *DAX1* gene was reported (14). She presented with primary amenorrhea, a small immature uterus, and gonadal dysgenesis without adrenal insufficiency. The deletion was also present in the patient's mother, who had a history of ovarian cysts, but was not found in 1184 controls. The authors suggested that loss of regulatory sequences may have resulted in an upregulation of DAX1 expression consistent with phenotypic consequences of *DAX1* duplication.

DAX1

DAX1 (DSS–AHC critical region on the X chromosome, gene 1) derives its name from its dual pathologic role in humans, that is, the DSS syndrome and adrenal hypoplasia congenita (AHC). AHC is a disease of the adrenal cortex and lethal if left untreated because of dehydration and electrolyte imbalance. Loss of DAX1 results in adrenal hypoplasia and hypogonadotropic hypogonadism and increased DAX1 lead to dosage-sensitive sex reversal and a female phenotype or ambiguous genitalia in XY genotypic males (15). Lin et al. studied the prevalence of *DAX1* and *SF1* mutations in 117 children and adults with primary adrenal failure of unknown etiology (i.e., not caused by CAH, adrenoleukodystrophy, or autoimmune disease). *DAX1* mutations were found in 58% (37 of 64) of 46,XY phenotypic boys referred with adrenal hypoplasia and in all boys (8 of 8) with hypogonadotropic hypogonadism and a family history suggestive of adrenal failure in males. SF1 mutations causing adrenal failure were found in only two patients with 46,XY gonadal dysgenesis. No DAX1 or SF1 mutations were identified in the adult-onset group (16). The authors concluded that DAX1 mutations are a relatively frequent cause of adrenal failure in this group of boys, whereas SF1 mutations causing adrenal failure in humans are rare and are more likely to be associated with significant under virilization and gonadal dysfunction in 46,XY individuals.

Wnt4

Wnt4 is "wingless-type MMTV integration site family, member 4". The *Wnt* gene family consists of structurally related genes encoding proteins that act as extracellular signalling factors. *Wnt* genes are implicated in a wide variety of biologic processes including cell fate determination and patterning in early embryos and in cell growth and/or differentiation in certain adult mammalian tissues.

In a woman with congenital absence of the vagina, normal female secondary sexual characteristics, rudimentary uterus in the form of bilateral and noncanaliculated muscular buds, normal tubes and ovaries, and normal endocrine and cytogenetic evaluations, a heterozygous mutation in the *Wnt4* gene was identified (17). The findings suggested a role for *Wnt4* in the development and maintenance of the female phenotype in women. Recently, a novel autosomal recessive syndrome designated SERKAL syndrome on the basis of its manifestations: female-to-male sex reversal and kidney, adrenal, and lung dysgenesis were described (18). A disease-causing homozygous missense mutation in the *Wnt4* gene was defined, which resulted in downregulated inhibition of the degradation of beta-catenin, critical for the establishment and maintenance of epithelial layers, such as those lining organ surfaces.

AMH

AMH is produced from the testicular Sertoli cells at seven to eight weeks of gestation, when the testis has recognizable tubules. High ipsilateral concentrations of AMH and testosterone lead to Müllerian duct regression, which would otherwise differentiate into the uterus and fallopian tubes, and Wolffian duct preservation, respectively (19). Notably, there seems to be a window during development when Müllerian duct regression occurs in response to AMH between 8 to 12 weeks of gestation. Misra et al. examined the role of AMH in the evaluation of 65 phenotypic females with mild virilization (20). Among the 28 subjects with AMH concentration above normal female range, all had abnormal gonadal tissue: ovotestes in 11, testes in 7, dysgenetic gonads in 7, and AMH-secreting ovarian tumors in 3. Among the 37 children with serum concentrations in the normal female range, 19 had detectable AMH and 18 had immeasurable AMH. In the former group, 16 subjects had ovaries, 1 had an ovotestis, and 1 had dysgenetic gonads containing testicular elements. Of the18 children with undetectable AMH, 16 had ovaries and 2 had ovarian dysgenesis. The authors concluded that elevation of serum AMH above the normal female range was consistently associated with the presence of testicular tissue or AMH-secreting tumors, requiring additional evaluation and surgical exploration. The type of persistent Müllerian duct syndrome caused by mutation in the *AMH* gene is referred to as type I. A mutation in the AMH receptor (AMHR), which gives the same phenotype, is designated as type II.

SRD5A2

SRD5A2 (steroid-5α-reductase 2) converts testosterone to the more potent 5α-dihydrotestosterone (DHT) in target organs; external genitalia (scrotum and penis) as well as the prostate gland. Deficiency of DHT, consequently, leads to an insufficient male development of external organs but with normal male internal genitalia (21). A lack of this enzyme does not have a phenotype in women. The condition is an autosomal recessively inherited form of male pseudohermaphroditism and was first described in an isolated area in the Dominican Republic (22). Also in this form of male pseudohermaphroditism, there is a masculinization during puberty because of an alternative isoform of the enzyme (SRD5A1). The isoenzyme is not expressed in fetal tissue and only very shortly expressed in newborn skin; however, later in life, after puberty, it is expressed in liver and skin. The remaining physical stigmata in affected individuals even after puberty is a small prostate gland, less body hair, lack of acne, and a female frontal hairline. Because of an underdevelopment of the prostate gland, this disorder almost always leads to male infertility with a few exceptions (23,24). Different mutations cause different degree of impairment of the enzymatic activity due to different functional defects concerning ligand binding, cofactor binding, or half-life of the enzyme that explains the different severity of phenotypes of affected males (25). These patients will subsequently have a high testosterone/DHT ratio, accentuated after hCG-stimulation test that can be used for diagnostic purposes together with mutation analysis.

Defects in Androgen Biosynthesis and Action

The immediate precursor of the gonadal steroids, as well as with the adrenal steroids, is cholesterol.

The conversion of cholesterol to testosterone requires the action of five enzymes: (1) 3β-hydroxysteroid dehydrogenase (3β-HSD); (2) $\Delta^{5,4}$-isomerase; (3) 17α-hydroxylase; (4) $C_{17,20}$ lyase; and (5) 17β-hydroxysteroid dehydrogenase (17β-HSD). The rate-limiting step, as in the adrenals, is cholesterol side-chain cleavage. Mutations in the side-chain cleavage enzyme have never been identified, but instead in the associated steroidogenic acute regulatory (StAR) protein, which facilitates transport of cholesterol from the outer to the inner membrane of mitochondria and is described in the following section.

StAR

StAR plays a crucial role in the transport of cholesterol from the cytoplasm to the inner mitochondrial membrane, facilitating its conversion to pregnenolone. Its essential role in steroidogenesis was demonstrated after observing that *StAR* gene mutations gave rise to the potentially lethal disease lipoid CAH, in which virtually no steroids are produced (26). Lipoid CAH is common among the Japanese, Korean, and Palestinian Arab populations, but is rare elsewhere. Bose et al. described six patients with lipoid CAH (26). All had classical clinical presentations of normal female external genitalia in both genetic sexes, with severe glucocorticoid and mineralocorticoid deficiency presenting in the first month of life. Quite atypically, one patient had small adrenal glands shown by computed tomography scanning. The *StAR* gene was characterized in all six patients. Three of the Japanese patients were heterozygotes for the common Japanese mutation gln258ter in association with three different novel frameshift mutations; the fourth Japanese patient was homozygous for the mutation arg182leu, which is common among Palestinian patients, but had not been described previously in individuals from Japan. The Palestinian and Native American patients were each homozygous for novel frameshift mutations. The authors concluded that the tomography finding of small adrenals in a patient with genetically proven lipoid CAH due to a StAR mutation suggested a substantially broader spectrum of clinical findings in this disease than had been appreciated previously.

3β-HSD

3β-HSD isoenzymes are essential for the formation of progesterone, the precursor hormone for aldosterone, and 17-hydroxyprogesterone (17-OHP), the precursor hormone for cortisol in the adrenal cortex. It is also essential for the formation of androstenedione, testosterone, and oestrogen in the adrenals and gonads, thus catalysing a step in the formation of all classes of active steroid hormones. In humans, there are two 3β-HSD isoenzymes, which were chronologically designated type I and II encoded by the *HSD3B1* and *HSD3B2* gene, respectively. *HSD3B1* gene encodes the almost exclusive 3β-HSD isoenzyme expressed in the placenta and peripheral tissues, whereas *HSD3B2* gene encodes the predominant 3β-HSD isoenzyme expressed in the adrenal gland, ovary, and testis; 3β-HSD, type II deficiency, first described in 1962 is responsible for a rare form of CAH causing various degrees of salt wasting in both sexes and incomplete masculinization of the external genitalia in genetic males (27). Salt loss is a frequent cause of death and may occur even with adequate adrenal replacement therapy, perhaps because of enzyme deficiency in other organs. A milder, nonclassic variant of 3β-HSD deficiency has also been reported to be the cause of premature sexual hair growth in many young children and of hirsutism and menstrual disorders in a great number of adolescent and young women (28).

17ββ-HSD Type 3

17β-HSD type 3 (17β hydroxysteroid dehydrogenase) is the last enzyme during the synthesis pathway from androstenedione to testosterone in the fetal testes. HSD17B3 deficiency is an autosomal recessive disorder that manifests in males as undermasculinization characterized by hypoplastic to normal internal genitalia (epididymis, vas deferens, seminal vesicles, and ejaculatory ducts), but female external genitalia and the absence of a prostate. This phenotype is caused by inadequate testicular synthesis of testosterone, which, in turn, results in insufficient formation of 5α-dihydrotestosterone in the developing external genitalia and prostate during fetal life. At the expected time of puberty, there is a marked increase in plasma luteinizing hormone (LH) and consequently in testicular secretion of androstenedione. Hence, a diagnostic hallmark of this disorder is a decreased plasma testosterone-to-androstenedione ratio (29). There are three isoforms of the enzyme that probably explains the spontaneous masculinization at puberty and the initial fetal male development. The syndrome can, therefore, be suspected in male pseudohermaphrodites with high concentration of androstenedione, exhibiting masculinization during puberty. A high frequency of HSD17B3 deficiency in a highly inbred Arab community in the Gaza strip affecting more than 60 persons has been reported (30). In a single family, 24 affected persons, ranging in age from a few months to 80 years, were identified. The external genitalia were usually female at birth although mild to moderate ambiguity was occasionally present. Gonads were palpable in the inguinal canals or labial folds. Although raised as females, all affected persons developed male body habitués and normal male secondary sexual characteristics at puberty.

LH

During the critical period of sex differentiation, testosterone secretion by the Leydig cells is initially autonomous and thereafter, controlled by maternal choriogonadotropin [human chorionic gonadotropin (hCG)]. After establishment of the pituitary–gonadal axis, this task is accomplished by LH. Leydig cell hypoplasia is a disorder characterized of defect or even absent Leydig cells in the testes, resulting in a low rate of production or absence of testosterone and DHT, generally in combination with elevated levels of LH. In some individuals with Leydig cell hypoplasia, inactivating mutations were detected in the gene encoding the gene for LH (31). In other patients inactivating mutations of the LH receptor, through which both hCG and LH are signaling, were found. An inactivating mutation in the LH receptor of a 46,XY individual can result in phenotypes, ranging from completely female external genitalia to mildly affected individuals. A different form of mutation of the LH receptor gene is associated with male-limited, familial, gonadotropin-independent form of precocious puberty (testotoxicosis). The mutation resulted in a constitutively active LH receptor, which in turn yielded in continuous stimulation of Leydig cells in the absence of LH.

AR

The androgen insensitivity syndrome (AIS), a disorder of male sexual differentiation, is by far the most common identifiable cause of male disorder of sex differentiation (32). AIS is an X-linked recessive disorder, only affecting individuals having a 46,XY karyotype and caused by an absent or dysfunctional androgen receptor (AR). The phenotype encompasses a wide spectrum of genital ambiguities from completely female phenotype to slightly undervirilized males. Both testosterone and DHT bind to the AR and consequently, any defect in the *AR* gene will in the most severe cases, with complete AIS (CAIS), lead to female external appearance, including female external genitalia. Generally, normal but immature testes are present and as differentiation of the embryonic Wolffian ducts occur in response to androgens, Wolffian ducts are absent in individuals with CAIS. Müllerian ducts are usually also absent, as AMH action in the fetus is normal. Usually affected subjects lack pubic and auxiliary hair as well.

At puberty, the androgen resistance results in high LH level in the circulation and subsequently increased testosterone level. Testosterone is in turn peripherally aromatized to oestradiol, which in individuals with AIS is observed as normal breast development and feminization of the body contours. Patients with CAIS come under medical attention at various stages of life, a few being diagnosed soon after birth and some with development of inguinal hernia containing a testis during infancy. A portion of individuals, undiagnosed throughout childhood, present after puberty with primary amenorrhoea.

In the partial form of AIS (PAIS), the genital phenotype in affected individuals varies widely, from predominantly female appearance (cases with female external genitalia and development of pubic hair in puberty, or with slight labial fusion and/or mild clitoromegaly) to subjects with ambiguous genitalia, or cases with predominantly male phenotype. Wolffian duct–derived structures may be fully developed or rudimentary in partial form of AIS, dependent on residual androgen activity. Thus, the epididymides, vasa deferens, and seminal vesicles may develop to a variable extent, from rudimentary to fully formed. At puberty, in general, the degree of feminization is less as compared to individuals with CAIS.

Diagnosis of AIS relies in demonstration of a 46,XY karyotype and functional testes, which are able to synthesize and metabolise androgens normally. Once a CAIS diagnosis has been made, the gonads often are removed, if possible before puberty, because of risk of malignancy. Although some mutations were found several times in unrelated individuals, no major hotspots for mutations exist in the *AR* gene (AR mutation database: http://www.mcgill.ca/androgendb/). In situations where there is a limited family history of the disorder, precise information may be obtained only by sequencing the *AR* gene for the causative mutation.

CLASSIFICATION OF DISORDERS OF SEX DEVELOPMENT

In 2006, a new classification system for what previously was called intersex disorders was proposed by the Lawson Wilkins Pediatric Endocrine Society (LWPES) and the European Society for Paediatric Endocrinology (ESPE). The term disorders of sex development (DSD), defined as congenital conditions in which development of chromosomal, gonadal, or anatomical sex is atypical was proposed to replace the term intersex. A new nomenclature for classifying different forms for DSD was also suggested (33,34). In the new nomenclature, the karyotype is used to prefix the category of DSD and the disorders have been divided into three categories: 46,XY DSD, 46,XX DSD, and sex chromosomal DSD, which are replacing the former terminology that included male and female pseudohermaphroditism and true hermaphroditism (Table 1).

CLINICAL ASSESSMENT

Disorders of male sex development comprise a heterogeneous group of conditions. The modes of presentation are diverse. Patients can come to attention at birth, presenting with

a. ambiguous genitalia;
b. severe hypospadias, with or without undescended testes, micropenis or bifid scrotum;
c. undescended testis with otherwise normal male development;
d. female infant with inguinal hernia;
e. genital anomalies associated with other syndromes.

Presentation in puberty includes virilization of a female, delayed or incomplete pubertal development, primary amenorrhea, and gynecomastia. In adults, hypogonadism and infertility are common modes of presentation.

EXAMINATION

A detailed family history and information about potential exposure to exogenous and endogenous androgens and estrogens are needed. Physical examination should record the palpable gonads and their position, phallic size, site of the urethral opening, one or two openings on the perineum, development of labioscrotal folds, and other anomalies.

LABORATORY STUDIES

The initial management of a child with ambiguous genitalia is focused on establishing a diagnosis allowing early sex assignment. Many schedules for laboratory investigations and imaging of the newborn infant with ambiguous genitalia have been presented. A range of investigations are usually performed as initial diagnostic work-up (Table 2). In most cases, these investigations lead to a functional diagnosis and allow early sex assignment.

CASE STORY

In 2004, a newborn baby was considered to be a girl with a suspected hypertrophic clitoris. Subsequently, the child was found to have a bifid scrotum and both testes were localized in the pelvic cavity by ultrasound and magnetic resonance tomography. A karyotyping was performed, showing 46,XY. Furthermore, ureterography disclosed a short but male-type urethra and the gender assignment was changed to a male with micropenis and hypospadias. A hCG test (1500 IU, IM) resulted in a rise in serum testosterone from 2.2 to 8.8 nM and 5α-dihydrotestosterone (DHT) from 0.08 to 0.34 nM. A swelling of the genitals was noted at inspection.

The pregnancy was normal and the mother of the boy was healthy during the whole period. There was no consanguinity between the parents. The father had a normal boy from a previous marriage. Blood samples were available from both the mother and grandmother.

The molecular work-up showed that the boy had a mutation in the androgen receptor gene, which was inherited from his mother and grandmother. The same mutation was shortly,

Table 2 Investigations Used in the Clinical Assessment of Children with Ambiguous Genitalia

Laboratory investigations
Genetics
FISH with X centromeric and SRY probes
Karyotype
Mutation analysis
Endocrine
17OH-progesterone, 11 deoxycortisol, renin, electrolytes, cortisol
Testosterone androstenedione, DHT
LH, FSH
AMH, inhibin-B
hCG stimulation test
24-hour urinary steroids
Imaging
Pelvic ultrasound
MRI
Other
Cystouretroscopy
Laparoscopy with gonadal biposies
Genital skin biopsies

Abbreviations: FISH, fluorescent in situ hybridization; SRY, sex-determining region of the Y chromosome; DHT, 5α-dihydrotestosterone; LH, luteinizing hormone; FSH, follicle-stimulating hormone; AMH, anti-Müllerian hormone; hCG, human chorionic gonadotropin; MRI, magnetic resonance imaging.

thereafter, also found in a normal man with cryptorchidism in childhood as the only manifestation of reduced androgen sensitivity. Bearing this in mind and since the newborn boy showed significant response to hCG stimulation, treatment with 1% DHT ointment was initiated during his first month of life and resulted in penile growth to 20 mm within two months, which was normal size for age (35).

In complete androgen insensitivity, there is no doubt regarding the gender of the child at birth since the child has female external genitalia. However, in children with disturbed sex differentiation and when there is a mismatch between genotype and phenotype, the management of these patients requires a multidisciplinary practice provided to the patient from birth to adulthood. An overview of normal male sex differentiation, clinical and genetic causes of disturbances in this process, as well as a description of the management of these patients is given in the chapter.

First-line testing includes the following:

1. Karyotyping with fluorescent in situ hybridization (FISH) using an X chromosome centromeric probe and probe for the *SRY* gene. A full karyotype is also needed to confirm the results from the FISH analysis and to rule out mosaicism.
2. Measurement of 17OH-progesterone is a reliable test for 21-hydroxylase deficiency and is mandatory in the initial investigation, especially in children without palpable gonads. The most common cause of ambiguous genitalia is congenital adrenal hyperplasia due to 21-hydroxylase deficiency, resulting in virilization of female infants.
3. In children with XY or XY/XO karyotypes, further investigations aim to assess the presence of testes and if present, their localisation and function.
4. A central test to evaluate the gonads' capacity to secrete androgens is the hCG test, in which Leydig cells are stimulated with hCG (1500 IU, IM, daily for three consecutive days) (36). Testosterone, androstenedione, and DHT are analysed before start of and 24 hours after the last hCG injection. A 2- to 10-fold increase in testosterone is expected. If there is no response to this short hCG-test, a prolonged test over three weeks (1000 IU, IM, twice weekly) can be performed (37). A testosterone-to-androstenedione ratio of less than 0.8 after hCG stimulation indicates 17β-hydroxysteroid dehydrogenase deficiency. A 24-hour urine output collection after the hCG test can be performed for a urinary steroid profile and used for the diagnosis of 5α-reductase deficiency, but is not helpful in the diagnosis of 17β-hydroxysteroid dehydrogenase deficiency (38).
5. Sertoli cell function can be assessed by measurements of AMH and inhibin B. Both proteins are elevated in serum during infancy. AMH levels are increased in children with androgen insensitivity but low in disorders with gonadal dysgenesis. An undetectable value of AMH and inhibin B indicates anorchia (4).
6. Imaging with ultrasound and magnetic resonance imaging is used to elucidate the internal genital anatomy. In addition, laparoscopy with gonadal biopsies is in a large proportion of cases required for diagnosis.

MANAGEMENT

Management of children and adolescents with DSD is complex and includes, as mentioned in the previous sections, establishment of a functional diagnosis allowing sex assignment, surgical correction of genital anomalies such as hypospadias and undescended testes, extirpation of gonads at risk for development of gonadal tumors, hormone replacement therapy during puberty and adulthood, and treatment of infertility. The management of these patients requires a multidisciplinary practice provided to the patient from birth to adulthood. A multidisciplinary team managing children and adolescents with DSD optimally includes an experienced pediatric endocrinologist, pediatric surgeons, and/or urologist, gynecologist, psychologist, geneticist, and social care is preferably performed at specialised tertiary care centers (34).

REFERENCES

1. Jost A. Recherches sur la differenciation sexuelle de l'embryon de lapin. Arch Anat Microsc Morphol Exp 1947; 36:271–315.

2. Chang HJ, Clark RD, Bachman H. The phenotype of 45,X/46,XY mosaicism: An analysis of 92 prenatally diagnosed cases. Am J Hum Genet 1990; 46:156–167.
3. Loojenga LH, Hersmus R, Oosterhuis JW, et al. Tumor risk in disorders of sex development (DSD). Best Pract Res Clin Endocrinol Metab 2007; 21:480–495.
4. Rey RA, Belville C, Nihoul-Fékété C, et al. Evaluation of gonadal function in 107 intersex patients by means of serum antimüllerian hormone measurement. J Clin Endocrinol Metab 1999; 84:627–631.
5. Uehara S, Sato K, Nata M, et al. Complete XY gonadal dysgenesis and aspects of the SRY genotype and gonadal tumor formation. J Hum Genet 2002; 47:279–284.
6. Achermann JC, Ito M, Hindmarsh PC, et al. A mutation in the gene encoding steroidogenic factor-1 causes XY sex reversal and adrenal failure in humans. Nat Genet 1999; 22:125–126.
7. Coutant R, Mallet D, Lahlou N, et al. Heterozygous mutation of steroidogenic factor-1 in 46,XY subjects may mimic partial androgen insensitivity syndrome. J Clin Endocrinol Metab 2007; 92:2868–2873.
8. Lin L, Philibert P, Ferraz-de-Souza B, et al. Heterozygous missense mutations in steroidogenic factor 1 (SF1/Ad4BP, NR5A1) are associated with 46,XY disorders of sex development with normal adrenal function. J Clin Endocrinol Metab 2007; 92:991–999.
9. Little M, Wells C. A clinical overview of WT1 gene mutations. Hum Mutat 1997; 9:209–225.
10. Francke U, Holmes LB, Atkins L, et al. Aniridia-Wilms' tumor association: Evidence for specific deletion of 11p13. Cytogenet Cell Genet 1979; 24:185–192.
11. Pelletier J, Bruening W, Kashtan CE, et al. Germline mutations in the Wilms' tumor suppressor gene disrupt urogenital development in humans. Cell 1991; 67:437–447.
12. Foster JW, Dominguez-Steglich MA, Guioli S, et al. Campomelic dysplasia and autosomal sex reversal caused by mutations in an SRY-related gene. Nature 1994; 372:525–530.
13. Bardoni B, Zanaria E, Guioli G, et al. A dosage sensitive locus at chromosome Xp21 is involved in male to female sex reversal. Nat Genet 1994; 7:497–501.
14. Smyk M, Berg JS, Pursley A, et al. Male-to-female sex reversal associated with an approximately 250 kb deletion upstream of NR0B1 (DAX1). Hum Genet 2007; 122:63–70.
15. Muscatelli F, Strom TM, Walker AP, et al. Mutations in the DAX-1 gene give rise to both X-linked adrenal hypoplasia congenita and hypogonadotropic hypogonadism. Nature 1994; 372:672–676.
16. Lin L, Gu WX, Ozisik G, et al. Analysis of DAX1 (NR0B1) and steroidogenic factor-1 (NR5A1) in children and adults with primary adrenal failure: ten years' experience. J Clin Endocrinol Metab 2006; 91:3048–3054.
17. Biason-Lauber A, Konrad D, Navratil F, et al. A WNT4 mutation associated with Müllerian-duct regression and virilization in a 46,XX woman. N Engl J Med 2004; 351:792–798.
18. Mandel H, Shemer R, Borochowitz ZU, et al. SERKAL syndrome: An autosomal-recessive disorder caused by a loss-of-function mutation in WNT4. Am J Hum Genet 2008; 82:39–47.
19. Josso N, Picarf JY, Tran D. The anti-Müllerian hormone. Recent Prog Horm Res 1977; 33:117–160.
20. Misra M, MacLaughlin DT, Donahoe PK, et al. The role of Müllerian inhibiting substance in the evaluation of phenotypic female patients with mild degrees of virilization. J Clin Endocrinol Metab 2003; 88:787–792.
21. Wilson JD, Griffin JE, Russell DW. Steroid 5-alphereductase 2 deficiency. Endocr Rev 1993; 14:577–593.
22. Imperato-McGinley J, Guerrero L, Gautier T, et al. Steroid 5à-reductase deficiency in man: An inherited form of male pseudohermaphroditism. Science 1974; 186:1213–1215.
23. Katz MD, Kligman I, Cai LQ, et al. Paternity by intrauterine insemination with sperm from a man with 5alpha-reductase-2 deficiency. N Engl J Med 1997; 336:994–997.
24. Nordenskjold A, Ivarsson SA. Molecular characterization of 5 alpha-reductase type 2 deficiency and fertility in a Swedish family. J Clin Endocrinol Metab 1998; 83:3236–3238.
25. Wigley WC, Prihoda JS, Mowszowicz I, et al. Natural mutagenesis study of the human steroid 5 alpha-reductase 2 isozyme. Biochemistry 1994; 33:1265–1270.
26. Bose HS, Sato S, Aisenberg J, et al. Mutations in the steroidogenic acute regulatory protein (StAR) in six patients with congenital lipoid adrenal hyperplasia. J Clin Endocrinol Metab 2000; 85:3636–3639.
27. Bongiovanni AM. The adrenogenital syndrome with deficiency of 3 beta-hydroxysteroid dehydrogenase. J Clin Invest 1962; 41:2086–2092.
28. Nayak S, Lee PA, Witchel SF. Variants of the type II 3beta-hydroxysteroid dehydrogenase gene in children with premature pubic hair and hyperandrogenic adolescents. Mol Genet Metab 1998; 64:184–192.
29. Geissler WM, Davis DL, Wu L, et al. Male pseudohermaphroditism caused by mutations of testicular 17beta-hydroxysteroid dehydrogenase 3. Nat Genet 1994; 7: 34–39.
30. Rosler A, Kohn G. Male Pseudo-hermaphroditism due to 17-beta-hydroxysteroid dehydrogenase-deficiency—Studies on the natural-history of the defect and effect of androgens on gender role. J Steroid Biochem Mol Biol 1983; 19:663–674.
31. Latronico AC, Anasti J, Arnhold IJ, et al. A novel mutation of the luteinizing hormone receptor gene causing male gonadotropin-independent precocious puberty. J Clin Endocrinol Metab 1995; 80:2490–2494.

32. Quigley CA, De Bellis A, Marschke KB, et al. Androgen receptor defects: Historical, clinical, and molecular perspectives. Endocr Rev 1995; 16:271–321.
33. Hughes IA. Disorders of sex development: A new definition and classification. Best Pract Res Clin Endocrinol Metab 2008; 22:119–134.
34. Hughes IA, Houk C, Ahmed SF, et al. Consensus statement on management of intersex disorders. Arch Dis Child 2006a; 91:554–563.
35. Giwercman YL, Ivarsson SA, Richthoff J, et al. A novel mutation in the D-box of the androgen receptor gene (S597R) in two unrelated individuals is associated with both normal phenotype and severe PAIS. Hormone Research 2004; 61:58–62.
36. Hughes IA, Debb A. Androgen resistance. Best Pract Res Clin Endocrinol Metab 2006; 20:577–598.
37. Honour JW, Savage MO. Endocrine function of the testis. In: Ranke MB, ed. Diagnosis of Endocrine Function in Children and Adolescents. Basel, Switzerland: Karger, 2003:339–355.
38. Faisal Ahmed S, Iqbal A, Hughes IA. The testosterone: Androstenedione ratio in male undermasculinization. Clin Endocrinol (Oxf) 2000; 53:697–702.

26 Disturbances in male pubertal development

Olle Söder

KEY POINTS (LEVEL OF EVIDENCE)

- According to Tanner, assessment of pubertal development in boys should be based on family history, the longitudinal growth chart, and clinical examination with staging of puberty.
- The first signs of puberty in boys are usually enlargement of testicular volume, initiation of the pubertal growth spurt, and evidence of skin puberty (pubic hair growth, apocrine sweating).
- Delayed puberty is the most common disorder of puberty in boys and most frequent because of a hereditary component in otherwise healthy boys. If treatment is required, testosterone in different formulations is an effective treatment to induce puberty in most cases.
- Precocious puberty in boys is more rare and more often because of an organic cause. Gonadotropin releasing hormone (GnRH) agonists are effective treatment to halt pubertal development in cases with central precocious puberty.

PHYSIOLOGY OF PUBERTY

Puberty is the transition period between childhood and adulthood during which reproductive function is attained. It is a developmental continuum and not a one-stage event and includes endocrine, physical, psychological, and psychosocial changes. In contrast to all other species, puberty in humans lasts for an extended period of time, lasting four to six years, and encompasses an important phase of psychosocial development during adolescence. This maturational phase seems important for adaptation to societal needs and must be a recent addition to evolution. Final height is reached after a phase of increased growth velocity, referred to as the pubertal growth spurt.

The clinical signs observed at the onset of puberty are due to the awakening of the hypothalamic–pituitary–gonadal (HPG) axis and the endocrine effects of sex hormones appearing in the circulation. This results in growth and maturational development of the genital organs and the appearance of the secondary sex characteristics. Typical first signs are testicular enlargement in males, breast development in females, and pubic/axillary hair growth in both sexes. Menarche in girls, usually appearing at mean age 12.5 years of Western societies, and spermarche in boys (release of mature sperm; mean age 13.5 years) are precise events when it comes to determination of their first appearance, although assessment of spermarche requires urine sampling and cannot be recorded from patients' reports.

The existence of a hypothalamic pulse generator is well established, which triggers GnRH pulsatile secretion by hypothalamic neurons and activates gonadotropin secretion by the pituitary. However, the nature of this pulse generator and the detailed signaling mechanisms, setting the pubertal clock to trigger the onset of puberty at a certain predetermined time point, are largely unknown. Humans share the fundamental principles of the regulation of pubertal activation with other vertebrate animals including nonhuman primates, but the set of neuroendocrine mediators involved seem to differ between species. However, a common principle seems to be that the pulse generator is intrinsically active and must be reversibly suppressed by inhibitory signals from neurotransmitters such as GABA. In humans, the hypothalamic pulse generator is functional and shows sexual dimorphism already in the fetal stage. Postnatally it becomes more active during the first months of life in boys ("baby puberty") and is then dampened to quiescence during childhood. At start of puberty, nightly reactivation of the GnRH pulse generator results in elevated levels of pulsatile LH secretion, triggering gonadal production and endocrine actions of the sex steroids. For reviews, see (1,2).

REGULATION OF PUBERTAL TIMING

Several factors have been shown to be related to the onset of puberty in humans, but large gaps still remain in our understanding of the genetic and environmental mechanisms involved in the control of onset of puberty. There are also notable differences between the sexes in the regulation of puberty, which, at least partially, is due to the obvious gender dimorphism in reproductive function. Factors that have been suggested to be associated with the timing of the onset of puberty are listed in Table 1. Historically, a secular trend to an earlier onset of puberty has been observed during the last centuries, generally believed to be due to improvement in general health status and psychosocial burdens of children. This trend, which has subtracted several years to the age of menarche during the last three centuries, is still observed in developing countries but should not be mixed up with the more recent findings of earlier onset of puberty of girls observed in the USA (3,4). In boys, the timing of puberty does not seem to have changed and is considered normal when it starts between 9.5 and 14 years of age (5,6).

Twin studies have shown that heritable factors account for more than 70% of the observed variability in pubertal timing. Clinically this is reflected by the observation that both delayed and precocious puberty most often show a familial pattern and that there are also well-described ethnic differences. However,

Table 1 Factors Related to the Timing of Onset of Puberty in Humans

Factor	Clinical and epidemiological correlate
Genetic	Familial delayed and precocius puberty, ethnicity
Health	Secular trend, infection, inflammatory disorders
Nutrition	Calorie malnutrition, anorexia nervosa, excessive labor
Psychosocial	Secular trend, adoption, earlier societal exposure to sexuality
Environmental	Exposure to endocrine disruptors, chemotherapy, endocrine drugs

the genetic structure of the trait is still poorly understood. Independent of these factors, gender is the most established determinant behind age differences at puberty onset. Thus, girls are on average two years earlier than boys in their normal pubertal development, which of course, needs to be accounted for when defining reference values for precocious and delayed puberty (7).

NUTRITIONAL FACTORS AND PUBERTY ONSET

There are common hypothalamic regulator mechanisms controlling the energy balance and food intake and the onset of puberty, which act through redundant pathways. Leptin and kisspeptin/GPR54 are the recently discovered mediators in this field, attracting considerable attention (7,8). At the population level, differences in energy intake may add to the physiological variations in timing of puberty, but such link may be more complex. It is obvious that an optimal nutritional status is of benefit for fetal survival (i.e., for female reproduction), which may be reflected by the earlier onset of puberty found in overweight girls (3,9). For males such link to calorie supply may not be beneficial or may even be negative, which may relate to the observation that obese boys often show late puberty. This may be compared with the situation in children with calorie malnutrition, as in many developing countries and in diagnoses such as anorexia nervosa and short bowel disorders, as well as in certain sports with high energy costs, where affected individuals often show late puberty.

CLINICAL SIGNS OF PUBERTY

The specific pubertal signs in boys usually show a certain order of appearance, although individual differences are common. The following ordered series of events is common:

1. Increased testicular volume
2. Start of longitudinal growth spurt
3. Pubic hair
4. Apocrine sweating and acne
5. Penile enlargement and muscular hypertrophy
6. Voice break

Endocrine effects of androgens are responsible for most of these pubertal signs, including penile growth, longitudinal growth spurt, muscular hypertrophy, androgen-dependent hair growth, activation of sebaceous glands with greasy skin and acne, and voice break due to growth of the larynx and the vocal cords.

Testicular growth is usually the first sign of puberty in boys and constitutes an integrated measure of a successful endocrine action of gonadotropins and paracrine effect of androgen on the testis, resulting in the start of spermatogenesis. This process increases the volume of the testis to >3 mL., which is easily determined by the use of a Prader orchidometer (Fig. 1). The penis has an average prepubertal length of 6 cm and increases to approximately 13 cm, measured from os pubis to tip of the glans penis in the stretched flaccid state. Other early signs of onset of puberty are the appearance of an apocrine sweat scent and an increased velocity of longitudinal growth, announcing the start of the pubertal growth spurt. It is not uncommon that boys are referred to the pediatric endocrinologist with a request for work up and treatment of short stature, although the real problem is delayed puberty with yet no recorded accelerated growth velocity, indicative of the onset of the pubertal growth spurt. Such boys retain their prepubertal growth velocity, resulting in a drop in growth channels, when compared with the age-matched normative growth pattern. Therefore, a properly plotted growth chart must always be at hand when growth and pubertal problems are to be investigated, to judge if the pubertal growth spurt has started (see Case Presentation and Fig. 2). Final height is gained after completion of the pubertal growth spurt, which is obvious from the individual growth charts, when growth velocity is approaching null. This reflects terminal differentiation and closure of the epiphyseal growth plates, which can be monitored by radiological

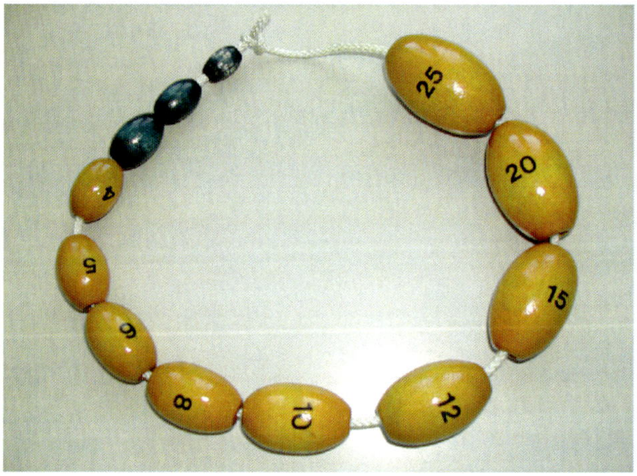

Figure 1 Prader orchidometer used as reference for testicular volume. Volumes 1 to 3 mL (blue color) represents prepubertal status and 4 mL onset of puberty.

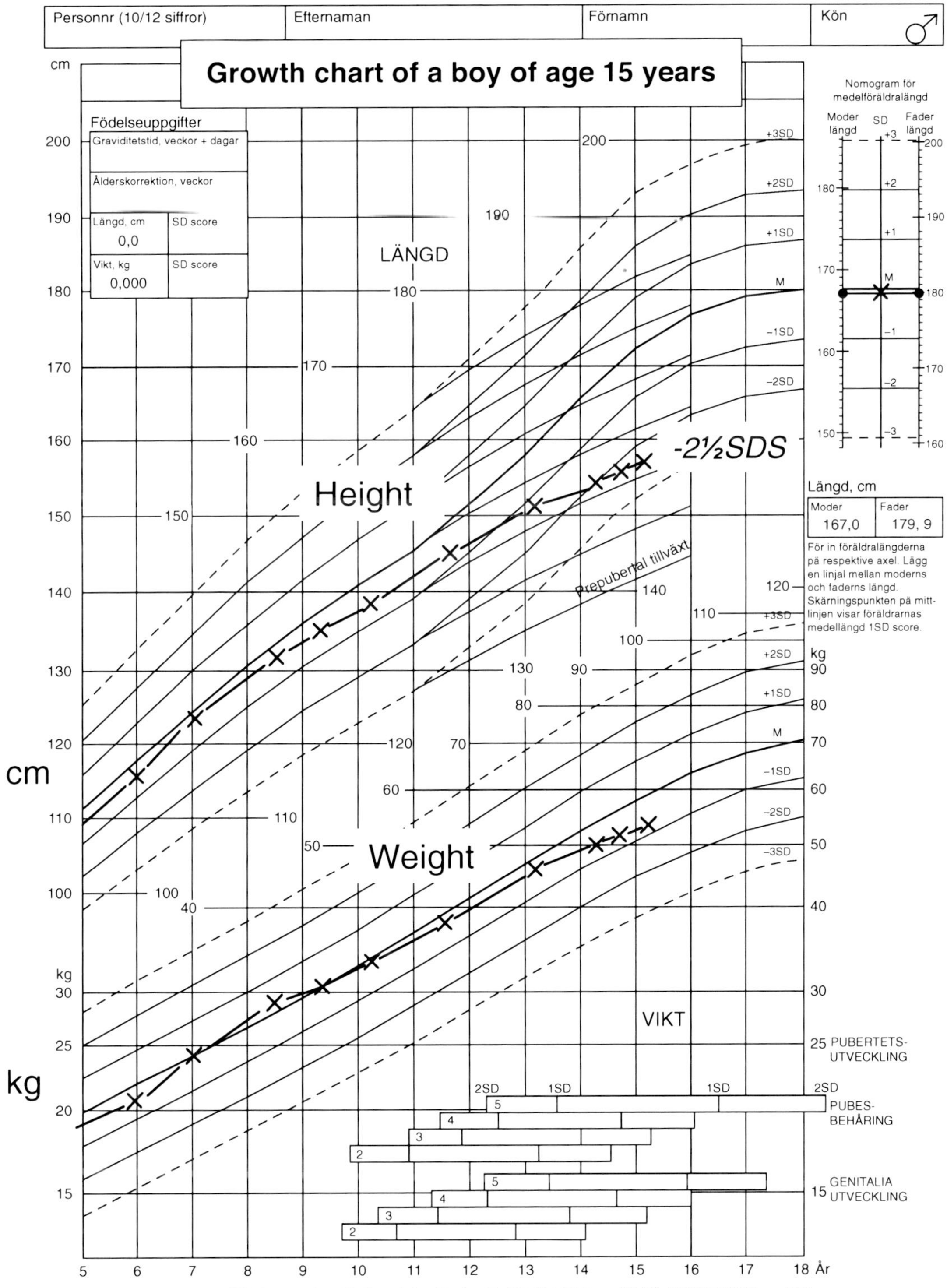

Figure 2 Growth chart of a boy referred as a result of short stature (see Case Presentation).

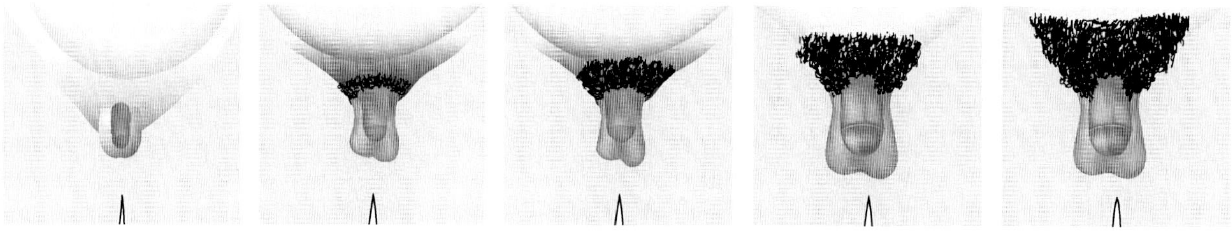

Figure 3 Tanner stages of male pubertal development. Genital (G) and pubic hair (PH) status are scored 1 to 5 independently, where score 1 represents prepubertal status and score 5 full adult development. Note that G and PH status are not always parallel events.

examination of the skeleton. X-ray examination of the left hand is used for calculation of the status of prepubertal bone maturation (bone age), which should be equal to chronological age if normal. Patients with precious puberty typically show advanced bone age whereas delayed puberty is characterized by retarded bone age.

TANNER STAGING

Tanner stages define physical measures of pubertal development on a 5-grade scale and include staging of pubic hair growth and the appearance of external genitalia, that is, size and maturational markers (skin color, wrinkles) of penis and scrotum, the latter also reflecting testicular size, which should be recorded separately. Although Tanner staging always includes a subjective component, it is important when judging puberty, as the tempo of pubertal development may also vary considerably. Tanner stage 1 refers to the prepubertal status whereas stage 5 represents the final adult outcome (Fig. 3).

Pubic hair in boys usually appear initially on the scrotum and at the base of the penis. Facial hair appear initially on the corners of the upper lip and the upper cheeks and spread to the rest of the face and chin. All skin puberty effects are due to increased levels of sex steroids from the gonads and a small contribution from adrenal cortex. Pubertal growth spurt occurs during Tanner stages 3 to 4 of puberty, and is completed by stage 5 in most boys.

DISORDERS OF PUBERTY

Diagnosis of Pubertal Disorders

Normal age of puberty is statistically defined and has a strong heritable component. Delayed puberty is much more common in boys than girls (10:1) and is defined as absence of pubertal signs before age 14 or later in boys and a corresponding delay of Tanner staging at appropriate later age. Precocious puberty is much less common in boys than girls (1:10) and is diagnosed if two pubertal signs appear before age 9 in boys.

Pubertal disorders should be diagnosed by use of family and clinical history, physical examination with Tanner staging, and growth chart, covering the whole period from birth to present age. Thus, precious and delayed puberty are clinical diagnoses and hormonal analyses are not needed for verification. However, a work-up including laboratory analyses and radiological examinations is often required to reveal the underlying cause of the disorder, although most cases are idiopathic with no obvious underlying pathology, representing outlayers of the statistical distribution curve of normal pubertal timing. A substantial number of idiopathic cases may still require treatment and follow-up and are, therefore, important to investigate thoroughly.

Delayed Puberty

Delayed puberty is the most common pubertal disorder in boys and is most often because of familial delay of unknown genetic cause. Typically, short stature is also a prominent component. This condition is referred to as constitutional delay of growth and puberty (CDGP) and is, by definition, transitory, albeit treatment may still be important, particularly in cases associated with psychosocial problems. There are also a number of other less common causes of delayed puberty that need to be excluded before treatment, if any, is initiated. Table 2 lists the most frequent causes of delayed puberty in boys divided into central and peripheral failure. Most common is central delayed puberty, also referred to as hypogonadotropic (or secondary) hypogonadism. In such case, the HPG axis is not activated and hormonal levels remain at prepubertal level. If a specific cause is not detected, it may be hard to discriminate hypogonadotropic hypogonadism from CDGP. However, the latter condition should always come with a family history and be self-limiting with spontaneous onset of puberty at later age, although this may occasionally occur as late as in the early twenties.

In gonadal failure, gonadotropin levels are elevated, which is an important diagnostic measure. This is much less common except for cases with a diagnostic medical history, for example, bilateral cryptorchidism with poor treatment outcome.

Clinical Work-up of Delayed Puberty

As stated above, delayed puberty is a clinical diagnosis but determining what specific level of the HPG axis that is engaged requires an endocrine laboratory work-up, guided by the

Table 2 Causes of Delayed Puberty in Boys

Hypogonadotropic hypogonadism (central failure)
Idiopatic
Familial (constitutional delay of growth and puberty; 85%)
Isolated gonadotropin deficiency
Panhypopituitarism
Genetic, syndromes
Kallman (KAL-1, FGFR1)
KiSS/GPR54
GnRH-R
Prader-Willi
Leptin, Leptin-R
Disorder of sex development (DSD)
Tumor
Craniopharyngeoma
Hypothalamic tumor
Prolactinoma
Negative calorie balance
Chronic illness, inflammation
Short bowel
Anorexia nervosa
Psychogenic
Excessive physical activity
Iatrogenic
Survivors of childhood cancer
CNS irradiation
Brain surgery
Total body irradiation
Chemotherapy
Hypergonadotropic hypogonadism (gonadal failure)
Chromosomal, genetic
Klinefelter
Other
Undescended testes
Bilateral, untreated
Testicular atrophy
Testicular agenesis
Torsion
Unknown cause
Iatrogenic
Gonadal irradiation
Other
Defects in androgen biosynthesis

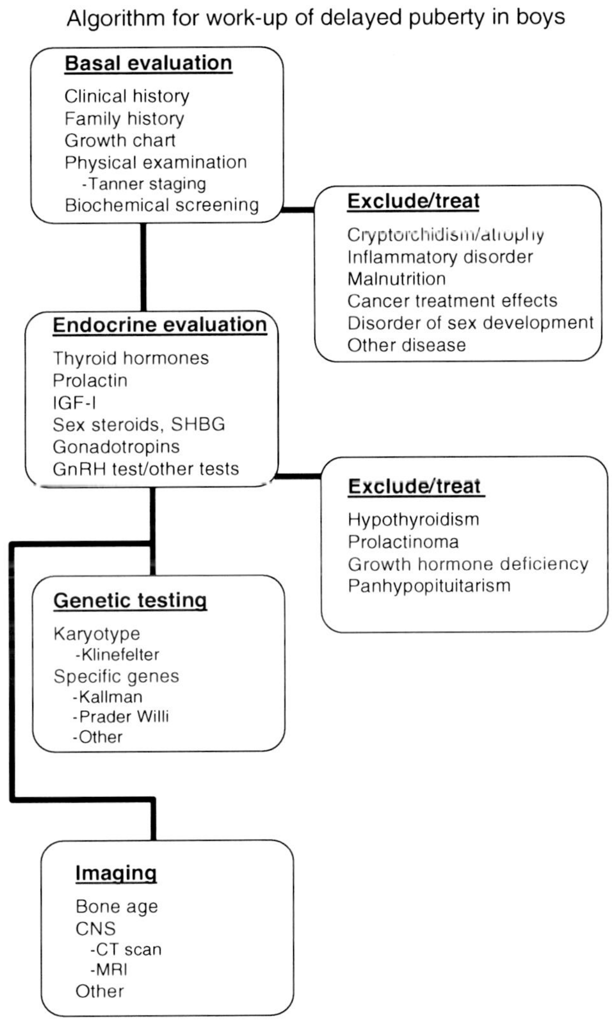

Flowchart I Basic algorithm for work-up of boys with delayed puberty. Careful phenotyping at the first step (clinical evaluation) is most important and should guide the following steps. The most common diagnosis is constitutional delay in growth and puberty. By definition, this diagnosis is self-limiting, but may need transient treatment for psychosocial reasons.

clinical observations. Flowchart I suggests an algorithm for work-up of boys with delayed puberty.

Treatment of Delayed Puberty

Treatment of delayed puberty should be causal, if possible, but androgen replacement therapy may be required for short period or permanently, depending on the specific diagnosis. In boys with transient delay of pubertal development such as in CDGP, which is the most common cause, counseling without pharmacological intervention is the preferred action. This is mostly accepted by the affected boy and his parents because of the familial nature of the disorder and identification of other affected family members. However, many boys with delayed puberty suffer from psychosocial pressure due to bullying and exclusion by peers from sports and social activities, which may lead to low self-esteem, isolation, and depression. Such cases are also underreported to the parents and must be actively explored by the physician, since many boys are hesitant to reveal their psychosocial situation.

In selected cases of CDGP and more frequently in boys with other causes of delayed puberty, treatment with androgen should be installed. The strategy should be to mimic endogenous androgen production in puberty by delivering androgen at low initial dose. Testosterone in depot formulations (e.g., as propionate ester) is usually effective and well tolerated (6,10). Other formulations such as transdermal patches and gel compositions may also be tried, especially in subjects with aversion against injection needles. For young patients requiring a short period of pubertal induction, long-acting androgen depot formulations such as undecanoate esters are less desirable since short-term fine-tuning of the dosing is not possible.

The recommended initial monthly single dose is 75 to 125 mg, to be increased gradually to adult replacement dose if permanent treatment is required. For induction of puberty in naïve patients, a treatment period of at least six months is recommended. The patient should then be re-examined to document the results. The expected outcome is appearance of pubertal signs such as pubic hair, growth of genitalia, and others, which should be documented in the records with reference to Tanner stages. Testicular enlargement is not a sign of the action of exogenous androgen but rather a record of the desired endogenous activation due to action of gonadotropins. In some patients an additional period of treatment of three to –six months may be needed. If signs of endogenous pubertal activity are recorded, that is, the testicular growth, the androgen replacement should be reconsidered and tapered to allow release from negative feedback exerted by the exogenous androgens and to invite a more rapid endogenous activation. Treatment of children with gonadotropin formulations to increase gonadal size and help possible future function, including fertility, has been studied but is still considered experimental (11).

Although individual sensitivity to androgen treatment may be seen and requires differential dosing, all boys with normal genital anatomy respond to androgen treatment. Poor responders may be found among patients with genital anomalies such as severe hypospadia and bilateral cryptorchidism, indicating partial androgen insensitivity.

If endogenous puberty does not start and progress well after induction of puberty by androgen therapy, the diagnosis of CDGP should be reconsidered and the patient should be subjected to work-up by a specialist to find an alternative diagnosis.

Precocious Puberty

Precocious puberty is much less common in boys than in girls and is more often associated with concomitant pathology than delayed puberty in boys. Still, similar to delayed puberty, most cases are familiar and thought to be due to an early but otherwise normal activation of the "pubertal clock" in affected cases and families. Central and peripheral causes of precocious puberty can be distinguished. Table 3 lists common causes of precocious puberty in boys. Central or gonadotropin-dependent precocious puberty is most common. It is characterized by hypothalamic activation of GnRH neurons and pulsatile secretion of pituitary gonadotropins, activating testicular androgen production and spermatogenesis. Peripheral or gonadotropin-independent precocious puberty (GIPP) is much less common and accounts for less than 10% of cases (12–14).

Table 3 Common Causes of Precocious Puberty in Boys

Hypergonadotropic hypergonadism (central)
Idiopatic
Familial
Tumor cerebri
Hamartoma
Other
CNS lesion
Hydrocephalus
Hypogonadotropic hypergonadism (peripheral)
Congenital adrenal hyperplasia (CAH)
21-OH-deficiency
Other
Steroid-producing tumor
Adrenal
Gonadal
Ectopic gonadotropin secretion
Activating LH receptor mutation
McCune Albright syndrome
Exogenous
Iatrogenic
Accidental exposure to hormones
Environmental factors with endocrine action (EDCs)

Abbreviations: EDCs, endocrine disrupting compounds.

Clinical Work-up of Precocious Puberty

Given the higher prevalence of associated pathology in boys with precocious puberty, the work-up should be more aggressive than for delayed puberty, particularly with younger age and in the absence of familiar history. Flowchart II shows an algorithm for work-up in boys with precocious puberty. The use of endocrine tests and imaging procedures should be guided by the clinical signs and the outcomes of screening tests.

Treatment of Precocious Puberty

Causal treatment is the aim in cases with organic causes of precocious puberty, if possible. Such cases include, for example, hydrocephalus, CNS tumors, and conditions with ectopic production of gonadotropins. In idiopathic central precious puberty (CPP), high dose long-acting depot GnRH agonist is the preferred treatment (13). The desirable action of such treatment is suppression of the pulsatile gonadotropin secretion by the pituitary, which is typically achieved after monthly dosing for a period of 2 months. Boys with precocious puberty may also be under psychosocial pressure, which is an important indication for treatment. Compromised adult final height is another

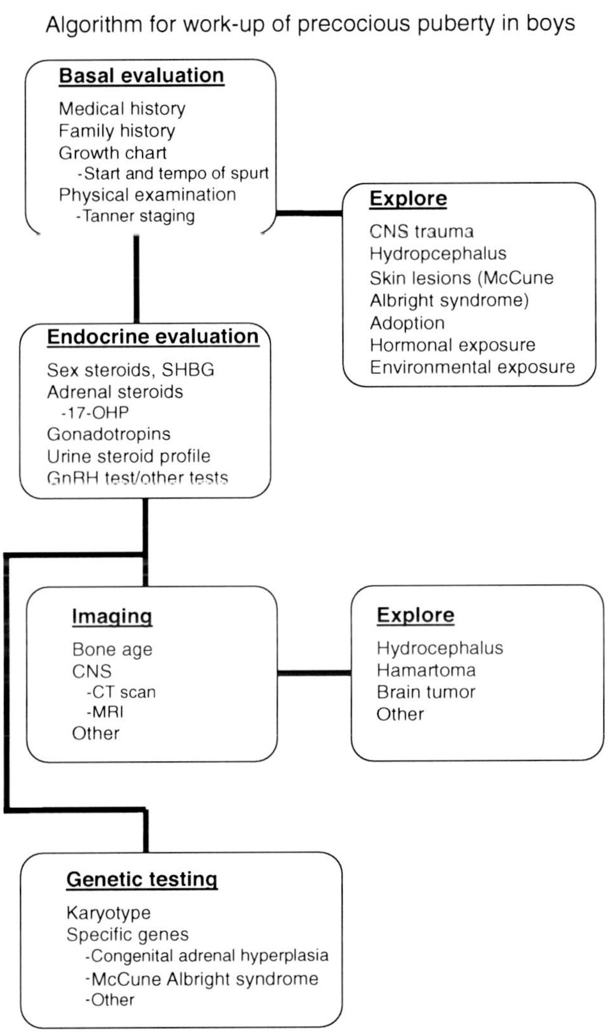

Flowchart II Basic algorithm for work-up of boys with precocious puberty. Careful phenotyping at the first step (clinical evaluation) is most important and should guide the following steps. Precocius puberty in boys is much less common than delayed puberty and should alert the physician to investigate a possible organic background.

indication for treatment and is evaluated by determination of bone age and calculation of projected final height.

In cases of peripheral (gonadotropin independent) precocious puberty (GIPP), treatment options are less favorable since GnRH agonists do not function. Causal treatment, by increasing corticosteroid and mineralocorticoid dosing thus suppressing adrenal androgen production, is preferable and usually successful in congenital adrenal hyperplasia (CAH). Symptomatic treatment options are androgen receptor antagonists such as flutamide, bicalutamide, and cyproterone.

The duration of treatment is to be discussed with the family but is most often determined by the chronological age of the patient with proposed termination at the desired age of puberty.

CASE PRESENTATION

Peter, age 15, comes with his parents to see the pediatric endocrinologist for short stature. There is an uneventful medical history and the boy is performing well in school. Hereditary background reveals a midparental height or a target height at –0.2 standard deviation (SD) from the mean height of the appropriate growth chart [often referred to as –0.2 SD scores (SDS)]. Peter's older sister, now age 17, is of normal stature (height +0.5 SDS) and had her menarche at age 14.5. The mother reports she had her menarche at age 13 and the father recalls he started growth spurt very late as compared to his schoolmates. It was found that Peter has been growing at the expected midparental height (MPH) channel until age 10, when his growth pace started lagging, resulting in today's stature of –2.5 SDS (Fig. 2). The actual growth velocity was calculated to 5 cm/yr on the basis of the two measurements: at present visit and 8 months earlier. The father told that Peter was a leading player in the school's football team when he was younger, but recently quitted the team "because it is not fun anymore." Physical examination revealed normal body proportions, thin musculature, and no signs of any disorder. Pubertal status showed Tanner 2 with a testicular volume of 5 mL on both sides. Routine biochemistry was normal and basal gonadotropins were low.

The diagnosis is delayed puberty and this is an illustration of a typical case at the pediatric endocrinologist's office. The family history reveals delayed puberty (father, sister) and physical examination indicates early signs of start of puberty (increased testicular volume). In cases with high psychosocial pressure, treatment with testosterone for three to—six months may be offered, which most often resolves the problem. The dose should be lower than that used for adult replacement therapy, for example, 75 to 125 mg of testosterone propionate monthly.

REFERENCES

1. Roth CL, Ojeda SR. Genes involved in the neuroendocrine control of normal puberty and abnormal puberty of central origin. Pediatr Endocrinol Rev 2005; 3:67–76.
2. Grumbach MM. The neuroendocrinology of human puberty revisited. Horm Res 2002; 57(suppl 2):2–14.
3. Kaplowitz PB, Slora EJ, Wasserman RC, et al. Earlier onset of puberty in girls: relation to increased body mass index and race. Pediatrics 2001; 108:347–353.
4. Lee JM, Appugliese D, Kaciroti N, et al. Weight status in young girls and the onset of puberty. Pediatrics 2007; 119:624–630.
5. Gluckman PD, Hanson MA. Evolution, development and timing of puberty. Trends Endocrinol Metab 2006; 17: 7–12.

6. Richmond EJ, Rogol AD. Male pubertal development and the role of androgen therapy. Nat Clin Pract Endocrinol Metab 2007; 3:338–344.
7. Ghizzoni L., Street ME, Marchesi M, et al. Normal and abnormal puberty. In: New M, ed. Pediatric Endocrinology. 2007:chap 13. Endotext.com. http://www.endotext.org/pediatrics/pediatrics13/pediatricsframe13.htm. Accessed March 1, 2010.
8. Tena-Sempere M. KiSS-1 and reproduction: focus on its role in the metabolic regulation of fertility. Neuroendocrinology 2006; 83:275–281.
9. Kaplowitz PB. Link between body fat and the timing of puberty. Pediatrics 2008; 121(suppl 3):S208–S217.
10. Rogol AD. Pubertal androgen therapy in boys. Pediatr Endocrinol Rev 2005; 2:383–390.
11. Hayes FJ, Pitteloud N. Hypogonadotropic hypogonadism (HH) and gonadotropin therapy. In: McLachlan R, ed. Endocrinology of male reproduction. 2004:chap 5. Endotext.com. http://www.endotext.org/male/male5/maleframe5.htm. Accessed March 1, 2010.
12. Muir A. Precocius puberty. Pediatr Rev 2006; 23:373–381.
13. Tuvemo T. Treatment of central precocious puberty. Expert Opin Investig Drugs 2006; 15:495–505.
14. Papathanasiou A, Hadjiathanasiou C. Precocious puberty. Pediatr Endocrinol Rev 2006; 3(suppl 1):182–7.

27 Clinical investigation and laboratory analyses in male hypogonadism

Gianni Forti, Giovanni Corona, and Mario Maggi

DEFINITION OF MALE HYPOGONADISM

Any situation of testicular failure, that is, impairment/lack of either (or both) of the two main functions of the testes: testosterone secretion and/or sperm formation. Testicular failure can result from disease of the testes (primary hypogonadism) or disease of the pituitary or hypothalamus (secondary hypogonadism).

SUMMARY: DIAGNOSIS OF MALE HYPOGONADISM

In prepubertal age, the diagnosis of male hypogonadism is difficult because testes are physiologically quiescent. No specific symptom is present and hormone assays are in the normal range.

In a **postpubertal/adult male**, impairment of testosterone secretion by the testes can be suspected on the basis of history taking and physical examination.

- Clinical history: symptoms of androgen deficiency are lack or reduced libido, erectile dysfunction, poor beard growth, reduced or absent ejaculate, low energy, asthenia, depressed mood.
- Clinical examination: objective findings of androgen deficiency are dependent on whether the disease has a prepubertal or postpubertal onset. Prepubertal onset implies eunuchoid proportions, infantile genitalia (penis and testes), gynecomastia, lack or reduced facial and pubic/axillary hair, small prostate. In subjects with normal pubertal development, the body proportions and genital development are normal, but the subjects may have a reduced muscle mass, gynecomastia, and/or female fat distribution.

The diagnosis will be confirmed by the **laboratory finding of low testosterone** levels. In primary and secondary hypogonadism, high and low/normal levels of LH and follicle-stimulating hormone (FSH) will be found, respectively.

Blood karyotyping and imaging techniques (NMR of the pituitary region) can be useful to complete the diagnostic procedure. In men with congenital hypogonadotropic hypogonadism, the sense of smell should also be checked since anosmia/hyposmia is a part of Kallmann syndrome (see below).

INTRODUCTION: ROLE OF THE HUMAN TESTIS FROM FETAL TO ADULT LIFE

The differentiation of the bivalent gonad into a testis starts around the sixth week of fetal life and is dependent on the presence of a normal Y chromosome and the activity of a network of genes (1,2). The secretion of testosterone (T) by the fetal testis in the first trimester is regulated by the chorionic gonadotropin (hCG) produced by the placenta and begins around the eighth to ninth week. Circulating T levels in male fetus reach values comparable to those of adult males around 12th to 14th week. Between the 8th and the 12th week of gestation, T induces the differentiation of Wolffian ducts into epididymis, vas deferens, and seminal vesicles, whereas Mullerian duct regression is induced by the Mullerian-inhibiting hormone secreted by the Sertoli cells. In the same period of fetal life, external genitalia differentiate into scrotum and penis because of the effects of locally produced dihydrotestosterone, which is also the main inducer of prostate development (3). In the second and third trimester of pregnancy the secretion of T by the fetal testis decreases but is still important for the testicular descent into the scrotum and the penile growth.

At birth after the withdrawal of gestational steroids, FSH and LH rise and in males T levels increase to nearly adult levels for—two to three months, but after six months of age infancy is characterized by the almost complete functional quiescence of the testis and T levels in boys overlap those of girls.

At puberty, due to the reactivation of the hypothalamic–pituitary axis, increased secretion of GnRH and pituitary gonadotropins stimulate Leydig cells (LH) and seminiferous tubules (FSH): The increased levels of T induce the differentiation of male secondary sex characteristics (development of external genitalia, sex accessory glands, body and facial hair growth, muscle development, libido) and in combination with FSH induce the multiplication of Sertoli cells and the initiation of spermatogenesis (3). Reduced levels of testosterone with aging induce some regression of the masculinization. (Fig. 1)

It is now well known that some of the effects of T are due to its transformation in dihydrotestosterone (hair growth, penile, and scrotal growth) and oestradiol (epiphyseal cartilages closure after the growth spurt) see Fig. 2.

During the adult life the testis has two main functions: (a) the production of mature sperm (100–200 millions/24 hr); (b) the maintenance of secondary sex characteristics by the secretion of testosterone: libido, hair growth, and muscle and bone mass.

CAUSES OF MALE HYPOGONADISM

Hypogonadism in a male can result either from a disease of the testis involving T and/or sperm production (primary hypogonadism) or from a disease of the pituitary or the hypothalamus usually involving both testicular functions (secondary hypogonadism).

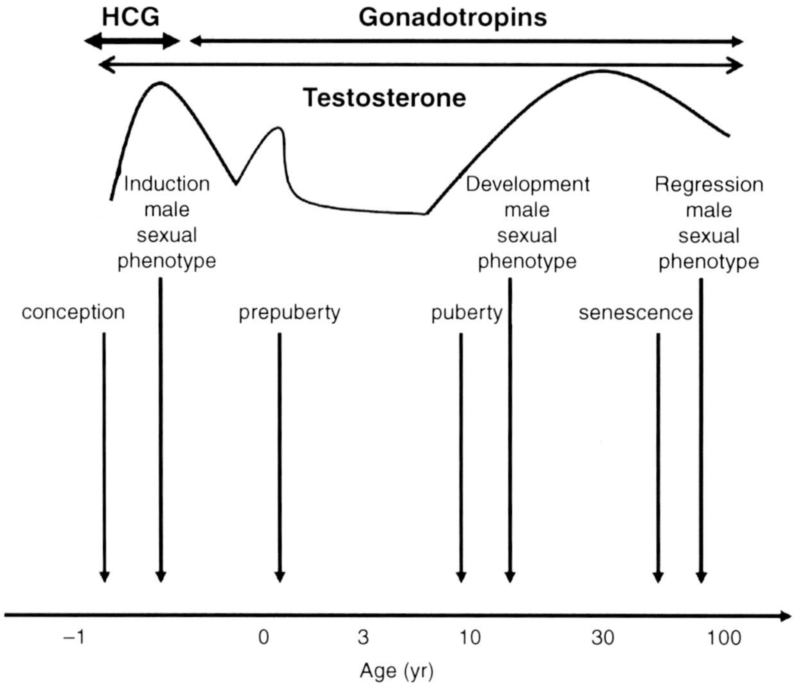

Figure 1 Schematic representation of testosterone levels and their biological effects on the male phenotype during the different phases of life. Secretion of testosterone during the first trimester of fetal life (under hCG control) is necessary for the differentiation of the internal and external male genitalia. The biological effects of the high levels of testosterone during the first—three to four months of life is unknown. Testosterone secretion at puberty is important for the completion of the differentiation of the male phenotype. Some regression of the male phenotype occurs with aging due to the reduced levels of testosterone.

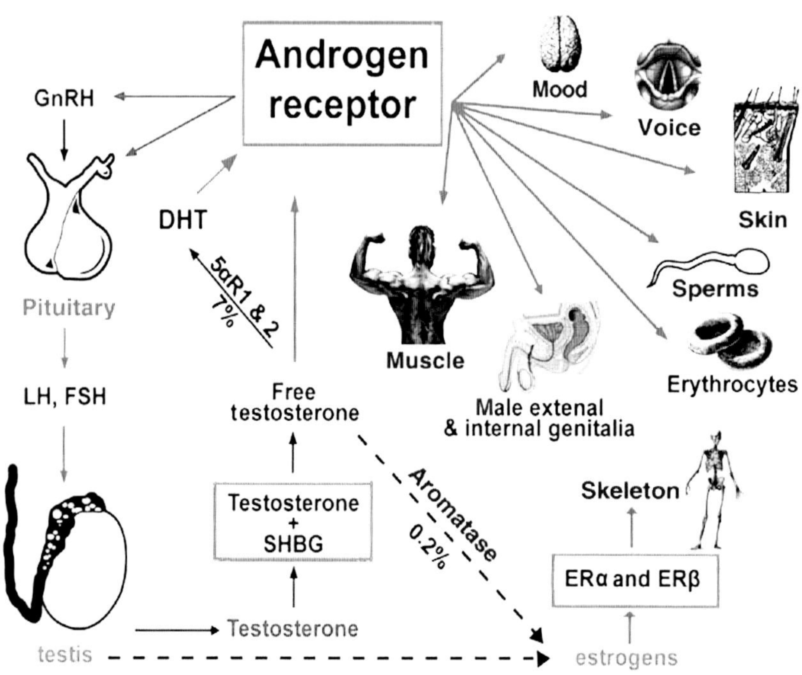

Figure 2 Testosterone formation and activity in the male. *Abbreviations:* DHT, dihydrotestosterone; SHBG, sex hormone–binding globulin; ER, estrogen receptor, 5αR1 & 2, 5α reductase type 1 and 5α reductase type 2; FSH, follicle stimulating hormone receptor.

Table 1 Causes of Primary Hypogonadism

Testicular diseases (↑ gonadotrophins ± ↓ testosterone)

Congenital

- **Klinefelter syndrome (1:500 male new borns)**
- Defects of testosterone biosynthesis (STAR, 20–22 desmolase, 3β-HSD, 17α-HSD, 17–20 desmolase, 17β-HSD: rare)
- Pure gonadal dysgenesis (46 XX and 46 XY, rare)
- Congenital anorchia (rare)
- Leydig cell hypoplasia (including type I and II for LH/hCG receptor mutations, rare)
- Myotonic dystrophy (including type I and II)
- **Cryptorchidism (1:100 male new borns)**
- Germinal aplasia (Del Castillo syndrome, sertoli-cell only syndrome)
- **Y Chromosome microdeletions (from 5 to 15: 100 in azoospermic and severely oligozoospermic males)**
- **Autosomal translocations (1:100 severely oligospermic males)**
- Follicule stimulating hormone receptor (FSHR) mutations (rare)
- Adrenoleukodystrophy

Acquired

- Orchitis (including mumps and autoimmune disorders), bilateral torsion trauma
- Chemotherapy (alkylating agents, metotrexate) and testicular irradiation
- Inhibitors of testosterone synthesis (ketoconazole, aminoglutethimide, mitotane metyrapone)
- **Varicocele (15:100)**
- **General diseases (including renal failure, liver cirrhosis, diabetes mellitus)**
- **Aging**

Table 2 Causes of Secondary Male Hypogonadism

A) Hypothalamic diseases (↓ gonadotrophins, ↓ testosterone)
- **Congenital (1:10000 male new borns)**
  - Kallmann syndrome (including KAL 1, FGFR1, PROK2, PROKR2 mutations)
  - Leptin and Leptin receptor mutation
  - GPR-54 mutation
  - DAX-1 mutation
  - SF-1 mutation
  - Prader–Willi syndrome
  - Laurence–Moon syndrome
  - Bardet–Biedl syndrome
- Acquired (rare)
  - (a) Hypothalamic tumors (germinomas, gliomas, astrocytomas, craniopharyngiomas, meningioma, metastases)
  - (b) Infiltrative and infective disorders (rare)
  - Langerhans' histiocytosis
  - Sarcoidosis and tuberculosis, syphilis
  - Encephalitis
  - (c) **Head trauma (10–15% of men after traumatic brain injury)**
  - (d) Idiopathic
  - (e) **Functional disorders**
  - **Hyperprolactinemia (prolactinoma, hypothyroidism, antidopaminergic and serotonergic drug–induced, opiates-induced)**
  - Nutritional
  - Critical illness
  - Excessive exercise (rare)
  - **Diabetes mellitus (30:100 of men with type 2 diabetes)**
  - **Metabolic syndrome (20–30:100 of men in western countries)**
  - **Aging**
  - Cushing disease (rare)
  - (f) Drugs (estrogens, anabolic steroids, progestogens)

B) Pituitary diseases (↓ gonadotrophins, ↓ testosterone)
- Congenital
  - Multiple hormone deficiency (including Prop1, LHX3, DAX-1 mutations, rare)
  - GnRHR mutations
  - FSHβ and LHβ mutations
  - Pituitary aplasia or hypoplasia
  - Hemochromatosis
- Acquired
  - (a) Pituitary tumors (functional and nonfunctional adenomas, craniopharyngiomas, metastases)
  - (b) Infiltrative and infectious diseases (primary hypophysitis, sarcoidosis, tuberculosis, syphilis, parasites, and fungal)
  - (c) **Head trauma**
  - (d) Empty sella
  - (e) Vascular
  - (f) Drugs (GnRH agonists and antagonists), estrogens, anabolic steroids, progestogens
  - (g) X-irradiation

The main causes of primary and secondary hypogonadism and their incidence are reported in Tables 1 and 2, respectively. For obvious reasons we will focus only on the most prevalent forms (given in bold in the tables).

CLINICAL FEATURES OF MALE HYPOGONADISM

The clinical features of male hypogonadism depend mainly on the time of onset of the impairment of testicular function (4).

(a) *Fetal hypogonadism (very early hypogonadism):* Ambiguous or completely feminine genitalia can be observed in a male infant with a normal karyotype 46XY but with a defective secretion/action of testosterone during the first trimester of fetal life usually because of genetic disorders, most commonly the *androgen insensitivity syndrome* (AIS) (for further details see chap. 26). These patients are rare and are usually seen by pediatricians. In boys with ambiguous external genitalia, urologists can be consulted for surgery of external genitalia for sex assignment or reassignment. The subjects with complete AIS having 46,XY karyotype but fully feminine external genitalia can be referred, at the age of puberty, either to a gynecologist or to an

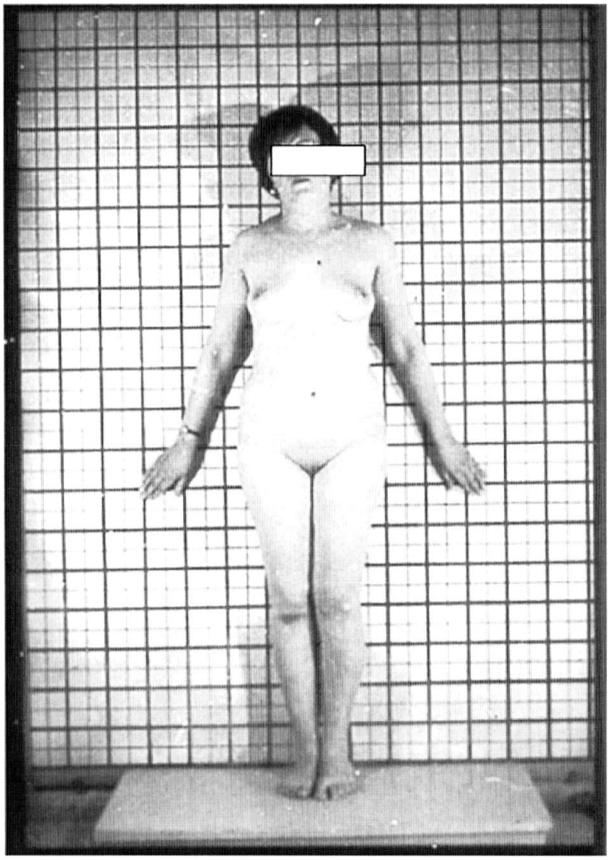

Figure 3 46,XY male with complete androgen insensitivity syndrome due to androgen receptor gene mutation: the phenotype is fully feminine (incidence: 1:50,000). Lack of pubic and axillary hair is typical of the complete form of the syndrome.

endocrinologist because of primary amenorrhea (Fig. 3). Another typical cause of referral for these subjects is uni- or bilateral inguinal hernia, which is uncommon in chromosomally normal females. In the AIS subjects, the hernia is caused by abnormal localization of the testes.

(b) *Prepubertal and peripubertal hypogonadism (early hypogonadism):* If hypogonadism occurs in infancy (e.g., because of vanishing testes, bilateral testicular torsion, sequelae of some types of cancer—for example, a craniopharyngioma that destroys the pituitary gonadotrophs, leukemia with testicular infiltrates) or is due to congenital causes (for instance, the Klinefelter syndrome (KS) or congenital hypogonadotropic hypogonadism) very few clinical symptoms can be observed, as infancy is a condition characterized "per se" by substantially quiescent testes. According to the different causes and severity, occurrence of Leydig cell dysfunction in the peripubertal age induces a complete or incomplete failure to undergo a normal pubertal development, with lack of or only partial virilization. The prevalence of early hypogonadism ranges around 1:500 male newborns (KS) to 1:10,000 for congenital hypogonadotropic hypogonadism (normosmic or with anosmia)

(c) *Adult hypogonadism:* In men with a previous history of normal virilization and/or fertility, symptoms of T deficiency are relatively mild even if T levels are very low (<5–6 nmol/L) due to, for instance, a pituitary macroadenoma. However, reduced libido, sexual dysfunction, asthenia, low energy, depressed humor, and more specific symptoms such as reduced volume of the ejaculate and poor growth of facial hair are often present in these patients. If hypogonadism has a duration of many months/years, a reduced volume of the testes as well as of the prostate can be objectively assessed. In men with sexual dysfunction a brief 12-item structured interview providing scores useful for detecting hypogonadism, defined as low total T (<10.4 nmol/L, 300 ng/dL) with a sensitivity and specificity of 68% and 65%, respectively, (Androtest) has been recently developed (5).

(d) *Late onset hypogonadism (LOH):* In addition to severe late-onset hypogonadism due to specific causes, there is a more frequent form or milder hypogonadism, the hypogonadism occurring with age in a consistent proportion of elderly men (6–9). This form of hypogonadism is discussed in chapter 28.

The prevalence and the clinical phenotype of very early, early, adult onset, and LOH are reported in Figure 4. Intersex states, mainly due to very early (fetal) hypogonadism are rare and will not be discussed in the present chapter as they are seen mainly by pediatricians.

CLINICAL INVESTIGATION IN MALE HYPOGONADISM

The diagnosis of hypogonadism is based on

- clinical symptoms and signs of androgen deficiency
- hormone measurements
- semen analysis

History taking is an important issue in the diagnosis of hypogonadism:

- Lack of or low libido,
- Erectile dysfunction,
- Poor beard growth,
- All the previous symptoms from libido to ejaculate are closely related to low testosterone levels. An important symptom is hyposmia/anosmia, which should be searched when congenital hypogonadotropic hypogonadism is suspected.

Less specific symptoms of androgen deficiency are

- decreased muscle mass and strength,
- increased body fat,
- osteoporosis,
- low energy,

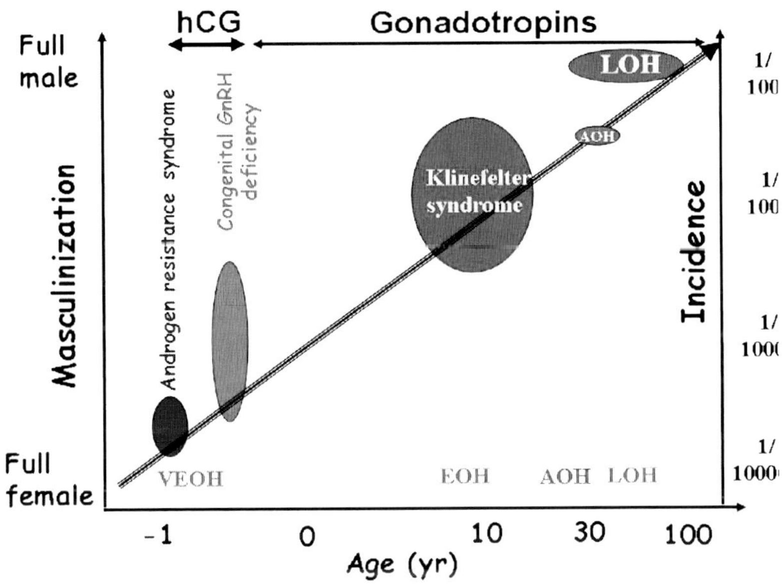

Figure 4 Schematic representation of male hypogonadism according to the age of onset of the disease and the patient's phenotype. *Abscissa* (log scale): age of onset and *ordinate* (log scale): incidence (right axis) or level of masculinization (from full female to full male phenotype, left axis, arbitrary unit). *VEOH:* very early onset hypogonadism, that is, starting during fetal life for absence of testosterone formation or activity (i.e., 17beta-hydroxysteroid dehydrogenase-3 defect or complete androgen insensitivity syndrome) or congenital impaired secretion or activity of GnRH. *EOH:* early onset hypogonadism [i.e., peripubertal onset, as in KS). *AOH:* adult onset hypogonadism due to organic causes. *LOH:* LOH, that is, a milder form of hypogonadism related to the aging process (also termed andropause)]. *Source:* Adapted with modifications from Ref. 4.

- decreased vitality, and
- depressed mood.

At clinical examination typical signs of testosterone deficiency are

- eunuchoid proportions (arm spam > height),
- underdeveloped genitalia,
- sparse low hair,
- gynecomastia,
- a small prostate and
- a low testicular volume.

Primary hypogonadism is more frequently characterized by gynecomastia, probably due to the stimulatory effect of high concentrations of FSH and LH on testicular aromatase activity and the higher concentrations of T, the main precursor of oestradiol.

Obviously symptoms of androgen deficiency are more evident in early onset than in adult onset hypogonadism.

In a man with symptoms/signs of hypogonadism laboratory investigation is needed to confirm the diagnosis.

LABORATORY INVESTIGATION IN MALE HYPOGONADISM

Endocrine Function

Testosterone and Sex Hormone–Binding Globulin

T is the main androgen in males. As 95% of secreted T comes from Leydig cells, which are stimulated by LH produced by the pituitary gonadotrophs under GnRH control, there is no need to measure other androgens or steroids with few exceptions such as in congenital disorders of steroidogenesis or in steroid-secreting tumors. In normal men only 2% of total T circulates free in the blood, as 45% is bound to sex hormone–binding globulin (SHBG, a protein produced by the liver, which is also able to bind dihydrotestosterone and estradiol) and 53% to albumin. The binding affinity of T to SHBG is 100 times higher compared to albumin, therefore, even if the amount of SHBG is much lower than that of albumin, the binding capacity of both proteins for T is approximately the same. There is a general agreement that T bound to albumin can easily dissociate from the protein in the capillary bed of many organs. Therefore, the amount of the so-called "bioavailable" T is approximately 50% of the total. However, as it is well known for thyroid hormones, when SHBG levels increase in normal men with an intact hypothalamic–pituitary axis, the consequent decrease of free T induces an activation of the secretion of LH with the achievement of normal levels of free T and increased levels of total T.

The measurement of total T in the past was usually done with immunoassays (Radioimmuno assay or Chemiluminescent immunoassay after extraction and chromatography of steroids). These methods are time consuming and cumbersome but give reliable result. Today, due to the large numbers of samples to be analyzed, the majority of laboratories use direct, often automated methods, which have several limits and pitfalls, especially at levels lower than 10.4 nmoles/L (300 ng/dL). Recent guidelines by the Endocrine Society in fact suggest not to use these methods in women and prepubertal boys (10).

Bioavailable and free T can also be measured by reliable but complex methods (equilibrium dialysis, precipitation of SHBG with ammonium sulfate), which cannot be used in a routine laboratory. Due to these problems, calculation of free T with formulae is now the most used method to estimate free or bioavailable T in plasma. The calculation depends on the measurement of total T, total SHBG, and total albumin, and the use of the equilibrium dissociation constants (K_d) for the binding of SHBG and T and albumin and T (11). When total T and SHBG levels are available, a calculator for free and bioavailable T can be found online at *http://www.issam.ch/freetesto.htm.*

In the majority of laboratories normal levels of total T for adult males range between 10 and 35 nmoles/L. No consensus is still present on normal levels of (calculated) free T and the lower threshold has been reported to range between 300 and 170 pmoles/L (8,9).

Due to considerable diurnal variation in T levels, the blood sample for this analysis should be obtained in the morning, preferably before 10 a.m.

Luteinizing Hormone

In men with low T (confirmed by a second measurement), luteinizing hormone (LH) levels must be also assessed to establish the cause of hypogonadism (high levels of LH are present in primary hypogonadism, low/normal levels in secondary hypogonadism).

Prolactin

The levels of this hormone should also be measured if LH levels are low/normal in men with subnormal T, in order to rule out the possibility of a prolactin-secreting pituitary adenoma.

The GnRH Stimulation Test

This test usually does not add very much information to the basal levels of the two gonadotropins and should be performed only in selected patients such as in the differential diagnosis between GnRH-dependent (normal response) and GnRH-independent precocious puberty (no response).

Human Chorionic Gonadotropin Stimulation Test

As hCG has a biologic action comparable to that of LH, the hCG stimulation test (1000– 2000 IU/day for 3–5 days) has been used to assess the functional reserve of Leydig cells, but in clinical practice the test has very few indications such as the differential diagnosis between bilateral anorchia (no increase of T levels) and bilateral cryptorchidism (increase of T to levels of normal adults) in prepubertal boys.

Spermatogenetic Function

Semen Analysis

Semen analysis should be offered to men with symptoms of testosterone deficiency who want to get information about their (potential) fertility or complain also for couple infertility.

Follicle-Stimulating Hormone and Inhibin B

Measurement of levels of these hormones can give indirect information about the efficiency of spermatogenic function. Primary hypogonadism is more frequently characterized by a decreased/absent sperm production than by decreased T production. Many infertile men have a low sperm count with normal/high FSH, but normal T concentration. Men with secondary hypogonadism usually have a combined reduction of T concentration and sperm production. For further details please look at chapters on male infertility (see chap. 1).

Genetic Assessment

Leukocyte blood karyotyping is indicated when Klinefelter syndrome is suspected and in men with azoospermia or severe oligozoospermia due to tubular damage (see below). A normal testicular volume and normal levels of FSH are usually found in men with obstructive azoospermia: if vas deferens and seminal vesicles agenesis is also present, mutations of the CFTR gene should be evaluated (12).

In the last few years, several monogenic disorders have been reported to be the cause of isolated or anosmia/hyposmia-coupled hypogonadotropic hypogonadism (Kallmann syndrome). Loss-of-function mutations in the genes encoding anosmin-1 (*KAL1*) and fibroblast growth factor receptor 1 (*FGFR1*) have been described in the X-linked and autosomal dominant forms of this syndrome, respectively. Two years ago, several heterozygous, homozygous, or compound heterozygous mutations in the G protein–coupled prokineticin receptor-2 (*PROKR2*) and of its ligand prokineticin-2 (*PROK2*) were reported in Kallmann syndrome.

In isolated hypogonadotropic hypogonadism without olfactory abnormalities, loss-of-function mutations in the gonadotropin-releasing hormone (GnRH) receptor (*GnRH-R*) or the G protein–coupled receptor 54 (*GPR54*) genes, both encoding transmembrane receptors, and FGFR1 mutations have been reported (13). More recently, mutations of several isoforms of fibroblast growth factor 8 have also been reported to cause congenital hypogonadotropic hypogonadism with/without hypo/anosmia (14). Only a few research laboratories, however, can assess the presence of mutations in these genes.

Finally, mutations of the beta subunit of LH (15–17) have been described in a few undervirilized males, whereas normal virilization was usually present in subjects with mutations of the beta subunit of FSH (18) (see also chap. 23).

Imaging in Male Hypogonadism

Ultrasound Examination of the Testis

This examination is very important, mainly in male infertility, to assess testicular volume as well as the presence of epididymal abnormalities, varicocele, and to rule out the presence of testicular tumors, which are much more frequent in infertile patients (1:200) versus a reported incidence of one to eight new reported cases per 100,000 men/yr in the general population (19). Presence of the so-called microlithiasis may be indicative of increased risk of testicular carcinoma in-situ, although the clinical consequences of microlithiasis finding are still debatable.

Magnetic Resonance Imaging/Computed Tomography
Computed tomography (CT) [if Magnetic Resonance Imaging (MRI) is not available] imaging of the pituitary region is indicated when an organic lesion (usually a tumor) of the hypothalamic pituitary region is suspected in a male with hypogonadotropic hypogonadism.

MOST COMMON FORMS OF HYPOGONADISM

Klinefelter Syndrome

With a prevalence of nearly 0.2% in the general male population (20), the syndrome is the most common form of male hypogonadism and chromosome aneuploidy. About 85% to 90% of cases are due to the congenital chromosome aberration 47,XXY, whereas the remaining 10% to 15% have 46,XY/47,XXY mosaicism or higher-grade chromosomal aneuploidies (48,XXXY, 48,XXYY) (21). Due to the relative mild phenotype, it has been estimated that approximately 65% of men with the syndrome are undiagnosed (22). Recent studies (23) suggest that the supranumerary X chromosome can be derived either from the father or the mother with the same probability.

The clinical picture of patients with KS (Fig. 5) varies with age: before puberty only a few signs (very small testes, long legs) can suggest hypogonadism. In many subjects puberty starts normally but there is no growth of testes so that after puberty, small firm testes [<3–4 mL each with the Prader orchidometer (Fig. 6) and ultrasound] and variable symptoms of androgen deficiency are found in most subjects.

T levels below 12 nmol/L have been reported in 63% of cases, with high levels of FSH and LH in virtually all subjects. A history of *maldescended testes* is nearly threefold more frequent in comparison to normal controls (19,24). In contrast to typical eunuchoid subjects, patients with KS are usually *taller than controls,* but their mean arm span has been reported to be equal to height in 138 subjects (23). *Decreased libido and potency* has been reported in more than 2/3 of patients and normal beard growth is present only in 1/5 (19,24). As a consequence of T deficiency, *osteoporosis and reduced muscle strength* are frequent in these patients (25,26). Recent research on the role of androgen receptor and, in particular, on the length of the CAG repeat of exon 1, which is inversely related to the receptor transcriptional activity, has shown that CAG repeat length is positively associated with the presence of tall stature and gynecomastia and negatively associated with stable relationships. These findings suggest a modulation of androgen effects via the CAG repeat polymorphism (27).

Varicose veins and increased thromboembolic risk, obesity, and reduced glucose tolerance has been reported in these patients (28–30). *Gynecomastia* of varying degree is present in 30% to 50% of subjects (24,31) but the risk of developing mammary carcinoma is no higher than in normal men (32). The reported increased frequencies of hematological malignancies or midline germ cell tumors were not confirmed in a large series (23).

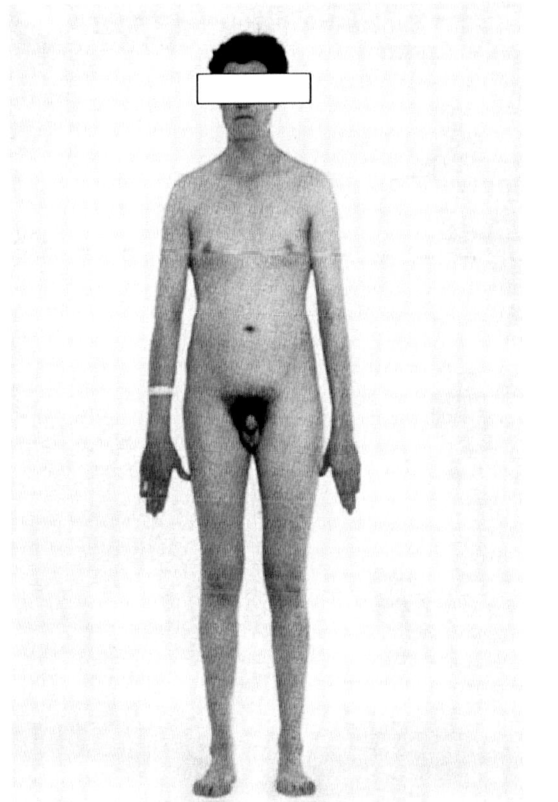

Figure 5 Patient with Klinefelter syndrome (47,XXY karyotype): A mild undervirilization is present (gynecomastia, poor hair and beard development, slightly eunuchoid proportions). *Source:* Modified from Ref. 80.

Children and adolescents with KS have been reported to show deficits in language processing including a learning disability in reading and spelling (33,34). Adult patients with KS have been reported to score significantly below controls in language skills, verbal processing speed, verbal and nonverbal executive abilities, and motor dexterity (35).

Recent studies performed with neuroimaging techniques (double-spin-echo brain magnetic resonance) showed that patients with KS, in comparison to age-matched controls, have a significant enlargement of ventricular volume, bilateral reduction of cerebellar hemispheres, and a significant reduction of left temporal lobe volume, thus suggesting a neurobiological substrate for cognitive deficits in these patients (36).

Prospective studies on chromosome surveys did not confirm a previously reported increased risk of psychiatric disturbances, criminal behavior, and mental retardation (37). A longitudinal study performed in a cohort of boys with KS that was identified at birth reported that the majority of boys had

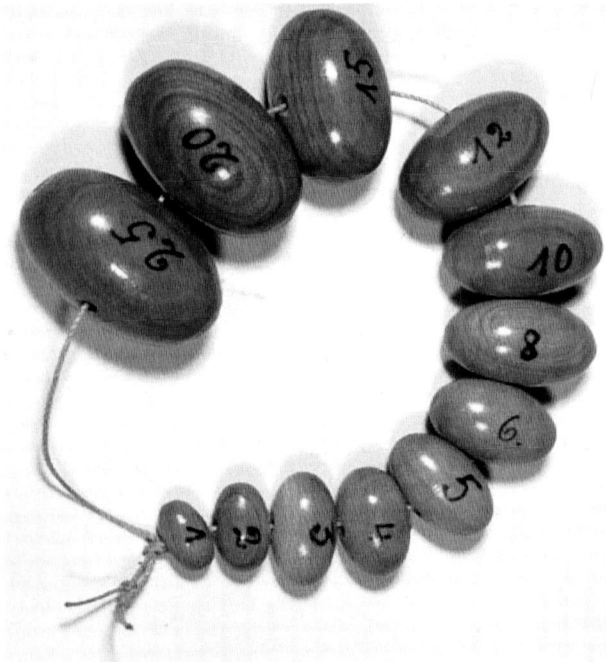

Figure 6 Prader Orchidometer: Normal testicular volume for an adult male is between 15 and 25 mL.

medical, psychological, or social problems. Standardized mortality ratio assessed in 3518 patients followed for more than 40 years and with 461 deaths was significantly raised (1.5) in comparison to normal controls. In particular, the standardized mortality ratio was raised to 5.8, 7.2, 5.7, 7.9, 5.0, and 39.4 for diabetes, epilepsy, pulmonary embolism, peripheral vascular disease, renal disease, and femoral fracture, respectively. Only mortality from ischemic heart disease was significantly decreased (SMR = 0.7) (38).

Nearly all patients with 47,XXY Karyotype are azoospermic, with sperm found only in rare cases and exceptional cases of spontaneous paternity (24,39).

Patients with chromosome mosaicism 46,XY/47,XXY have milder phenotype and hormone abnormalities and may have normal testis size with sperm in the ejaculate. The 46,XX karyotype is considered a variant of Klinefelter karyotype; however, a recent study has shown that the incidence of cryptorchidism and gynecomastia was more frequent in 46,XX males. Furthermore the 46,XX males were significantly smaller than patients with KS or healthy men, resembling female controls in height and weight (40).

In men with three or more X chromosome (48,XXXY or 49,XXXXY), the severity of the phenotype increases with the number of X chromosomes.

However, as approximately two-thirds of men with KS are not diagnosed, the clinical picture observed in published studies could be biased showing only the most severe cases, whereas the majority of these patients could have a normal life except for infertility.

Diagnosis of KS is difficult in prepubertal boys as no specific symptoms/signs are present. In adults, the diagnosis can be suspected on a clinical basis in a man complaining for infertility and azoospermia and/or symptoms of T deficiency (low libido, reduced potency, poor beard growth) if small firm testes (<3–4 mL with the Prader orchidometer) can be observed. The diagnosis is also suggested by the presence of low/normal total T levels and high levels of the two gonadotropins, especially FSH. Estradiol level can be higher than in normal men and serum SHBG is often high, causing a further decrease in biologically active free T. Inhibin B levels are normal in boys and low in adults with KS, but its measurement is of little value for the diagnosis. Blood leukocyte karyotyping will confirm the diagnosis.

Chronic T treatment is indicated in the majority of patients with KS, as most of them have total or calculated free T in low or in the low/normal range. Early treatment in adolescent patients has a beneficial effect on mood, behavior, and self-esteem on one hand and results in increased muscle strength, libido, bone density, and body hair on the other hand. Among the different T preparations, long-acting preparations for IM injection such as T enanthate, cypionate, and in particular, T undecanoate, acting for about three months seems to be largely preferable in younger patients with KS in comparison to short-acting forms requesting daily administration (oral T undecanoate, buccal T, transdermal T in patches or gels).

T treatment has no effect on fertility; however, successful recovery of spermatozoa from azoospermic patients with KS by means of testicular sperm extraction from multiple testicular biopsies can be obtained and several term pregnancies with newborns with normal karyotype have been reported after intracytoplasmic sperm injection procedures, with a success rate that in some centers was reported to be close to that obtained in men with unselected nonobstructive azoospermia (41,42,43). Preimplantation genetic diagnosis and genetic counseling should be obviously offered to these men and their partners.

Cryptorchidism

Isolated cryptorchidism can affect one or both testes and has an incidence of 3% in male newborns. Several causes (prematurity, anatomic defects, fetal T deficiency, environmental toxicants) can induce cryptorchidism (44,45) but in the majority of cases the reason for the lack of testicular descent is unknown.

INSL3 and its receptor, LGR8, are essential for the first phase of testicular descent as homozygous loss of either of the two genes leads to cryptorchidism in mice. Mutations in both homologous human genes are not a common cause of cryptorchidism: to date, only one missense mutation at codon 222 (T222P) of the LGR8 gene has been proposed as causative mutation for cryptorchidism in humans (46) but this finding was not confirmed by another recent study (47).

In two-thirds of boys cryptorchid at birth, spontaneous testicular descent occurs in the first four to six months of life so that only 0.8% to 1% of infants are really cryptorchid at one year of age. Surgery is indicated in the first years of life as medical treatment with GnRH or hCG is effective only in 20% of cases and less if retractile testes are excluded. In recent years, a number of potentially serious side effects of medical therapy have also been reported. Therefore, the general use of hCG and GnRH in the treatment of cryptorchidism cannot be further recommended (48)

Clinical consequences of cryptorchidism depend upon whether one or both testes are undescended: in monolateral cryptorchidism, the sperm count will be subnormal in 25% to 35% of cases, whereas T levels are usually normal. In bilateral cryptorchidism, the sperm count is usually severely impaired (49) and serum T may also be reduced. Another clinical consequence of cryptorchidism is a 3- to 10-fold increase in risk of testicular cancer. Some recent data suggest that orchiopexy before puberty decreases such risk (50,51), but this issue is still debatable (52).

Male Infertility

Infertility, defined as the lack of pregnancy after one year of unprotected intercourse, affects about 15% of couples and that in approximately 50% of infertile couples there is a male factor (in 20% as main cause and in 30% as a cocause) (53). So we can expect that approximately 6% to 7% of men have fertility problems. Infertile/subfertile males, however, usually do not show signs or symptoms of androgen deficiency and testosterone levels are normal in the majority of them. An important clinical finding to assess in infertile males is the testicular volume (Fig. 6), which is inversely related to sperm output. LH levels are usually normal in infertile men, whereas FSH levels are increased only when a severe oligozoospermia is present (sperm concentration <5 millions/mL) (54). Inhibin B levels are inversely related to FSH, but this measurement is of low clinical value (55).

Abnormalities of sex chromosomes and abnormalities of autosomes (translocations) are present in 15% of males with nonobstructive azoospermia and in 5% to 6% of men with oligozoospermia (sperm concentration <10 millions/mL), respectively. These figures are approximately 10 fold higher than those found in normal controls (56). In men with nonobstructive azoospermia or severe oligozoospermia, Y chromosome microdeletions are present in approximately 10% and 5% (57–59). Therefore, genetic assessment is now very important in the diagnostic management of the infertile male.

Issues related with male infertility, however, are covered in more detail in other chapters of this book (see chap. 1).

Varicocele

Idiopathic left varicocele is still a disputed cause of male infertility; however, in a large WHO multicentee study, including 7094 male partners of infertile couples, the prevalence of varicocele in men with abnormal and normal semen was 25.4% and 11.7%, respectively (60). A recent metaanalysis of nine randomized controlled clinical trials has shown that varicocele treatment has no benefit over expectant management in improving the chances of conception in couples with otherwise unexplained subfertility (61).

Even if several studies have reported subtle abnormalities of hormone parameters (gonadotropin responsiveness to GnRH, inihibin B levels), T and LH levels are usually in the normal range in men with isolated varicocele (62).

Acquired Primary Hypogonadism

An impairment of spermatogenesis and/or T secretion can occur because of many causes (testicular torsion, trauma, radiation, mumps, orchitis, chemotherapy with alkylating and antineoplastic drugs, therapy with inhibitors of steroidogenesis, such as ketoconazole, chronic treatment with glucocorticoids, work exposure to pesticides, such as dibromochloropropane): the degree of testicular failure depends on the entity of testicular damage: generally the cells of the spermatogenetic lineage are more fragile than Leydig cells (63).

Many chronic systemic illness, such as liver cirrhosis, chronic renal failure, or HIV infection can also cause hypogonadism. The mechanisms explaining hypogonadism in systemic disease are not completely understood, but these conditions are likely caused by a combination of stress, nonspecific weight loss, inflammation, and medications that often act both at the testicular and hypothalamic–pituitary level (64). Effective treatment of the systemic disease (renal transplantation in chronic renal failure, for instance) is followed by improvement of hypogonadism.

Congenital Gonadotropin-Releasing Hormone Deficiency

Congenital GnRH deficiency is a rare disorder occurring in approximately 1:10,000 male newborns. Micropenis and/or cryptorchidism are frequent in these subjects; however, during infancy and childhood the diagnosis is difficult unless anosmia/hyposmia or skeletal abnormalities such as cleft lip/cleft palate are present (see below). At pubertal age, there is no sexual maturation, nor a clear-cut growth spurt. In some cases there is some degree of pubertal development that then stops. In a few cases GnRH deficiency occurs in adult age, following a completely normal pubertal development (adult onset hypogonadotropic hypogonadism) (65).

In untreated adolescent patients the body proportions are often eunuchoidal, with arm span exceeding height, due to the lack of closure of the epiphyses of the long bones because of testosterone deficiency. Beard and body hair growth is very poor, if any, with exception in some cases of axillary hair due to adrenarche. Muscle mass does not show a significant development and external genitalia maintain the size of prepubertal boys with testicular volume usually <4 mL. Gynecomastia is not typical in these patients because testosterone levels are very low, and estradiol in men is mainly derived from aromatization of T. Furthermore, the low levels of LH results in low testicular aromatase activity and therefore little estrogen secretion by the testis. These patients usually have low libido and have no or just a few drops of ejaculate because seminal fluid is produced by seminal vesicles and prostate under control of adult levels of T. In patients with congenital GnRH deficiency, hyposmia or anosmia and other several congenital abnormalities as cleft lip/palate, syndactylia, unilateral renal agenesis can be observed. The presence of hyposmia/anosmia coupled to congenital GnRH deficiency is called *Kallmann syndrome*, whereas if normosmia is present, it is called idiopathic hypogonadotropic hypogonadism. A milder phenotype with some virilization and low-normal testicular volume with sperm in the ejaculate can be seen in cases where a partial pubertal development has occurred, and, obviously, in the rare forms of adult onset. Spontaneous recovery has been very recently described in a minority of patients (66) and can be considered as case of extremely delayed onset of puberty. The phenotype of men with congenital GnRH deficiency is similar to the phenotype of men with mutations of the GnRH receptor or LH beta subunit genes. Some genetic causes of Kallmann syndrome are given above.

Usually in the complete form of congenital GnRH deficiency, the phenotype is much less virilized than that found in subjects with KS because T levels are much lower (Fig. 7).

Hypogonadotropic hypogonadism can also be due to lack of action of gonadotropins because of mutations of LH beta subunit gene (14,15,16). Hypogonadotropic hypogonadism can be also found coupled to other pituitary hormone deficiencies because of mutations in genes, such as Prop1, HESX 1, or LHX3, and in rare congenital syndromes due to monogenic disorders as in DAX1 mutations where hypogonadism is associated with adrenal insufficiency (adrenal hypoplasia congenita) (67). It is also linked with obesity in patients with mutations of leptin and its receptor (68). Hypogonadotropic hypogonadism can also be found in complex chromosomal disorders such as Prader–Willi, Laurence–Moon, and Bardet–Biedl syndrome. In these syndromes, the diagnosis is usually established in pediatric age because of other symptoms, such as hypotonia; short stature; hyperphagia; and obesity in Prader–Willi syndrome, which is caused by the absence of certain paternally inherited genes on the long arm of chromosome 15 and results in a complete absence of the active copy of the genetic information in this region (69). Bardet–Biedl syndrome is a genetically heterogeneous autosomal recessive disorder mapping to eight known loci with the cardinal features of obesity, retinitis pygmentosa, polydactyly, hypogenitalism, renal abnormalities, and developmental delay (70,71) whereas spastic paraplegia and retinitis pygmentosa are features of the Laurence–Moon syndrome (71).

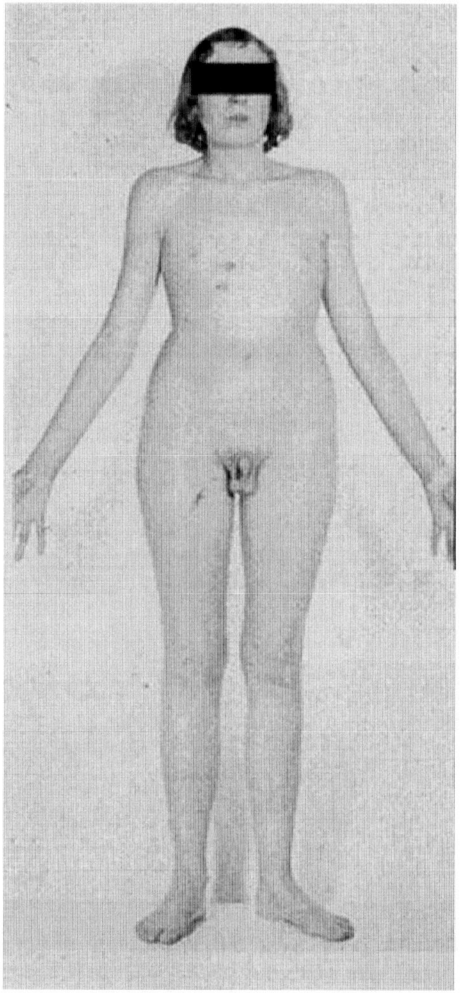

Figure 7 Patient with Kallmann Syndrome (congenital hypogonadotropic hypogonadism + anosmia): Severe undervirilization is present (eunuchoid body proportions, infantile external genitalia, no hair and beard development). *Source:* Modified from Ref. 81.

Acquired Secondary Hypogonadism

Infiltrative disorders, tumors of the hypothalamic region, and traumas can induce acquired hypogonadotropic hypogonadism because of GnRH deficiency, which can be coupled to other pituitary hormone deficiencies. In the recent years, it has been demonstrated that subjects undergoing head trauma have a 10% to 15% risk of hypopituitarism, which is often undiagnosed so that, due the very many cases of traumatic brain injuries (100–300 cases per 100,000 inhabitants worldwide), thousands of individuals experience low quality of life, and possibly impaired life expectancy (72).

Hypogonadotropic hypogonadism can be induced by hyperprolactinemia due to a prolacting-secreting pituitary macroadenoma (more frequent than microprolactinoma in males) with a double mechanism: reduced GnRH secretion and damage to the pituitary gonadotropes (73). Hyperprolactinemia can also be induced by primary hypothyroidism, antidopaminergic drugs, and opiates.

Other pituitary causes of reduced gonadotropin secretion are secreting or nonsecreting pituitary macroadenomas, pituitary metastases or infiltrative disorders (hemochromatosis for instance), and irradiation. Reversible hypogonadotropic hypogonadism can also be induced by treatment with GnRH agonists, estrogens, progestogens, and supraphysiological doses of T and/ or anabolic androgens.

A milder form of functional hypogonadotropic hypogonadism (T levels <10.4 nM/L) can also be found in a significant percentage of men with type 2 diabetes and in men with metabolic syndrome (74,75,76,77).

Testosterone Deficiency of the Aging Male (Late Onset Hypogonadism)

This topic will be discussed in detail in a specific chapter of the book (see chap. 28). To give the reader a preliminary idea, we will only remind that the decrease of total and, in particular, free testosterone levels with aging in males is a well-known phenomenon, partly due to reduced testicular responsiveness to LH and partly due to other factors (obesity, diabetes, and other comorbidities, medications). According to different established thresholds for total or free T, the prevalence of LOH based just on low testosterone levels varied from 20% to 50% in 60- to 90-year-old men. Recent guidelines have recommended combining clinical symptoms with a low total (78,79,80) or free (78) T level to provide a more accurate diagnosis of LOH. According to these guidelines and using different groups of clinical symptoms and different thresholds for total T and/or free T, crude prevalence of LOH was estimated to range between 5% and 6% in men 30 to 70 years old (8,9), with an increasing incidence with age (8,9). Diagnosis, treatment, and monitoring of LOH in males should be performed according to the above-mentioned guidelines.

CONCLUSION

In conclusion, the clinical approach to males suspected of testicular failure relies first on the clinical history focused on symptoms such as reduced libido and nocturnal erections, low energy, depressed mood, reduced volume of ejaculate and beard growth, abnormal sense of smell, and past history of cryptorchidism, orchitis, or testicular trauma. Clinical history should be followed by a careful objective examination looking at body proportions, muscle mass, hair abundance and distribution, presence of gynecomastia, testicular and penis size as well as prostate volume by digital rectal examination. Among laboratory assays, total serum T is the most important androgen to measure, followed by LH and FSH measurement to establish whether the hypogonadism is primary or secondary. If testosterone is low and LH and FSH are low/normal, prolactin should be also measured to rule out functional or organic hyperprolactinemia as well as other pituitary disorders (Fig. 8). If total T is borderline, SHBG and calculated free T can be of help.

Semen analysis can establish the presence of spermatogenic failure and FSH measurement is important in severely oligozoospermic and azoospermic men. Inhibin B measurement is a complementary assay.

Karyotyping is important to confirm the presence of KS and to rule out other chromosomal abnormalities in males with severe oligozoospermia or azoospermia.

Monogenic abnormalities such as those recently reported in congenital hypogonadotropic hypogonadism can be assessed only in research laboratories.

LEVELS OF EVIDENCE AND GRADE OF CLINICAL RECOMMENDATIONS

1. Use of automated methods for testosterone analysis is not recommended for measurements in women and prepubertal boys (10) (grade 3/A).
2. Due to considerable diurnal variation in testosterone levels, the blood sample for the analysis should be obtained in the morning, preferably before 10 am (grade 3/B).
3. In men with low T (confirmed by a second measurement), LH levels must also be assessed to establish the cause of hypogonadism (high levels of LH are present in primary hypogonadism, low/normal levels in secondary hypogonadism) (grade 3/B).
4. The levels of prolactin should also be measured if LH levels are low/normal in men with subnormal testosterone, in order to rule out the possibility of a prolactin-secreting pituitary adenoma (grade 3/B).
5. Early androgen replacement in adolescent patients with KS has a beneficial effect on mood, behavior, and self-esteem on one hand and results in increased muscle strength, libido, bone density, and body hair on the other hand (grade 3/B).
6. The general use of hCG and GnRH in the treatment of cryptorchidism cannot be further recommended (grade 1a).

CLINICAL CASE 1

A 42-year-old man consulting for infertility.

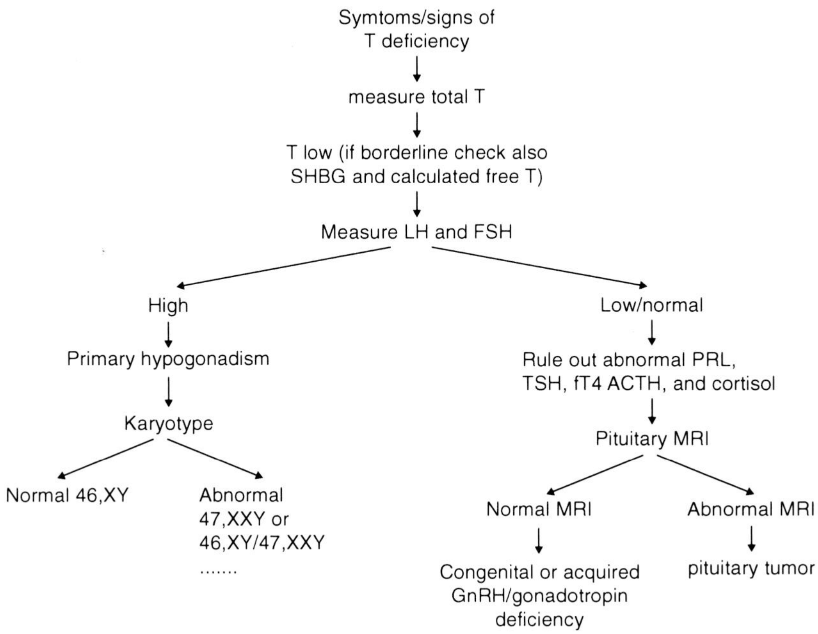

Figure 8 Algorithm for the clinical approach to a male suspected to be hypogonadal.

Medical History

Normal pubertal development and military duty. Masters degree in economy. Manager in a pharmaceutical industry. Twenty cigarettes per day. No major health problems or surgery either in infancy or adult life.

Married for 5 years with a regularly menstruating woman aged 38. The couple had protected intercourse for 2 years followed by unprotected intercourse for 3 years but no conception occurred. A recent semen analysis revealed azoospermia.

Clinical Examination

Height 184 cm, weight 95 kg. BMI = 28. Pulse rate 84/min, BP 135/90. Normal body proportions and normal virilization and hair distribution. Slight left gynecomastia. Normal penis. Small firm testes (testicular volume with Prader orchidometer 3 mL for each testis; normal 15–25 mL)

Comment

The finding of very small firm testes in an azoospermic otherwise normal man in apparent good health strongly suggests the presence of Klinefelter syndrome (KS), the most frequent chromosomal abnormality in humans (1:500 male newborns) due to a 47,XXY Karyotype (90% of cases) or its variants (mosaicism 46,XY/47,XXY; 48, XXXY). The phenotype of these men is characterized by variable levels of undervirilization. A nearly costant feature of the syndrome is the lack of sperm in the ejaculate.

LABORATORY ANALYSES

Total testosterone: 7.9 nmoles/L (normal 10–35 nmoles/L)
FSH: 40.8 U/L (normal 1.5–9.0 U/L)
LH: 15.9 U/L (normal 1.0–8.0 U/L)
Blood karyotype: 47XXY

Comment

Subnormal levels of testosterone are frequent in men with KS; however, normal levels can also be observed. FSH is always higher than LH.

CLINICAL CASE 2

A 19 years and 5 months old man consulting for delayed puberty.

Medical History

Adopted when he was three years old. Secondary school degree. Exempted from military duty because of testicular hypoplasia. Nonsmoker, works as a photographer. Normal smell. Reason of consultation is the lack of pubertal development and virilization.

Clinical Examination

Height 175 cm, weight 73 kg, BMI = 24.5, pulse rate 76, blood pressure 125/75. Arm span 177 cm (i.e., 2 cm > height): slightly eunuchoidal habitus. Penile length 5.5 cm (normal 10 $\pm$ 2); testicular volume (Prader orchidometer) 4 mL for each testis (normal 15–25 mL). No gynecomastia. Pubic hair: P2, no axillary hair.

Comment

The lack of pubertal development after 18 years of age is diagnosed as hypogonadism. The medical history and clinical examination suggest congenital isolated hypogonadotropic hypogonadism, but other forms of hypogonadism are also possible.

Laboratory Analyses

Total testosterone: 1.94 nmoles/L (normal 10–35 nmoles/L)
FSH : 2.5 U/L (normal 1.5–7.0 U/L)
LH : 0.7 U/L (normal 1.0–8.0 U/L)
Semen analysis: not feasible because the patient has no ejaculate

Comment

These findings seem to support the diagnosis of isolated congenital hypogonadotropic hypogonadism. However, the diagnosis must be confirmed by the evaluation of other pituitary hormones and by imaging of the pituitary region to rule out other pituitary deficiencies and organic causes (for instance a macroprolactinoma or a craniopharingioma).

Other Laboratory Analyses

Normal values of PRL, TSH, free thyroxine, ACTH, and cortisol
MRI of pituitary region: no abnormalities

Comment

These findings seemed to confirm the diagnosis. DNA samples for research of gene mutations were sent to different laboratories. Testosterone treatment was started for four months with testosterone enanthate 250 mg every three weeks. After a two months stop of therapy, the testosterone and gonadotropin levels were rechecked and the following was found:

Testosterone: 1.9 ng/mL (2.4–11.0 ng/mL)
FSH: 4.1 U/L (2.0–14.0 U/L)
LH: 7.2 U/L(1.0–8.0 U/L)
Testicular volume: 8 mL each testis
These findings suggested the activation of the hypoyhalamic–pituitary–testicular axis.

FINAL DIAGNOSIS: (VERY MUCH) DELAYED PUBERTY

Final Comment

Brief discontinuation of hormonal therapy to assess the reversibility of hypogonadotropic hypogonadism is suggested.

REFERENCES

1. MacLaughlin DT, Donahoe PK. Sex determination and differentiation. N Engl J Med 2004; 350(4):367–378. Erratum in: N Engl J Med 2004; 351(3):306.
2. Grumbach MM, Hughes IA, Conte FA. Disorders of sex differentiation. In: Larsen PR, Kronenberg HM, Melmed S, Polonsky KS, eds. Williams Textbook of Endocrinology, Philadelphia, PA: Saunders. 2003:842–1003.
3. Grumbach MM, Styne DM. Puberty: ontogeny, neuroendocrinology, physiology, and disorders. In: Larsen PR, Kronenberg HM, Melmed S, Polonsky KS, eds. Williams Textbook of Endocrinology, Philadelphia, PA: Saunders. 2003:1115–1286.
4. Morelli A, Corona G, Filippi S, et al. Which patients with sexual dysfunction are suitable for testosterone replacement therapy? J Endocrinol Invest 2007; 30(10):880–888.
5. Corona G, Mannucci E, Petrone L, et al. ANDROTEST: a structured interview for the screening of hypogonadism in patients with sexual dysfunction. J Sex Med 2006; 3(4):706–715.
6. Harman SM, Metter EJ, Tobin JD, et al. Longitudinal effects of aging on serum total and free testosterone levels in healthy men. J Clin Endocrinol Metab 2001; 86(2):724–731.
7. Smith KW, Feldman HA, McKinlay JB. Construction and field validation of a self-administered screener for testosterone deficiency (hypogonadism) in ageing men. Clin Endocrinol (Oxf) 2000; 53(6):703–711.
8. Araujo AB, O'Donnell AB, Brambilla DJ, et al. Prevalence and incidence of androgen deficiency in middle-aged and older men: estimates from the Massachusetts Male Aging Study. J Clin Endocrinol Metab 2004; 89(12):5920–5926.
9. Araujo AB, Esche GR, Kupelian V, et al. Prevalence of symptomatic androgen deficiency in men. J Clin Endocrinol Metab 2007; 92(11):4241–4247.
10. Rosner W, Auchus RJ, Azziz R, et al. Position statement: Utility, limitations, and pitfalls in measuring testosterone: an Endocrine Society position statement. J Clin Endocrinol Metab 2007; 92(2):405–413.
11. Vermeulen A, Verdonck L, Kaufman JM. A critical evaluation of simple methods for the estimation of free testosterone in serum. J Clin Endocrinol Metab 1999; 84(10):3666–3672.
12. Aittomäki K, Wennerholm UB, Bergh C, et al. Safety issues in assisted reproduction technology: should ICSI patients have genetic testing before treatment? A practical proposition to help patient information. Hum Reprod 2004 19(3):472–476.
13. Trarbach EB, Silveira LG, Latronico AC. Genetic insights into human isolated gonadotropin deficiency. Pituitary 2007; 10(4):381–391.
14. Falardeau J, Chung WC, Beenken A, et al. Decreased FGF8 signaling causes deficiency of gonadotropin-releasing hormone in humans and mice. J Clin Invest 2008; 118(8):2822–2831.
15. Lofrano-Porto A, Barra GB, Giacomini LA, et al. Luteinizing hormone beta mutation and hypogonadism in men and women. N Engl J Med 2007; 357(9):897–904.
16. Weiss J, Axelrod L, Whitcomb RW, et al. Hypogonadism caused by a single amino acid substitution in the β subunit of luteinizing hormone. N Engl J Med 1992; 326:179–183.
17. Valdes-Socin H, Salvi R, Daly AF, et al. Hypogonadism in a patient with a mutation in the luteinizing hormone beta-subunit gene. N Engl J Med 2004; 351(25):2619–2625.

18. Lofrano-Porto A, Casulari LA, Nascimento PP, et al. Effects of follicle-stimulating hormone and human chorionic gonadotropin on gonadal steroidogenesis in two siblings with a follicle-stimulating hormone beta subunit mutation. Fertil Steril 2007.
19. Nieschlag E, Behre HM, Meschede D, et al. Disorders at the testicular level. In: Nieschlag E, Behre HM, Nieschag S, eds. Andrology: male reproductive health and dysfunction. 2nd ed. Berlin, Heidelberg, New York, NY: Springer, 2000:144–172.
20. Morris JK, Alberman E, Scott C, et al. Is the prevalence of Klinefelter syndrome increasing? Eur J Hum Genet 2007.
21. Bojesen A, Juul S, Gravholt CH. Prenatal and postnatal prevalence of Klinefelter syndrome: a national registry study. J Clin Endocrinol Metab 2003; 88(2):622–626.
22. Abramsky L, Chapple J. 47,XXY (Klinefelter syndrome) and 47,XYY: estimated rates of and indication for postnatal diagnosis with implications for prenatal counselling. Prenat Diagn 1997; 17(4):363–368
23. Lanfranco F, Kamischke A, Zitzmann M. et al. (Klinefelter's syndrome. Lancet 2004; 364 (9430): 273–283.
24. Kamischke A, Baumgardt A, Horst J, et al. Clinical and diagnostic features of patients with suspected Klinefelter syndrome. J Androl 2003; 24(1):49–50.
25. Breuil V, Euller-Ziegler L. Gonadal dysgenesis and bone metabolism. Joint Bone Spine 2001; 68(1):26–33.
26. van den Bergh JP, Hermus AR, Spruyt AI, et al. Bone mineral density and quantitative ultrasound parameters in patients with Klinefelter's syndrome after long-term testosterone substitution. Osteoporos Int 2001; 12(1):55–62.
27. Zitzmann M, Depenbusch M, Gromoll J, et al. X-chromosome inactivation patterns and androgen receptor functionality influence phenotype and social characteristics as well as pharmacogenetics of testosterone therapy in Klinefelter patients. J Clin Endocrinol Metab 2004; 89(12):6208–6217.
28. Zollner TM, Veraart JC, Wolter M, et al. Leg ulcers in Klinefelter's syndrome–further evidence for an involvement of plasminogen activator inhibitor-1. Br J Dermatol 1997; 136(3):341–344.
29. Igawa K, Nishioka K. Leg ulcer in Klinefelter's syndrome J Eur Acad Dermatol Venereol 2003; 17(1):62–64.
30. Ota K, Suehiro T, Ikeda Y, et al. Diabetes mellitus associated with Klinefelter's syndrome: a case report and review in Japan. Intern Med 2002; 41(10):842–847.
31. Ratcliffe S. Long-term outcome in children of sex chromosome abnormalities. Arch Dis Child 1999; 80(2):192–195.
32. Hasle H, Mellemgaard A, Nielsen J, et al. Cancer incidence in men with Klinefelter syndrome. Br J Cancer 1995; 71(2):416–420.
33. Geschwind DH, Boone KB, Miller BL, et al. Neurobehavioral phenotype of Klinefelter syndrome. Ment Retard Dev Disabil Res Rev 2000; 6(2):107–116.
34. Temple CM, Sanfilippo PM. Executive skills in Klinefelter's syndrome. Neuropsychologia 2003; 41(11):1547–1559.
35. Boone KB, Swerdloff RS, Miller BL, et al. Neuropsychological profiles of adults with Klinefelter syndrome. J Int Neuropsychol Soc 2001; 7(4):446–456.
36. Itti E, Gaw Gonzalo IT, Pawlikowska-Haddal A, et al. The structural brain correlates of cognitive deficits in adults with Klinefelter's syndrome. J Clin Endocrinol Metab 2006; 91(4):1423–1427.
37. Götz MJ, Johnstone EC, Ratcliffe SG. Criminality and antisocial behaviour in unselected men with sex chromosome abnormalities. Psychol Med 1999; 29(4):953–962.
38. Swerdlow AJ, Higgins CD, Schoemaker MJ, et al; on behalf of the United Kingdom Clinical Cytogenetics Group. Mortality in Patients with Klinefelter Syndrome in Britain: A Cohort Study. J Clin Endocrinol Metab 2005; 90(12):6516–6522
39. Terzoli G, Lalatta F, Lobbiani A, et al. Fertility in a 47,XXY patient: assessment of biological paternity by deoxyribonucleic acid fingerprinting. Fertil Steril 1992; 58(4):821–822.
40. Vorona E, Zitzmann M, Gromoll J, et al. Clinical, endocrinological, and epigenetic features of the 46,XX male syndrome, compared with 47,XXY Klinefelter patients. J Clin Endocrinol Metab 2007; 92(9):3458–3465.
41. Palermo GD, Schlegel PN, Sills ES, et al. Births after intracytoplasmic injection of sperm obtained by testicular extraction from men with nonmosaic Klinefelter's syndrome. N Engl J Med 1998; 338(9):588–590.
42. Vernaeve V, Staessen C, Verheyen G, et al. Can biological or clinical parameters predict testicular sperm recovery in 47,XXY Klinefelter's syndrome patients? Hum Reprod 2004; 19(5):1135–1139.
43. Schiff JD, Palermo GD, Veeck LL, et al. Success of testicular sperm extraction [corrected] and intracytoplasmic sperm injection in men with Klinefelter syndrome. J Clin Endocrinol Metab 2005; 90(11):6263–6267.
44. Richiardi L, Pettersson A, Akre O. Genetic and environmental risk factors for testicular cancer. Int J Androl 2007; 30(4):230–240; discussion 240–241.
45. Virtanen HE, Cortes D, Rajpert-De Meyts E,et al. Development and descent of the testis in relation to cryptorchidism. Acta Paediatr 2007; 96(5):622–627.
46. Bogatcheva NV, Ferlin A, Feng S, et al. T222P mutation of the insulin-like 3 hormone receptor LGR8 is associated with testicular maldescent and hinders receptor expression on the cell surface membrane. Am J Physiol Endocrinol Metab 2007; 292(1):E138–E144.
47. Nuti F, Marinari E, Erdei E, et al. The leucine-rich repeat-containing G protein-coupled receptor 8 gene T222P mutation does not cause cryptorchidism. J Clin Endocrinol Metab 2008; 93(3):1072–1076.
48. Thorsson AV, Christiansen P, Ritzén M. Efficacy and safety of hormonal treatment of cryptorchidism: current state of the art. Acta Paediatr 2007; 96(5):628–630.

49. Murphy F, Paran TS, Puri P. Orchidopexy and its impact on fertility. Pediatr Surg Int 2007; 23(7):625–632.
50. Walsh TJ, Dall'Era MA, Croughan MS, et al. Prepubertal orchiopexy for cryptorchidism may be associated with lower risk of testicular cancer. J Urol 2007; 178(4Pt 1):1440–1446.
51. Pettersson A, Richiardi L, Nordenskjold A, et al. Age at surgery for undescended testis and risk of testicular cancer. N Engl J Med 2007; 356(18):1835–1841.
52. Hack WW, Sijstermans K, van der Voort-Doedens LM. Correction of Cryptorchidism and testicular cancer. N Engl J Med 2007; 357:825–827.
53. Crosignani PG, Rubin B. The ESHRE Capri Workshop. Guidelines to the prevalence, diagnosis, treatment and management of infertility. Hum Reprod 1996; 11:1775–1807.
54. Bergmann M, Behre HM, Nieschlag E. Serum FSH and testicular morphology in male infertility. Clin Endocrinol (Oxf) 1994; 40(1):133–136.
55. Pierik FH, Vreeburg JT, Stijnen T, et al. Serum inhibin B as a marker of spermatogenesis. J Clin Endocrinol Metab 1998; 83(9):3110–3114.
56. Vincent MC, Daudin M, De MP, et al. Cytogenetic investigations of infertile men with low sperm counts: a 25-year experience. J Androl 2002; 23(1):18–22.
57. Krausz C, Rajpert-De Meyts E, Frydelund-Larsen L, et al. Double-blind Y chromosome microdeletion analysis in men with known sperm parameters and reproductive hormone profiles: microdeletions are specific for spermatogenic failure. J Clin Endocrinol Metab 2001; 86(6):2638–2642.
58. Krausz C, Forti G, McElreavey K. The Y chromosome and male fertility and infertility. Int J Androl 2003; 26(2):70–75.
59. Krausz C, Degl'Innocenti S. Y chromosome and male infertility: update 2006. Front Biosci 2006; 11:3049–3061.
60. No authors listed] The influence of varicocele on parameters of fertility in a large group of men presenting to infertility clinics. World Health Organization. Fertil Steril 1992; 57(6):1289–1293.
61. Evers JL, Collins JA. Surgery or embolisation for varicocele in subfertile men. Cochrane Database Syst Rev 2004; (3):CD000479
62. Forti G, Krausz C, Cilotti A, et al. Varicocele and infertility. J Endocrinol Invest 2003; 26(6):564–569.
63. Handelsman DJ. Testicular dysfunction in systemic disease Endocrinol Metab Clin North Am 1994; 23(4):839–856.
64. Kalyani RR, Gavini S, Dobs AS. Male hypogonadism in systemic disease. Endocrinol Metab Clin North Am 2007; 36(2):333–348.
65. Nachtigall LB, Boepple PA, Pralong FP, et al. Adult-onset idiopathic hypogonadotropic hypogonadism—A treatable form of male infertility. N Engl J Med 1997; 336(6):410–415.
66. Raivio T, Falardeau J, Dwyer A, et al. Reversal of idiopathic hypogonadotropic hypogonadism. N Engl J Med 2007; 357(9):863–873.
67. Layman LC. Hypogonadotropic hypogonadism. Endocrinol Metab Clin North Am 2007; 36(2):283–296.
68. Farooqi IS, Wangensteen T, Collins S, et al. Clinical and molecular genetic spectrum of congenital deficiency of the leptin receptor. N Engl J Med 2007; 356(3):237–247.
69. Chen C, Visootsak J, Dills S, et al. Prader-Willi syndrome: an update and review for the primary pediatrician. Clin Pediatr (Phila) 2007; 46(7):580–591.
70. Sheffield VC. Use of isolated populations in the study of a human obesity syndrome, the Bardet-Biedl syndrome. Pediatr Res 2004; 55(6):908–911.
71. Aimaretti G, Ghigo E. Should every patient with traumatic brain injury be referred to an endocrinologist? Nat Clin Pract Endocrinol Metab 2007; 3(4):318–319.
72. Corona G, Mannucci E, Fisher AD, et al. Effect of hyperprolactinemia in male patients consulting for sexual dysfunction. J Sex Med 2007; 4(5):1485–1493.
73. Corona G, Mannucci E, Petrone L, et al. A comparison of NCEP-ATPIII and IDF metabolic syndrome definitions with relation to metabolic syndrome-associated sexual dysfunction. J Sex Med 2007; 4(3):789–796.
74. Corona G, Mannucci E, Schulman C, et al. Psychobiologic correlates of the metabolic syndrome and associated sexual dysfunction [published online ahead of print March 13, 2006]. Eur Urol 2006; 50(3):595–604; discussion 604.
75. Corona G, Mannucci E, Petrone L, et al. NCEP-ATPIII-defined metabolic syndrome, type 2 diabetes mellitus, and prevalence of hypogonadism in male patients with sexual dysfunction. J Sex Med 2007; 4(4Pt 1):1038–1045.
76. Kalyani RR, Dobs AS. Androgen deficiency, diabetes, and the metabolic syndrome in men. Curr Opin Endocrinol Diabetes Obes 2007; 14(3):226–234.
77. Wang C, Nieschlag E, Swerdloff R, et al. Investigation, treatment and monitoring of late-onset hypogonadism in males. Int J Androl 2008.
78. [No authors listed] Testosterone replacement therapy for male aging: ASA position statement. J Androl 2006; 27(2):133–134.
79. Bhasin S, Cunningham GR, Hayes FJ, et a. Testosterone therapy in adult men with androgen deficiency syndromes: an endocrine society clinical practice guideline. J Clin Endocrinol Metab 2006; 91(6):1995–2010.
80. Hall R, Evered D, Greene R. A Colour Atlas of Endocrinology. London: Wolfe Medical Publications Ltd, 1979.
81. Besser GM, Thorner MO, eds. Slide Atlas of Clinical Endocrinology. St. Louis: Mosby-Wolfe, 1994.

28 Testosterone deficiency syndrome

Stefan Arver

TESTOSTERONE DEFICIENCY—TERMINOLOGY

Hypogonadism is a clinical syndrome complex that comprises symptoms and signs as well as biochemical evidence of testosterone deficiency.

Male hypogonadism is classically related to relatively rare disorders of the hypothalamic–pituitary–gonadal axis. Thus the classical diagnosis of hypogonadism involves disorders like Kallman's syndrome, pituitary tumors (secondary hypogonadism) and Klinefelter syndrome, and XX-males syndrome (primary hypogonadism), which will be covered in detail in another section. It is evident that low testosterone levels precipitating symptoms is far more prevalent than these disorders and that men with symptoms related to testosterone deficiency are regularly seen in most clinical settings, though without being identified as potential candidates for testosterone replacement therapy. Testosterone deficiency and hypogonadism may cause compromised function in multiple organ systems and be a modifiable cause of hampered quality of life as well as facilitating different disease processes. The classical underlying diseases causing hypogonadism are thus not responsible for the majority of testosterone deficiency in men. There is a need to make the diagnosis of hypogonadism less challenging and more familiar to physicians in a wider range of specialities. Men with severe hypogonadism are easily diagnosed in a straightforward way, whereas men with less severe deficiency without a definite or clearly identifiable cause are more of a challenge. In these cases, a combination of primary (testicular) and secondary (hypothalamic/pituitary) failure is often at hand, indicating that concomitant morbidity may affect both hypothalamic and pituitary function as well as testicular capacity to respond to gonadotropin stimulation and decreased capacity to produce testosterone.

LATE ONSET HYPOGONADISM OR SIMPLY TESTOSTERONE DEFICIENCY SYNDROME?

The terminology regarding hypogonadism has drifted over the years and in an effort to distinguish the more common forms of hypogonadism from the classical etiologies various nomenclatures have been put forward especially related to the increased prevalence of testosterone deficiency in elderly men, that is, PADAM (partial androgen deficiency in aging men), ADAM (androgen deficiency in aging men), and LOH (late onset hypogonadism). These proposed names have also been launched as an alternative form to label the conditions occurring from time to time as male climacterium. Male climacterium or andropause is conceptually misleading and refers to a phenomenon that does not occur in men, the predetermined loss of gonadal function. It is important to emphasize that a majority of healthy men retain normal testosterone levels throughout life and do not have testosterone levels in the hypogonadal range (1). On the other hand, men who become overweight attain an increased risk to develop hypogonadism. This seems especially pronounced if obesity also causes development of metabolic and vascular disease. In the current text the term testosterone deficiency or testosterone deficiency syndrome (TDS) is used as a synonym to hypogonadism and includes the combination of low testosterone levels and the presence of clinical symptoms attributed to low testosterone levels. LOH has become a commonly used term and has been introduced to clearly identify hypogonadism occurring in aging men. The definition is similar to general hypogonadism but also includes the age aspect. In the recommendations for management of LOH (2) the definition reads: "A clinical and biochemical syndrome associated with advancing age and characterized by typical symptoms and a deficiency in serum testosterone levels. It may result in significant detriment in the quality of life and adversely affect the function of multiple organs" (3). There is no clear definition of the age that defines advancing age, though taken from the context of the recommendations, one may interpret that as men over 60 years of age. In this chapter it is suggested that that the term TDS is used due to the fact that in testosterone deficiency, irrespective of whether a man is 40 or 70 years of age, he faces the same clinical problems and requires the same androgen levels for adequate stimulation of androgen-dependent functions. The relevance of the age distinction is the increased prevalence of low testosterone levels in elderly men and that our knowledge and experience of risks and benefits of testosterone therapy in that group is limited. Most of our current knowledge and understanding of signs and symptoms of hypogonadism are based on experiences from clinical observations and substitution therapy in younger men. It remains to be clarified what symptoms are precipitated in elderly men by testosterone deficiency and whether these regress with substitution therapy or not. An important contribution to this understanding was the recent demonstration that the androgen-stimulated increment in lean body mass showed the same dose-response relationship in young as well as elderly men (4). Hypogonadism in aging men is often associated with increased body mass index (BMI), which to some extent reflects obesity and also the presence of concomitant medical disorders. The endocrine mechanism causing declined testosterone levels may include either hypothalamic–pituitary dysfunction, testicular dysfunction, or a combination of both.

PRIMARY, SECONDARY, OR MIXED HYPOGONADISM

The classification of hypogonadism into primary or secondary etiology is defined by the level within the hypothalamic–pituitary–testicular axis that malfunctions. Levels of luteinising hormone (LH) are the simple laboratory assessment that clarifies the etiology. If testosterone is low and LH is high, the condition is classified as primary hypogonadism; if LH levels are low, it is classified as secondary hypogonadism. A common clinical situation in elderly men is the presence of midnormal LH levels and low testosterone levels indicating an inability of the pituitary to respond to the low testosterone level. This could be regarded as an insufficient hypothalamic or pituitary response to a low circulating testosterone level and thus a secondary hypogonadism. At the same time the testicular response to LH stimulation may be weakened indicating a primary component. These cases may be referred to as a state of mixed hypogonadism with both a primary and a secondary component. Although a substantial number of middle age and elderly men presents with the sign of classical primary hypogonadism i.e. low testosterone and elevated LH levels (EMAS study).

It is well documented that testosterone replacement therapy in hypogonadal men improve muscle mass and strength, bone mineral density, mood, sexual function (libido and erectile function) as well as general appreciation of increased energy. Identifying eligible men for testosterone therapy is based on a combination of measurement serum testosterone assessment and clinical evaluation of hypogonadal symptoms.

SYMPTOMS AND SIGNS OF TESTOSTERONE DEFICIENCY

The clinical presentation of hypogonadism depends on four main factors (*i*) age at onset of androgen deficiency, (*ii*) duration of androgen deficiency, (*iii*) the profoundness of the deficiency, and (*iv*) genetic factors controlling androgen receptor responsiveness (androgen receptor polymorphism and mutations) and probably also post receptor regulatory mechanisms and signaling. Thus it is evident that serum testosterone assessment or determination of subfractions of testosterone in blood (free or SHBG-bound testosterone) are coarse methods of more indicative than clearly defining assessments. The clinical evaluation remains of utmost importance in the decision making.

Adult men who experience a decline in testosterone levels have undergone normal virilization at puberty and for a longer or shorter period maintained normal levels of testosterone and thus also normal androgen-dependent functions. Symptoms develop gradually as testosterone levels decrease and different androgen-dependent processes have different "dose-response" relations. The gradual loss of function has been demonstrated in a cohort of men referred for androgen deficiency evaluation (5) with increased prevalence of hypogonadal symptoms appearing at different androgen levels. Prepubertal onset of hypogonadism results in lack of virilization, sustained height increase without closure of the epiphysis, lack of pubertal growth spurt, incomplete sexual development, and aspermia. Adult onset results in loss of function of androgen-dependent pathways and symptoms and signs are often nonspecific and subject to the influence of comorbidity, age, and other factors. Androgen deficiency related symptoms and signs in the adult include reduced libido and reduced sexual activity, loss of spontaneous erections and erectile dysfunction, loss of body hair, reduced need to shave, reduced muscle mass and strength, and also flushes and sweating. Gynecomastia signifies a decrease in testosterone levels as well as low trauma fractures and finding a very small testis (<5 mL). These symptoms are regarded as more specific to testosterone deficiency than other symptoms that are also reported to occur as a consequence of lowered testosterone levels. These symptoms include depressed mood and dysthymia, poor ability to concentrate and poor memory, decreased energy, initiative, and self-confidence. Also irritability or aggressiveness is seen as a result of testosterone deficiency as well as a shift in body composition with increased body fat and BMI and diminished physical performance (6).

In the Endocrine Society guidelines, symptoms are separated into two groups, group A suggestive of hypogonadism and group B of less specific symptoms (4) (Table 1).

Table 1 Endocrine Society's Clinical Guidelines Classification of Symptoms and Signs of Androgen Deficiency

A. Symptoms and signs suggestive of androgen deficiency in men, incomplete sexual development, eunuchoidism, aspermia
   - Reduced sexual desire (libido) and activity
   - Decreased spontaneous erections
   - Breast discomfort, gynecomastia
   - Loss of body (axillar and pubic) hair, reduced shaving
   - Very small or shrinking testis (especially <5 mL)
   - Inability to father children, low or zero sperm count
   - Height loss, low trauma fracture, low bone mineral density
   - Reduced muscle mass and strength
   - Hot flushes, sweats
B. Symptoms and signs associated with androgen deficiency that are less specific than those in group A
   - Decreased energy, motivation, initiative, aggressiveness, self-confidence
   - Feeling sad or blue, depressed mood, dysthymia
   - Poor concentration and memory
   - Sleep disturbance, increased sleepiness
   - Mild anemia (normochromic, normocytic, in the female range)
   - Increased body fat, body mass index
   - Diminished physical or work performance

The selection of symptoms indicating androgen deficiency is based on clinical observations of hypogonadal men and intervention studies with testosterone substitution therapy. There are no population-based symptom surveys relating symptoms to testosterone levels. There are few symptoms that are pathognomonic for hypogonadism, though lack of pubertal development (voice deepening, genital organ maturation, development of secondary hair, and muscle accretion) is a strong indicator of hypogonadism in a person of postpubertal age. Whether loss of libido or spontaneous erection is more suggestive then decreased energy or dysthymia of hypogonadism could be questioned. The complete spectrum of symptoms, potentially related to androgen deficiency, need to be assessed where hypogonadism is part of the differential diagnosis. Loss of body hair requires a long duration of hypogonadism and a beard may stay for decades in a severely hypogonadal man. Changes in hair growth and shaving frequency may be a more specific and sensitive indicator of testosterone deficiency (see Fig. 1).

The onset of symptoms seems to be related to prevailing testosterone levels (6). There is evidence that the symptoms of hypogonadism are precipitated at different testosterone levels. This implies that there may be different thresholds for specific androgen-dependent pathways. Loss of libido and vigor becomes significant below a serum testosterone level of 15 nmol/L, whereas erectile dysfunction and flushes are significantly related to a testosterone level below 8 nmol/L. In the same study, type 2 diabetes and depressive symptom became significantly more common when testosterone levels were below 10 nmol/L (5).

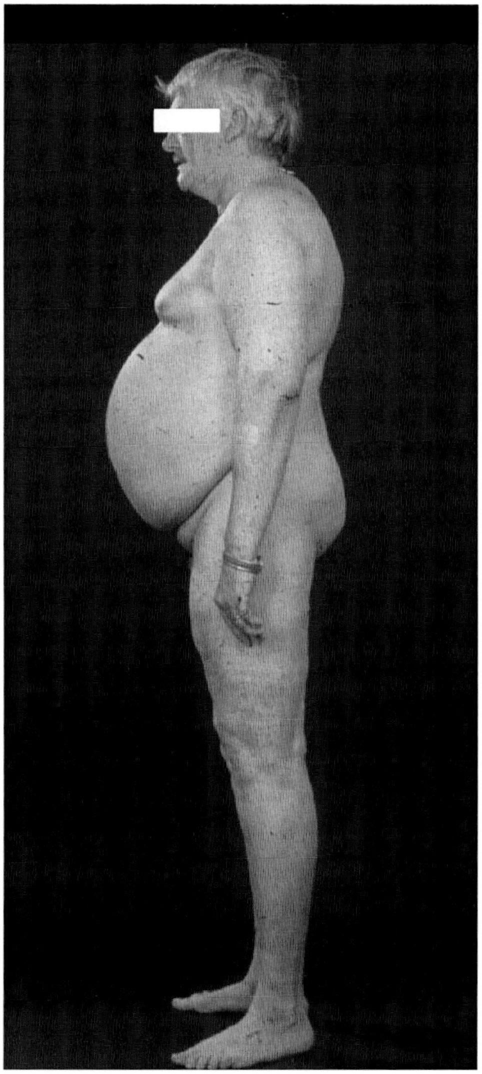

Figure 1 A 56-year-old male, presenting with muscle and joint pain, anemia, loss of body hair, tiredness, and with low bone mineral density (−2SD). S-testosterone 3.2 nmol/L and S-LH 15. Other pituitary hormones normal. Small atrophic testis. Probable etiology: bilateral orchitis at the age of 35.

QUESTIONNAIRES AND INTERVIEW INSTRUMENTS FOR HYPOGONADISM DIAGNOSIS

Questionnaires and a structured interview for screening of male hypogonadism have been proposed and four different tools with some validation are currently available. Their limited specificity makes them unsuitable for general screening. The Androtest (7) has the best specificity at the cost of lower sensitivity (Table 2) while the AMS (8) scale has met the widest use. These scales serve the purpose of strengthening the diagnostic criteria for hypogonadism and help in fulfilling the clinical requirement of symptoms in addition to analyzing low serum testosterone levels.

Table 2 Sensitivity and Specificity of Interview and Screening Questionnaires

	Sensitivity (%)	Specificity (%)
ADAM (8)	97	30
MMAS (9)	60	59
AMS (7)	83	39
Androtest (6)	68	65

Symptoms related to comorbidities, psychological influence, and age will influence and confound the diagnosis of hypogonadism. This is further compounded by the knowledge that there are no clear-cut levels where hypogonadal symptoms occur. All of these factors significantly affect the overall assessment and decision making in the diagnosis of hypogonadism. It is becoming clear, however, that certain patient groups with specific comorbidities should have an increased awareness of hypogonadism as it is an additional factor afflicting the patients' physical and psychological status. Such conditions include, but are not limited to, metabolic syndrome, type 2 diabetes, cardiovascular disease, chronic obstructive pulmonary disease, and depression.

Another valuable use of these questionnaires is the evaluation of treatment effects. Until we have access to instruments with higher specificity and sensitivity, preferably in the 90% range, they cannot be used for general screening in unselected patient populations

ADAM questionnaire (9)

1. Do you have a decrease in libido (sex drive)?
2. Do you have a lack of energy?
3. Do you have a decrease in strength and/or endurance?
4. Have you lost height?
5. Have you noticed a decrease in enjoyment of life?
6. Are you sad and/or grumpy?
7. Are your erections less strong?
8. Have you noticed a recent deterioration in your ability to perform sports?
9. Are you falling asleep after dinner?
10. Has there been a recent deterioration in your work performance?

If you answered YES to questions 1 or 7 or any 3 other questions, you may have a low testosterone level.

The AMS evaluation (Fig. 2) is summarized in a total score and as psychological (Q 6, 7, 8, 11, and 13), sexual (Q12, 14–17), and somatic (Q 1–5, 9, 10) subscales.

ANDROTEST© is a structured interview for the screening of hypogonadism (total testosterone <10.4 nmol/L or 300 ng/dL in patients with sexual dysfunction). The test is applicable only to patients reporting at least one incidence of sexual intercourse during the past 3 months.

The interview is composed of 12 key items. The interviewer should ask the questions written in bold, using the exact words proposed. The further questions written in normal characters can be used to clarify the patient's answers, if needed. The patient should be permitted to answer freely, using his own words.

The patient's answers are codified on a 0 to 3 scale by the interviewer, following detailed instructions reported after each item. For some of the items, the answers had a yes/no format.

The order in which the questions are presented should be observed, as alterations in this sequence could theoretically modify the patient's answers.

(1) **Age**

After asking the patient how old he is, rank a progressive score as a function of patient's age at the time of the visit.

0 <40 years
1 40–49 years
2 50–59 years
3 >59 years

(2) **When did you undergo your sexual development (puberty)?**

At what age did you undergo your sexual development? Did you experience puberty at the same time as your schoolmates? Did you notice that pubic hairs and the development of genitalia happened to you as well as to your schoolmates?

Rank 0 if patient reports a sexual development at the same time or before that of his schoolmates; 3 if patients reported a delayed puberty.

0 9–14 years (normal)
3 >14 years (delayed)

(3) **Have you ever had a pituitary disease?**

Have you ever undergone surgery for pituitary disease? Have you ever been treated with medical therapy for pituitary disease?

The score will be 0 if patients did not report a pituitary disease and 3 for an affirmative response.

0 No
3 Yes

(4) **Have you ever had a diagnosis of undescended testes (cryptorchidism)?**

Have you ever undergone surgery for cryptorchidism? Have you ever been treated with medical therapy for cryptorchidism?

The score will be 0 if patients did not report a history of cryptorchidism (even monolateral) and 3 for an affirmative response.

0 No
3 Yes

(5) **Describe what happens during sexual intercourse: how often do you have lack of an erection?**

The description of the problems refers to the last 3 months. Sometimes = <25%, quite often = 25% to 49%, often = 50% to 74%, and always = >75% of cases.

0 Sometimes
1 Quite often
2 Often
3 Always

(6) **Do you ever wake up with an erection?**

How often has it happened in the last 3 months?

Rank 0 if patient reports spontaneous nocturnal/morning erection with the same frequency previously observed: 1 nocturnal/morning erections are present, but their frequency during the last 3 months is somewhat lower than that observed previously; 2 if the frequency of nocturnal/morning erections of the last 3 months is reduced by at least 50%; 3 if nocturnal/morning erections are not present.

0 Yes, regularly
1 Less frequently than in the past
2 Only occasionally
3 Never

AMS Questionnaire

Which of the following symptoms apply to you at this time? Please, mark the appropriate box for each symptom. For symptoms that do not apply, please mark "none".

	Symptoms:	none	mild	moderate	severe	extremely severe
	Score =	1	2	3	4	5
1	**Decline in your feeling of general well-being** (general state of health, subjective feeling)	☐	☐	☐	☐	☐
2	**Joint pain and muscular ache** (lower back pain, joint pain, pain in a limb, general back ache)	☐	☐	☐	☐	☐
3	**Excessive sweating** (unexpected/sudden episodes of sweating, hot flushes independent of strain)	☐	☐	☐	☐	☐
4	**Sleep problems** (difficulty in falling asleep, difficulty in sleeping through, waking up early and feeling tired, poor sleep, sleeplessness)	☐	☐	☐	☐	☐
5	**Increased need for sleep, often feeling tired**	☐	☐	☐	☐	☐
6	**Irritability** (feeling aggressive, easily upset about little things, moody)	☐	☐	☐	☐	☐
7	**Nervousness** (inner tension, restlessness, feeling fidgety)	☐	☐	☐	☐	☐
8	**Anxiety** (feeling panicky)	☐	☐	☐	☐	☐
9	**Physical exhaustion / lacking vitality** (general decrease in performance, reduced activity, lacking interest in leisure activities, feeling of getting less done, of achieving less, of having to force oneself to undertake activities)	☐	☐	☐	☐	☐
10	**Decrease in muscular strength** (feeling of weakness)	☐	☐	☐	☐	☐
11	**Depressive mood** (feeling down, sad, on the verge of tears, lack of drive, mood swings, feeling nothing is of any use)	☐	☐	☐	☐	☐
12	**Feeling that you have passed your peak**	☐	☐	☐	☐	☐
13	**Feeling burnt out, having hit rock-bottom**	☐	☐	☐	☐	☐
14	**Decrease in beard growth**	☐	☐	☐	☐	☐
15	**Decrease in ability/frequency to perform sexually**	☐	☐	☐	☐	☐
16	**Decrease in the number of morning erections**	☐	☐	☐	☐	☐
17	**Decrease in sexual desire/libido** (lacking pleasure in sex, lacking desire for sexual intercourse)	☐	☐	☐	☐	☐

Have you got any other major symptoms? Yes ☐ No ☐

If Yes, please describe: ______________________________

Figure 2 AMS questionnaire (8).

(7) **How often have you practiced autoerotism (masturbation) in the last 3 months?**

0 >8 times/month
1 3–7 times/month
2 1–2 times/month
3 Never

If the patient does not practice autoerotism (answer 3), the following question (#8) is not applicable. In this case assign rank 1 to question 8 and continue with question #9.

(8) **How do you feel during autoerotism?**
After asking the question above, rank with the following score:

0 Well
1 With a little sense of guilt
2 With a big sense of guilt
3 With a very big sense of guilt

(9) **Have you had more or less desire to make love in the last 3 months?**
Has your desire increased or reduced in comparison to the past?

Rank 0 when the patient's desire is unmodified or increased; 1 if desire is reduced.

0 Unmodified or increased desire
1 Reduced desire

(10) **Have you noticed a reduction of the quantity of the volume of ejaculate?**
Rank 0 when the patient did not notice any modification of the volume of ejaculate; 1 when the patient has the feeling

that the volume of ejaculate could be slightly reduced; 2 when the volume of ejaculate is markedly reduced; 3 when no ejaculation occurs.

0 No modification
1 Slightly reduced
2 Markedly reduced
3 Ejaculation absent

(11) **In the last 3 months, has it been difficult to ejaculate (or to achieve climax) during sexual intercourse?**
Are you able to ejaculate during sexual intercourse with penetration or only with manual or oral stimulation by your partner?

Rank 0 if patient did not report difficulties in ejaculating or, as in some rare cases, if ejaculation and climax could be obtained but only with autoerotism conducted in the absence of the partner or if it could not be obtained at all; 1 if ejaculation and climax were still possible, but only with great effort and after prolonged intercourse or if they were possible only with autoerotism, although in the presence of the partner, but not during coitus.

0 No
1 Yes

(12) **How much do you weigh and how tall are you?**
After asking the patient his weight and height, the interviewer should rank a progressive score as a function of the calculation (body mass index = weight [kg]/height [m^2]).

0 <25 kg/m^2
1 25–29.9 kg/m^2
2 30–34.9 kg/m^2
3 >34.9 kg/m^2

MEASUREMENT OF SERUM TESTOSTERONE

Measurement of serum testosterone is of key importance in the diagnosis of hypogonadism. Generally good testosterone assays are available at most hospital laboratories that reliably distinguish low and normal testosterone levels in men. Total testosterone levels are affected by circadian variation, in some areas circannual variation and also by concomitant medical conditions and some medical treatments (opiates and glucocorticoids). Due to the circadian variation, serum samples should be drawn between 7 and 10 in the morning after a normal nights sleep and without prior exposure to vigorous physical activity. Fasting samples are preferred as the glucose load suppresses testosterone levels. Low serum level should be confirmed especially in men with borderline levels. In healthy young men, as much as 15% of randomly taken serum testosterone samples show levels in the hypogonadal range (11).

Most of testosterone in blood is bound to SHBG (sex hormone–binding globulin) and to albumin with only some 0.5% to 3% being unbound or free. The pool of albumin-bound testosterone is freely dissociated and participates in tissue interaction while the SHBG-bound fraction is tightly bound and is considered not available for tissue interaction. Determination of nonSHBG-bound testosterone can be made in different ways. Ammonium precipitation (of the testosterone–SHBG complex) prior to testosterone measurement directly measures the nonSHBG-bound testosterone fraction (12). Methods to calculate the available pool of testosterone, commonly referred to as nonSHBG-bound testosterone or bioavailable testosterone ("Bio-T") are readily available even on the internet (www.ISSAM.ch and www.him-link.com) and some laboratories also provide these calculated values. Measurement of free testosterone can only be done with equilibrium dialysis and is only reliably available in a few research laboratories worldwide. Free testosterone assays based on analogue methods are readily available but should be avoided and are considered incorrect (13) In clinical practice, assessment of total testosterone is most often sufficient. In some cases SHBG levels may be exceedingly high or low and then estimation of the nonSHBG-bound fraction adds valuable information.

What to Measure: Total Testosterone, Free T, or Bioavailable T

The value of assessment of bioavailable testosterone has been convincingly demonstrated in men with type 2 diabetes (14) where hypogonadal symptoms and sexual dysfunction were closely related to nonSHBG-bound testosterone or calculated free testosterone levels (taking SHBG into consideration) than to total testosterone. Whether Bio-T is more discriminating than total testosterone in all circumstances remains to be elucidated. First line analysis include testosterone and SHBG assay; if the results show low levels of testosterone, a repeat sample should be taken and LH and prolactin should also be included. The latter will be helpful to distinguish primary from secondary hypogonadism and the eventual need for further endocrine evaluation.

General screening of testosterone levels is not indicated and should so far be limited to men who seek medical attention with symptoms suggestive of testosterone deficiency and in some groups of men with specific underlying disorders known to have a high prevalence of hypogonadism. These conditions include, but are not limited to, men with suspected pituitary tumor or disease in the pituitary hypothalamic region, osteoporosis, or low trauma fracture, moderate to severe chronic obstructive disease, catabolic conditions with wasting (e.g., HIV infection), and men treated with medication that interferes with testosterone production or metabolism, such as glucocorticoids, opiates, and ketoconazole.

INTERPRETATION OF TESTOSTERONE ASSESSMENT

There is no clear level of testosterone that unambiguously separates normal men from hypogonadal men, and there is no uniform threshold where symptoms start to occur (2,5). There is no level beyond which androgen therapy results in improvement of health in all men. The interpretation of data thus relies on clinical assessment of symptoms and signs, taking into

Table 3 Conditions that influence SHBG levels (6)

Conditions with high SHBG levels	Conditions with low SHBG levels
Aging	Obesity, hyperinsulinemia, metabolic syndrome, type 2 diabetes
Catabolic conditions (general disease, malnutrition, malabsorption, HIV infection)	Use of ANABOLIC Steroids, progestins, and glucocorticoids
Medication (anticonvulsants and estrogen)	Hypothyroidism
Hepatic cirrhosis, hyperthyroidism, acromegaly	Nephrotic syndrome

account SHBG levels. Genotype differences also play a role in the evaluation of patients and may also be of importance in management of androgen replacement therapy. Variation in CAG repeat length on exon 1 of the androgen receptor determines the transactivation activity of the receptor. Shorter CAG repeats codes for a more active receptor while long CAG repeats codes for a less active and thus less androgenic receptor. Clinical use of CAG repeat length determination may be a part of androgen evaluation but more data is needed. CAG repeat length may, however, be of direct value in dose adjustment of testosterone therapy (15).

A practical approach (2) to clinical evaluation of testosterone determination is to recognize the different thresholds and the variability in androgen sensitivity and thus regard (*i*) levels below 8 nmol/L as suggestive of testosterone deficiency, (*ii*) level between 8 to 12 nmol/L as a grey zone in which individuals may be testosterone deficient or replete, and (*iii*) levels >12 nmol/L as most likely normal and not related to any androgen-dependent symptoms (6). Although there are data that suggests that some androgen-dependent symptoms become significant even in the range up to 15 nmol/L, however, no recommendation so far have stretched the lower limit of normal testosterone to that level. Thus a male without symptoms of hypogonadism and a testosterone level of 8 nmol/L is considered normal while a male with such symptoms and a testosterone level of 11 nmol/L is considered a likely candidate for androgen therapy. Note that the reference values are not age dependent and testosterone effects on body composition and muscle mass remain the same in young and elderly men (4). Current guidelines do not support the use of age-adjusted reference ranges as there is no evidence suggesting that elderly men should have a reduced testosterone requirement (2,5)). In the current recommendations issued by the International Society of Andrology (ISA), International Society for the Study of the Aging Male (ISSAM), European Academy of Andrology (EAA), and the European Urology Association (EUA), cut-off levels of testosterone are suggested clearly.

EVALUATION OF SUSPICIOUS SECONDARY HYPOGONADISM

Hypogonadism has a complex and varied pathogenesis and a definitive etiological diagnosis is not always attainable. Most cases of clinical hypogonadism in middle age and elderly men have a combination of primary and secondary hypogonadism, known as mixed hypogonadism (Table 4).

An important question is when to extend the investigation when a patient presents with hypogonadal symptoms and low testosterone levels in combination with low or normal gonadotropin levels, that is, secondary hypogonadism. In secondary hypogonadism, adequate stimulation of testicular Leydig cells by LH from the pituitary is lacking due to either hypothalamic or pituitary failure. Secondary hypogonadism or contribution by a relative gonadotropin deficiency becomes more prevalent as we age and a mixed etiology with both a primary and a secondary component seems to be the overall most common background to hypogonadism. In the vast majority of these cases, there is no pituitary tumor or other underlying diseases processes that need specific treatment. Though it is important not to overlook the presence of treatable underlying disorders. Assessment to pituitary function and evaluation of the local topography in the pituitary and hypothalamic region with imaging (MRI) is clearly indicated, if testosterone levels are very low, that is, <5 nmol/L and LH levels below the midreference range according to the local laboratory (5,16,17). If there is a suspicion of pituitary failure, gonadotropin levels that are low or lower than expected for the level of testosterone, which often is below 5 nmol/L, should raise the suspicion of hypothalamic or pituitary hypogonadism. The most frequent causes in adults are pituitary adenomas, both secreting and not secreting adenomas. Metastases in the pituitary or/and hypophyseal stalk, postoperative states, and post-radiotherapy of the area can cause secondary hypogonadism. Other causes are iron overload (hemochromatosis), sarcoidosis, and other infiltration disorders. Idiopathic hypogonadotropic hypogonadism is a diagnosis made after exclusion of other causes of hypogonadotropic hypogonadism.

DIAGNOSIS OF SECONDARY HYPOGONADISM

Modern imaging techniques with magnetic resonance technique (MRI) and computerized tomography (CT) have made diagnosis of pituitary tumors much easier. Endocrine evaluation of the anterior pituitary function with LH, FSH, prolactin,

Table 4 Causes of Mixed Hypogonadism

Aging
Alcohol abuse
Diabetes mellitus/metabolic cluster syndrome
Drugs (glucocorticoids, opioids, and ketoconazol)
Chronic infections (HIV) and autoimmune disease
Systemic disease (liver failure, uremia, sickle cell disease, hemochromatosis)

TSH, ACTH, and GH and their corresponding peripheral hormones testosterone, cortisol, thyroid hormone, and IGF should be assessed in order to clarify the extent of pituitary dysfunction and thus the need for substitution therapy. In depth presentation for insight into hypothalamic and pituitary diseases is found in Chapter 27.

Large pituitary adenomas may cause partial or complete hypopituitarism by impinging of neighboring structures (e.g., adjacent normal gland, pituitary stalk). Compression of the optic chiasm by mass effect is also associated with disturbance of vision. The chiasm is found at variable distance above the diaphragma sella and in some subject the distance is less than 10 mm. Approximately 90% of neuronal axons in the chiasma are responsible for central vision and its is not uncommon to find an early disturbance by visual examination (e.g., foggy vision). The most common visual disorder caused by large pituitary adenoma or other diseases causing mass effect in this area is bitemporal hemianopia or bilateral scotoma rather than hemianopia. If the mass expands laterally, it can also affect the sinus cavernous and paralyze the occulomotor nerve without visual field defects. If the mass expands further laterally, the fourth, fifth, and sixth cranial nerve may be involved. It is therefore of importance that all patients with adenoma larger than 10 mm (macroadenomas) are carefully evaluated for visual impairment.

SUMMARY

Hypogonadism is a clinical syndrome complex, which consists of the presence of symptoms and signs and biochemical confirmation of testosterone deficiency. Classical diagnosis of pituitary or testicular disease represents a minority of men with hypogonadism. The observed increase in hypogonadism with age seem to be more related to comorbidity and increments in BMI than age per se. Cohorts of men with various medical disorders, for example, metabolic syndrome, type 2 diabetes, cardiovascular disease, COPD, chronic infections, rheumatoid diseases, are all associated with a high prevalence of low testosterone levels and symptoms related to androgen deficiency. Diagnostic work-up includes review of symptoms, laboratory assessments, clarification of etiological background, and screening for potential absolute and relative contraindications. Symptom assessment questionnaires may be used to assist in symptom assessment and as a reference for evaluating therapeutic intervention. Laboratory analysis of serum testosterone is readily available but with some limitations. The lack of definitive levels defining testosterone deficiency and the difference in symptom precipitating threshold levels for different testosterone-dependent pathways strongly underline the need for a careful clinical assessment of the patient. In general, testosterone levels below 8 nmol/L probably signify a deficiency while levels above 12 nmol/L are most likely normal. Testosterone levels between 8 and 12 nmol/L may be further scrutinized with determination of free or bioavailable testosterone. In the absence of contraindications, patients may be given a limited trial period of adequate testosterone replacement therapy. Monitoring testosterone therapy includes prostate (PSA and digital examination) and hematological (hematocrit) safety assessment after the initial three, six, nine, and twelve months of therapy and on a yearly basis thereafter. Evaluation of efficacy endpoints may include subjective symptoms and signs and assessment of bone mineral density.

REFERENCES

1. Harkonen K, Huhtaniemi I, Makinen J, et al. The polymorphic androgen receptor gene CAG repeat, pituitary-testicular function and andropausal symptoms in ageing men. Int J Androl 2003; 26(3):187–194.
2. Nieschlag E, Swerdloff R, Behre HM, et al. Investigation, treatment, and monitoring of late-onset hypogonadism in males: ISA, ISSAM, and EAU recommendations. J Androl 2006; 27(2):135–137.
3. Wang C, Nieschlag E, Swerdloff R, et al. Investigation, treatment and monitoring of late-onset hypogonadism in males: ISA, ISSAM, EAU, EAA and ASA recommendations. Eur J Endocrinol 2008; 159(5):507–514.
4. Bhasin S, Woodhouse L, Casaburi R, et al. Older men are as responsive as young men to the anabolic effects of graded doses of testosterone on the skeletal muscle. J Clin Endocrinol Metab 2005; 90(2):678–688.
5. Zitzmann M, Faber S, Nieschlag E. Association of specific symptoms and metabolic risks with serum testosterone in older men. J Clin Endocrinol Metab 2006; 91(11):4335–4343.
6. Bhasin S, Cunningham GR, Hayes FJ, et al. Testosterone therapy in adult men with androgen deficiency syndromes: an endocrine society clinical practice guideline. J Clin Endocrinol Metab 2006; 91(6):1995–2010.
7. Corona G, Mannucci E, Petrone L, et al. ANDROTEST: a structured interview for the screening of hypogonadism in patients with sexual dysfunction. J Sex Med 2006; 3(4):706–715.
8. Heinemann LAJ, Zimmerman T, Vermeulen A, et al. A new aging male symptoms (AMS) rating scale. Aging Male, 1998(2):105e–114e.
9. Morley JE, Charlton E, Patrick P, et al. Validation of a screening questionnaire for androgen deficiency in aging males. Metabolism 2000; 49(9):1239–1242.
10. Smith KW, Feldman HA, McKinlay JB. Construction and field validation of a self-administered screener for testosterone deficiency (hypogonadism) in ageing men. Clin Endocrinol (Oxf) 2000; 53(6):703–711.
11. Spratt DI, O'Dea LS, Schoenfeld D, et al. Neuroendocrine-gonadal axis in men: frequent sampling of LH, FSH, and testosterone. Am J Physiol 1988; 254(5Pt 1):E658–E66.
12. Tremblay RR, Dube JY. Plasma concentrations of free and non-TeBG bound testosterone in women on oral contraceptives. Contraception 1974; 10(6):599–605.

13. Vermeulen A, Verdonck L, Kaufman JM. A critical evaluation of simple methods for the estimation of free testosterone in serum. J Clin Endocrinol Metab 1999; 84(10):3666–3672.
14. Kapoor D, Aldred H, Clark S, et al. Clinical and biochemical assessment of hypogonadism in men with type 2 diabetes: correlations with bioavailable testosterone and visceral adiposity. Diabetes Care 2007; 30(4):911–917.
15. Zitzmann M. Mechanisms of disease: pharmacogenetics of testosterone therapy in hypogonadal men. Nat Clin Pract Urol 2007; 4(3):161–166.
16. Citron JT, Ettinger B, Rubinoff H, et al. Prevalence of hypothalamic-pituitary imaging abnormalities in impotent men with secondary hypogonadism. J Urol 1996; 155(2):529–533.
17. Buvat J, Lemaire A. Endocrine screening in 1,022 men with erectile dysfunction: clinical significance and cost-effective strategy. J Urol 1997; 158(5):1764–1767.

29 Androgen replacement—indications and principles

Fotios Dimitriadis, Evlalia Vlachopoulou, Stavros Gratsias, Dimitrios Baltogiannis, Dimitrios Giannakis, Panagiota Tsounapi, Michael Rimikis, Nikolaos Pardalidis, Takeshi Watanabe, Motoaki Saito, Ikuo Miyagawa, and Nikolaos Sofikitis

INDICATIONS FOR ANDROGEN ADMINISTRATION

A distinction should be made between androgen administration to compensate for androgen deficiency in primary or secondary hypogonadism and androgen administration for other reasons. Compensation for a deficit is known as **replacement.**

WIDELY ACCEPTED INDICATIONS FOR ANDROGEN REPLACEMENT

Primary and Secondary Hypogonadism

Primary and secondary forms of hypogonadism are the classical indications for testosterone replacement (Table 1). After establishing the diagnosis and repeatedly obtaining low serum testosterone levels, androgen deficiency should be corrected, provided that there are no absolute contraindications to androgen replacement. Apart from correction of current symptoms of androgen deficiency (e.g., inadequate virilization, loss of libido and potency, muscle atrophy, androgen deficiency anemia), the aim of testosterone administration is to prevent long-term sequelae of hypogonadism (such as osteoporosis).

Expected Effects of Androgen Replacement in Hypogonadal Men

Patients frequently demonstrate an increase or restoration of libido or potency as the first sign. Most men demonstrate normal libido and erections after only three to five months of testosterone replacement therapy (11). Testosterone stimulates seminal vesicular secretions and prostatic secretions. Thus, the volume of the ejaculate increases too. Testosterone administration has a beneficial effect on emotional state, self-confidence, and activity (1–4).

Testosterone replacement has been demonstrated to have a beneficial effect on musculature. Within 6 to 12 months from the beginning of the therapy, there is a significant increase in overall muscle mass attributable to an increase in the size of individual muscle cells, although the number of cells remains the same. The overall result is a functional increase in muscle strength and capacity (12,13). In addition, there is a decrease in fat tissue and increase in lean body tissue. Men with hypogonadism demonstrate a relative increase in fat mass. This is normalized by testosterone administration. Serum testosterone levels inversely correlate with the mass of visceral adipose tissue and plasma HDL cholesterol levels (14–16). Bone mass is enhanced by testosterone replacement. When testosterone is given, the lower the initial bone density, the greater is the increase in bone mass (8,17,18). Since the bone anabolic effect is largely caused by aromatization of testosterone to estradiol, aromatizable androgens should be given to obtain this effect. For this reason, nonaromatizable androgens are not suitable for treating hypogonadism and osteoporosis.

The skin is an important target for androgens. Sebum production ceases when there is androgen deficiency. Thus, skin becomes dry and sensitive and growth of secondary male hair occurs slowly. Testosterone administration rapidly causes an increase in sebaceous gland activity.

During testosterone replacement, the prostate increases in size. Increased prostatic growth is not anticipated at normal replacement doses. Benign hyperplasia or, more rarely, carcinoma of the prostate may occur in older men on testosterone replacement. Although it has not been shown that testosterone replacement per se can cause these pathologies, recommendations for prostate screening apply to men on androgen replacement (see in the following section) (19).

It should be mentioned that the penis of an adult male rarely increases in size when testosterone is administered. In addition, the testes may shrink as a result of the negative feedback, which testosterone and its metabolite estradiol exert on the gonadotropins. Some studies tend to suggest that there may be an increase in the size of penis in children (20,21). Another study has suggested that the lack of androgens in adult male hamsters has resulted in shortening of penile spines. Administration of androgens partially restored the size of penile spines in this animal model (22).

Androgen deficiency anemia usually responds well to testosterone replacement, and the red cell count increases within a few months (23). If red cell count, hematocrit, and hemoglobin do not increase after testosterone administration, different causes of anemia must be considered. Testosterone administration usually causes a change in lipid metabolism (24,25). During the preexisting phase of hypogonadism, serum HDL cholesterol levels are often high. Testosterone causes a slight decrease in HDL cholesterol and occasionally increases LDL cholesterol. However, this testosterone effect cannot be unequivocally accepted.

Table 1 Widely Accepted Indications for Androgen Replacement

- Primary or secondary hypogonadism in men (1–4)
- Induction of puberty in boys (5,6)
- Excessive constitutional growth in boys (7)
- Transsexuality (female to male) (8)
- Late-onset hypogonadism (9,10)

Androgens such as mesterolone, which do not aromatize, have the same effect as testosterone and its esters on serum cholesterol (24,26).

Testosterone administration does not promote fertility. Although low doses of testosterone undecanoate combined with tamoxifen citrate have been suggested to serve as a treatment of oligospermia, this treatment cannot be considered as *evidence based* (27). If men with secondary hypogonadism want to have children, pulsatile GnRH or recombinant FSH and recombinant LH treatment can stimulate spermatogenesis. Men with primary hypogonadism wishing to have children should be referred for assisted reproduction technology (for more details see chapters 11, 27, and 28).

The level of evidence suggesting a therapeutic effect of testosterone replacement on men with deficiency in the satisfaction with erectile function is 1a (28,29). The level of evidence supporting that testosterone replacement in aging males causes an increase in bone mass, an enhancement in erythropoiesis, and an increase in lean body is 1a (30,31). Furthermore, the level of evidence indicating a therapeutic role of testosterone replacement on men with refractory depression is 1b (4). Additionally, the level of evidence supporting a beneficial effect of testosterone administration in men with secondary hypogonadism due to AIDS wasting syndrome is 1b (32,33).

Induction of Puberty in Boys

Please see chapter 26.

Excessive Growth

If a patient is suffering from psychological or emotional problems due to his excessive height, this is an indication that the excessive growth in height should be halted. Boys are treated with, for example, 500 mg testosterone enanthate intramuscularly one to two times a week. Testosterone treatment should start before a bone age of 14 years if a significant reduction in height is to be achieved (Table 1).

Transsexuality (Female to Male)

Transsexuality is the situation in which patients with normal genetic and phenotypical gender differentiation are convinced or believe that they belong to the opposite sex. They usually have an urgent desire for their body to match their psychological gender (Table 1).

It is usually recommended that patients first live in the role of the opposite sex for one to two years prior to the beginning of hormonal therapy. Then a one- to two-year period of hormonal administration follows before sex-change surgery is performed (mastectomy, removal of ovaries, hysterectomy, and phalloplasty).

In women, hormonal therapy comprises 250 mg testosterone enanthate intramuscularly every 2 weeks or testosterone undecanoate, also intramuscularly, 1000 mg every 12 weeks. This causes suppression of gonadotropins. In addition, this treatment stops ovulation. Menstruation also stops.

Testosterone therapy causes virilization and increased growth of secondary hair. Over the course of several years, this will resemble that of a normal male. Shaving will be necessary (8).

Late-Onset Hypogonadism

Testosterone **replacement** in men with late-onset hypogonadism is expected to have a beneficial effect on bone metabolism, musculature, erythropoiesis, libido, sexual satisfaction, and general mood (Table 1).

Studies of the effect of testosterone replacement on bone metabolism in older men demonstrate a reduction in bone loss and reduced excretion of bone degradation parameters (hydroxyproline, pyridinoline) (9,10).

Even short-term testosterone therapy in older men causes a slight increase in muscle mass of approximately 3% to 8% resulting in a functional increase in muscle strength (34). However, some studies have resulted in different findings. Testosterone administration in older hypogonadal men maintains body composition at the level of younger eugonadal men (35).

New experimental studies have shown that testosterone has an acute vasodilatory effect. Intracoronary administration of testosterone during coronary angiography in relatively old men (61 ± 11 years old) with coronary heart disease (CHD) has demonstrated an acute vasodilatory effect. It has also increased coronary blood flow (36). The above vascular effects of testosterone should be taken into careful consideration when testosterone is to be administered in relatively old men. While acute administration (37) appears to decrease vascular tone, the long-term net effect of androgens appears to be vasoconstrictive. Furthermore, androgens cause cardiac hypertrophy, promote atherosclerosis, and stimulate prohypertensive processes involving the renin–angiotensin–aldosterone system. The latter effects of androgen administration to older men should be carefully evaluated.

Testosterone stimulates erythropoiesis directly through its effect on stem cell proliferation. In addition, testosterone administration results in an enhanced renal production of the hematopoietic growth factor erythropoietin. Testosterone administration in young men with hypogonadism causes an increase in red cell count, hemoglobin concentration, and hematocrit (23). Erythropoiesis is enhanced by testosterone replacement in older men. In one study, an increase in hematocrit of around 3% to 7% has been demonstrated (34). The increased ability to transfer oxygen through the capillaries to the cell may be associated with an improvement in physical capacity and individual organ function (23).

There are some studies indicating a beneficial effect of androgen therapy on mood and mental well-being in men with late-onset hypogonadism. Studies in hypogonadal men demonstrated an improvement in mood and emotional well-being during testosterone replacement (38).

A recent clinical trial in men with refractory depression and low or borderline serum testosterone levels confirmed the clinical experience (4). In a randomized, placebo-controlled study, subjects receiving testosterone gel for eight weeks had significantly larger scores on the Hamilton Depression Rating Scale than subjects receiving placebo. Men with late-onset depression responded considerably better to the testosterone replacement than men with early-onset depression (4). Thus, testosterone appears to be able to particularly improve depression in the elderly men (4).

There are specific aspects of treating older subjects with testosterone [e.g., the relationship of testosterone with prostate cancer and benign prostatic hyperplasia (BPH)]. It is interesting that testosterone production reduces in the developmental stage of BPH. On the other hand, androgens, specifically dihydrotestosterone (DHT), play an important role in the development of BPH; decreasing systemic concentrations of androgens causes BPH to recede (39). The metabolism of androgens to DHT and estradiol is very important for the development of BPH (33,39). When there is an absolute indication for surgery in men with BPH, testosterone supplementation is not recommended.

On the other hand, the administration of testosterone to older men with testosterone deficiency does not appear to promote the de novo generation of malignant cells (40,41). However, there may be a risk that testosterone administration may promote the growth of existing malignant cells (42). Androgens appear to play a permissive role in the development of prostatic malignant cells. However, they do not induce malignancy. It is not known whether androgens promote the progression of preclinical foci to clinical prostatic cancer (42,43). In contrast, the fact that established prostatic carcinoma is dependent on testosterone for growth has been documented. It has been suggested (44) that there is an increased prevalence of prostate cancer among hypogonadal men with prostate-specific antigen (PSA) levels of 4.0 ng/mL or less. In another study (45), it has been suggested that there is a little reason to withhold testosterone replacement therapy from men with favorable outcomes after definitive treatment for prostatic cancer. On the basis of available data nowadays, testosterone may be available in older men provided that prostate screening will be performed as mentioned earlier (for more details see chap. 24).

POSSIBLE INDICATIONS FOR ANDROGEN ADMINISTRATION

Primary and Secondary Osteoporosis

It is widely accepted that men with primary or secondary hypogonadism have a benefit from testosterone replacement (17). The osteoanabolic effect of androgens in postmenopausal women is well known. However, this therapy has been largely abandoned in favor of other medications because of the virilization that occurs in a subpopulation of female patients. It should be emphasized that only androgens that are aromatizable produce an osteoanabolic effect. In men, similarly, estrogens that are formed in the peripheral tissues (e.g., adipose tissue) and bones from testosterone (and other androgens as well) stimulate the bone growth (Table 2) (46).

Table 2 Probable Indications for Androgen Replacement

- Primary and secondary osteoporosis in men (46)
- Weight loss in consumptive diseases (32)
- Hereditary angioedema (47)
- Male contraception (48)
- Aplastic and renal anemia (49,50)
- Micropenis in the newborn (20,21)

Weight Loss in Consumptive diseases

In a randomized, placebo-controlled study, the intramuscular administration of 300 mg testosterone enanthate every three weeks caused a reversal in weight loss in men with HIV disease and an increase in body weight, lean body mass, and muscle mass (32). This was manifested as an increase in physical capacity and improved quality of life (32). As the prognosis for HIV patients has considerably improved, testosterone treatment may be recommended in all patients with AIDS-associated weight loss (Table 2).

Hereditary Angioedema

Hereditary angioedema is attributable to a genetic deficiency in the C1 esterase inhibitor. It causes recurrent edema of the skin, gastrointestinal tract, and respiratory tract. Alkylated androgens such as danazol, stanozolol, or mestanolone enanthate, which stimulate hepatic production of the C1 esterase inhibitor, can be administered prophylactically, however, not during the acute phase (Table 2).

Male Contraception

Administration of high testosterone doses suppresses the hypophyseal production of the gonadotropins FSH and LH through negative feedback. As a result, the testes are not stimulated by gonadotropins and testicular endocrine and exocrine function stops. Azoospermia is the final result. However, this result is only achieved in 66% Caucasian males (51,52), whereas the effect is more distinct in Asians (almost 100% develop azoospermia). This lack of efficiency as safe contraceptives is one of the reasons why, so far, use of androgens for contraception is limited to clinical trials (Table 2).

Aplastic and Renal Anemia

Testosterone promotes renal and extrarenal generation of erythropoietin and directly promotes differentiation of pluripotent stem cells to erythropoietic precursor cells. Numerous case reports demonstrate an improvement in hematopoiesis in individuals with aplastic anemia, Fanconi anemia, hemolytic anemias, myelofibrosis, and sickle cell anemia. In the pathophysiology of hemochromatosis with androgen deficiency, testosterone replacement results in increased hematopoiesis (49). Nowadays erythropoietin, to a high degree, has replaced the usage of testosterone in patients with renal anemia. As previously mentioned, administration of erythropoietin in anemic animals with chronic renal failure increasing the hematocrit improves the health of the animals including their testicular function (Table 2) (50,53). In fact, the above pharmaceutical treatment in animals with chronic renal failure has improved both the steroidogenic and spermatogenic function of the testis (50,53). Improvement in Sertoli cellular secretory function has been demonstrated as well (50,53).

Abnormally Small Penis (Micropenis) in the Newborn

A micropenis is considered as a penis of normal structure and shape but which is too small. The penis of a healthy newborn male is 3.9 ± 0.8 cm when extended. A penis, which is smaller than 2 cm in length, is considered to be a micropenis. This condition is occasionally caused by primary or secondary hypogonadism, chromosome defects, or rare syndromes.

The success of testosterone or DHT therapy in boys with abnormally small penises is controversial. If it is necessary to increase the length of the penis, androgen therapy should be started before the onset of puberty (20,21). A dose of 25 mg testosterone enanthate intramuscularly every two weeks may be sufficient to cause significant growth in the penis of a newborn (20,21). However, there is a risk of systemic side effects due to virilizing effects of androgens. An alternative is to administer DHT topically (Table 2).

Testosterone and Erectile Dysfunction

Testosterone plays a crucial role for the achievement of penile erection (54–58). Indeed, androgen ablation results in a consistent impairment in corpora cavernosa (CC) relaxation and inhibits penile erection. Penile erection is promptly restored by testosterone supplementation (Table 2). Physiological values of androgens are required for a normal libido. Testosterone supplementation was reported to enhance sexual desire and rigidity of nocturnal penile tumescence (59). In addition, it appears that the main action of testosterone in CC is to allow an adequate formation of nitric oxide. Indeed, both acetylcholine and electrical field stimulation relax CC strips by favoring nitric oxide formation and release.

An androgen regulation of nitric oxide formation has been documented by several experimental trials, recently reviewed elsewhere (57). Essentially, these studies demonstrate that testosterone, or its metabolite DHT, upregulate neuronal or endothelial isoforms of nitric oxide synthase. However, erectile activity may be present even in conditions where nitric oxide formation is reduced, such as castration or prepuberty period. In these conditions, it appears that the decreased penile cGMP formation is somehow counteracted by the simultaneous reduction in penile cGMP degradation (58). Therefore, in hypoandrogenic status, penile erections are still possible. Thus, testosterone should be regarded as a hormone acting on the penile tissue with a dual, apparently antithetic, activity. On one hand, it increases penile cGMP formation while on the other hand it favors cGMP degradation (60).

Testosterone has been shown to restore diabetes-induced erectile dysfunction and penile responses to sildenafil in two distinct animal models of diabetes. It was shown that testosterone supplementation completely reverses neural nitric oxide synthase deficiency in the rabbit or rat model of diabetes (58). Administration of sildenafil alone is not effective in ameliorating diabetes-associated erectile dysfunction, most probably because of the diabetes-induced androgen deficiency.

Medical (56) or surgical (58) castration produces a significant decrease in the expression and activity of phosphodiesterase type 5 (PDE5) in rabbit, rat, and even human CC. It has become clear that both *PDE5* gene and PDE5 protein expression as well as the conversion of cGMP to its metabolites are substantially reduced by decreasing androgen milieu.

Combined therapy with PDE5 inhibitors and testosterone often results in a significant improvement in potency and sexual activity. In patients with erectile dysfunction in whom PDE5 inhibitor monotherapy has failed, testosterone salvage might temporarily restore the positive clinical erectile response (61). It may be suggested that testosterone administration rescues the sildenafil effect. Short-term testosterone administration has improved penile arterial inflow and ameliorated penile response to sildenafil. Similarly, sildenafil plus testosterone replacement treatment is more effective in improving sleep-related erections than sildenafil treatment alone or testosterone treatment alone. Thus, a synergic effect between testosterone and sildenafil on the induction of sleep-related erections may be suggested. Following testosterone supplementation, changes in hemodynamic penile parameters are observed. The overall result of testosterone administration is a higher capacity of cavernous smooth muscle to relax completely during sexual intercourse. Thus, in patients with erectile dysfunction demonstrating testosterone levels in the lower values of the normal range who are not responding to sildenafil because of low penile arterial blood flow, short-term testosterone therapy leads to increased circulating androgen levels, higher arterial inflow to the penis, and finally improves the penile erectile response to sildenafil (61). It has also been suggested that androgens may act on penile sensation and the autonomic nervous system innervation of penile vascular structures (62).

Testosterone deficiency results in an atrophy of the penile musculature architecture (63). In fact, testosterone stimulates cavernous smooth muscle cell growth (64) and its deprivation results in penile atrophy (65,66). In addition, some investigators have demonstrated that testosterone promotes the commitment of pluripotent stem cells into the myogenic lineage

(64–66). Furthermore, testosterone inhibits the differentiation of pluripotent stem cells in adipogenic lineage (67–69). The overall result is an increased ratio of smooth muscle fibers to collagen fibers in the CC. The level of evidence supporting the beneficial effect of testosterone on sexual function in men is 1a (28,60).

CONTRAINDICATIONS FOR ANDROGEN REPLACEMENT

Absolute Contraindications

Confirmed *prostatic carcinoma* is an absolute contraindication for androgen therapy. In addition to PSA testing and digital rectal examination, transrectal ultrasonography is recommended in men older than 45 years to determine prostatic size and evaluate any focal changes in the prostate. It is not known whether androgens may be administered several years after removal of a T1 stage prostatic carcinoma. However, it may not be appropriate to withhold testosterone replacement from men with definite successful treatment of prostate cancer (Table 3).

Mammary carcinoma in men represents another absolute contraindication. Androgens are aromatized to estrogens and therefore, the growth of estrogen receptor-positive mammary carcinomas may be promoted by androgen replacement. On the other hand, hypogonadism-induced gynecomastia is not a contraindication for testosterone replacement.

Relative Contraindications

Benign hypertrophy of the prostate is a relative contraindication. If there is already significant hypertrophy with residual urine in the bladder, caution should be raised.

If there is high hemoglobin with increased hematocrit and a high red cell count, a general laboratory examination should be carried out first and appropriate treatment administered before androgen administration. Androgens stimulate erythropoiesis and increase hemoglobin, resulting in lower blood flow and a risk of thrombosis.

Table 3 Absolute and Relative Contraindications to Androgen Therapy

Absolute contraindications	Relative contraindications
• Prostate carcinoma (70) • Mammary carcinoma (71) • **Sleep apnea (particularly in obstructive pulmonary disease in overweight persons or heavy smokers)** (71)	• Obstructive benign hyperplasia of the prostate (71) • Liver dysfunction (71) • Gynecomastia (71) • Wishing to father a child (high doses of androgens are contraindicated) (71) • Cardiovascular diseases such as congestive heart failure, severe hypertension, and peripheral edema • Dyslipidemia (71) • **Polyglobulism** (72)

In addition, the presence of liver dysfunction, gynecomastia, severe hypertension, sleep apnea, and immediate desire to father a child represent relative contraindications for testosterone replacement (Table 3).

Men having fertility wish should be informed that androgen replacement may cause azoospermia due to suppression of gonadotropin secretion (negative feedback).

EVALUATION PROCEDURES BEFORE AND DURING TREATMENT WITH ANDROGENS

Baseline Evaluation

Prior to testosterone administration, the diagnosis of hypogonadism should be confirmed.

In patients at risk or suspected of hypogonadism, a thorough physical and biochemical work-up is necessary (level 4, grade A). Transient decreases of serum testosterone levels such as those due to acute illnesses should be excluded by careful clinical evaluations and repeated hormone measurement. Hypogonadism (primary or secondary) can occur at all ages including elderly men. Risk factors for hypogonadism in older men may include chronic illnesses (including diabetes mellitus, chronic obstructive lung disease, inflammatory arthritic disease, renal disease, and HIV-related disease), obesity, metabolic syndrome, and hemochromatosis (18). Such chronic diseases should be investigated and treated (level 4, grade A).

A serum sample for total testosterone determination should be obtained between 0700 and 1100 hours (level 2a, grade A) (34). The most widely accepted parameter to establish the presence of hypogonadism is the measurement of serum total testosterone. There are no generally accepted lower limits of normal. There is, however, general agreement that the total testosterone level greater than 12 nmol/L (350 ng/dL) does not require substitution. Similarly, on the basis of the data of younger men, there is a consensus that patients with serum total testosterone levels lower than 8 nmol/L (230 ng/dL) will usually benefit from testosterone treatment. If the serum total testosterone level is between 8 and 12 nmol/L, repeating the measurement of total testosterone with sex hormone-binding globulin (SHBG) to calculate free testosterone or free testosterone by equilibrium dialysis may be helpful (level 2b, grade A).

Measurements of serum luteinizing hormone will assist in differentiating between primary and secondary hypogonadism, and serum prolactin is indicated when the serum testosterone is lower than 5.2 nmol/L (150 ng/dL) (35–38) or when secondary hypogonadism is suspected (18,39,40) (level 3, grade B).

Since there are known variations between assay methods, it is imperative that the practitioners utilize reliable laboratories and are acquainted with the reference ranges for testosterone from their local laboratory (41–44) (level 2b, grade A).

Alterations in other endocrine systems occur in association with aging [i.e., estradiol, growth hormone (GH), and dehydroepiandrosterone (DHEA)] but the significance of these changes is not well understood. Determinations of estradiol, thyroid hormones, cortisol, DHEA, sulfate ester of dehydroepiandrosterone (DHEA-S), melatonin, growth hormone, and insulinlike growth factor I are not indicated unless other endocrine disorders are suspected based on the clinical signs and symptoms of the patient (18) (level 2, grade A).

Then serum LH profiles, blood pressure, blood count, liver transaminases (glutamyl oxaloacetic transaminase (GOT) and glutamic-pyruvic transaminase (GPT)), lipidemic profile, bilirubin, and in men older than 45 years, PSA should be evaluated. In addition, baseline voiding history and history (if present) of sleep apnea should be obtained. After the age of 45 years, digital rectal examination and transrectal ultrasound of the prostate are included in the pretherapeutic evaluation since focal changes in the prostatic gland should be evaluated before androgen administration. Physical examination should evaluate the androgen target organs as well. Secondary hair growth, musculature, body shape, reproductive tract, and the voice should be evaluated. Dual energy X-ray absorptiometry (DEXA) scan should be carried out to determine bone mineralization in men with hypogonadism (Table 4).

Table 4 Evaluation Procedures Before and Under Androgen Replacement (73–75)

	Evaluation
Baseline	• Medical history • Examination (hair, skin, sexuality, mood, chest) • Determine baseline voiding history or use standardized questionnaire • Determine history of sleep apnea • Perform blood tests for baseline total testosterone levels, free testosterone levels, LH, and estradiol • Perform blood tests for baseline blood count, hematocrit, or hemoglobin and lipids; in addition, assess bone density (**DEXA scan**) • Perform blood tests for baseline transaminase values • Perform digital rectal examination (DRE) and prostate-specific antigen (PSA) measurement (in men older than **45** years); ultrasonographical evaluation of the prostate is recommended
Follow-up	• Case history • Examination (hair, skin, sexuality, mood) every 3 months for the first year and yearly thereafter • Perform efficacy evaluation with dosage adjustment for suboptimal response at 3 months • Perform monitoring of blood viscosity every 3 months for the first year and yearly thereafter • Assess urinary symptoms and presence or exacerbation of sleep apnea or gynecomastia every 3 months for the first year and yearly thereafter • Perform blood tests for baseline total testosterone levels, free testosterone levels, estradiol, LH, blood count, and transaminases every 3 months for the first year and yearly thereafter • Perform blood tests for lipids at 3 and 6 months for the first year and yearly thereafter • Assessment of bone density 12 months after the therapy initiation and every one or two years thereafter • Perform DRE and PSA measurement (in men older than **45** years) every 3 months for the first year and yearly thereafter • Ultrasonographical evaluation of prostate

Follow-up Evaluation

The first follow-up examination should be scheduled three months following testosterone administration. The patient should be asked about his physical capacity, libido, potency, and general well-being. Physical examination should evaluate the androgen target organs. In order to adjust the testosterone dose, it is important to evaluate carefully the consequences of the initial dose of testosterone. In patients with primary hypogonadism, serum LH should be determined (76). Ideally, if LH was increased prior to testosterone administration, it should have been normalized during testosterone replacement. However, this may not necessarily occur when testosterone is administered percutaneously or orally, but more often with intramuscular testosterone administration. After appreciating the testosterone levels, serum LH, and blood count and the clinical effect on androgen-dependent organs simultaneously, the dose of testosterone or administration interval can be adjusted (Table 4).

Thus, as a general recommendation, three months after initiation of the replacement therapy, the patient should return for an efficacy assessment. This includes a voiding history, sexual function history, blood pressure evaluation, digital rectal examination, blood tests [including measurement of PSA (if age 45 years or more), transaminases, lipids, cholesterol, and bilirubin], and morning total testosterone level for patch users.

The patient should specifically be asked if he has noticed improvements in the symptoms that led to the diagnosis of hypogonadism (i.e., sexual function, energy level, or muscle mass). If the patient has noticed improvements in his overall symptomatology, he can be followed every three months during the first year and thereafter, once a year.

Bone density measurements can be performed yearly, starting at one year after the initiation of treatment. It is important to keep in mind that monitoring must be tailored to the individual. Sexual function history should be obtained. Transrectal ultrasonographical evaluation of the prostate may be performed as well. There is no target level for replacement, and the patient's answer to questionnaires regarding the effectiveness of the therapy is generally a reliable indicator of success. Once testosterone replacement therapy is initiated, the treatment is likely to be lifelong (77).

It is important to monitor PSA levels every three months during the first year of treatment. The role of testosterone in development or progression of prostate cancer is a controversial issue. Androgens are known to play a role in BPH (76,78). Some have

Table 5 Time Needed for Improvement of Symptoms During Testosterone Replacement

Indication for replacement	Testosterone replacement results in	Route of administration	Testosterone form	Time needed
Primary and secondary hypogonadism	Restoration of libido or potency	IM	TE	3–12 mo (11)
	Amelioration of emotional status, self-confidence, and activity	IM	TE	1–1.5 mo (1–3)
		SL	T cyclodextrin	1–1.5 mo (1,3)
		SC (implant)	MENT acetate	1.5 mo (2)
		Gel	T	2 mo (4)
	Increased lean muscle and decreased adipose tissue	IM	TE or T cypionate	6–12 mo (12,13)
	Increased bone density	IM	TE or T cypionate	6 mo (10)
			Sustanon	12 mo (83)
		Patch	T	36 mo (84)
	Increased hematocrit	IM	Mesterolone, TU, TE	3–5 mo (23)
		SC implant	T	3–5 mo (23)
Induction of puberty in boys		IM	TE	6 mo (85)
Excessive growth in boys		IM	TE	3–6 mo (86)
Transsexuality (female to male)	Cessation of menses	Orally	TU	1,5–5 mo (87)
	Elongation of the clitoris	IM	TC	12 mo (88)
	Hirsutism	IM	Sustanon 250	>12 mo (89)
	Increased sebum production	IM	Sustanon 250	4–12 mo (89)
Late-onset hypogonadism	Increased bone density	IM	TE or TC	12–36 mo (10)
			Sustanon 250	6–18 mo (83)
		Patch	T	36 mo (84)
	Increased musculature, decreased adipose tissue	IM	TE	6–12 mo (90)
	Vascular alterations	IM	TC	2 mo (91)
	Erythropoiesis	IM	TE	3–12 mo (34)
			TC	12 mo (92)
	Mental well-being and positive cognitive activities	Gel	T	6 mo (26)
		Patch	T	6 mo (26)
Primary and secondary osteoporosis	Increased bone density	IM	Sustanon 250	6–12 mo (83,93,94)
Weight loss in consumptive diseases	Increase in weight	IM	TE	6 mo (32)
Hereditary angioedema	Orally	Stanozolol	12 mo (95)	
Male contraception	Oligospermia/azoospermia	IM	TE	6–12 mo (51)
Aplastic and renal anemia	Increase in hematocrit	IM	Nandrolone decanoate	2–4 mo (11,96)
Abnormally small penis (micropenis) in the newborn		IM	TE	1–2 mo (20)

Abbreviations: T, testosterone; TE, testosterone enanthate; MENT, 7alpha-methyl-19-nortestosterone; TU, testosterone undecanoate; TC, testosterone cypionate; IM, intramuscular; SC, subcutaneous; SL, sublingual; Sustanon 250, trade name for an oil-based injectable blend of four esterized testosterone compounds including 30 mg testosterone propionate, 60 mg testosterone phenylpropionate, 60 mg testosterone isocaproate, and 100 mg testosterone decanoate.

suggested that occult prostate cancer might progress rapidly in the presence of exogenous androgens, (42,79) but others refute this (80,81). In addition, digital rectal examination should be performed and prostate-related symptoms should be assessed every three months. An increase in PSA to a level ≥4.0 ng/mL or rapidly increasing PSA levels are widely accepted standards for urologic referral and/or prostate biopsy considering discontinuing testosterone administration (depending on the biopsy outcome). Annual PSA increases ≥1 ng/mL should prompt prostate biopsy, whereas annual increases of 0.7 to 0.9 ng/mL should trigger repeat measurements in three to six months, with biopsy if there are further increases (73).

For patients under testosterone gel therapy, it is recommended to collect blood specimen one month after the beginning of the treatment and approximately every three months after the initial gel application as well. Because of the risk of contamination of the blood sample with the transdermally applied testosterone, leading to falsely high serum testosterone levels, it is recommended that in these patients the blood sample is obtained in the morning, prior to the administration of the gel.

For patients using daily application of one testosterone patch, a blood specimen for testosterone evaluation should be collected a month after the first patch application. Clinical examinations and additional blood sample collections should be performed every three months after the first appli-cation (82).

For men receiving intramuscular injections, blood samples should be taken at the end of an injection interval immediately before the next dose when serum testosterone should be at the lower limit of normal range.

After evaluating the testosterone trough level, serum LH, blood count, clinical effects, and studying the outcome of questionnaires, the dose of testosterone or administration interval can be adjusted. For any type of hypogonadism, the desired goal of testosterone administration is serum trough testosterone levels to be in the lower third of the normal range (12–18 nmol/L), but the clinical symptomatology for individualization of the therapy should also be considered. Interruption of the administration of a specific testosterone preparation should be recommended in cases of failure to (a) achieve the above-described blood testosterone levels (switching to another testosterone preparation is considered), (b) improve specific hypogonadism-related symptoms (switching to another testosterone preparation is considered) (Table 5), and in addition, (c) in cases of intolerable adverse reactions (Table 6). Indications for switching from one testosterone preparation to another (Table 7) is (a) failure to achieve the desirable already described testosterone levels, (b) achievement of desired serum trough testosterone levels that are not accompanied by an improvement in the symptoms, and (c) significant fluctuation in the levels of serum testosterone over a specific period of time.

Some men exhibit a marked increase in red blood cell production that requires testosterone therapy be stopped, be significantly titrated, or can even require phlebotomy or blood donation (71). The risk appears to be higher with intramuscular preparations (73) and may be due to the supraphysiologic levels that are sometimes seen. This risk is also higher in men who have comorbidities known to increase hematocrit levels such as chronic obstructive lung disease.

Table 6 Side effects of Androgen Administration (12,51,73,79,89)

Male reproductive tract
- Testicular atrophy
- Oligospermia, azoospermia
- Infertility
- Gynecomastia
- Low intratesticular testosterone

Female reproductive system
- Masculine secondary hair growth
- Oligomenorrhea, amenorrhea
- Infertility
- Virilization, male appearance
- Pitch of voice drops
- Hypertrophy of the clitoris

Blood
- Erythrocytosis
- Polyglobulism
- Risk of thrombosis

Liver
- Cholestatic jaundice
- Peliosis hepatitis
- Hepatocellular adenoma and carcinoma; this does not refer to testosterone replacement but only to some of the synthetic androgens

Skin
- Acne
- Androgenic alopecia

Cardiovascular
- Myocardial hypertrophy
- Disturbed contractility
- Increased blood pressure

Metabolism
- Occasional reduction of HDL cholesterol
- Occasional increase in LDL cholesterol

Musculoskeletal
- Premature epiphyseal closing with reduced final height

Psychological
- Euphoric effect with risk of developing dependence to testosterone
- Depression when drug discontinued
- Mood swings

Abbreviations: LDL, low-density lipoprotein; HDL, high-density lipoprotein.

Failure to benefit clinical manifestations within a reasonable time interval (three to six months is adequate for libido and sexual function, muscle function, and improved body fat; improvement in bone mineral density requires a longer interval to show improvement) should result in discontinuation of treatment. Further investigation for other causes of symptoms is then mandatory (level 1b, grade A).

Table 7 Types of Androgen Preparations--Advantages and Disadvantages

- Intramuscular testosterone undecanoate (3-monthly injection)
  - Advantages: stable testosterone levels within normal range over months, easily accepted by the patient, no problems with compliance, very good efficacy, low cost
  - Disadvantages: pain at the site of injection and the need for frequent medical visits for administration of the injections
- Intramuscular testosterone enanthate (3-weekly injection)
  - Advantages: inexpensive, hardly any problems with compliance
  - Disadvantages: frequent painful intramuscular injections, moderate pharmacokinetics with unpleasant fluctuations for patients
- Testosterone pellets (subcutaneous)
  - Advantages: good pharmacokinetics and pharmacodynamics with stable physiological T levels, longest duration of effect of all preparations, easily accepted by the patient (71)
  - Disadvantages: cost for implantation process, local infections, substantial hepatotoxicity
- Testosterone gel
  - Advantages: very good pharmacokinetics, no fluctuation in testosterone levels, good efficacy, suitable approach if there are contraindications to injections, few side effects, individual dosing, discrete application
  - Disadvantages: inadequate long-term experience, risk for interperson contamination if not properly dried
- Testosterone patches
  - Advantages: good pharmacokinetics with uniform levels, suitable when there are contraindications to injections, easy to use and maintenance of relatively uniform serum testosterone levels over time (26,97)
  - Disadvantages: scrotal patches—DHT increase, very expensive; nonscrotal patches—frequent, pronounced skin irritations, expensive
- Oral testosterone undecanoate
  - Advantages: for patients who do not tolerate patches and when intramuscular injections are refused
  - Disadvantages: poor bioavailability, very expensive, substantial hepatotoxicity; usage of these agents is discouraged because of their potential toxicity (73)

Abbreviations: T, testosterone; DHT, dihydrotestosterone.

CASE REPORT

A 32-year-old azoospermic man visited our institute because of inability to impregnate his wife. Peripheral serum FSH, LH, prolactin, estradiol, free testosterone, and total testosterone profiles were normal. Three semen analyses demonstrated azoospermia. Clinical examination demonstrated two testicles of normal volume. However, the left testis exhibited during palpation a hard region. Ultrasonographical evaluation showed a region suspicious for left testicle cancer. α-Fetoprotein and β-hCG were evaluated. Both of them were found to be elevated. Pelvic and abdominal CT scanning did not show enlarged lymph nodes. The patient was operated. During the operation, he underwent multiple left testicular biopsies that revealed testicular carcinoma. Left orchidectomy was performed. At that time, he underwent right testicular biopsy to exclude the presence of contralateral testicular cancer and to recover and freeze right testicular spermatozoa. After a four-year period, this man underwent for the same reason (i.e., presence of testicular cancer) right orchidectomy. After right orchidectomy, the patient achieved a pregnancy via assisted reproduction technology using frozen/thawed right testicular spermatozoa. Then he received lifelong **replacement** with testosterone undecanoate (1000 mg, IM) every 12 weeks. This example refers to primary hypogonadism as a result of acquired anorchidism due to bilateral malignancy, which requires lifelong androgen **replacement**. Permanent **replacement** is possible with long-acting preparations **known to have a beneficial effect on erectile function** (Table 8). **Testosterone gel or testosterone patches also offer a therapeutic possibility for this man.**

Table 8 Effects of Androgens on Cavernosal Tissue (38,54–60)

- Regulation of nitric oxide synthase isoforms, expression, and activity
- Regulation of phosphodiesterase-5 expression and activity
- Regulation of smooth muscle cell growth and response to vasodilators
- Maintenance of penile neural structure and function
- Regulation of the alpha-adrenoreceptor expression and function
- Regulation of penile connective tissue metabolism
- Regulation of differentiation of progenitor vascular stroma cells into myogenic and adipogenic lineages

REFERENCES

1. Alexander GM, Swerdloff RS, Wang C, et al. Androgen-behavior correlations in hypogonadal men and eugonadal men. I. Mood and response to auditory sexual stimuli. Horm Behav 1997; 31:110–119.
2. Anderson RA, Martin CW, Kung AW, et al. 7Alpha-methyl-19-nortestosterone maintains sexual behavior and mood in hypogonadal men. J Clin Endocrinol Metab 1999; 84:3556–3562.
3. Wang C, Alexander G, Berman N, et al. Testosterone replacement therapy improves mood in hypogonadal men–A clinical research center study. J Clin Endocrinol Metab 1996; 81:3578–3583.
4. Pope HG Jr, Cohane GH, Kanayama G, et al. Testosterone gel supplementation for men with refractory depression: A randomized, placebo-controlled trial. Am J Psychiatry 2003; 160:105–111.
5. Brown DC, Butler GE, Kelnar CJ, et al. A double blind, placebo controlled study of the effects of low dose testosterone undecanoate on the growth of small for age, prepubertal boys. Arch Dis Child 1995; 73:131–135.
6. Finkelstein JS, Neer RM, Biller BM, et al. Osteopenia in men with a history of delayed puberty. N Engl J Med 1992; 326:600–604.
7. Nieschlag E. Current status of testosterone substitution therapy. Int J Androl 1982; 5:225–228.
8. van Kesteren P, Lips P, Gooren LJ, et al. Long-term follow-up of bone mineral density and bone metabolism in transsexuals treated with cross-sex hormones. Clin Endocrinol (Oxf) 1998; 48:347–354.
9. Tanaka S, Haji M, Nishi Y, et al. Aromatase activity in human osteoblast-like osteosarcoma cell. Calcif Tissue Int 1993; 52:107–109.
10. Katznelson L, Finkelstein JS, Schoenfeld DA, et al. Increase in bone density and lean body mass during testosterone administration in men with acquired hypogonadism. J Clin Endocrinol Metab 1996; 81:4358–4365.
11. Burris AS, Banks SM, Carter CS, et al. A long-term, prospective study of the physiologic and behavioral effects of hormone replacement in untreated hypogonadal men. J Androl 1992; 13:297–304.
12. Bhasin S, Storer TW, Berman N, et al. The effects of supraphysiologic doses of testosterone on muscle size and strength in normal men. N Engl J Med 1996; 335: 1–7.
13. Brodsky IG, Balagopal P, Nair KS. Effects of testosterone replacement on muscle mass and muscle protein synthesis in hypogonadal men–A clinical research center study. J Clin Endocrinol Metab 1996; 81:3469–3475.
14. Barrett-Connor E, Khaw KT. Endogenous sex hormones and cardiovascular disease in men. A prospective population-based study. Circulation 1988; 78:539–545.
15. Marin P. Testosterone and regional fat distribution. Obes Res 1995; 3(suppl 4):609S–612S.
16. Bjorntorp P, Marin P, Holmang S. Still too early for androgen therapy of abdominal obesity in males—Inspite of good results [in Swedish]. Lakartidningen 1992; 89:1568–1569.
17. Behre HM, Kliesch S, Leifke E, et al. Long-term effect of testosterone therapy on bone mineral density in hypogonadal men. J Clin Endocrinol Metab 1997; 82:2386–2390.
18. Finkelstein JS, Klibanski A, Neer RM, et al. Increases in bone density during treatment of men with idiopathic hypogonadotropic hypogonadism. J Clin Endocrinol Metab 1989; 69:776–783.
19. Jackson JA, Waxman J, Spiekerman AM. Prostatic complications of testosterone replacement therapy. Arch Intern Med 1989; 149:2365–2366.
20. Aaronson IA. Micropenis: Medical and surgical implications. J Urol 1994; 152:4–14.
21. McMahon DR, Kramer SA, Husmann DA. Micropenis: Does early treatment with testosterone do more harm than good? J Urol 1995; 154:825–829.
22. Arteaga-Silva M, Vigueras-Villasenor RM, Retana-Marquez S, et al. Testosterone, androstenedione, and 5alpha-dihydrotestosterone on male sexual behavior and penile spines in the hamster. Physiol Behav 2008; 94:412–421.
23. Jockenhovel F, Vogel E, Reinhardt W, et al. Effects of various modes of androgen substitution therapy on erythropoiesis. Eur J Med Res 1997; 2:293–298.
24. Jockenhovel F, Bullmann C, Schubert M, et al. Influence of various modes of androgen substitution on serum lipids and lipoproteins in hypogonadal men. Metabolism 1999; 48:590–596.
25. Zgliczynski S, Ossowski M, Slowinska-Srzednicka J, et al. Effect of testosterone replacement therapy on lipids and lipoproteins in hypogonadal and elderly men. Atherosclerosis 1996; 121:35–43.
26. Wang C, Swerdloff RS, Iranmanesh A, et al. Transdermal testosterone gel improves sexual function, mood, muscle strength, and body composition parameters in hypogonadal men. J Clin Endocrinol Metab 2000; 85:2839–2853.
27. Adamopoulos DA, Pappa A, Billa E, et al. Effectiveness of combined tamoxifen citrate and testosterone undecanoate treatment in men with idiopathic oligozoospermia. Fertil Steril 2003; 80:914–920.
28. Perleth M. Testosterone–a "fountain of youth" for ageing men? Brief assessment of the efficacy and safety of androgen substitution in healthy men. Z Arztl Fortbild Qualitatssich 2007; 101(7):487–497
29. Bolona E, Uraga M, Haddad R, et al. Testosterone use in men with sexual dysfunction: A systematic review and meta-analysis of randomized placebo-controlled trials. Mayo Clin Proc 2007; 82:20–28.
30. Krause W. Testosterone substitution in aging males. Which questions are answered? [in German]. Urologe A 2004; 43:1097–1100.

31. Isidori AM, Giannetta E, Greco EA, et al. Effects of testosterone on body composition, bone metabolism and serum lipid profile in middle-aged men: A meta-analysis. Clin Endocrinol (Oxf) 2005; 63:280–293.
32. Grinspoon S, Corcoran C, Askari H, et al. Effects of androgen administration in men with the AIDS wasting syndrome. A randomized, double-blind, placebo-controlled trial. Ann Intern Med 1998; 129:18–26.
33. Levine AC. Pathogenesis and medical management of benign prostatic hyperplasia. Trends Endocrinol Metab 1995; 6:128–132.
34. Morley JE, Perry HM III, Kaiser FE, et al. Effects of testosterone replacement therapy in old hypogonadal males: A preliminary study. J Am Geriatr Soc 1993; 41:149–152.
35. Rolf C, von Eckardstein S, Koken U, et al. Testosterone substitution of hypogonadal men prevents the age-dependent increases in body mass index, body fat and leptin seen in healthy ageing men: Results of a cross-sectional study. Eur J Endocrinol 2002; 146:505–511.
36. Webb CM, McNeill JG, Hayward CS, et al. Effects of testosterone on coronary vasomotor regulation in men with coronary heart disease. Circulation 1999; 100:1690–1696.
37. Kienitz T, Quinkler M. Testosterone and blood pressure regulation. Kidney Blood Press Res 2008; 31:71–79.
38. Jain P, Rademaker AW, McVary KT. Testosterone supplementation for erectile dysfunction: Results of a meta-analysis. J Urol 2000; 164:371–375.
39. Pryor JL. Androgen supplementation causes BPH. In: Bhasin S, Gabelnick HL, Spieler JM, Swerdloff RS, Wang C, Kelly C, eds. Pharmacology, Biology, and Clinical Applications of Androgens. New York: John Wiley & Sons, 1996:111–114.
40. Griffiths K. Estrogens and prostatic disease. International Prostate Health Council Study Group. Prostate 2000; 45:87–100.
41. Signoretti S, Loda M. Estrogen receptor beta in prostate cancer: Brake pedal or accelerator? Am J Pathol 2001; 159:13–16.
42. Slater S, Oliver RT. Testosterone: Its role in development of prostate cancer and potential risk from use as hormone replacement therapy. Drugs Aging 2000; 17:431–439.
43. Cunningham GR. Overview of androgens on the normal and abnormal prostate. In: Bhasin D, Gabelnick HL, Spieler JM, Swerdloff RS, Wang C, Kelly C, eds. Pharmacology, Biology, and Clinical Applications of Androgens. New York: John Wiley & Sons, 1996:79–93.
44. Morgentaler A, Rhoden EL. Prevalence of prostate cancer among hypogonadal men with prostate-specific antigen levels of 4.0 ng/mL or less. Urology 2006; 68:1263–1267.
45. Morgentaler A. Testosterone therapy for men at risk for or with history of prostate cancer. Curr Treat Options Oncol 2006; 7:363–369.
46. Riggs BL, Khosla S, Melton LJ III. Sex steroids and the construction and conservation of the adult skeleton. Endocr Rev 2002; 23:279–302.
47. Birjmohun RS, Kees Hovingh G, Stroes ES, et al. Effects of short-term and long-term danazol treatment on lipoproteins, coagulation, and progression of atherosclerosis: Two clinical trials in healthy volunteers and patients with hereditary angioedema. Clin Ther 2008; 30:2314–2323.
48. Sofikitis N, Ono K, Yamamoto Y, et al. Influence of the male reproductive tract on the reproductive potential of round spermatids abnormally released from the seminiferous epithelium. Hum Reprod 1999; 14:1998–2006.
49. Ammus SS. The role of androgens in the treatment of hematologic disorders. Adv Intern Med 1989; 34:191–208.
50. Yamamoto Y, Sofikitis N, Miyagawa I. Effects of erythropoietin, bromocryptine and hydralazine on testicular function in rats with chronic renal failure. Andrologia 1997; 29:141–144.
51. WHO. Contraceptive efficacy of testosterone-induced azoospermia in normal men. World Health Organization Task Force on methods for the regulation of male fertility. Lancet 1990; 336:955–959.
52. WHO. Contraceptive efficacy of testosterone-induced azoospermia and oligozoospermia in normal men. Fertil Steril 1996; 65:821–829.
53. Yamamoto Y, Sofikitis N, Miyagawa I. Effects of chronic renal failure on hypothalamo-pituitary-testicular axis function and fertility in rats. Int J Urol 1996; 3:484–490.
54. Filippi S, Luconi M, Granchi S, et al. Endothelium-dependency of yohimbine-induced corpus cavernosum relaxation. Int J Impot Res 2002; 14:295–307.
55. Filippi S, Luconi M, Granchi S, et al. Estrogens, but not androgens, regulate expression and functional activity of oxytocin receptor in rabbit epididymis. Endocrinology 2002; 143:4271–4280.
56. Morelli A, Filippi S, Mancina R, et al. Androgens regulate phosphodiesterase type 5 expression and functional activity in corpora cavernosa. Endocrinology 2004; 145:2253–2263.
57. Vignozzi L, Corona G, Petrone L, et al. Testosterone and sexual activity. J Endocrinol Invest 2005; 28:39–44.
58. Zhang XH, Morelli A, Luconi M, et al. Testosterone regulates PDE5 expression and in vivo responsiveness to tadalafil in rat corpus cavernosum. Eur Urol 2005; 47:409–416; discussion 416.
59. Shamloul R, Ghanem H, Fahmy I, et al. Testosterone therapy can enhance erectile function response to sildenafil in patients with PADAM: A pilot study. J Sex Med 2005; 2:559–564.
60. Isidori AM, Giannetta E, Gianfrilli D, et al. Effects of testosterone on sexual function in men: Results of a meta-analysis. Clin Endocrinol (Oxf) 2005; 63:381–394.
61. Aversa A, Isidori AM, Spera G, et al. Androgens improve cavernous vasodilation and response to sildenafil in

patients with erectile dysfunction. Clin Endocrinol (Oxf) 2003; 58:632–638.

62. Davidson JM, Kwan M, Greenleaf WJ. Hormonal replacement and sexuality in men. Clin Endocrinol Metab 1982; 11:599–623.
63. Aversa A, Isidori AM, Greco EA, et al. Hormonal supplementation and erectile dysfunction. Eur Urol 2004; 45:535–538.
64. Crescioli C, Maggi M, Vannelli GB, et al. Expression of functional estrogen receptors in human fetal male external genitalia. J Clin Endocrinol Metab 2003; 88:1815–1824.
65. Mills TM, Lewis RW. The role of androgens in the erectile response: A 1999 perspective. Mol Urol 1999;3:75–86.
66. Traish AM, Park K, Dhir V, et al. Effects of castration and androgen replacement on erectile function in a rabbit model. Endocrinology 1999; 140:1861–1868.
67. Bhasin S, Taylor WE, Singh R, et al. The mechanisms of androgen effects on body composition: Mesenchymal pluripotent cell as the target of androgen action. J Gerontol A Biol Sci Med Sci 2003; 58:M1103–M1110.
68. Singh R, Artaza JN, Taylor WE, et al. Testosterone inhibits adipogenic differentiation in 3T3-L1 cells: Nuclear translocation of androgen receptor complex with beta-catenin and T-cell factor 4 may bypass canonical Wnt signaling to down-regulate adipogenic transcription factors. Endocrinology 2006; 147:141–154.
69. Singh R, Artaza JN, Taylor WE, et al. Androgens stimulate myogenic differentiation and inhibit adipogenesis in C3H 10T1/2 pluripotent cells through an androgen receptor-mediated pathway. Endocrinology 2003; 144:5081–5088.
70. Schröder FH. The prostate and androgens: The risk of supplementation. In: Oddens B, Vermeulen A, eds. Androgens and the Aging Male. New York: Parthenon Publishing, 1996:223–231.
71. Vermeulen A. Androgen replacement therapy in the aging male—A critical evaluation. J Clin Endocrinol Metab 2001; 86:2380–2390.
72. Gasser RW. Androgen therapy from the viewpoint of the internal medicine physician [in German]. Wien Med Wochenschr 2001; 151:444–447.
73. Rhoden EL, Morgentaler A. Risks of testosterone-replacement therapy and recommendations for monitoring. N Engl J Med 2004; 350:482–492.
74. McGriff NJ, Csako G, Kabbani M, et al. Treatment options for a patient experiencing pruritic rash associated with transdermal testosterone: A review of the literature. Pharmacotherapy 2001; 21:1425–1435.
75. Nieschlag E. Testosterone treatment comes of age: New options for hypogonadal men. Clin Endocrinol (Oxf) 2006; 65:275–281.
76. Morales A, Bain J, Ruijs A, et al. Clinical practice guidelines for screening and monitoring male patients receiving testosterone supplementation therapy. Int J Impot Res 1996; 8:95–97.
77. Ohl DA, Quallich SA. Clinical hypogonadism and androgen replacement therapy: An overview. Urol Nurs 2006; 26:253–259, 269; quiz 260.
78. Nolten WE. Androgen deficiency in the aging male: When to evaluate and when to treat. Curr Urol Rep 2000; 1:313–319.
79. Rolf C, Nieschlag E. Potential adverse effects of long-term testosterone therapy. Baillieres Clin Endocrinol Metab 1998; 12:521–534.
80. Hajjar RR, Kaiser FE, Morley JE. Outcomes of long-term testosterone replacement in older hypogonadal males: A retrospective analysis. J Clin Endocrinol Metab 1997; 82:3793–3796.
81. Snyder PJ, Peachey H, Berlin JA, et al. Effects of testosterone replacement in hypogonadal men. J Clin Endocrinol Metab 2000; 85:2670–2677.
82. Behre HM, von Eckardstein S, Kliesch S, et al. Long-term substitution therapy of hypogonadal men with transscrotal testosterone over 7–10 years. Clin Endocrinol (Oxf) 1999; 50:629–635.
83. Reid IR, Wattie DJ, Evans MC, et al. Testosterone therapy in glucocorticoid-treated men. Arch Intern Med 1996; 156:1173–1177.
84. Snyder PJ, Peachey H, Hannoush P, et al. Effect of testosterone treatment on body composition and muscle strength in men over 65 years of age. J Clin Endocrinol Metab 1999; 84:2647–2653.
85. Soliman AT, Khadir MM, Asfour M. Testosterone treatment in adolescent boys with constitutional delay of growth and development. Metabolism 1995; 44:1013–1015.
86. Bramswig JH, von Lengerke HJ, Schmidt H, et al. The results of short-term (6 months) high-dose testosterone treatment on bone age and adult height in boys of excessively tall stature. Eur J Pediatr 1988; 148:104–106.
87. Scheele F, Hompes PG, Gooren LJ, et al. The effect of 6 weeks of testosterone treatment on pulsatile luteinizing hormone secretion in eugonadal female-to-male transsexuals. Fertil Steril 1991; 55:608–611.
88. Meyer WJ III, Webb A, Stuart CA, et al. Physical and hormonal evaluation of transsexual patients: A longitudinal study. Arch Sex Behav 1986; 15:121–138.
89. Giltay EJ, Gooren LJ. Effects of sex steroid deprivation/administration on hair growth and skin sebum production in transsexual males and females. J Clin Endocrinol Metab 2000; 85:2913–2921.
90. Tenover JS. Effects of testosterone supplementation in the aging male. J Clin Endocrinol Metab 1992; 75:1092–1098.
91. Jaffe MD. Effect of testosterone cypionate on postexercise ST segment depression. Br Heart J 1977; 39:1217–1222.
92. Sih R, Morley JE, Kaiser FE, et al. Testosterone replacement in older hypogonadal men: A 12-month randomized controlled trial. J Clin Endocrinol Metab 1997; 82:1661–1667.
93. Anderson FH, Francis RM, Peaston RT, et al. Androgen supplementation in eugonadal men with osteoporosis:

Effects of six months' treatment on markers of bone formation and resorption. J Bone Miner Res 1997; 12:472–478.

94. Pechersky AV, Mazurov VI, Semiglazov VF, et al. Androgen administration in middle-aged and ageing men: Effects of oral testosterone undecanoate on dihydrotestosterone, oestradiol and prostate volume. Int J Androl 2002; 25: 119–125.

95. Sheffer AL, Fearon DT, Austen KF. Clinical and biochemical effects of stanozolol therapy for hereditary angioedema. J Allergy Clin Immunol 1981; 68:181–187.

96. Ballal SH, Domoto DT, Polack DC, et al. Androgens potentiate the effects of erythropoietin in the treatment of anemia of end-stage renal disease. Am J Kidney Dis 1991; 17:29–33.

97. Comhaire FH. Andropause: Hormone replacement therapy in the ageing male. Eur Urol 2000; 38:655–662.

30 Androgen deficiency in cancer-treated men

Jakob Eberhard, Patrik Romerius, and Aleksander Giwercman

CASE STORY

42-year-old man referred from the Department of Oncology for hormonal evaluation. Two years earlier treated for seminoma in the left testis. No metastases were detected. However, biopsy from the right testis showed carcinoma-in-situ, which was subsequently treated by localized irradiation, 16 Gray given to the testis in eight fractions. Following the cancer treatment, the patient observed profound changes in the mood and also developed a tendency for sweating and hot flushes. He noted reduced libido and sexual function. He was referred to a psychologist for a "post cancer syndrome." Hormone analysis a couple of months later revealed a serum testosterone of 3.2 nmol/L (normal range: 10–30 nmol/L), SHBG of 56 nmol/L, and LH of 17 IU/L (normal range: 1–10 IU/L). Replacement therapy with testosterone enanthate injections, 250 mg every third week, was initiated. The patient came to the outpatient clinic 3 months later. He was whistling and glad and felt psychologically complete in his habitual shape.

Over the past few decades, the survival rates for a number of malignant diseases have significantly increased. This is, in particular, true for some of the malignancies affecting young individuals. Thus, among patients having testicular germ cell cancer (TGCC), 95% or more are now cured for their diseases (1). For malignant lymphomas, the figure is 65% to 80% with even higher survival rate in young adults and children. The same is true for childhood cancer and it has been estimated that 1 out of 600 adults has been treated for a malignant disease during childhood.

This significant improvement in the outcome of a number of malignant diseases means that while dealing with these patients just focusing on the question of survival is no longer enough. Attention should also be given to the quality of life in these subjects post treatment.

One of the important issues of the quality of life in cancer survivors is the question of their reproductive function. Many studies have shown that the fear of impairment of reproductive ability, as a consequence of cancer treatment, is one of the most pronounced fears of young cancer survivors.

In men, normal reproductive function means preserving the ability to father children. However, another important aspect is related to normal androgen production, namely the ability to have a normal sexual life and also the general well being dependent on sufficient testosterone levels.

The issue of preservation of fertility in oncologically treated men has attracted a lot of attention and freezing sperms prior to cancer therapy is now a well-established routine in many centers. However, the issue of the risk of hypogonadism (androgen deficiency) in males treated for cancer has been relatively less acknowledged. This means that a significant proportion of male patients treated for cancer might be hypogonadal without being diagnosed as such.

MECHANISMS OF CANCER TREATMENT–RELATED MALE HYPOGONADISM

Men who have been treated for cancer may develop hypogonadism by one, or both, of the following mechanisms:

a. *Primary hypogonadism*—due to impairment of Leydig cell function;
b. *Secondary hypogonadism*—testosterone production is reduced because of impairment of hypothalamic and/or pituitary function, leading to reduced secretion of luteinizing hormone (LH).

Primary hypogonadism may be caused by:

I. *Cancer disease per se*: The typical example is represented by patients with TGCC. It has been found that these men have a Leydig cell dysfunction, which may be related to the etiology of the disease (2). It is believed that TGCC has a fetal origin and is part of a syndrome involving Sertoli, as well as Leydig cell dysfunction (3). Thus TGCC patients may be hypogonadal even before cancer has been diagnosed.
II. *Surgery*: Uni- or bilateral orchidectomy leads to reduced total Leydig cell number and subsequently androgen deficiency. The major patient group within this category is men treated for TGCC. Orchidectomy is routinely done in these men. Both testes are removed if the disease is bilateral, the tumors occurring synchronously or the second tumor diagnosed some years after the occurrence of the first—if no contralateral biopsy for diagnosis of carcinoma-in-situ (CIS) has been done. Available data indicate that contralateral CIS can be found in up to 5% to 6% of TGCC cases (4).
III. *Chemotherapy*: Intense cytotoxic drug treatment may also have harmful effects on Leydig cell function. In TGCC patients, such an effect was seen in those who had received three to four cycles of chemotherapy (5). However, this effect was transient. There is only scarce information considering the impact of different types of cytotoxic drugs on androgen secretion. However, alkylating drugs seem to have profound effects, not only on sperm production but even on the endocrine function of

the testis (6). Other chemotherapeutic agents should also be considered as potentially harmful. It is now known that even cancer treatment given in the prepubertal age can imply a permanent Leydig cell damage.

IV. *Irradiation:* Radiation treatment has a negative impact on Leydig cells. This is, in particular, true if the irradiation is given directly to the testis(es) as is true in TGCC men with CIS in the contralateral testis, as part of total body irradiation prior to bone marrow transplantation, or in some boys with acute lymphoblastic leukemia. Even irradiation directed against other parts of the body near the testis may imply impairment of Leydig cell function. Leydig cells are more resistant to damage from radiotherapy. Significant rises in LH have been demonstrated with single-dose radiation doses of above 0.75 Gray (Gy) (7) and fractionated doses of above 2 Gy (8). However, no change in testosterone level was seen at these doses, and LH values showed a gradual return to normal levels over 30 months. Higher testicular radiation doses, however, result in more marked Leydig cell insufficiency. A dose of 16 to 20 Gy given in 8 to 10 fractions for CIS in the remaining testis resulted in a significant increase in mean LH levels within the first 3 months with a decrease in mean serum testosterone levels (9). Similar results were observed (10) in adults treated with high dose (30 Gy) of testicular irradiation following unilateral orchidectomy. In addition, more marked abnormalities were observed in a group of men treated with the same testicular dose of irradiation during childhood, suggesting that the prepubertal testis is much more vulnerable to radiation-induced Leydig cell damage (10).

Secondary hypogonadism in cancer survivors is related to treatment of cancer in the hypothalamus, the pituitary region, or other parts of the brain. It could also be pharmacologically induced as in the treatment of advanced prostatic cancer in middle-aged or older men. However, in this category of men hypogonadism is the goal and not side effect of the treatment.

The types of treatment related to the risk of secondary hypogonadism are

I. *Surgery*, for example, hypophysectomy
II. *Irradiation.*

It should be kept in mind that some patients may have a combined primary and secondary hypogonadism.

These mechanisms of action are summarized in Figure 1.

AGE RELATED RISK OF HYPOGONADISM

In males, the serum concentration of total testosterone is subject to age-related decline. In average, the magnitude of this decrease in serum testosterone levels is about 0.015 nmol/L (11) annually. Parallel with the decrease in testosterone levels, the sex hormone–binding globulin (SHBG) concentration increases, implying that the age-related reduction in the amount is more pronounced for free testosterone than is for total testosterone. It is unknown whether the decline in androgen levels in cancer survivors is more pronounced, or of the same magnitude, as that in the general male population.

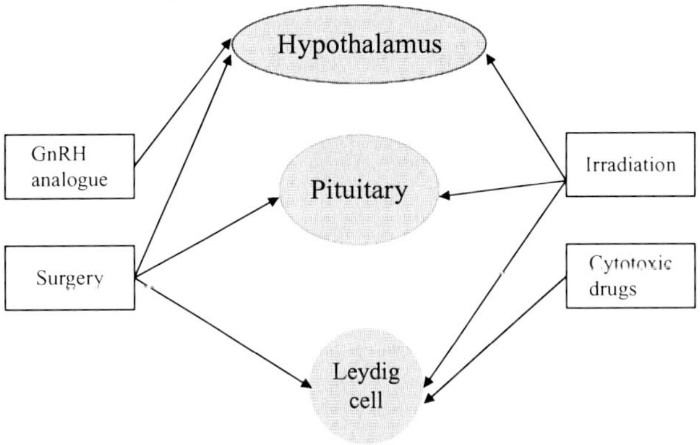

Figure 1 Schematic illustration of possible targets of different types of cancer treatment in relation to Leydig cell function.

This age-related decrease regarding testosterone concentration has some implications for cancer survivors. Men having low normal androgens shortly after termination of oncological treatment may be more prone to become hypogonadal by age. The question whether these alterations may hypothetically influence further prognosis cannot be answered until today. In untreated men the risks for prostate cancer seems not to be associated with endogenous hormone levels (12).

CONSEQUENCES OF ANDROGEN DEFICIENCY

The symptoms of hypogonadism because of cancer and its treatment are partly dependent on whether the androgen deficiency has started in the prepubertal or pubertal age (Table 1). Roughly, the symptoms of hypogonadism do not differ from those of other forms of hypogonadism and are as follows:

Apart of the immediate symptoms related to androgen deficiency, male hypogonadism may have long-term consequences leading to:

Decreased insulin sensitivity
Type II diabetes
Metabolic syndrome
Cardiovascular disease

CLINICAL GUIDELINES

At Cancer Diagnosis

Prepubertal Boys

Apart from the first three to six months after birth, Leydig cells are inactive until puberty. Therefore, there is no possibility of assessing the precancer treatment status of the testicular

Table 1 Clinical Signs of Hypogonadism—Based on Whether it Initiates Pre- or Postpubertally

	Prepubertal	Postpubertal
Larynx	No pubertal voice change	–
Hair	Horizontal pubic hair border Reduced beard growth Reduced beard growth Straight frontal hairline	Reduced secondary body hair
Skin	No sebum, acne, or skin wrinkling	Less sebum, acne, or skin wrinkling
Bones	Eunuchoid body proportions Osteoporosis	Osteoporosis
Bone marrow	Slight anemia	Slight anemia
Muscles	Underdeveloped	Atrophy
Prostate	Underdeveloped	Atrophy
Penis	Infantile	No change of size
Testes	Small volume	Atrophic/small volume
Spermatogenesis	Not developed	Involuted
Libido	Not developed	Reduced
Sexual function	Not developed	Reduced

Source: Adapted from Ref. 13.

endocrine function in these subjects. Furthermore, apart from shielding the testes to avoid scattered irradiation of the gonads, there are no means of protecting the Leydig cells from the potential harmful effects of cancer therapy.

Postpubertal Men

These patients will typically be referred for semen cryopreservation. In such case, the status of the Leydig cell function should be assessed in order to be able to detect possible deterioration attributable to treatment. Hormone analyses should include serum levels of

- Testosterone (free and total)
- LH
- SHBG
- Oestradiol (optional)

The blood sampling should be performed between 8 and 10 a.m. (see chap. 27). In TGCC patients, the ultrasonographic appearance of microcalcifications in the contralateral testicle should be examined, since it can predispose for posttreatment hypogonadism (optional).

After Cancer Treatment

Prepubertal Boys

These patients should be carefully followed for signs of delayed puberty (see chap. 26).

Postpubertal Men

Men treated for cancer in childhood or adulthood should, as a part of follow-up, be offered investigation aiming to disclose any signs of androgen deficiency. In childhood cancer survivors it should be done after completion of puberty. In case of malignancy in adulthood, it should be done 6 to 12 months after completing cancer treatment, if hypogonadism is not expected immediately after the therapy has been given (e.g., following bilateral orchidectomy or hypophysectomy and/or radiotherapy to the testes or the pituitary gland). The symptoms of male hypogonadism, which are rather uncharacteristic, can develop slowly and gradually. Therefore the symptoms may be overseen by the patient as well as by a doctor not specifically focusing on the possibility of androgen deficiency.

Diagnosis of androgen deficiency in adult patients previously treated for cancer is based on traditional criteria of male hypogonadism (see above)

√ Symptoms of androgen deficiency in males (see also Chapter 27)
√ Low serum testosterone (<10 nmol/L or significantly lower than pretreatment) and/or
√ High serum LH (>10 IU/L)*

* Not applicable if secondary hypogonadism is suspected

If the patient has no clear symptoms of hypogonadism and testosterone levels are in the lower end of the normal range and/or LH is in the upper normal range, a reinvestigation should be offered in one to five years, and even longer follow-up should be considered. *Androgen replacement* should be given according to the standard guidelines (see chap. 29). Note that prostate cancer and breast cancer in males are contraindications of treatment with androgens.

LEVELS OF EVIDENCE

1. *Cancer and cancer treatment can lead to hypogonadism: Level 1b*
2. *Male hypogonadism leading to cardiovascular and metabolic disturbances: Level 3*
3. *Androgen replacement in cancer-treated men prevents cardiovascular and metabolic disease: Level 4*

REFERENCES

1. Schmoll HJ, Souchon R, Krege S, et al. European consensus on diagnosis and treatment of germ cell cancer: a report of the European Germ Cell Cancer Consensus Group (EGCCCG). Ann Oncol 2004; 15:1377–1399
2. Willemse PHB, Sleijfer DTh, Sluiter WJ, et al. Altered Leydig cell function in patients with testicular cancer: evidence for a bilateral testicular defect. Acta Endocrinol 1983; 102:616–624.

3. Skakkebæk NE, Rajpert-De Meyts E, Main KM. Testicular dysgenesis syndrome: an increasingly common developmental disorder with environmental aspects. Hum.Reprod 2001; 16:972–978.
4. von der Maase H, Giwercman A, Müller J, et al. Management of carcinoma-in-situ of the testis. Int J Androl 1987; 10:209–220.
5. Eberhard J, Stahl A, Cwikiel M, et al. Risk factors for post-treatment hypogonadism in testicular cancer patients. Eur J Endocrinol 2008; 158:561–570.
6. Howell SJ,.Shalet SM. Effect of cancer therapy on pituitary-testicular axis. Int J Androl 2002; 25:269–276.
7. Rowley MJ, Leach DR, Warner GA, et al. Effect of graded doses of ionizing radiation on the human testis. Radiat Res 1974; 59:665–678.
8. Shapiro E, Kinsella TJ, Makuch RW, et al. Effects of fractionaed irradiation on endocrine aspects of testicular function. J Clin Oncol 1985; 3:1232–1239.
9. Petersen PM, Giwercman A, Daugaard G, et al. Effect of graded testicular doses of radiotherapy in patients treated for carcinoma-in-situ in the testis. J Clin Oncol 2002; 20:1537–1543.
10. Shalet SM, Tsatsoulis A, Whitehead E, et al. Vulnerablity of the human Leydig cell to radiation damage is dependent upon age. J Endocrinol 1989; 120:161–165.
11. Wu FC, Tajar A, Pye SR, et al. Hypothalamic-pituitary-testicular axis disruptions in older men are differentially linked to age and modifiable risk factors. J Clin Endocrinol Metab 2008; 93:2737–2745.
12. Endogenous hormones and prostate cancer collaborative group. Endogenous sex hormones and prostate cancer: a collaborative analysis of 18 prospective studies. J Nat Cancer Inst 2008; 100:170–183.
13. Nieschlag E, Behre HM (eds). Andrology: Male Reproductive Health and Dysfunction, 2nd Edition. Berlin Heidelberg: Springer Verlag, 2009.

31 Gynecomastia

Niels Jørgensen, Niels Kroman, Jens-Jørgen Elberg, and Anders Juul

INTRODUCTION

Gynecomastia is a benign proliferation of glandular tissue of the breast in males, which results in concentric enlargement of one or both mammary regions. Mammary tissue is present in children of both sexes, and development of breasts depends on hormonal stimulation. The growth and differentiation of mammary tissue in the male is controlled by stimulatory and inhibitory hormones (1). Estradiol binds to estrogen receptors (ERα and ERβ) and stimulates glandular cell growth, whereas testosterone binds to the androgen receptor (AR), which seem to inhibit growth and differentiation of breast tissue (2). Gynecomastia may be the result of increased estradiol levels that may occur from direct gonadal or adrenal sources, or from peripheral conversion of androgens (3,4). Thus, the principal determinant of breast development is the balance between androgenic and estrogenic stimulation. Testosterone is converted enzymatically to estradiol by aromatase (encoded by the CYP19 gene). Likewise androstenedione is aromatized to estrone by aromatase. Any changes in the ratio between testosterone and estradiol (either from decreased testosterone or increased estradiol) may stimulate dormant mammary gland tissue to proliferate and lead to the development of gynecomastia (1). Familial cases of gynecomastia due to aromatase excess syndrome have been described (5,6), but in many cases the testosterone-to-estradiol ratio is normal in circulation. Aromatase activity is present in gonads, adipose tissue, and breast tissue. Most likely local aromatase activity in breast tissue may be increased in patients with gynecomastia (4). Clearly marked differences in the sensitivity of breast tissue to estrogens exist between subjects. Other hormones like growth hormone (GH) and insulin-like growth factor I (IGF-I) seem to have permissive effects increasing the activity of other hormones on breast tissue. Thus, development of gynecomastia is a well-known side effect of GH treatment in adult males in some cases (7). Thyroxine increases sex hormone binding globulin (SHBG) and subsequently lowers free testosterone levels which may result in increased glandular growth (8). Prolactin stimulates lactation, but it is not directly related to breast development. Indirectly, however, prolactin decreases gonadotropin secretion and lowers testosterone, which in turn may stimulate male breast development. Thus, in some cases hyperprolactinemia may result in gynecomastia (9).

CLINICAL EVALUATION OF PATIENTS WITH GYNECOMASTIA

It may be troublesome to distinguish glandular breast tissue from fat tissue (lipomastia) especially in obese subjects. Successful palpation is most likely if the tissue is squeezed between the thumb and forefinger in a patient in the sitting position. The examiner should try to find an edge, hereby distinguishing the outer limits of the gynecomastia. The distance between thumb and forefinger should be recorded as precisely as possible (10). This may often be difficult, and the diagnosis of gynecomastia may be subject to some clinical judgement. Some authors define pathological gynecomastia when the diameter is more than 4 cm, or more than 2 cm if the tissue is tender upon palpation. Tenderness of the breast tissue may be considered a sign of recent hormone stimulation. Staging of the degree of breast development can be performed using the 5 breast stages described by Tanner (11). Breast stage 1 denotes no gynecomastia, whereas breast stage 2 denotes breast budding (glandular tissue can be palpated within the areolar area). Breast stages 3–4 are more advanced breast stages (Fig. 1), and breast stage 5 denotes the mature breast of an adult female. The gynecomastia may be unilateral or bilateral which should be recorded.

In few cases radiological mammography (or ultrasound) is warranted if the diagnosis is questionable (Figs. 2 and 3), especially if a breast tumour is suspected (12). Importantly, if a firm swelling (usually painless) is present, especially in an excentric position, one should not hesitate to perform a biopsy to rule out breast cancer.

A complete physical examination of patients with gynecomastia is not confined to the breast, but includes a full clinical evaluation and laboratory investigations (Table 1).

Height, weight, and body mass index should be recorded. Body proportions (determined by sitting height to standard height ratio) to quantify any degree of eunuchoidism (longleggedness) as well as fat distribution should be recorded. The degree of virilization should be recorded which include evaluation of the presence of beard and body hair, acne, and baldness. Genital development includes evaluation of penile size, scrotal development, pubic hair, and testicular size. Testicular volume can be determined by the use of an orchidometer or by ultrasonography. Testicular palpation is mandatory and should preferably be accompanied by testicular ultrasound examination to rule out the presence of germ cell or Leydig cell tumors (Fig. 4) because the diagnosis of small tumors may be missed by palpation. Finally, signs of hepatic, renal, and other systemic disease should be ruled out.

The patient should be asked about the time course of the development of the gynecomastia in detail, whether it is *(i)* persistent pubertal gynecomastia, *(ii)* a long-lasting problem

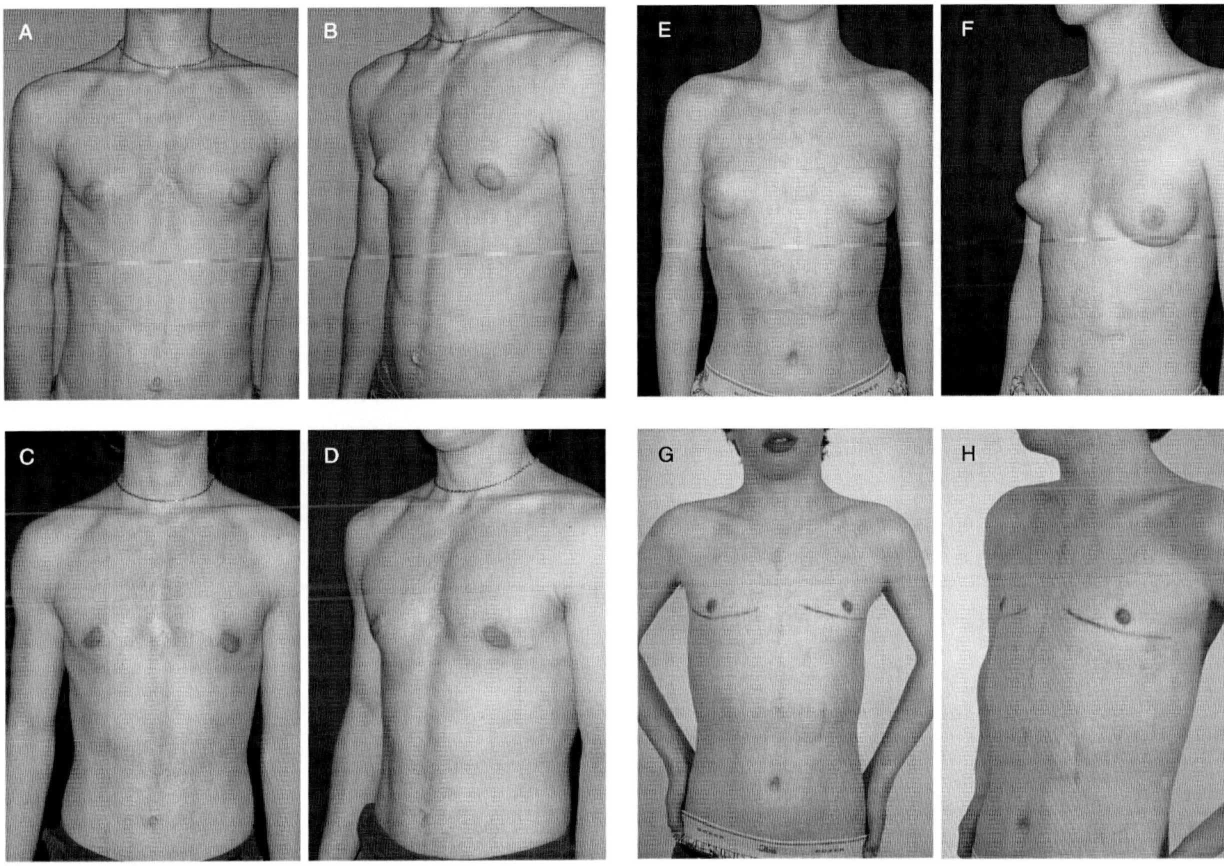

Figure 1 Two young men with gynaecomastia of different severity. Panels A and B show an 18-year-old man with a slight and bilateral gynaecomastia (Tanner stage B2-B3) of unknown reason. Panels C and D the same man after liposuction. Panels E and F show a more pronounced gynaecomastia (Tanner stage B4) of a 16-year-old man having a congenital heart failure for which he was treated by spironolactone. He was treated by a subcutaneous mastectomy, skin resection and transplantation of the nipple-areola complex (G and H).

(for years), or *(iii)* a new and rapidly developing condition. Furthermore, the patient should be asked for signs of hypogonadism like decreased libido, tiredness, sweats and hot flushes, mood changes, and erectile dysfunction. Because many types of medicine may cause gynecomastia, any intake of medication should be recorded (Table 2).

Laboratory investigations should be individualized depending on the clinical presentation and medical history. If a diagnosis of adolescent gynecomastia seems obvious or if the gynecomastia is mild and nonprogressive, there may not be a need for blood sampling. However, in most cases laboratory investigations are needed and include determination of testosterone, estradiol, SHBG, follicle stimulating hormone (FSH), luteinizing hormone (LH), prolactin, thyroid stimulating hormone, human chorionic gonadotropin (hCG), α-foetoprotein, and hepatic and renal function tests. In some cases inhibin B, karyotyping, and DNA analyses may be useful.

PHYSIOLOGICAL GYNECOMASTIA

There are physiological forms of gynecomastia in different periods of life.

In newborns exposure to the high levels of sex steroids in utero may stimulate breast tissue that may persist several weeks after birth. Furthermore, exposure to estrogen in breast milk may result in varying degrees of palpable breast tissue.

In infancy the pituitary–gonadal axis is very active at three months of age resulting in pubertal levels of FSH, LH, testosterone, and estradiol in all boys (this phenomenon is also termed "minipuberty") (13). The reason for this first activation of the pituitary–gonadal axis remains unknown, but insufficient secretion of testosterone during this period (as seen in newborns with hypogonadotropic hypogonadism) is associated with decreased penile growth. Furthermore, boys born with cryptorchidism often exhibit spontaneous descent of testes at three months of age, when testosterone levels are high. Altogether, these findings

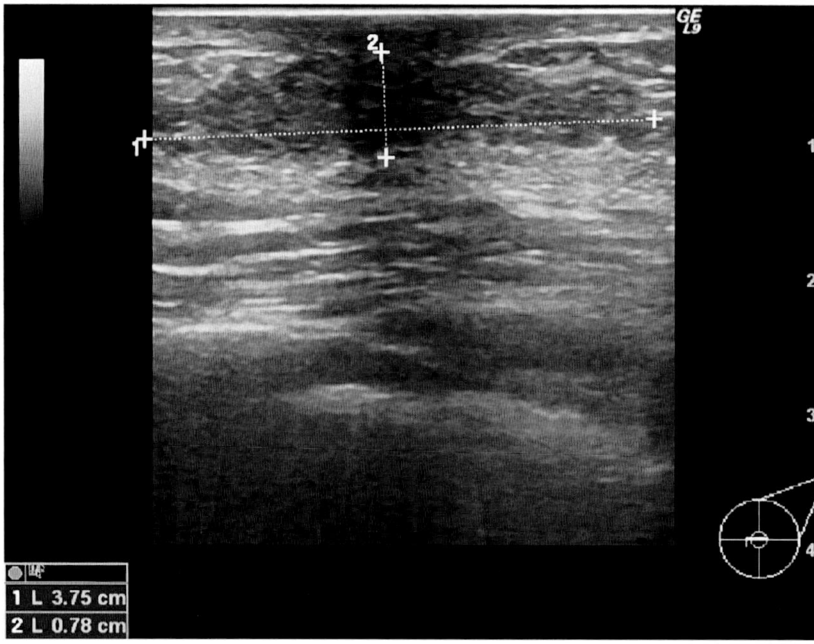

Figure 2 Ultrasound examination of breast tissue of a 71-year-old man showing a well-defined hypoechoic discoid area compatible with gynaecomastia 3.75 cm in width (line 1) and 0.78 cm in depth (line 2). Neither ultrasound examination nor mammography is usually needed in the routine work-up of patients, but should be restricted to situations where there is doubt whether an enlargement of the breast tissue represents gynaecomastia or lipomastia. If a breast cancer is suspected a biopsy should be performed.

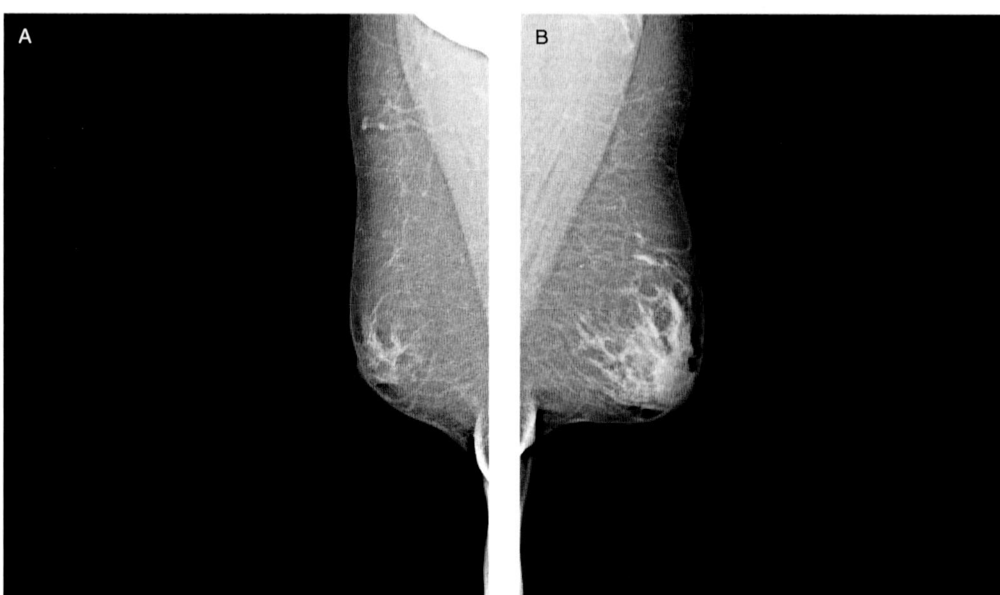

Figure 3 Mammography of a 63-year-old man with breast enlargement. Panels A and B show the right and left mammary regions, respectively. The gynaecomastia on the left side was significantly larger than on the right side. On both sides significant amounts of fat tissue are seen. At the physical examination it was difficult to distinguish mammary tissue from fat tissue. As noted for Figure 2, mammography should not routinely be used in the diagnostic procedure of gynaecomastia.

Table 1 Suggestions for Primary Evaluation of Men with Gynecomastia. It is Our Experience that the History, Physical Examination, and Initial Laboratory Investigations in the Majority of Cases will be Sufficient to Reach a Conclusion Regarding the Underlying Cause(s)

History
- Duration of gynecomastia (uni- or bilateral), tenderness
- Previous gynecomastia
- Previous or current cryptorchidism, fertility status
- Symptoms of hypogonadism, hyperthyroidism, or other systemic illness
- Complete list of medication, use of recreational drugs, and/or supplements

Physical examination
- Gynecomastia (uni- or bilateral), size, tenderness
- Height, weight, and body mass index
- Goiter
- Testicular size, cryptorchidism, palpation for tumor
- Ultrasound examination of testicles

Initial laboratory investigations
- Testosterone, LH, estradiol, SHBG, (FSH and Inhibin-B)
- hCG
- TSH, thyroxine, (free-thyroxine)
- Prolactin
- Liver and kidney parameters

Additional laboratory investigations, depending on the results of the initial investigations
- Adrenal androgens (DHEA, DHEA-sulfate, androstendione)
- Estrone
- Karyotype
- DNA (e.g., for androgen receptor analysis)

Abbreviations: LH, luteinizing hormone; SHBG, sex hormone binding globulin; FSH, follicle stimulating hormone; hCG, human chorionic gonadotropin; TSH, thyroid stimulating hormone; DHEA, dehydroepiandrosterone.

suggest that this brief pituitary–gonadal activation may play a role for postnatal genital development. Breast tissue can frequently be palpated in three-month old boys, and seems to be related to circulating estradiol concentrations (14).

Adolescent gynecomastia is seen in a large proportion of normal adolescent boys who may develop palpable and sore glandular tissue (> 0.5 cm in diameter), which, however, regresses spontaneously within 6 to 12 months in the majority of boys (15). This is assumed to be due to a skewed androgen-to-estrogen balance, although circulating testosterone and estradiol levels are usually no different from similar aged boys without palpable gynecomastia. The incidence of adolescent physiological gynecomastia varies in different studies from 4% to as much as 60%, which may depend on study design as well as differences in the adolescent age groups studied (10–12 years vs. 10–18 years) (16). It usually appears in midpuberty (genital Tanner stages 3–4) and can be considered a normal variation in most cases and usually does not require detailed investigations or treatment. Most boys should just be checked again after 6 months and be reassured that it will most likely disappear spontaneously (17). However, in some cases it may cause considerable cosmetic and psychological distress. Thus, adolescent gynecomastia may have a negative impact on self-esteem and lead to decreased participation in social activities like swimming and showering after gymnastics. In some boys the adolescent gynecomastia does not disappear. If gynecomastia persists for more than 2 to 3 years it is not likely to disappear spontaneously (18). The development of gynecomastia in adolescent boys without any other signs of puberty must raise suspicion of an underlying endocrinopathy including hormone-producing tumor, and warrant further evaluation.

PATHOLOGICAL GYNECOMASTIA

If a diagnosis of physiological gynecomastia is not obvious, pathological conditions resulting in gynecomastia must be ruled

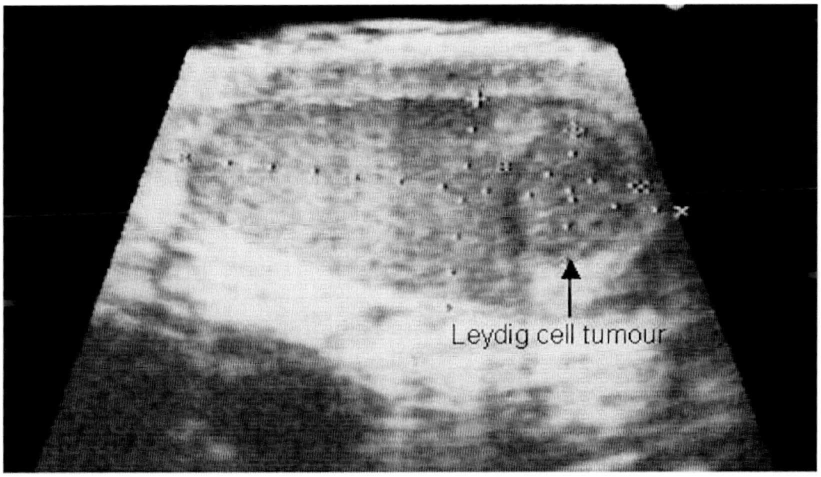

Figure 4 Ultrasound examination of the left testis of a 45-year-old man referred due to gynaecomastia. The ultrasound examination clearly showed a tumor formation 1.3 cm in diameter and well defined from the surrounding normal looking tissue close to the bottom of the testis (arrow). Using the Prader ochidometer the testis was estimated to be approximately 12–15 ml in size. It was soft in consistency but without palpable tumor. Sex hormone levels indicated the presence of a Leydig cell tumor, which was confirmed after isolated removal of the tumor. Following operation sex hormone levels normalized and gynaecomastia regressed.

Table 2 Commonly Used Drugs Associated with Development of Gynecomastia

Sex steroid modulating agents

- Androgens and anabolic steroids
- Estrogens
- Clomiphene
- Human chorionic gonadotropin
- 5-α-reductase inhibitors
- Cyproterone
- Ketoconazole and metronidazole
- Spironolactone and H2-receptor antagonists

Cardiovascular drugs

- Angiotensin converting enzyme (ACE) inhibitors
- Calcium antagonists
- Digoxin

Psychoactive drugs

- Phenytoin
- Serotonin reuptake inhibitors
- Tricyclic antidepressants

Antiviral agents

- Zidovudine
- Stavudine

out. An underlying endocrine disorder is the most likely cause. Such endocrinopathy may be associated with estrogen excess, androgen deficiency, impaired androgen action, or imbalanced estrogen/testosterone ratio, all of which conditions may lead to gynecomastia.

Obese men have increased risk of gynecomastia. Excess truncal fat deposition result in lipomastia (pseudogynecomastia). In addition increased peripheral conversion of testosterone to estradiol in fat tissues may often result in real glandular tissue.

Elderly men often show some degree of gynecomastia. In this age group systemic diseases, increased adiposity, medication, or late-onset hypogonadism are more likely to play a pathogenetic role for the development of gynecomastia.

Endocrine Disorders

Almost all conditions associated with lowered testosterone are associated with gynecomastia at a high frequency (for review see (19). Hypogonadism may be of primary/testicular (hypergonadotropic) or secondary/pituitary (hypogonadotropic) origin.

Primary Gonadal Failure

Primary testicular failure is associated with increased LH levels, which in turn stimulates testicular estradiol secretion in excess of androgens. Patients with bilateral cryptorchidism may have impaired Leydig cell function resulting in hypogonadism. Other forms of primary testicular insufficiency (orchitis following mumps, granulomatous orchitis) may result in hypogonadism resulting in gynecomastia. Patients with Klinefelter syndrome (47,XXY) or SRY-positive karyotypes have gynecomastia in 50% to 70% of cases (20) as a consequence of their relative hypogonadism (low-normal testosterone and elevated LH and in some cases elevated estradiol) (21). In addition to gynecomastia, Klinefelter patients may exhibit eunuchoid body proportions, increased height, and all have small testes. Patients who have unilateral orchiectomy performed (e.g., due to torsion or testicular cancer) usually maintain a sufficient testosterone production from the remaining testis. However, some patients develop subtle clinical signs of hypogonadism over time, which is reflected in declining testosterone levels (and increased LH). If the remaining testis receives irradiation (due to carcinoma in situ), approximately 50% of patients will develop overt hypogonadism (22) and risk of gynecomastia.

Thyrotoxicosis may lead to gynecomastia and is associated with increased estradiol and SHBG levels, which diminish free bioavailable testosterone levels.

Hypogonadotropic Hypogonadism

Isolated hypogonadotropic hypogonadism (IHH) is commonly associated with gynecomastia (23). It can occur in a congenital form like Kallmans syndrome (KAL-1 mutations) or due to mutations in the GPR54 or FGFR1 genes. Hypogonadotropic hypogonadism may also be acquired following hyperprolactinemia due to a pituitary prolactinoma (micro- or macroadenoma), medication-induced hyperprolactinemia (e.g., antidepressants), or idiopathic. Hemochromatosis may result in isolated hypogonadotropic hypogonadism.

Androgen Resistance

Complete androgen resistance results in the development of breast tissue in a genetic male with phenotypic appearance of a female (Morris syndrome). However, partial androgen insensitivity may result in a phenotypic male with gynecomastia (24). Androgen sensitivity may be influenced by the number of CAG repeats in the AR gene. In case of Kennedy syndrome, an increased number of CAG repeats in the AR gene results in signs of hypogonadism including gynecomastia in addition to the neurodegenerative findings (muscular weakness, atrophy, and fasciculations), which typically present from 40 to 50 years of age.

Endocrine Active Tumors

Testicular tumors may produce estrogenic hormones, which lead to gynecomastia. These tumors may be of germ cell, Leydig cell (Fig. 4), or Sertoli cell origin. Germ cell tumors may or may not be palpable depending on their size, whereas Leydig cell or Sertoli cell tumors are usually very small at the time of referral for gynecomastia and can only be detected by testicular ultrasonography. An increase in aromatase activity in the gonadal tumors is responsible for the estrogen excess and development of gynecomastia (25).

Choriocarcinomas of the testis may produce hCG which stimulates local testicular production of testosterone and estradiol. Extragonadal (e.g., mediastinal) germ cell tumors may also produce hCG which stimulates testicular hormone productions.

Gynecomastia is seen in patients with Sertoli cell tumors. *Peutz-Jeghers syndrome,* which is an autosomal dominant disorder, characterized by melanocytic macules of the lips, buccal mucosa and digits, and multiple gastrointestinal hamartomatous polyps. The testicular lesions seen in patients with Peutz-Jeghers syndrome mostly represent multifocal intratubular neoplasia of large Sertoli cells with unique morphology.

Ectopic production of hCG may occur in tumors in the liver, stomach, lung, and kidney. Thus, if hCG is elevated and no testicular tumor is found upon palpation and ultrasound, X ray of thorax as well as CT of abdomen is warranted.

In cases of testicular or ectopic hCG production, testosterone levels are usually high-normal and FSH and LH levels are usually completely suppressed.

Adrenal tumors (adenomas or adenocarcinomas) may produce estradiol or androgenic estrogen precursors like dehydroepiandrosterone (DHEA), DHEA sulfate (DHEAS), or androstenedione. Patients harboring an adrenal tumor may present with hypertension and elevated urinary excretion of ketosteroids.

Systemic Diseases with Gynecomastia

Patients with chronic renal failure often present with hypogonadism and lowered testosterone that may result in hypogonadism. Chronic liver disease commonly results in gynecomastia due to increased aromatization of testosterone to estradiol in the liver. Furthermore, alcohol inhibits testicular steroidogenesis resulting in lowered testosterone. In general, chronic diseases are commonly associated with gynecomastia and often associated with treatment with various drugs.

Medication

Numerous medications may result in gynecomastia (Table 2). Thus, a detailed list of medication used by the patient is needed in the clinical work-up. Alternative treatments should be considered if possible when the patient develops gynecomastia.

Exogenous Exposure to Estrogens

Unintended exposure to estrogen may occur during intercourse with women using vaginal estrogen cream or from women using transdermal estrogen treatment, i.e., by applying estrogen gel to the skin. Boys with gynecomastia who have ingested their mothers' oral contraceptives by mistake have also been described.

Illegal use of anabolic steroids often result in gynecomastia (26). There may be several reasons for this. Some anabolic steroids may aromatize to estrogens, which stimulate breast tissue directly. Consequently, some bodybuilders use estrogen receptor antagonists to prevent this. However, many anabolic steroids do not aromatize to estrogens, but result in hypogonadotropic hypogonadism after cessation of use, which in turn leads to gynecomastia. The hypogonadism following illegal use of anabolic steroids may be long lasting (several years) and some illegal users of anabolic steroids try to circumvent this by using hCG injections after stopping with anabolic steroids. HCG is known to cause gynecomastia itself. Thus, long-lasting hypogonadism and gynecomastia together with life-threatening hepatic and cardiac side effects are frequent features following illegal use of anabolic steroids and hCG. In our mind, such patients should be helped and treated like any other drug addicts. Treatment includes psychological support, regular monitoring of drug misuse (urine samples), and in cases of persistent hypogonadism androgen substitution should be offered.

An important differential diagnosis to gynecomastia is male breast cancer.

Breast Cancer

Breast cancer in men is a rare disease with an incidence about 200-fold lower compared to women in the Western world. However, men are aware that they can contract breast cancer and are quite often concerned whether a gynecomastia may represent cancer. In case of a suspicious tumor in a male breast, the diagnostic approach is to perform a core biopsy. In general there is no need to perform imaging if there is agreement between the clinical appearance and the result of the biopsy. Ultrasound sonography can be used in case of uncertainty. In case of malignancy, diagnostic work, surgical treatment, and adjuvant treatment should follow the guidelines for the disease in women.

TREATMENT

Any underlying pathology should be treated or corrected if possible. In case of systemic disease where gynecomastia can be attributed to medications, the suspected drug should be changed if possible. In case of hypogonadism, substitution with testosterone should be initiated. In some cases this will result in regression of gynecomastia.

Medical treatment with aromatase inhibitors or estrogen receptor blockade (like Tamoxifen) have proven efficient in some studies, but cannot be considered standard treatment (27).

Surgical Treatment

Approximately, 85% of men with inconvenience from gynecomastia will experience spontaneous regression (1,28). Thus, in general, surgical treatment should not be offered before a period of observation, especially in pubertal boys. If cancer is a concern for the patient, a biopsy can be performed. The patient will generally accept after assurance of benign conditions. The classical surgical treatment is nipple-sparing subcutaneous mastectomy. However, suction lipectomy has proved helpful for tapering the edges and in mild gynecomastia it may be used as the sole procedure. The incision should be periareolar. It is important to preserve a button of tissue under the areolar complex to maintain a sufficient blood supply and to prevent the nipple from sticking on the chest wall and retracting (29). In severe gynecomastia, skin resection is often necessary in combination with transposition of the nipple–areola complex (Fig. 1). The most frequent complication after surgery is numbness of the nipple and adherence of the areola to the pectoral muscle.

ACKNOWLEDGMENT

We thank the clinic for mammography screening (Mammografiscreeningsklinikken) at the department of Diagnostic Radiology, Rigshospitalet, Copenhagen, Denmark, for providing Figures 2 and 3.

REFERENCES

1. Mathur R, Braunstein GD. Gynecomastia: pathomechanisms and treatment strategies. Horm Res 1997; 48:95–102.
2. Rochefort H, Garcia M. The estrogenic and antiestrogenic activities of androgens in female target tissues. Pharmacol Ther 1983; 23:193–216.
3. Carlson HE, Kane P, Lei ZM, et al. Presence of luteinizing hormone/human chorionic gonadotropin receptors in male breast tissues. J Clin Endocrinol Metab 2004; 89:4119–4123.
4. Sasano H, Kimura M, Shizawa S, et al. Aromatase and steroid receptors in gynecomastia and male breast carcinoma: an immunohistochemical study. J Clin Endocrinol Metab 1996; 81:3063–3067.
5. Binder G, Iliev DI, Dufke A, et al. Dominant transmission of prepubertal gynecomastia due to serum estrone excess: hormonal, biochemical, and genetic analysis in a large kindred. J Clin Endocrinol Metab 2005; 90:484–492.
6. Shozu M, Sebastian S, Takayama K, et al. Estrogen excess associated with novel gain-of-function mutations affecting the aromatase gene. N Engl J Med 2003; 348:1855–1865.
7. Cohn L, Feller AG, Draper MW, et al. Carpal tunnel syndrome and gynaecomastia during growth hormone treatment of elderly men with low circulating IGF-I concentrations. Clin Endocrinol (Oxf) 1993; 39:417–425.
8. Kidd GS, Glass AR, Vigersky RA. The hypothalamic-pituitary-testicular axis in thyrotoxicosis. J Clin Endocrinol Metab 1979; 48:798–802.
9. Kaneda Y, Fujii A, Yamaoka T, et al. Neither gynecomastia nor galactorrhea is a common side effect of neuroleptics in male patients. Neuro Endocrinol Lett 2000; 21:447–451.
10. Braunstein GD. Clinical practice. Gynecomastia. N Engl J Med 2007; 357:1229–1237.
11. Marshall WA, Tanner JM. Variations in pattern of pubertal changes in girls. Arch Dis Child 1969; 44:291–303.
12. Hines SL, Tan WW, Yasrebi M, et al. The role of mammography in male patients with breast symptoms. Mayo Clin Proc 2007; 82:297–300.
13. Andersson AM, Toppari J, Haavisto AM, et al. Longitudinal reproductive hormone profiles in infants: peak of inhibin B levels in infant boys exceeds levels in adult men. J Clin Endocrinol Metab 1998; 83:675–681.
14. Schmidt IM, Chellakooty M, Haavisto AM, et al. Gender difference in breast tissue size in infancy: correlation with serum estradiol. Pediatr Res 2002; 52:682–686.
15. Biro FM, Lucky AW, Huster GA, et al. Hormonal studies and physical maturation in adolescent gynecomastia. J Pediatr 1990; 116:450–455.
16. Kumanov P, Deepinder F, Robeva R, et al. Relationship of adolescent gynecomastia with varicocele and somatometric parameters: a cross-sectional study in 6200 healthy boys. J Adolesc Health 2007; 41:126–131.
17. Moore DC, Schlaepfer LV, Paunier L, et al. Hormonal changes during puberty: V. Transient pubertal gynecomastia: abnormal androgen-estrogen ratios. J Clin Endocrinol Metab 1984; 58:492–499.
18. Bannayan GA, Hajdu SI. Gynecomastia: clinicopathologic study of 351 cases. Am J Clin Pathol 1972; 57:431–437.
19. Braunstein GD. Gynecomastia. N Engl J Med 1993; 328:490–495.
20. Bojesen A, Gravholt CH. Klinefelter syndrome in clinical practice. Nat Clin Pract Urol 2007; 4:192–204.
21. Aksglaede L, Andersson AM, Jorgensen N, et al. Primary testicular failure in Klinefelter's syndrome: the use of bivariate luteinizing hormone-testosterone reference charts. Clin Endocrinol (Oxf) 2007; 66:276–281.
22. Petersen PM, Giwercman A, Daugaard G, et al. Effect of graded testicular doses of radiotherapy in patients treated for carcinoma-in-situ in the testis. J Clin Oncol 2002; 20:1537–1543.
23. Males JL, Townsend JL, Schneider RA. Hypogonadotropic hypogonadism with anosmia–Kallmann's syndrome. A disorder of olfactory and hypothalamic function. Arch Intern Med 1973; 131:501–507.
24. Giwercman A, Kledal T, Schwartz M, et al. Preserved male fertility despite decreased androgen sensitivity caused by a mutation in the ligand-binding domain of the androgen receptor gene. J Clin Endocrinol Metab 2000; 85:2253–2259.
25. Ulbright TM, Amin MB, Young RH. Intratubular large cell hyalinizing sertoli cell neoplasia of the testis: a report of 8 cases of a distinctive lesion of the Peutz-Jeghers syndrome. Am J Surg Pathol 2007; 31:827–835.
26. Maravelias C, Dona A, Stefanidou M, et al. Adverse effects of anabolic steroids in athletes. A constant threat. Toxicol Lett 2005; 158:167–175.
27. Shulman DI, Francis GL, Palmert MR, et al. Use of aromatase inhibitors in children and adolescents with disorders of growth and adolescent development. Pediatrics 2008; 121:e975–e983.
28. Treves N. Gynecomastia; the origins of mammary swelling in the male: an analysis of 406 patients with breast hypertrophy, 525 with testicular tumors, and 13 with adrenal neoplasms. Cancer 1958; 11:1083–1102.
29. Boljanovic S, Axelsson CK, Elberg JJ. Surgical treatment of gynecomastia: liposuction combined with subcutaneous mastectomy. Scand J Surg 2003; 92:160–162.

32 Male infertility in chronic urogenital infections and inflammation with special reference to ejaculate findings

Wolfgang Weidner, Thorsten Diemer, and Florian M. E. Wagenlehner

CASE REPORT

Mr S.R. who is 41 years old attended our special outpatient consultation for urogenital infections. He complained of an infertile partnership of 24 months although he had ovulation-optimized intercourse. His 32-year-old spouse was apparently healthy (as shown by the results of the gynecological examination). He reported a history of bacterial prostatitis with several courses of antibiotic therapy. The last diagnosis was chronic prostatitis/chronic pelvic pain syndrome (CP/CPPS) NIH III b at the urological examination. The first clinical examination demonstrated a swollen caput epididymidis on both sides (palpation, sonography), normal testicular volumes and normal testosterone (T), follicle stimulating hormone (FSH), and luteinizing hormone (LH). The ejaculate analysis (twice) according to WHO demonstrated the following three key point results: oligozoospermia with <10 million spermatozoa/mL (twice), leukocytospermia ($>1\times10^6$ PPL/mL), elastase in seminal plasma >1000 ng/mL. Ejaculate culture was sterile.

INTRODUCTION

There is no current consensus concerning the influence of urogenital infections and inflammation on the reproductive situation of the male. This is due to several factors: (*i*) the complicated situation for diagnosis of the following different entities: chronic urethritis, prostatitis, epididymitis, and orchitis; (*ii*) the necessity to consider these infections and/or inflammatory disorders as functional units because of the special anatomic situation with confluent seminal pathways, and (*iii*) the lack of evidence-based clinical data to define the interactions in detail.

This confuse situation resulted in the definition of an obscure entity by the WHO (1)—male accessory gland infection (MAGI)—followed by much urological criticism concerning the definition and the criteria for classification (2,3) initiating an ongoing debate on the acceptance of MAGI as a clinical truth.

Based on this background this chapter focuses on spermatological alterations, e.g., azoospermia or asthenozoospermia in association with defined infections and inflammatory entities of the urogenital tract.

EPIDEMIOLOGY

Epidemiologically, urogenital infections and inflammation are accepted causes of male infertility. The percentage of infectious and inflammatory causes is 6.9% in the WHO study of 1987 (4) and 8.0% in *Nieschlag's* report in 2002 (5). The recent analysis of the diagnosed causes of infertility in our Giessen Reproductive Center demonstrated infections and inflammation in 155 of 1834 (8.5%) men examined for infertility (Fig. 1).

CLASSIFICATION OF CHRONIC UROGENITAL INFECTIONS AND INFLAMMATION

For simplification, the classification criteria are shortly summarized for chronic urethritis, bacterial prostatitis and inflammatory CP/CPPS, chronic epididymitis, and orchitis. MAGI is discussed as a separate point.

Chronic Urethritis

The definition of chronic urethritis is not really clear. Patients, without urethral discharge, are suffering from burning and urethral itching during voiding. Chlamydial and gonococcal infections are typical etiological causes (6). Normally, the diagnosis is based on the evidence of leukocytes in the first voided urine and PCR findings of the mentioned microorganisms. Though sexually transmitted infections are the predominant cause for chronic urethritis, also noninfectious causes (physical, postendoscopy) have to be considered (7).

Prostatitis/CP/CPPS

The andrological relevance of the consensus findings of the 6th International Consultation on New Developments in Prostate Cancer and Prostate Diseases (8) has been discussed recently (2). The authors have thoroughly evaluated the consensus summary statement of the Paris expert group with particular focus on the feasibility of suggested diagnostic procedures and therapeutic trials in our andrological experience. Although not accepted worldwide in andrology, all statements and suggestions are based on the National Institutes of Health (NIH) classification of prostatitis syndromes (Table 1).

Chronic Epididymitis

Chronic epididymitis is a narrowly defined clinical entity that is typified by the clinical signs of an enlarged epididymis, painful sensation during palpation, and positive semen cultures for pathogenic bacteria in about 50% of cases (9). Chronic infectious events in the epididymis have been frequently associated with distinct spermatological alterations, sperm morphology such as "tapering" of sperm tails, and differences in tail coloring according to strict criteria (10). To date there is no evidence that pharmacotherapy exerts a positive effect of treatment on fertility outcomes (11).

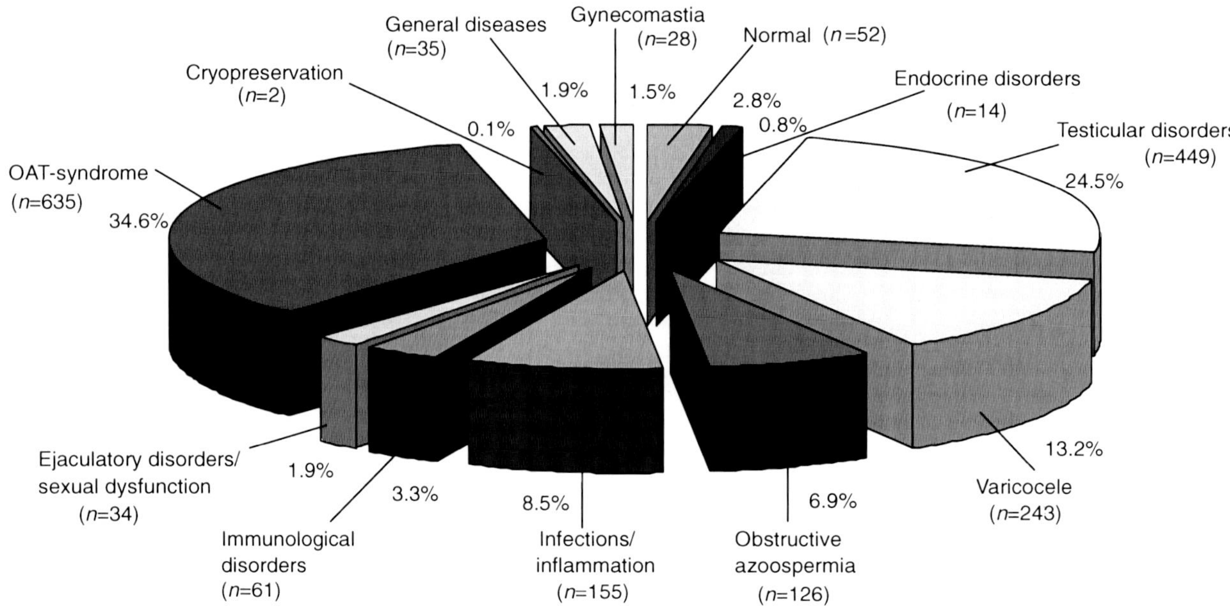

Figure 1 Diagram of diagnosis of consecutive 1834 men with fertility problems (Giessen Reproductive Center).

Orchitis

Bacterial orchitis and epididymo-orchitis are induced by certain enterobacteria, chlamydia, mycoplasma, gonococci, and other bacterial species. The epididymis appears to be the primary site of infection (via canalicular pathway) but the testis is severely affected if antibiotic treatment is delayed or fails. Subacute or chronic torpid inflammations in the testis remain asymptomatic in the majority of patients (12). The testicular innate immune defense against the antigens or toxins of the microorganisms is one major hypothesis for reduced spermatogenesis in these cases (13). Persistent infection can lead to fibrosis and hyalinization of seminiferous tubules and eventually cause different grades of spermatogenic defects, such as spermatogenic arrest. Bacterial infections of hematogenous origin such as tuberculosis are known to induce necrosis and calcification of the testicular tissue (11).

Several viruses including mumps may localize within the testis to induce a primary viral orchitis (14). Mumps orchitis represents the only clinically significant entity among the viral forms of orchitis frequently resulting in testicular defects such as fibrosis and hyalinization of the tubular compartment. A clinical hallmark of mumps orchitis is an isolated orchitis (without epididymitis) with high fever resistant to antibiotic treatment usually involving both testes in the majority of cases. Patients present with the classical signs of systemic infection, as simultaneous parotitis, are rare.

Table 1 Prostatitis NIH Classification

I. ABP
II. CBP
III. CP/CPPS
  (a) inflammatory
  (b) noninflammatory
IV. Asymptomatic, inflammatory

Abbreviations: NIH, National Institutes of Health; ABP, Acute Bacterial Prostatitis; CBP, Chronic Bacterial Prostatitis; CP, Chronic Prostatitis; CPPS, Chronic Pelvic Pain Syndrome.

MALE ACCESSORY GLAND INFECTION

The WHO (1) suggests that two of the following criteria are required to diagnose male accessory gland infection (MAGI) in men with oligo-, astheno-, or teratozoospermia: (*i*) history or physical signs of UTI, epididymitis, or abnormal rectal examination; (*ii*) abnormal urine after prostatic massage (describing the 4-glass test); or (*iii*) elevated numbers of peroxidase-positive white blood cells (WBCs), high numbers of bacteria in semen, *C. trachomatis* findings, and/or abnormal biochemistry or elevated inflammatory markers in the seminal fluid. Analysis of prostatic fluid is not recommended. It is our opinion that this suggested classification does not clearly differentiate between prostatitis, epididymitis, and other inflammatory alterations of the urethral compartment (2,3).

ALTERED EJACULATE PARAMETERS

Ejaculate Volume and pH

Well-designed studies concerning both parameters are lacking. After chronic urethritis, the development of obstruction either as normal stricture or at the level of the verumontanum has

Table 2 OAT-syndrome in Men with CBP (NIH II) and CP/CPPS (NIH III)

			Significant changes to controls		
Cohort (*n*)	Reference	NIH Groups	Sperm count	Motility	Morphology
276	19	II, IIIa, IIIb	NS	NS	NS
44	20	IIIa, IIIb	NS	NS	NS
112	16	IIIa, IIIb	NS	NS	NS
30	15	IIIb	NS	$P < 001$[a]	NS

[a] $P < 001$ motility improved.
Abbreviation: NS, not significant.

been discussed as a cause of decreased ejaculate volume. Publications are rare and describe single cases. A proven reduction of ejaculatory volume has never been shown (11). Studies analyzing the ejaculate pH with association to the described entities are not published. Available data on prostatitis do not demonstrate reduced ejaculatory volume in men with noninflammatory CP/CPPS (15); this is similar to data of our group demonstrating no reduced ejaculate volume in men with inflammatory signs in the ejaculate (16).

Sperm Count, Motility, Morphology, Evidence of OAT-syndrome

In men with evidence of DNA from sexually transmitted infectious pathogens in semen, a decrease of sperm concentration and motility has been observed (17). Urethritis, per se, seems not to be a major problem (11) and HIV infections have a negative impact on testicular function with progression of immunodeficiency, although the percentage of OAT-syndrome is not described in detail (18). In this context, especially data for CP/CPPS are of high importance. Our own examinations reconfirm earlier findings that these ejaculate parameters in prostatic infections are unlikely to be affected (16). Table 2 summarizes recent study data demonstrating no significant effect on sperm count and morphology in infectious and inflammatory prostatitis (NIH II and NIH IIIa).

From an andrological point of view, the development of epididymo-orchitis is of particular concern. In unilateral epididymitis a significant decrease of ejaculate quality (sperm density, motility, and morphology) has been demonstrated, indicating testicular involvement despite adequate antimicrobial therapy. Although ejaculate quality normalizes after 3 months in most patients, severe oligoasthenoteratozoospermia and azoospermia persisted in 15% and 8%, respectively. Obstructive azoospermia following bilateral epididymitis accounts for 20% of all cases with obstructive azoospermia and normally requires microsurgical tubulovasostomy (19).

Precise data concerning the andrological impact of orchitis are lacking. As urologists and andrologists will mostly be concerned with mumps orchitis, we are discussing in this chapter the risks for a disturbed spermatogenesis for this entity. Chronic inflammatory conditions of the testis, in chronic epididymitis, epididymo-orchitis, and orchitis appear to be similar (10,12). The risk of development of azoospermia is obvious, but the true prevalence of male infertility as a consequence of chronic orchitis/epididymitis seems to be unknown till today. Depending on severity, sperm quality may be affected only temporarily and may recover without treatment (10,19,20).

MORPHOLOGICAL ALTERATIONS

Special Sperm Morphology According to "Strict Criteria"

The possible negative effect of infections and inflammations on sperm morphology has been highlighted in chapter 34. Our data, using strict criteria, provide evidence that a negative effect is present in inflammatory CP/CPPS (21). In cases with chronic epididymitis, increased numbers of macrophages and disturbed epididymal maturation seem predominant, as indicated by blue immobilized flagella in SHORR stain (10,20). The clinical impact of these findings remains unclear.

Morphological Findings Affecting the Acrosome Reaction

It is evident that microorganisms adhere to spermatozoal membranes resulting in ultrastructural alterations and damage of the plasma membrane also involving the head of the spermatozoa including acrosomal structures (22). Evidence of leukocytes has been discussed for a long time as cause for abnormal morphology and midpiece abnormalities not depending upon the underlying entity (23). Unfortunately clear study results are not available; in inflammatory CP/CPPS, associated with leukocytospermia, significant morphological alterations are not detectable (24). Our own data in inflammatory and noninflammatory CP/CPPS demonstrate poorer sperm morphology compared to controls and a significantly reduced acrosomal inducibility (25).

Seminal Plasma Alterations

The first demonstration that infections of the sex glands could impair their excretory function was made in the late 1960s. Decreased quantities of citric acid, phosphatase, fructose concentration, zinc, and α-glutamyltransferase (α-γ-GT) activity have been evaluated as disturbed prostatic secretory parameters, and reduced fructose concentration as indicator of disturbed vesicular function (11). Furthermore, epididymitis reduces the quantity of the epididymal marker α-glucosidase (26), thus indicating the possible biological role of these alterations in the whole inflammatory process. Fructose has been found reduced in men with chronic prostatitis, in asymptomatic men with leukocytospermia, and in severe prostatovesiculitis (11). Our own data in inflammatory CP/CPPS provide evidence that in cases with elevated numbers of granulocytes in expressed prostatic secretions (EPS), secretory damage of the prostate gland is detectable (16).

Antisperm Antibodies (ASA)

The relevance of seminal plasma antibodies in genitourinary infections is still debatable. Some authors suggest an association between increased levels of sperm antibodies and prostatitis (27,28). Also associations in semen between chlamydial infections and sperm antibodies have been described (29). The prevalence of MAGI in patients with a positive mixed antiglobulin (MAR) test seems to be in the range of 20%, whereby it is generally accepted that only antibodies bound to surface antigen of vital spermatozoa are clinically significant (30). Own data in chronic urethritis, epididymitis, and CP/CPPS do not demonstrate an association between proven inflammatory/infectious diseases of the male reproductive tract and the presence of ASA (31).

Cytokines

Cytokines are inflammatory mediators secreted by activated leukocytes or other immunocompetent cells in semen; the role of these cytokines (IL-6, 8) is decisive for the course of the inflammatory reaction (32). The deleterious effects of these proinflammatory cytokines on the motility and the function of spermatozoa have been observed in experimental and clinical studies (33). The proinflammatory cytokines also affect Leydig cells, which produce the gonadal steroids; this effect has been verified after the induction of bacterial lipopolysaccharide in mice, causing immediate degradation of steroidogenesis (34). Since recent studies demonstrate a high correlation between IL-8 levels and elastase in seminal plasma (35), the measurement of one of these inflammatory parameters seems to us mandatory in the suspected inflammatory situation of the urogenital tract.

Bacteriospermia

After exclusion of urethritis and bladder infection, the presence of $\geq$1,000,000 peroxidase-positive WBC/mL ejaculate indicates an inflammatory process (11). In these cases a culture for common urinary tract pathogens, especially gram-negative bacteria, should be performed. A concentration $\geq$1000 CFU/mL of urinary tract pathogens in the ejaculate is regarded as significant bacteriospermia (11). It must be kept in mind that the ejaculate analysis does not allow a definitive localization of the infectious process, because the ejaculate represents a mixture of different genital secretions and is usually contaminated by flora of the anterior urethra. Cleaning of the forceps and the glans reduces the bacterial content. Nevertheless, we know that about 70% of randomized semen samples are contaminated with nonpathogenic bacteria, so bacteriospermia does not inevitably mean infection (36). On the other hand, bacteriospermia is significantly represented ($>$ 50%) in patients with bacterial prostatitis (2).

DIRECT INTERACTIONS BETWEEN SPERMATOZOA AND BACTERIA

Some pathogenic microorganisms have the ability to directly interact with spermatozoa. These interactions are typified by attachments between bacteria and spermatozoa, agglutination phenomena, and morphological alterations of spermatozoa. The majority of observations of these phenomena are derived from experimental in vitro studies and their significance for in vivo infections has been questioned. Among bacterial species that interact with spermatozoa are well-established causative pathogens of genitourinary infections such as *E. coli*, *Ureaplasma urealyticum*, *Mycoplasma hominis*, and *C. trachomatis*. *E. coli* likely represents the most frequently isolated microorganism in cases of genitourinary infections. *E. coli* rapidly adheres to human spermatozoa in vitro, resulting in agglutination of spermatozoa (37). A profound decline in sperm motility is evident over time caused by severe alterations in sperm morphology. Morphological alterations involve both defects of the plasma membrane and degeneration of acrosomes (22,38). *U. urealyticum* also attaches to plasma membranes of spermatozoa and affects motility. Specific defects localized to heads of spermatozoa including acrosomal structures have been observed for *C. trachomatis*. Bacterial concentrations utilized in in vitro experiments undoubtedly are much higher than are ever recoverable from ejaculate specimens. This condition might contribute considerably to the outcome of the studies. Similar discrepancies have been observed in tests for the inducibility of the acrosome reaction in artificially infected semen samples. None of these phenomena, evident in vitro clearly, has been documented in semen specimens of patients with MAGI. As bacterial concentrations required for affecting sperm motility, morphology, and function are considerably high, the clinical impact remains debatable (37).

C. TRACHOMATIS IN SEMEN

The diagnostic difficulty with *C. trachomatis* infections has provoked researchers to develop new molecular methods to detect this microorganism in semen. However, until now no "ideal" diagnostic test for *C. trachomatis* in semen has been established (39). In contrast to serological findings in women, antibody tests for *C. trachomatis* in seminal plasma are nonindicative if no type-specific methods are used. Unfortunately, the high frequency of serum antibodies and seminal plasma activity in both infertile and healthy men, hampers a clear differentiation. This problem is also the cause for the debate on the association of chlamydial antibodies with leukocytospermia. Questionable, the interaction between IL-8 and anti-chlamydial mucosal Ig-A in the ejaculate provides a new chance for a better, clear

Table 3 Evidence of *C. trachomatis* Infections in the Epididymis/Testicle Impact on Ejaculate Parameters

	Decreasing evidence			
	+++	++	+	−
Detection in the testicle	+			
Detection in the epididymis	+			
Detection in sperms	+			
Obstructive azoospermia		+		
Leukocytospermia			+	
ASA formation				−
Heat shock protein activation	+			

Source: Modified from Ref. 41.

diagnosis (40). Numerous publications cover the problem—*C. trachomatis* infections and influence on sperm quality (41). The debated effects are summarized in Table 3.

There is only one new study based on serological findings, demonstrating a decrease of sperm concentration and motility (42).

LEUKOCYTOSPERMIA

The clinical significance of an increased concentration of WBC in the ejaculate is highly controversial (43). It is generally accepted that only an increased number of leukocytes (particularly polymorphonuclear granulocytes) and their products secreted into the seminal fluid (e.g., leukocyte elastase) are an indicator of inflammation. According to WHO classification, the presence of $\geq 1 \times 1000{,}000$ WBC/mL is defined as leukocytospermia. The great majority of leukocytes are neutrophilic granulocytes, as suggested by the specific staining of the peroxidase reaction. Although most authors consider leukocytospermia to be a sign of bacterial-induced inflammation, this condition is not necessarily associated with bacterial or viral infections. This is in accordance with earlier findings that elevated leukocyte numbers are not a natural cause of male infertility. Only few studies have analyzed alterations of WBC in the ejaculate of patients with proven prostatitis (2), demonstrating a higher number of leukocytes in men with bacterial infections. There is also an obvious resolution of leukocytospermia after antibiotic therapy (44). In spite of the data, the influence of leukocytospermia on sperm function is complex and will be covered in chapter 33. It is the suggestion of the authors to re-establish leukocytospermia using elastase and/or IL-8 determination. In case of a proven inflammatory situation, exclusion of a bacterial infection including chronic bacterial prostatitis and epididymitis seems to be mandatory. Table 4 summarizes current inflammatory cut-points in EPS and ejaculate for routineuse (45).

REACTIVE OXYGEN SPECIES

The reactive oxygen species (ROS) source in semen are the polymorphonuclear granulocytes and the seminal macrophages as response to cytokine-stimulating factors, enhanced in the presence of cytokines and lipopolysaccharide. In a normal situation, the antioxidant mechanisms of seminal plasma are likely to quench these ROS and protect against any spermatozoal damage. However, during infection/inflammation these antioxidant mechanisms may create a situation called "oxidative stress" due to the elevated levels of ROS beyond the available total antioxidant capacity in the semen (46) (see chapter 36 for details).

Table 4 Cutpoints for Expressed Prostatic Secretions (EPS), Urine after Prostatic Massage (VB3) and Ejaculate/Seminal Plasma Indicative for Inflammation.

	Parameter	Cutpoint
EPS	leukocytes	≥ 10–20/1000 ×
VB3	leukocytes	$\geq 10/mm^3$
Semen	PPL	$\geq 0.113 \times 10^6$/mL
Seminal plasma	elastase	≥ 280 ng/mL
Seminal plasma	IL-8	> 10600 pg/mL

Source: From Refs. 2, 8, and 45.

INFECTION-RELATED THERAPY AND INTERACTIONS TO SPERM QUALITY

Therapy in infectious diseases of the urogenital tract is normally targeted to relieve symptoms (2,47). Andrologically, targets of therapy regarding altered semen composition in male adnexitis include: *(i)* eradication or reduction of microorganisms in prostatic secretions and in semen, *(ii)* if possible, normalization of inflammatory parameters such as leukocytes and inflammatory secretory parameters, and *(iii)* if possible, improvement of sperm parameters to counteract impaired fertility.

Modalities of therapy include surgical procedures, antibiotics, antiphlogistic drugs, normalization of urine flow, physical therapy, and changes in general and sexual behavior (8). Transurethral surgery in chronic bacterial prostatitis means radical transurethral resection of the prostate (TURP). It is generally accepted that only patients with a stubborn resistance to long-term medical treatment, remaining symptomatic with a concomitant obstruction can be considered for radical resection, e.g., including the removal of prostatic calculi that act as permanent foci of infection. This therapy results in permanent retrograde ejaculation. Surgical therapy in chronic epididymitis is discussed under urological auspices in cases with recurrent symptomatic episodes and ongoing scrotal pain. There is no andrological relevance of these procedures. Bilateral epididymectomy results in azoospermia.

Unfortunately, until now only the antibiotic therapy of chronic bacterial prostatitis has proved to be really efficacious in providing symptomatic relief, eradication of microorganisms, and a decrease in cellular and humoral inflammatory parameters in urogenital secretions (2,8). Although antibiotic therapy provides an improvement in male sperm quality in many studies, therapy does not regularly enhance the probability of conception. Why is it so difficult to demonstrate an antibiotic

Table 5 Cumulative Bacteriologic Cure (eradication of pathogens) in Patients with Chronic Bacterial Prostatitis (CBP) Treated with Fluoroquinolones. Only those Studies Are Listed in Which the Diagnosis Was Derived from Application of the Meares and Stamey Technique and a Follow-up of at least 6 Months Was Available

Quinolone	Daily dosage (mg)	Duration of therapy (days)	Bacteriologic cure (%)	Duration of follow-up (months)
Norfloxacin	800	28	64	6
Norfloxacin	4–800	174	69	8
Ofloxacin	400	14	67	12
Ciprofloxacin	1000	14	60	12
Ciprofloxacin	1000	28	63	21–36
Ciprofloxacin	1000	60–150	86	12
Ciprofloxacin	1000	28	76	6
Ciprofloxacin	1000	28	72	6
Lomefloxacin	400	28	63	6
Ciprofloxacin	1000	28	77	6
Levofloxacin	500	28	75	6
Levofloxacin	500	28	84	6

effect on sperm quality in cases with prostatitis, if this infection is a major factor for this disorder? It has been hypothesized that only men with a chronic active infection, "where the pathological organism is still present and where the degree of damage is still limited," may benefit from a suitable therapy. However, when focusing on prostatitis, only chronic bacterial prostatitis (CBP) is a type of infection, which may correctly fit into this category. This is a type of infection that is present in only 5% to –10% of prostatitis patients (8). Modern fluoroquinolones are ideal therapeutic substances and show bacteriologic cure rates between 60% to 86% (Table 5) (45). On the other hand, we do not consider that common antibiotic substances in normal "in-vivo" dosage really affect spermatogenesis and sperm function Therefore, it seems to us absolutely necessary to re-analyze the influence of antibacterial treatment on sperm quality, sperm function, and secretory disorders following the new classification proposal of prostatitis (2)

Antibiotic treatment of epididymitis follows the different etiologies. In sexually active men, who are at risk of *C. trachomatis* or Neisseria gonorrhoeae (*N. gonorrhoeae)* infections, a therapeutic regimen, which covers both pathogens, is mandatory. Antibiotic resistance in *N. gonorrhoeae* increased dramatically over the last years. The WHO surveillance of antibiotic resistance in *N. gonorrhoeae* revealed resistance rates of penicillins and quinolones up to 100%, and of tetracyclines up to 80% in some countries (48). The CDC therefore adapted to this resistance trend and now recommend ceftriaxone as first-line agent for the treatment of epididymitis caused by N. gonorrhoeae. Additional treatment of nongonococcal agents is also recommended, which can be a tetracycline agent. In men where uropathogens causing complicated urinary tract infections are

Table 6 Suggested Therapeutic Regimens to Treat Infectious/Inflammatory Diseases of the Urogenital Tract

Chronic urethritis	antichlamydial, antigonococcal
Chronic bacterial prostatitis (NIH II)	Fluoroquinolones
CP/CPPS (NIH IIIa, inflammatory)	α-blockers
Chronic epididymitis	antiphlogistic, antibiotic
Orchitis	Interferon-α 2 b

the causative source, empiric treatment is best done according to the local susceptibility patterns. If possible, fluoroquinolones should be favored, although clinical studies in this area have not been performed sufficiently (9).

Treatment of mumps orchitis is poorly evaluated. There is no specific antiviral therapy for mumps. Use of steroids should be avoided in the treatment of mumps orchitis because steroids can decrease testosterone concentrations and increase concentrations of FSH and LH, which could facilitate, rather than alleviate, testicular atrophy (49). Other treatments of mumps orchitis include subcutaneous administration of interferon alfa-2b (14) or the downregulation of spermatogenesis with gonadotropin releasing hormone analogues (50). Both treatment schedules cannot be considered as proven evidence.

In conclusion, data are lacking demonstrating that therapeutic effects in chronic urethritis, epididymitis, and infectious and inflammatory prostatitis do really improve the andrological situation. Therapy targeted against symptoms may eradicate microorganisms and may improve the inflammatory situation. Table 6 summarizes general therapeutic principles of drug treatment usually given by the authors.

CONCLUSIONS

Recommendations are given on the basis of evidence-based suggestions following the modification of the US Department of Health and Human Services 1992 (51). No recommendation can be given on a level 1 basis.

- OAT-syndrome seems not to be relevant in CBP and CP/CPPS (Level 2; Grade B)
- Increased sperm abnormal morphology is detectable in CP/CPPS (Level 3, Grade C)
- Bacteriospermia is common in CBP (Level 2; Grade B). The biological significance is different for different pathogens.
- Leukocytospermia is debatable in cut-points and relevance for bacteriospermia. Other, additional inflammatory parameters (e.g., IL-8, elastase) may improve inflammatory diagnosis (Level 4; Grade C)
- In inflammation, negative effects on sperm motility (Level 3; Grade B) and increased oxidative stress (Level 3; Grade C) have to be mentioned.
- Formation of ASA does not interact with urogenital infections (Level 2; Grade A)
- Seminal plasma alterations occur in CP/CPPS without evidence for significance.

REFERENCES

1. World Health Organization. WHO Manual for the Standardised Investigation and Diagnosis of the Infertile Couple. Cambridge, UK: Cambridge University Press, 1993.
2. Weidner W, Wagenlehner FME, Marconi M, et al. Acute bacterial prostatitis and chronic prostatitis/chronic pelvic pain syndrome: andrological implications. Andrologia 2008; 40:105–112.
3. Weidner W, Diemer T, Meinhardt A, et al. 12th Andrology Symposium/5th Symposium of the Hessian Center for Reproductive Medicine and EAA Center Giessen [editorial]. Andrologia 2008; 40:65.
4. WHO Task Force on The Diagnosis and Treatment of Infertility: Towards more objectivity in diagnosis and management of male infertility. Int J Androl 1987; (suppl 7): 1–53.
5. Nieschlag E. Nosologie andrologischer Krankheitsbilder. In Nieschlag E, Behre H, eds. Andrologie: Grundlagen und Klinik der reproduktiven Gesundheit des Mannes. Berlin: Springer, 2002, S91–S95.
6. Schiefer HG. Microbiology of male urethroadnexitis: diagnostic procedures and criteria for aetiologic classification. Andrologia 1998; 30:7–13.
7. Schneede P, Tenke P, Hofstetter AG: Sexually transmitted diseases – a synoptic overview for urologists. European Urology 2003; 44:1–7.
8. Schaeffer AJ, Anderson RU, Krieger JN, et al. The assessment and management of male pelvic pain syndrome including prostatitis. In: Mc Connel J, Abrams P, Denis L, Khoury S, Roehrborn C, eds. Male Lower Urinary Tract Dysfunction. Evaluation and Management, 6th International Consultation in Prostate Cancer and Prostate Diseases. Paris: Health Publications, 2006:343–385.
9. Tracy CR, Steers WD, Costabile RD. Diagnosis and management of epididymitis. Urol Clin North Am 2008; 35:101–108.
10. Haidl G, Allam JP, Schuppe HC. Chronic epididymitis – impact on semen parameters and therapeutic options. Andrologia 2008; 40:92–96.
11. Weidner W, Krause W, Ludwig M. Relevance of male accessory gland infection for subsequent fertility with special focus on prostatitis. Hum Reprod Update 1999; 5:421–432.
12. Schuppe HC, Meinhardt A, Allam JP, et al. Chronic orchitis: a neglected cause of male infertility ? Andrologia 1998; 40:84–91.
13. Bhushan S, Schuppe HC, Tchaltalbochev S, et al. Testicular innate immune defense against bacteria. Mol Cell Endocrinol 2009; 306:37–44.
14. Weidner W, Krause W. Orchitis. Encyclopedia Reprod 1999; 3:524–527.
15. Engeler DS, Hauri D, John H. Impact of Prostatitis NIH IIIB (Prostatodynia) on Ejaculate Parameters. Eur Urol 2003; 44:546–548.
16. Ludwig M, Vidal A, Diemer T, et al. Seminal Secretory Capacity of the Male Accessory Sex Glands in Chronic Pelvic Pain Syndrome (CPPS)/Chronic Prostatitis with Special Focus on the New Prostatitis Classification. Eur Urol 2002; 42:24–28.
17. Bezold G, Politch JA, Kiviat NB, et al. Prevalence of sexually transmissible pathogens in semen from asymptomatic male infertility patients with and without leukocytospermia. Fertil Steril 2007; 87:1087–1097.
18. Ochsendorf FR. Sexually transmitted infections: impact on male fertility. Andrologia 2008; 40:72–75.
19. Ludwig M. Diagnosis and therapy of acute prostatitis, epididymitis and orchitis. Andrologia 2008; 40:76–80.
20. Haidl G, Weidner W. Epididymitis and orchitis – andrological implications. Egypt J Androl Reprod 2003; 17: 3–15.
21. Menkveld R, Huwe P, Ludwig M, et al. Morphological sperm alternations in different types of prostatitis. Andrologia 2003; 35:288–293.
22. Diemer T, Huwe P, Michelmann HW, et al. Escherichia coli – induced alterations of human spermatozoa. An electron microscopic analysis. Int J Androl 2000; 23:178–186.
23. Thomas J, Fishel SB, Hall JA, et al. Increased polymorphonuclear granulocytes in seminal plasma in relation to sperm morphology. Hum Reprod 1997; 12:2418–2421.
24. Pasqualotto FF, Sharma RK, Potts JM, et al. Seminal oxidative stress in patients with chronic prostatitis. Urology 2000; 55:881–885.
25. Henkel R, Ludwig M, Schuppe H-C, et al. Chronic pelvic pain syndrome/chronic prostatitis affect the acrosome reaction in human spermatozoa. World J Urol 2006; 24: 39–44.
26. Cooper TG, Weidner W, Nieschlag E. The influence of inflammation of human genital tract on secretion of the seminal markers alpha-glucoside, glyceryl- phosphocholine, carnitine, fructose and citric acid. Int J Androl 1990; 13:329–336.
27. Bates CA. Antisperm antibodies and male subfertility. Br J Urol 1997; 80:691–697.
28. Hinting A, Soebadi DM, Santoso RI. Evaluation of the immunological cause of male infertility. Andrologia 1996; 123–126.
29. Dimitrova D, Kalaydjiev S, Hristov L, et al. Antichlamydial and antisperm antibodies in patients with chlamydial infections. Am J Reprod Immunol 2004; 52:330–336.
30. Mazumdar S, Levine A. Antisperm antibodies: etiology, pathogenesis, diagnosis and treatment. Fertil Steril 1998; 70:799–810.
31. Marconi M, Pilatz A, Wagenlehner F, et al. Are antisperm antibodies really associated with proven inflammatory, infectious diseases of the male reproductive tract: Eur Urol 2009; 56:708–715.
32. Zalata A, Hafez T, Van Hoecke MJ, et al. Evaluation of beta-endorphin and interleukin-6 in seminal plasma of

patients with certain andrological diseases. Hum Reprod 1995; 10:3161–3165.

33. Diemer T, Hales DB, Weidner W. Immuno-endocrine interactions and Leydig cell function: the role of cytokines. Andrologia 2003; 35:55–63.
34. Hales DB, Diemer T, Held Hales K. Role of Cytokines in testicular function. Endocrine 1999; 10:201–217.
35. Penna G, Mondaini N, Amuchastegin S, et al. Seminal plasma cytokines and chemokines in prostate inflammation: Interleukin 8 as a predictive biomarker in CP/CPPS and benign prostatic hyperplasia. Eur Urol 2007; 51:524–533.
36. Cotell E, Harrison RF, Mc Caffrey M, et al. Are seminal fluid microorganismus of significance or merely contaminants. Fertil Steril 2000; 74:465–470.
37. Diemer T, Ludwig M, Huwe P, et al. Influence of Urogenital infections on sperm function. Curr Opin Urol 2000; 10:39–44.
38. Diemer T, Huwe P, Ludwig M, et al. Urogenital infections and sperm motility. Andrologia 2003; 35:283–287.
39. Weidner W, Diemer T, Huwe P, et al. The role of C. trachomatis in Prostatitis. Int J Antimicrob Agents 2002; 19:466–470.
40. Mazzoli S, Lai T, Rupealta V, et al. Interleukin 8 and antichlamydia trachomatis mucosal Ig-A as urogenital immunological markers in patients with C. trachomatis prostatic infection. Eur Urol 2007; 51:1385–1993.
41. Gonzales GT, Munoz G, Sanchez R, et al. Update on the impact of C. trachomatis infection on male infertility. Andrologia 2004; 36:1–12.
42. Idahl A, Abramsson L, Kumlin U, et al. Male serum C. trachomatis If-A and If-f, but not heat shock protein 60 Igf, correlates with negatively affected semen characteristics and lower pregnancy rates in the infertile couple. Int J Androl 2007; 30:99–107.
43. Tomlinson MJ, Barratt CLR, Cooke ID. Prospective study of leukocytes and leukocyte subpopulations in semen suggests they are not a cause of male infertility. Fertil Steril 1993; 60:1069–1075.
44. Branigan EF, Muller CHH. Efficacy of treatment and recurrence rate of leukocytospermia in infertile men with Prostatitis. Fertil Steril 1994; 62:580–584.
45. Wagenlehner FME, Naber KG, Bschleipfer T, et al. Diagnostik und Therapie der Prostatitis und des männlichen Beckenschmerzsyndroms. Dtsch Ärzteblatt 2009; 106:175–183.
46. Agarwal A, Saleh H. Role of oxidants in male infertility: rationale, significance and treatment. Urol Clin North Am 2002; 29:817–827.
47. Weidner W, Ludwig M, Miller J. Therapy in male accessory gland infection what is fact, what is fiction? Andrologia 1998; 30(suppl):87–90.
48. The WHO Western Pacific Gonococcal Antimicrobial Surveillance Programme. Surveillance of antibiotic resistance in Neisseria gonorrhoeae in the WHO Western Pacific Region, 2005. Commun Dis Intell 30:430–433.
49. Hviid A, Rubin S, Mühlemann K. Mumps. Lancet 2008; 371:932–944.
50. Vicari E, Mongioi A. Andrology: Effectiveness of long-acting gonadotrophin-releasing hormone agonist treatment in combination with conventional therapy on testicular outcome in human orchitis/epididymo-orchitis. Hum Reprod 1995; 10:2072–2078.
51. US Department of Health and Human Services, Public Health Service, Agency for Health Care Policy and Research, 1992:115–127.

33 Inflammatory parameters of the ejaculate

Zsolt Kopa and Mihály Berényi

CASE REPORT

A 32-year-old patient was admitted to the andrology outpatient unit with two years of infertility problems. Physical examination showed normal genital status. Semen analysis revealed normal sperm concentration (42 million/mL.), motility parameters showed a light decrease according to the WHO criteria (a: 20%, b: 15%, c: 15%, d: 50%). Normal morphology was 12% using the WHO strict criteria. Peroxidase staining revealed 0.8 million/mL leukocytes in semen. Performing interleukin-6 (IL-6) and antisperm antibody (ASA) assays, highly elevated levels were detected. After antibiotic, antiphlogistic treatment a follow-up therapy was induced with vitamins, antioxidants, macromolecules and zinc. Control spermatogram found normal motility (morphology was unchanged). IL-6 level decreased to the normal range; ASA decreased but remained in pathologic range. After the treatment of the inflammation—which was detected by biochemical methods—a later succesful assisted reproductive technique (intrauterine insemination (IUI)) was indicated.

INTRODUCTION

The frequency of infections as a cause of male infertility is quoted to account for approximately 15% to 20%. Its harmful effect means primarily the impairment of spermatozoa function; the classical parameters of the ejaculate remain mostly unchanged. Inflammation is accompanied by a variety of chemical reactions giving the possibility to the more precise diagnosis. Today, the determination of standard ejaculate parameters according to WHO is not sufficient for diagnosis of the often silent genital tract inflammations, additional determination of biochemical markers are suggested.

This chapter deals with the updated measurable inflammatory markers of the ejaculate. These markers can be classified by their biological properties, so round cells; leukocytes and oxidative stress; enzymes, cytokines, and chemokines, small molecules; proteins and immune proteins, DNA; and chromatin condensation will be discussed.

ROUND CELLS IN SEMEN

White blood cells (WBCs) like round cells (RC) in the ejaculate are not always leukocytes. RCs can be classified as spermatogenic (spermatida etc.) and as nonspermatogenic origin cells. The nonspermatogenic round cells are made up of different types of leukocytes (polymorphonuclear granulocytes, macrophages, lymphocytes), epithelial cells from the prostate and seminal vesicles, and transitional cells originating from the bladder and the urethra, and squamous epithelial cells.

The normal ejaculate contains less than 5×10^6 RC per mL, while the number of WBCs should be less than 1×10^6 per mL according to the WHO recommendations.

Spermatogenesis often results in the release of immature germ cells in the semen sample. High number of spermatogonial cells reflects spermatogenetic failure or spermatogenetic arrest. Because round spermatids can be used for ICSI the differentiation has a grown importance.

Leukocytospermia has a harmful effect on the sperm function, so it is of real clinical importance to differentiate between round cells. Papanicolaou staining and the peroxidase staining can help in the differentiation. Additional special tests can also be used, e.g., specific antibody recognizing leukocyte antigens or flow cytometry, using monoclonal antibodies that enables to detect leukocytes in the semen sample.

LEUKOCYTOSPERMIA AND OXIDATIVE STRESS

According to the WHO classification, $>1 \times 10^6$ WBCs per mL have been defined as leukocytospermia. The clinical significance of an increased concentration of white blood cells or leukocytes in the ejaculate is still controversial. Infection is indicated only by an increased level of leukocytes (particularly PMN or polymorphonuclear leukocytes) and their products secreted into the seminal fluid. The great majority of the leukocytes in the ejaculate are neutrophilic granulocytes (60%–80%). Macrophages can be detected in 20% to 30%, the presence of T-lymphocytes is 2% to 5%, and B-lymphocytes and plasma cells are rare. Usefulness of the classification of leukocyte subtypes in the ejaculate is not exactly proven.

The impact of leukocytes depends upon the stages and sites at which WBCs enter the semen and the involvement of specific types and concentrations of leukocytes and their states of activation. As 90% of the ejaculate volume derives from seminal vesicles and prostate, higher numbers of leukocytes are detected in the seminal fluid during the inflammation of these organs. This is not the case in chronic inflammations of the epididymis, which are difficult to diagnose, but much more harmful to fertility.

Clinical symptoms do not always correlate with the presence or absence of WBCs. Elevated WBC count is not necessarily associated with infections, and antibiotic treatment does not significantly lower the extent of leukocytospermia. Leukocytospermia can be associated with subclinical or silent genital tract infection and can also be observed in absence of infection:

varicocele, smoking, drug abuse like marijuana, alcohol, exposure to irritants and toxins, abstinence, and in men with spinal cord injury.

For the diagnosis, a classical specific staining may be achieved by peroxidase reaction. Till recently flow cytometry using monoclonal antibodies was seen to be a simple, reproducible method that enables to detect WBC subpopulations.

Leukocytospermia was considered as being one of the causes of male infertility, but its deleterious effects on sperm density, motility, and morphology are under debate. Moreover, a few papers indicated a positive role for seminal leukocytes by elimination of morphological abnormal spermatozoa by phagocytosis. The most deleterious effect of leukocytospermia is the damage of spermatozoa function.

The pathogenesis leads from neutrophilic granulocytes, which specifically invade the lipid membrane of the pathogens by releasing reactive oxygen species (ROS). 30% to 40% of ejaculates from infertile men generate excessive levels of ROS. WBCs are mainly responsible for ROS production even when present at very low concentrations. The degree of WBC infiltration observed in infertile patients is still the subject of controversy, because their seminal WBC concentrations have been found to be in the normal-to-high range when compared with normal fertile controls. The results of recent studies confirm the need for a change of the threshold value of peroxidase-positive cells according to WHO definition to lower levels for definition of silent genital tract inflammation.

Measurement of these pro- and antioxidant markers leads to the correct evaluation of whether spermatozoa underwent an inflammatory functional damage. ROS and its impact on fertility are discussed in detail in chapter 36.

ENZYMES

Polymorphonuclear Elastase

Inflammation is accompanied by a variety of chemical reactions, such as the release of various enzymes from polymorphonuclear leucocytes. One of the main changes during the inflammatory process is the discharge of large amounts of proteolytic enzymes (proteases). The most important proteases produced by granulocytes are elastase, cathepsin G, and collagenase. Elastase has a major role in the diagnosis of silent genital tract inflammations. It is released from the neutrophil leucocytes during phagocytosis, degranulation, or cell death and may also lead to proteolytic damage of spermatozoa; on the contrary, the protease may serve as an objective indicator of granulocyte activity in semen. A seminal elastase-inhibitor complex (Ela/α_1-PI) has been proposed as a marker of male silent genital tract inflammation, measured by enzyme-linked immunoabsorbent assay.

Elastase level is higher in infertile population. It positively correlates with other inflammatory parameters of the ejaculate and can be decreased by antibiotic therapy. Elastase concentrations correlate with the number of peroxidase-positive cells; in addition, there are inverse correlations with the vitality of spermatozoa. No association can be found with the sperm count. Its correlation with sperm motility and morphology is under debate.

There is an association between silent genital tract inflammation as reflected by elevated levels of elastase and disturbed sperm DNA integrity, leading to decreased implantation and pregnancy rates in in vitro fertilization/intracytoplasmic sperm injection (IVF/ICSI), in addition a low blastocyst development rate was also observed. According to these findings; a screening for silent genital tract inflammations should be suggested in patients undergoing methods of artificial reproduction. Increased elastase levels can be observed in elderly men

An antielastase polypeptide, the secretory leukocyte protease inhibitor, found in fluids lining mucosal surfaces, is produced by prostatic epithelial cells. Its localization is possible with immunohistochemical method (ELISA, Western blotting). Secretory leukocyte protease inhibitor acts as an antiprotease, primarily against PMN elastase.

A direct influence of elastase on sperm function seems rather unlikely, other leukocyte-derived inflammatory factors like ROS or pro-inflammatory cytokines should also be considered with regard to their impact on sperm functions.

Screening for PMN elastase is an easy, reproducible, and reliable test for diagnosis and prognosis and follow-up of silent genital tract inflammation. Studies showed a correlation between levels of granulocyte elastase and the number of peroxidase-positive cells; however, in a considerable number of patients there were elevated concentrations of the biochemical markers despite peroxidase–positive cells below 1 million/mL, supporting the suggestion of a change of the normal value of peroxidase-positive cells in the seminal fluid considering the different origins of the components of seminal plasma.

Seminal α-glucosidase

Infections generate numerous seminal biochemical changes. One of these changes is focused on the neutral α-glucosidase (NAG).

Sperm function depends on epididymal transit where spermatozoa maturation occurs. The most important epididymal marker in the seminal plasma is the α-glucosidase, measured by its iso-enzyme, the neutral α-glucosidase produced mostly in the corpus and cauda of epididymis, but a small proportion is secreted by the seminal vesicles.

Measurement of α-glucosidase activity is a rapid and sensitive way to differentiate azoospermia types and to localize the site of obstruction and to identify partial obstruction at epididymal level.

Activity of NAG correlates positively with conventional sperm characteristics and with seminal ATP. The real correlation between NAG and sperm motility is not yet clear. α-glucosidase is negatively correlated with both ROS and the concentration of peroxidase-positive white blood cells, which are known to adversely affect fertilization in vivo and in vitro.

Low levels of NAG in semen may be related to epididymitis and have been associated with defective sperm maturation. Its low levels in seminal plasma of patients with oligozoospermia may reflect either varying degrees of epididymal obstruction (possible consequence of infection) or epididymal hypofunction, but functional disturbances at the level of the epididymis cannot be characterized by the NAG assay. A high level of NAG was correlated with strong binding capacity of the spermatozoa to the human zona pellucida and with a high probability of success following intrauterine insemination.

Acrosin

To evaluate the fertilizing capacity of human spermatozoa, determination of acrosin is a useful approach. Acrosin is the major enzyme required for the penetration of the oocytes's zona pellucida. Normal acrosin activity is observed in men with high fertilization rates and low acrosin activity in the case of poor fertilization.

Inflammation-caused oxidative stress is harmful for the sperm membrane fluidity, which regulates specific functions such as acrosome reaction and fusion with oocyte membrane, so the presence of oxidative stress with leukocytospermia and abnormal semen parameters associated with impaired sperm function can be proven by its acrosin activity.

γ-glutamyl Transpeptidase

γ-glutamyl transpeptidase (GGT) and membrane-bound dipeptidases supply amino acids for glutathione (GSH) synthesis and protein synthesis. GGT is expressed in many mammalian tissues and is essential for catalyzing secreted GSH. The generation of GSH is crucial for the protection of cells against oxidative stress and other forms of cellular injury resulting from cytotoxic and carcinogenic compounds. Thus, GSH acts as a major antioxidant in many physiological processes. GGT is expressed in the testis, seminal vesicle, and epididymis. The highest levels of GGT expression were found in the epididymis.

In GGT-deficient animals the testes, seminal vesicles, and epididymises are decreased in size, and severe oligo- or azoospermia occurs. In addition, sperm motility is completely abolished. Genital tract infection can be improved by systemic supplementation of GSH. GSH is also important for direct protection against oxidative stress. Glycosylation of seminal GGT is altered by accessory gland infection. The significant correlation between GGT and sperm motility is another sign for its function for cell protection against free radicals.

PROTEINS

Inflammatory Cytokines

A deleterious effect on sperm quality may be exerted through ROS, cytokines (interleukins [IL], tumor necrosis factors [TNF]) and their soluble receptors. Polymorphonuclear granulocytes in semen are the major source of ROS, and ROS production by these cells is enhanced by bacterial products and seminal cytokines. Cytokines are a heterogeneous group of peptides that are involved in numerous physiological and pathological processes. Cytokines particularly act in the mediation of inflammatory responses than in the immune system and intercellular communication. Inflammatory cytokines are produced by monocytes/macrophages, T cells, and neutrophils in response to foreign antigens and pathogens. Cytokines mainly act in the initiation of the immunoinflammatory cascade. Cytokine elevation may represent part of a nonspecific acute-phase response or may be due to specific interactions of microorganisms and the immune system. The pathophysiological significance of seminal cytokines in sperm function is still not completely understood.

Several studies evaluated the inflammatory significance of seminal cytokines: IL-1α, IL-2, IL-4, IL-6, IL-8, TNF-α, interferon-γ, granulocyte colony-stimulating factor (GCSF), macrophage CFS (MCSF). IL-8 and IL-6 might be used as the most sensitive marker for silent male genital tract infection. IL-6 seems to be highly sensitive but possesses lower specificity compared with elastase. The concentration of inflammatory cytokines, especially interleukin-6 and interleukin-8 is closely correlated with the number of peroxidase-positive leucocytes and ROS production. No association of interleukin concentrations with the bacterial colonization of semen samples and microorganisms was found. IL-6 concentrations are negatively correlated with the vitality of spermatozoa as determined by eosin staining.

Elevated levels of cytokines can be found in infertile patients compared with healthy controls, however no significant correlations between elevated cytokines and semen parameters were reported. By investigating a higher number of samples other studies revealed that elevated levels of both IL-6 and granulocyte elastase showed significant correlations with semen quality, and a significant association was observed between IL-6 levels and sperm motility, but there were no correlations with other semen parameters such as sperm count.

After cytokines the chemokines should be mentioned too. Chemokines constitute a large family of chemotactic cytokines that act at receptors to regulate diverse biological processes, e.g., leukocyte trafficking. A meaningful chemokine is the fractalkine, which regulates the chemotaxis in the seminal plasma. Fractalkine is produced by epithelial cells. Its small protein molecules stimulate and regulate the migration and accumulation of WBCs at the site of inflammation. Fractalkine shows a positive correlation with sperm motility. There is no correlation with WBC count in semen.

Chemokines are believed to be both beneficial in host defence against infectious agents and harmful in diseases marked by pathologic inflammation; however, actual clinical roles in these areas have not yet been established.

C3 Complement Component and Ceruloplasmin

Male accessory gland infections (MAGI) cause alterations in the blood–testis barrier resulting in barrier permeability. Levels of protein markers, primarily the complement component C3 and ceruloplasmin are a good sign of the inflammatory changes. Ceruloplasmin is a glycoprotein containing 6–8 copper atoms. C3 complement component is absent in seminal plasma or only detectable in traces. Its transudation from the blood is increased in the case of inflammation, elevated levels of C3 complement component and ceruloplasmin can be found only in such semen samples.

C3 concentrations are significantly correlated with leukocyte counts, but show no association with semen quality or with the bacterial colonization of semen samples. C3 complement determinations seem to be much more sensitive. C3 might be used as an additional marker for silent male genital tract infection, although its screening does not reveal any further information about semen quality or inflammation pathogenesis of the male genital tract.

Heat Shock Proteins

Heat shock proteins (HSP) are essential stress proteins in mammals and bacteria. They protect and repair the proteins and help to preserve cell survival. The HSP60 is produced in response to various stresses such as temperature elevation ("heat shock"), ischemia, toxic chemicals, metabolic disruption, free oxygen radicals, bacterial and viral infection, and inflammation mediators. The relationship with tubal factor infertility, ectopic pregnancy, and reduced IVF success is known. At the cellular level, the HSPs functioning as chaperones and important regulators of differentiation and apoptosis an essential reproductive factor. During an infection the microbial stress protein synthesis is enhanced and HSP induce cytokine release and provoke an immune response.

Members of the 10, 60, and 70 kDa HSP families have been recognized as antigens of many microbial pathogens, where IgA and IgG are the most important antigens; IgG does not show the acute infection. Chlamydial infection is one of the most frequent sexually transmitted diseases (STD) with infertility consequences. A significant relationship was found between IgA antibodies to human HSP60 with anti-chlamydial IgA, but there is no relationship in the same day serum samples. Serum antibody levels to HSP antigens are lower in subfertile population. The presence of HSP60 IgA antibody in seminal fluid correlates with leukocytospermia, with the presence of C3, and also with high interleukin levels in seminal plasma, but it is not related to the bacterial colonization and semen quality. Fertilizing capacity also shows no correlation with HSP60. The immune response to heat shock proteins in silent male genital tract infection plays an important role, but it has no association with standard parameters of semen quality.

Antisperm Antibodies and Immune Infertility

Sperms are not produced before puberty, so spermatozoa could appear as new antigens for the immune system. The blood–testis barrier protects the spermatozoa against the immune reaction. Due to inflammation, surgical intervention, or trauma the barrier will be injured; spermatozoa as actually "strange" can be exposed to the immune system. As a result, antibodies will be produced against the spermatozoa surface antigens. On the other hand, women can also produce antisperm antibodies. These antisperm antibodies (ASA) are the main cause of immunological infertility. ASA inhibit the penetration of the cervical mucus, the binding to the zona pellucida and the sperm–oocyte fusion thereby developing the immune infertility. ASA impair both sperm function and fertilization.

Table 1. Demonstrates the development of the immunological infertility.

ASA can be measured with the mixed antiglobulin reaction test (MAR test) or immunobead test.

A simple washing method will not suffice for removing ASA from the sperm surface. To reduce the ASA, using a swim-up technique with fetal cord serum is suggested. The method of choice to treat severe cases of immunological infertility is IVF/ICSI in which a pregnancy rate of 30% to 40% per cycle can be achieved.

SMALL MOLECULES

Malondialdehyde

Malondialdehyde (MDA) is an end product of lipid peroxidation and so an early marker of oxidative stress. Serum MDA level is correlated with viscosity and other oxidative stress parameters. MDA might be the cause of the viscosity changes by its protein crosslink effect. Determination of MDA is a widely used index of lipid peroxidation due to its simplicity. Increased seminal plasma MDA and protein carbonyl levels were found in infertile subjects.

Seminal MDA concentrations are negatively correlated with sperm concentration and motility; negative correlation can be found between MDA level and fertilization rate. MDA levels in seminal plasma may have a prognostic value for IVF success.

Isoprostanes

8-Isoprostane is a reliable index of lipid peroxidation. Isoprostanes are formed in situ in cell membranes, following free radical attack. They are not only markers of oxidative injury but active participants in the pathophysiology of some disorders.

Fructose

Fructose is really not an inflammatory marker but its seminal plasma level may be decreased due to bacteria. Fructose is produced by the seminal vesicles with a small contribution from the deferential duct. In vitro, fructose can function as an energy source for spermatozoa, while the in vivo function of seminal fructose is not clear. Fructose can also be used as a marker for seminal vesicular secretion and therefore indicate abnormal influence on the sperm chromatin stability (sperm chromatin stability in humans does depend on the correct ejaculation together with the zinc-rich prostatic secretion). In case of ejaculatory duct obstruction semen samples show low volume, low pH, and absence of fructose. Fructose levels are also

Table 1

Development of Immunological Infertility

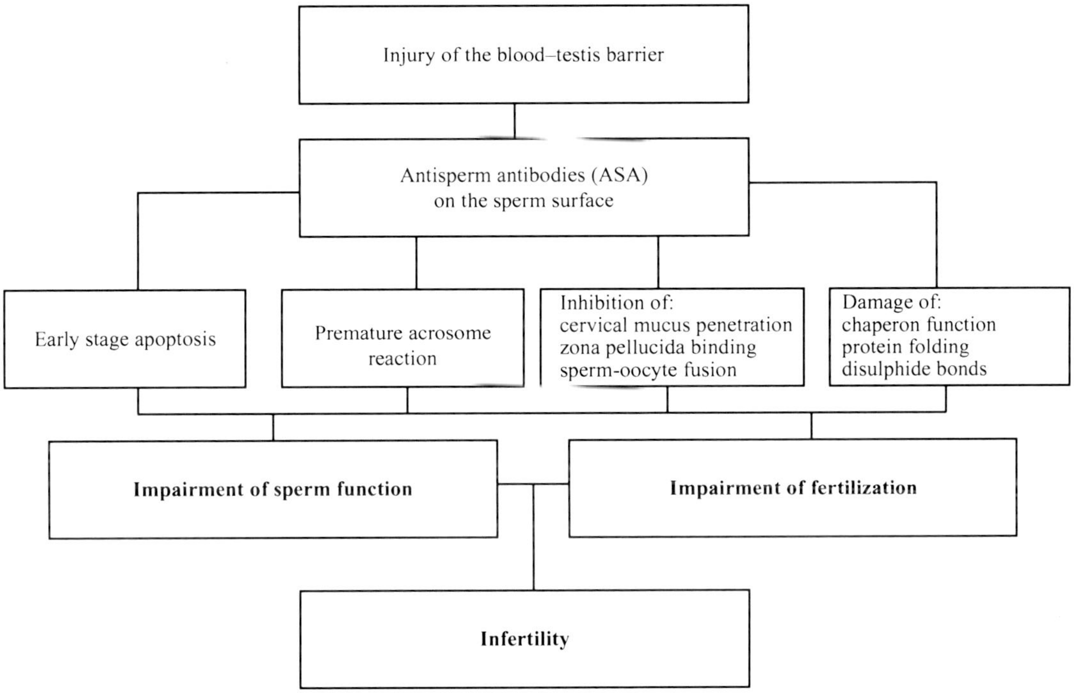

reduced in case of postinflammatory atrophy of the seminal vesicle epithelium or relative androgen deficiency. True corrected fructose has been shown to be a better marker of the seminal vesicle function.

Sperm DNA Fragmentation, Chromatin Condensation

Fertilization is an interaction of the sperm and oocyte, fusion of the cell membranes, and union of male and female gamete genomes. The completion of this process and the embryo development depend in part on the inherent integrity of the sperm DNA.

Sperm chromatin (DNA and nuclear proteins) is a double nucleoprotamine-nucleohistone structure. It is tightly packaged by protamines during spermiogenesis in the testis, but up to 15% of the DNA remains packaged by histones. Infertile men appear to have an increased sperm histone/protamine ratio, but this could also be due to histone staining having easier access to the inner parts of the chromatin in men with abnormal sperm chromatin condensation. Defects in the acrosome formation is often linked to abnormal chromatin decondensation. With a high percentage of sperm with abnormally stained DNA–usually classified as DNA damage or DNA fragmentation–the natural fertility rate is decreased.

Sperm DNA damage has been associated with high levels of reactive oxygen species, showing the influence of inflammations on the sperm DNA integrity. Leukocyte concentration in semen shows a correlation with chromatin alterations in immature and mature sperm.

Sperm DNA damage can also occur due to apoptosis, drugs, chemotherapy, and irradiation. Cigarette smoking, environmental toxins, testicular hyperthermia, varicocele, and hormonal deficiency can also be a cause of sperm chromatin defects.

Assisted reproductive technologies can use the DNA-damaged spermatozoa. Sperm DNA integrity in recent knowledge has no influence on reproductive outcomes of IVF/ICSI. There is no relation between sperm DNA damage and fertilization rates. Neither fertilization nor early embryo development is dependent on sperm DNA integrity, although, we know that IVF/ICSI is associated with an increased risk of birth defects and genetic abnormalities.

Prostatic Gland Secretion

Prostatic gland secretion offers several markers, including zinc, citric acid, and prostatic acid phosphatase. The determination of prostatic gland secretions is of no great diagnostic value to localize an obstruction for sperm transport. The assessment of the specific prostatic marker PSA may give information about inflammatory reactions and tumor cells in the prostate. PSA is used as a screening test for prostatic cancer or chronic inflammatory processes. Despite decreased prostatic secretory function

Table 2 Changes of the Inflammatory Markers of the Ejaculate in Inflammations

Markers	
Increasing	**Decreasing**
Round cells count (RCC)	intracellular ATP
White blood cells (WBCs)	total antioxidant capacity (TAC)
Reactive oxygene species (ROS)	superoxid dismutase (SOD)
Oxidative stress status (OSS)	catalase (CAT)
PMN elastase	glutathion peroxidase (GPX)
Cytokines (interleukins, TNF)	sulphhydryl groups
C3 complement component	carotenoids
Coeruloplasmin	secretory leukocyte protease inhibitor (SLPI)
Heath shock proteins (HSP)	neutral alpha-glucosidase
Antigens	acrosin
Antisperm antibodies (ASA)	glutathion (GSH)
Malondialdehyde (MDA)	gamma-glutamyl transpeptidase (GGT)
Isoprostanes	chemokines
DNA fragmentation	fructose
PSA	

by infectious agents, the total amount of markers in semen may be still within normal range.

Special infections are discussed in chapter 32.

CONCLUSION

Table 2 summarizes the changes of the inflammatory parameters discussed in this chapter.

The harmful effect of male genital tract inflammations must not be underestimated. Inflammations either with their cytotoxic effect or by promotion of genotoxic events or due to reactive oxygen species formation often impair several sperm functions like motility, acrosomal function, or sperm DNA integrity leading to impaired fertility. Components of seminal fluid produced by inflammatory processes mean an essential factor in the diagnosis of male factor infertility and lead to improved therapeutic consequences.

KEY MESSAGES

1. The frequency of infections as a cause of male infertility is quoted to account for approximately 15% to 20%.
2. Leukocytospermia has a harmful effect to the sperm function but clinical symptoms do not always correlate with the presence or absence of WBCs.
3. Infections generate numerous seminal biochemical changes shown by oxidative stress, enzymes (elastase, etc.), cytokines and chemokines (interleukins, fractalkine), small molecules (malondialdehyde), proteins, DNA fragmentation and chromatin condensation, and other markers.
4. Due to inflammation the blood–testis barrier can be injured; antisperm antibodies (ASA) will be produced as the main cause of immunological infertility impairing both sperm function and fertilization.
5. Components of seminal fluid produced by inflammatory processes are an essential factor in the diagnosis of male factor infertility and lead to improved therapeutic consequences.

FURTHER READING

Aitken RJ, Baker HW. Seminal leukocytes: passengers, terrorists or good samaritans? Hum Reprod 1995; 10(7):1736–1739.

Alvarez JG, Sharma RK, Ollero M, et al. Increased DNA damage in sperm from leukocytospermic semen samples as determined by the sperm chromatin structure assay. Fertil Steril 2002; 78(2):319–329.

Athayde KS, Cocuzza M, Agarwal A, et al. Development of normal reference values for seminal reactive oxygen species and their correlation with leukocytes and semen parameters in a fertile population. J Androl 2007; 28:613–620.

Aziz N, Agarwal A, Lewis-Jones I, et al. Novel associations between specific sperm morphological defects and leukocytospermia. Fertil Steril 2004; 82 (3):621–627.

Berényi M. Markers of andrological infections. STD and Genital Infectology (in Hungarian) 2007; 1(1):9–12.

Blenk H., Hofstetter A. Complement C3, coeruloplasmin and PMN-elastase in the ejaculate in chronic prostato-adnexitis and their diagnostic value. Infection.1991; 19(suppl 3):138–140.

Bohring C, Krause E, Habermann B, et al. Isolation and identification of sperm membrane antigens recognized by antisperm antibodies, and their possible role in immunological infertility disease. Mol Hum Reprod 2001; 7(2):113–118.

Bohring C, Krause W. Characterization of spermatozoa surface antigens by antisperm antibodies and its influence on acrosomal exocytosis. Am J Reprod Immunol 2003; 50(5):411–419.

Boit R, Petzoldt D, Klinga K, et al. C_3 in seminal plasma has no additional informative value in the diagnosis of infection/inflammation of the male genital tract. Andrologia 2003; 35(2):93–99.

Curi SM, Ariagno JI, Chenlo PH, et al. Asthenozoospermia: analysis of a large population. Arch Androl 2003; 49(5):343–349.

Diemer T, Hales DB, Weidner W. Immune-endocrine interactions and Leydig cell function: the role of cytokines. Andrologia 2003; 35(1):55–63.

Diemer T, Huwe P, Ludwig M, et al. Urogenital infection and sperm motility. Andrologia 2003; 35(5):283–287.

Dohle GR, Colpi GM, Hargreave TB, et al. EAU guidelines on male infertility. Eur Urol 2005; 48(5):703–711.

Eggert-Kruse W, Boit R, Rohr G, et al. Relationship of seminal plasma interleukin (IL) -8 and IL-6 with semen quality. Hum Reprod 2001; 16(3):517–528.

Eggert-Kruse W, Neuer A, Clussmann C, et al. Seminal antibodies to human 60 kd heat shock protein (HSP 60) in male partners of subfertile couples*. Hum Reprod 2002; 17(3):726–735.

Elzanaty S, Richthoff J, Malm JM, et al. The impact of epididymal and accessory sex gland function on sperm motility. Hum Reprod 2002; 17(11):2904–2911.

Erenpreiss J, Hlevicka S, Zalkalns J, et al. Effect of leukocytospermia on sperm DNA integrity: a negative effect in abnormal semen samples. J Androl 2002; 23(5):717–723.

Friebe K, Bohring C, Skrzypek J, et al. Levels of interleukin-6 and interleukin-8 in seminal fluid of men attending an andrological clinic. Andrologia 2003; 35(2):126–129.

Furuya Y, Akashi T, Fuse H. Soluble Fas and interleukin-6 and interleukin-8 levels in seminal plasma of infertile men. Arch Androl 2003; 49(6):449–452.

Glander H-J, Grunewald S, Paasch U, (eds). Biology of Male Germ Cells. Leipzig: Shaker Verlag, 2008.

Greco E, Scarselli F, Iacobelli M, et al. Efficient treatment of infertility due to sperm DNA damage by ICSI with testicular spermatozoa. Hum Reprod 2005; 20:226–230.

Gonzales GF, Munoz G, Sanchez R, et al. Update on the impact of Chlamydia trachomatis infection on male fertility. Andrologia 2004; 36(1):1–23.

Gruschwitz MS, Brezinschek R, Brezinschek HP. Cytokine levels in the seminal plasma of infertile males. J Androl 1996; 17(2):158–163.

Haidl G, Weidner W. Epididymitis and orchitis – andrological implications. Egypt J Androl Reprod 2003; 17:3–16.

Hammadeh ME, Stieber M, Haidl G, et al. Association between sperm cell chromatin condensation, morphology based on strict criteria, and fertilization, cleavage and pregnancy rates in an IVF program. Andrologia 1998; 30(1):29–35.

Henkel R, Kierspel E, Stalf T, et al. Effect of reactive oxygen species produced by spermatozoa and leucocytes on sperm functions in non-leukocytospermic patients. Fertil Steril 2005; 83:635–642.

Henkel R, Ludwig M, Schuppe HC, et al. Chronic pelvic pain syndrome/chronic prostatitis affect the acrosome reaction in human spermatozoa. World J Urol 2006; 24 (1):39–44.

Henkel R, Maab G, Jung A, et al. Age-related changes in seminal polymorphonuclear elastase in men with asymptomatic inflammation of the genital tract. Asian J Androl 2007; 9(3):299–304.

Hsieh YY, Chang CC, Lin CS. Seminal malondialdehyde concentration but not glutathione peroxidase activity is negatively correlated with seminal concentration and motility. Int J Biol Sci 2006; 2:23–29.

Jedrzejczak P, Fraczek M, Szumala- Kakol L, et al. Consequences of semen inflammation and lipid peroxidation on fertilization capacity of spermatozoa in in vitro conditions. Int J Androl 2003; 28(5):275–283.

Kaleli S, Oçer F, Irez T, et al. Does leukocytospermia associate with poor semen parameters and sperm functions in male infertility? The role of different seminal leukocyte concentrations. Eur J Obstet Gynecol Reprod Biol 2002; 89(2):185–191.

Karinen L, Pouta A, Hartikainen A-L, et al. Antibodies to Chlamydia trachomatis heat shock proteins Hsp60 and Hsp10 and subfertility in general population at age 31. Am J Reprod Immunol 2004; 52(5):291—297.

Khosrowbeygi A, Zarghami N. Levels of oxidative stress biomarkers in seminal plasma and their relationship with seminal parameters. BMC Clin Pathol 2007; 7(6):10–11.

Kopa Z, Wenzel J, Papp GK, et al. Role of granulocyte elastase and interleukin-6 in the diagnosis of male genital tract inflammation. Andrologia 2005; 37(5):188–194.

Krause W, Bohring C, Gueth A, et al. Cellular and biochemical markers in semen indicating male accessory gland inflammation. Andrologia 2003; 35(5):279–282.

LaVerda D, Albanese LN, Ruther EP, et al. Seroreactivity to Chlamydia trachomatis Hsp10 Correlates with Severity of Human Genital Tract Disease. Infect Immun 2000; 68 (1):303–1309.

Locati M, Murphy MP. Chemokines and chemokine receptors: biology and clinical relevance in inflammation and AIDS. Annu Rev Med 1999; 50:425–440.

Ludwig M, Vidal A, Diemer T, et al. Chronic prostatitis/chronic pelvic pain syndrome): seminal markers of inflammation. World J Urol 2003; 21(2):82–85.

Maegawa M, Kamada M, Irahara M, et al. A repertoire of cytokines in human seminal plasma. J Reprod Immunol 2002; 54(1–2):33–42.

Mahmoud MA, Geslevich J, Kint J, et al. Seminal plasma α-glucosidase activity and male infertility. Hum Reprod 1998; (13)3:591–595.

Menkveld R, Huwe P, Ludwig M, et al. Morphological sperm alternations in different types of prostatitis. Andrologia 2003; 35(5):288–293.

Munoz MG, Jeremias J, Witkin SS. The 60 kDa heat shock protein in human semen: relationship with antibodies to spermatozoa and Chlamydia trachomatis. Hum Reprod 1996; 11(12)2600—2603.

Munuce MJ, Bregni C, Carizza C, et al. Semen culture, leukocytospermia, and the presence of sperm antibodies in seminal hyperviscosity. Arch Androl 1999; 42(1):21–28.

Papp GK, Kopa Z, Szabó F, et al. Aetiology of haemospermia. Andrologia 2003; 35(5):317–320.

Pasqualotto FF, Sharma RK, Kobayashi H, et al. Oxidative stress in normospermic men undergoing infertility evaluation. J Androl 2001; 22(2):316–322.

Penna G, Mondaini N, Amuchastegui S, et al. Seminal plasma cytokines and chemokines in prostate inflammation: interleukin 8 as a predictive biomarker in chronic prostatitis/chronic pelvic pain syndrome and benign prostatic hyperplasia. Eur Urol 2007; 51(2):524–533.

Pentyala S, Lee J, Annam S, et al. Current perspectives on pyospermia: a review. Asian J Androl 2007; 9:593–600.

Perticarari S, Ricci G, Granzotto M, et al. A new multiparameter flow cytometric method for human semen analysis. Hum Reprod 2007; 22(2):485–494.

Potts JM, Pasqualotto FF. Seminal oxidative stress in patients with chronic prostatitis. Andrologia 2003; 35(5):304–308.

Punab M, Loivukene K, Kermes K, et al. The limit of leucocytospermia from the microbiological viewpoint. Andrologia 2003; 35:271–278.

Reinhardt A, Haidl G, Schill WB. Granulocyte elastase indicates silent male genital tract inflammation and appropriate anti-inflammatory treatment. Andrologia 1997; 29:187–192.

Rowe PJ, Comhaire FH, Hargreave TB, et al. WHO Manual for the Standardized Investigation, Diagnosis and Management of the Infertile Male. Cambridge, UK: Cambridge University Press, 2000.

Saleh RA, Agarwal A, Kandirali E, et al. Leukocytospermia is associated with increased reactive oxygen species production by human spermatozoa. Fertil Steril 2002; 78(6):1215–1224.

Schill WB, Henkel R. Advancement in biochemical assays in andrology. Asian J Androl 1999; 1:45–51.

Sharma RK, Pasqualotto AE, Nelson DR, et al. Relationship between seminal white blood cell counts and oxidative stress in men treated at an infertility clinic. J Androl 2001; 22 (4):575–583.

Vicari E. Seminal leukocyte concentration and related specific reactive oxygen species production in patients with male accessory gland infections. Hum Reprod 1999; 14(8):2025–2030.

Villegas J, Schulz M, Vallejos V, et al. Indirect immunofluorescence using monoclonal antibodies for the detection of leukocytospermia: comparison with peroxidase staining. Andrologia 2002; 34(2):69–73.

Wathes CD, Abayasekara DRE, Aitken JR. Polyunsaturated fatty acids in male and female reproduction. Biol Reprod 2007; 77:190–201.

Weidner W, Krause W, Ludwig M. Relevance of male accessory gland infection for subsequent fertility with special focus on prostatitis. Hum Reprod Update 1999; 5:421–432.

WHO Laboratory Manual for the Examination of Human Semen and Sperm–Cervical Mucus Interaction, 4th ed. Cambridge, UK: Cambridge University Press, 1999.

Zalata AA, Ahmed HA, Allamaneni SSR, et al. Relationship between acrosin activity of human spermatozoa and oxidative stress. Asian J Androl 2004; 6:313–318.

Zarghami N, Khosrowbeygi A. Seminal plasma levels of 15-F2-isoprostane, malondialdehyde and total homocysteine in normozoospermic and asthenozoospermic males. Indian J Clin Biochem 2005; 20(2):86–91.

Židovec S, Vujisić S. Cytokines in human seminal plasma and their effect on male fertility. J Reprod Contracept 2005; 16(2):107–126.

Zorn B, Sešek-Briški A, Osredkar J, et al. Semen polymorphonuclear neutrophil leukocyte elastase as a diagnostic and prognostic marker of genital tract inflammation – a review. Clin Chem Lab Med 2003; 41(1):2–12.

Zorn B, Virant-Klun I, Meden-Vrtovec H. Semen granulocyte elastase: its relevance for the diagnosis and prognosis of silent genital tract inflammation. Hum Reprod 2000; 15(9):1978–1984.

34 Sperm morphology in male urogenital tract infections

Roelof Menkveld

Male urogenital tract infections account for almost 15% of cases of male infertility (1). Acute or chronic male urogenital infections can negatively affect spermatogenesis, resulting in decreased sperm production, and can have a negative effect on the development and maturation of spermatozoa leading to impaired sperm functions due to the production of reactive oxygen species (ROS) by leukocytes and spermatozoa (2).

The clinical diagnosis of urogenital infections is a complex process (3). Clinical diagnoses are mostly made in combination with laboratory tests, or in many cases diagnoses can be based on laboratory tests alone (4). Although controversial, the presence of leukocytospermia in semen samples can now be regarded as a definite indicator of male urogenital tract infections (5,6). One of the main reasons why the presence of leukocytospermia i.e., more than 1×10^6 white blood cells/mL semen according to the WHO (7) manual, is controversial is due to the fact that no correlation exists between the outcome of semen cultures for microorganisms and leukocytospermia (8).

Another reason for the controversy surrounding the presence of leukocytospermia as a diagnostic indicator of male urogenital tract infections are the many different methods that exist for the detection of leukocytes, such as immunocytochemical (9,10), the use of monoclonal antibodies (11), the leukocyte peroxidase tests (7), and cytologically on semen smears (5,6). These different methods also identify different leukocyte subsets, adding more confusion to the role of leukocytospermia in male urogenital tract infections. Furthermore, it has been found that poor correlations exist between the different methods for the determination of leukocytes in semen (5).

Different reports have also been published on the effect of leukocytospermia on semen parameters. Most of the earlier articles have indicated that the presence of leukocytes have a negative effect on semen parameters (12). Recently more controversy resulted in the literature on the role of leukocytospermia on sperm morphology. In general it was believed that the presence of leukocytospermia was associated with a reduced sperm morphology quality (13,14), but thereafter a few papers have been published reporting that the presence of leukocytes had a positive effect on sperm morphology due to the phagocytosis of abnormal spermatozoa by the leukocytes (9,15). However, these groups all used advanced methods for identification of leukocyte subpopulations such as immunocytochemical assays (10) and the leukocyte peroxidase tests (15), while in those articles where cytological methods were used to detect leukocytes a negative effect on sperm morphology was reported (5,6). The majority of articles published recently reported a negative effect on semen parameters and sperm function and especially sperm morphology (8).

WHY IS SPERM MORPHOLOGY OF IMPORTANCE IN THE FERTILIZATION PROCESS?

The evaluation of sperm morphology according to strict criteria (16) together with the addition of the acrosome index is an uncomplicated way of gaining important data on the functional ability of a specific semen sample, based on sperm morphological functions (17). Therefore, sperm morphology still remains an important prognosticator for expected in vivo and in vitro fertilization outcome, and it underlines the important relationship between normal sperm morphology and normal sperm function, especially in a negative way. If sperm morphology is low, poor results for the different sperm functional tests, i.e., the zona pellucida-sperm binding test (18), acrosin activity (19), and DNA content may be expected. Therefore, normal sperm morphology is needed for normal sperm function.

HOW IS SPERM MORPHOLOGY EVALUATED?

There are several sperm morphology evaluation systems described in the literature where the best known are the early or liberal approach which evolved into the early WHO criteria of 1980 (20) and 1987 (21) before the 1999 WHO manual (7) adopted the strict criteria principals (16) for sperm morphology evaluation.

Liberal Approach and WHO Criteria

Most domestic animals generally reveal a morphological homogeneous looking sperm population. This homogeneous picture of sperm morphology made it possible to use the appearance of the dominant spermatozoon form, in proven fertile animals, as a model to describe the normal form for that specific species. The same approach was adopted unsuccessfully for the human male due to the extreme heterogeneity of sperm morphology in the human semen sample between and even within individual males. The so-called normal and abnormal sperm forms were depicted by inaccurate schematic drawings. With this system the normal spermatozoa were identified by default, as all spermatozoa that could not be identified as having an abnormality were considered as normal. This is reflected by the statement of MacLeod who stated, "we are not prepared at this time to classify any but the most distorted forms as truly abnormal" (22). The disadvantage of the so-called liberal approach was that no specific criteria were put forward to describe morphological normal spermatozoa and the so-called normal population will therefore, contain the truly normal spermatozoa and a fraction that, based on functionality and biological evidence, cannot be regarded as morphologically normal. With this approach "borderline" morphological normal spermatozoa are considered as abnormal (8). This may lead to an incorrect classification of a specific males' fertility potential, and the couples are then very likely to be classified as presenting with unexplained infertility as has been demonstrated by Oehninger et al. (23), who found that with the old WHO (liberal) criteria 40.4% of the couples were diagnosed with unexplained infertility as compared to only 11.5% when strict criteria was used to evaluate sperm morphology on the day of IVF. Therefore, when the liberal approach for spermatozoa morphology evaluation is applied, poor correlations with normal sperm functions and in vivo and in vitro fertilization rates can be expected (24).

The liberal approach methodology has been adopted by the two earliest WHO manuals of 1980 (20) and 1987 (21). In the first WHO manual of 1980 (20), very little attention was given for the description of the methodology for sperm morphology evaluation and criteria for sperm normality, except for some legends to the color plates. It was also stated that the classification of the germinal cells were based on the proposals by MacLeod, thus following the liberal approach. In the second WHO manual of 1987 (21) the same approach was followed although some more detail on sperm morphology evaluation was given. In both manuals it is stated that in case of spermatozoa with borderline morphology the spermatozoa must be classified as normal.

Strict Criteria for Sperm Morphology Evaluation

In the early 1980s a new concept for sperm morphology evaluation was put forward by Menkveld (25), where for the first time the description of a so-called normal spermatozoon was based on biological evidence for normality. Previous studies by Fredricsson and Björk (26) and Mortimer et al. (27) has shown that a strong selection for certain morphological types of spermatozoa occur with migration of spermatozoa through cervical mucus and that the morphological normality of these populations are significantly increased and of strong prognostic significance for expected in vivo fertilization (26). Menkveld used the appearance of these spermatozoa as a reference population to describe the ideal "normal" spermatozoon (25).

Strict (Tygerberg) criteria for an ideal morphological normal spermatozoon is therefore based on the morphology of postcoital spermatozoa found at the level of the internal cervical os, mostly consisting of an apparently homogeneous sperm population in contrast to the heterogeneous sperm populations found in the first or lower part of the endocervical canal. Probably the most important aspect of the evaluation criteria is that the range allowed for normal biological variations should be kept as small as possible to ensure repeatable evaluations and therefore spermatozoa with so-called borderline or slightly abnormal head forms are regarded as abnormal by strict criteria (16). Due to the stricter approach, the percentage of morphological normal spermatozoa obtained by this methodology will be considerably lower compared to the liberal approach. The 1999 WHO (7) manual now recommends that sperm morphology evaluation should be performed according to the strict (Tygerberg) criteria.

Teratozoospermia Index

The 1992 (28) and 1999 WHO (7) manuals recommend that spermatozoa should only be classified as normal or abnormal. The manuals state that a note should be made if a specific abnormality occurs in a frequency of >20%. However, an abnormal spermatozoon can have only one specific abnormality or any combination of two, three, or up to four abnormalities. These abnormalities can be one or more of the following: head abnormalities, neck/midpiece abnormalities, tail abnormalities, and the presence of cytoplasmic residues. To reflect this, the teratozoospermia index (TZI) was introduced as an indication of the mean number of abnormalities per abnormal spermatozoon. The TZI value will therefore always be between 1 and 4. However, in the 1999 WHO manual, cytoplasmic residues were omitted as an abnormality and the TZI value was indicated as between 1 and 3 but the manual provides the same cut-off value (7). This must be regarded as an error, because the presence of cytoplasmic residue material on spermatozoa is an important source of ROS production and must therefore be regarded as a sperm abnormality (8).

Acrosome Index

As an additional tool to normal sperm morphology, Menkveld et al. (19) described the acrosome index (AI) based on the size and form of the acrosomes as well as their staining characteristics. Results for the AI are expressed as the percentage of normal acrosomes. For the evaluation of the acrosome morphology the same principles are applicable as for the evaluation of normal sperm morphology according to strict criteria. The only exception is that the postacrosomal part of the sperm head can be abnormal but not the rest of the spermatozoa including the neck/midpiece and tails as well as the absence of cytoplasmic residues.

WHAT CAN BE REGARDED AS NORMAL SPERM MORPHOLOGY VALUES?

When evaluating sperm morphology, especially for research purposes, it is important not only to determine the percentage of morphological normal spermatozoa but also to do a more extensive sperm morphology evaluation, including the TZI, AI, and different types of head abnormalities, especially head elongations where male urogenital tract infections are concerned (6).

Many different so-called normal values are proposed by different authors and the WHO manuals (7,29). For the purpose of this chapter only the values proposed by the 1999 WHO manual (7) and those obtained by strict criteria will be presented (29). For strict criteria, normal values were laid down by Kruger

Table 1 Comparison of 1999 WHO (7) and Strict Criteria (5,29) Normal Values for Sperm Morphology Variables and Leukocytospermia

		Strict criteria	
Morphology parameter	WHO 1999 values	Fertile	Subfertile
Morphology (% normal)	$\geq 30^a$	≥ 4	≤ 3
Acrosome index (% normal acrosomes)	No value	≥ 8	≤ 3
TZI value	≤ 1.60	≤ 1.64	≥ 2.09
Elongated spermatozoa (%)	No value		7.0
Leukocytospermia	$> 1 \times 106$/mL		$\geq 0.20 \times 10^6$/mL

[a]WHO 1992 (28) value; no value given in WHO 1999 (7) manual.

et al. (30) with the following prognostic categories for in vitro fertilization outcome viz., the poor prognosis or P-group with $\leq$ 4% morphological normal spermatozoa, the good prognosis or G-group with 5% to 14% morphological normal spermatozoa and the normal group with $\geq$15% morphological normal spermatozoa. Cut-off values for the AI and TZI were calculated by Menkveld et al., based on the investigation of fertile and subfertile male populations (29). The cut-off point value of about 7% for elongated spermatozoa was obtained from the investigation of males with different localized urogenital infections and a normal control group (6). The different values are presented in Table 1.

WHAT ARE THE EFFECTS OF MALE UROGENITAL TRACT INFECTIONS ON SPERM MORPHOLOGY?

In the literature two types of articles are published with regards to leukocytospermia. The first is where there is reference to leukocytospermia as an entity on its own or a suggestion of the presence of male urogenital tract infections (5) and the second where male urogenital tract infections are based on clinical evidence and leukocytospermia is regarded as one of the symptoms for male urogenital tract infections (31).

What is Leukocytospermia?

Leukocytospermia is the presence of leukocytes (white blood cells) in semen. There are differences of opinion on the occurrence of leukocytes in semen. Some authors regard the presence of some leukocytes as a normal phenomenon (32). It is also stated by some authors that leukocytes are found throughout the male reproductive tract and in almost every human ejaculate (33), while others believe that no leukocytes should be present in semen samples at all (8). The WHO manual defines leukocytospermia as the presence of more than 1×10^6 WBC/mL semen. However this cut-off point may be too high. Several authors have suggested lower cut-off points, and it will therefore appear as if we can now regard leukocytospermia to be present when more than 0.2×10^6 WBC/mL semen is present (2,5).

Effects of Leukocytospermia on Sperm Morphology

Contradicting reports have been published in the literature on the effect of leukocytospermia on sperm morphology. Some earlier articles reported a negative effect of leukocytospermia on sperm morphology (13,14) while other authors reported a positive effect of leukocytes on sperm morphology due to phagocytosis of the morphological abnormal spermatozoa in the male reproductive tract (9,15), although, others did not find any effect on sperm morphology in the presence of leukocytospermia (34).

Sharma et al. (35) could not find any statistical significant effect of leukocytospermia on normal sperm morphology evaluated according to both the WHO (7) and strict criteria (16) approach, although normal sperm morphology values were lower in the leukocytospermia group compared to that of the nonleukocytospermia group. However, most of the more recently published articles reported the negative effects of leukocytospermia on sperm morphology. Although exact data is not always provided, several authors reported on negative correlations between increasing leukocyte concentrations and normal sperm morphology with values of $r = -0.225$, $P<0.001$; $r = -.358$, $P = 0.03$ and $r = -0.46$, $P = 0.05$, respectively (31,36,37), while in some articles actual data are presented. Bezold et al. (38) found a slight but statistical significant decrease in normal sperm morphology in a group of men with leukocytospermia compared to a control group of men without leukocytospermia with 48.0% and 52.0% morphological normal spermatozoa, respectively. Lackner et al. (32) found median sperm morphology values of 46.0% and 64.0% for men with and without leukocytospermia, respectively. Both studies evaluated sperm morphology according to the old WHO (liberal) approach.

Very few detailed morphological sperm assessments have been published. Thomas et al. (39) found a negative correlation between increasing leukocyte concentrations and the percentage of morphological normal spermatozoa. At two cut-off points (0.5 and 1.0×10^6 leukocytes/mL semen) the leukocytospermia group had a lower percentage of morphological normal spermatozoa compared to the nonleukocytospermia group. There was also a significant positive correlation between tail abnormalities and increasing leukocyte concentrations.

Menkveld and Kruger (5) investigated 150 consecutive semen samples of men attending an infertility clinic for leukocytospermia by means of the cytological examination of Papanicolaou stained semen smears as well as by the use of the leukocyte peroxidase test (7). Results from their study indicated that the presence of leukocytospermia, as diagnosed cytologically, may have a negative effect on sperm morphology parameters. There was a tendency for a decrease in the percentage morphological normal spermatozoa and an increase in sperm morphology abnormalities when the amount of WBC/HPF increased. This was applicable to all the types of morphological abnormalities investigated, like elongated and small heads, tail and neck abnormalities, and cytoplasmic residues. There was also a negative effect on acrosomal morphology as indicated by a decrease in the acrosome index. There was also a small but not statistically significant increase in the TZI. In the case where leukocytes were determined by the leukocyte peroxidase test as described in the WHO manual (7), a statistical significant differences was only found for a lower percentage of morphological normal spermatozoa and an increase in the percentage of spermatozoa with elongated heads in the leukocytospermia group compared to the leukocytospermia negative group (see Table 2 for detailed results). The question was asked by Menkveld and Kruger (5) if the presence of leukocytes in a semen smear as diagnosed microscopically might perhaps be of more clinical significance than the diagnosis of leukocytospermia by means of cytochemical methods.

Menkveld et al. (6) reported on a group of men who were investigated for chronic pelvic pain syndrome and diagnosed with either NIH IIIA (prostatitis) or NIH IIIB (prostatodynia, i.e., males with noninflammatory chronic pelvic pain syndrome). Men with NIH IIIA had lower normal sperm morphology values, as evaluated with both WHO and strict criteria, and lower TZI values (although $P > 0.05$), a lower acrosome index, and a higher percentage of elongated spermatozoa ($P < 0.05$) compared to the men in the NIH IIIB group, who presented on their part again with poorer sperm morphology values compared to a control group.

Aziz et al. (40) also showed that leukocytospermia was positively correlated with the percentage of morphologically abnormal spermatozoa with spermatozoa showing increased incidences of acrosomal damage, cytoplasmic residues, midpiece, and tail defects. The average value of the sperm abnormalities index (SDI) was higher for the leukocytospermia group compared to the nonleukocytospermia group. The SDI score is calculated by dividing the total number of deformities (sperm abnormalities) observed by the number of spermatozoa that are randomly selected and evaluated, irrespective of their morphological normality (see Table 2 for details). The results of the study by Gambera et al. (41) also confirmed that leukocytospermia has a negative effect on sperm morphology and especially on the presence and shape of the acrosomal complex and tail structure.

The negative effect of leukocytospermia on sperm morphology is not only confined to a decrease in semen parameters and normal sperm morphology parameters but also by the negative effects on certain sperm functional tests. Zalata et al, (42) found that the sperm acrosin activity index was significantly higher in patients without leukocytospermia compared to a matched group of men with leukocytospermia. Significant correlations were found between acrosin activity and normal sperm morphology ($r = 0.61$; $P = 0.001$), and between acrosin activity and leukocyte concentration ($r = -0.71$; $P = 0.001$).

WHAT ARE THE POSSIBLE CAUSES FOR SPERM MORPHOLOGICAL ABERRATIONS FOUND IN LEUKOCYTOSPERMIA?

From the previous section it is clear that leukocytospermia does not only have a negative effect on the percentage of morphologically normal spermatozoa (5,35,40) but also on the sperm shape and structure as well as the functional abilities of spermatozoa. Alternations in sperm form or shape include smaller sperm heads and elongation of the sperm heads (5,6). Sperm structural damage includes aberrations and damage of the acrosome structure (5,6,41), increased neck/midpiece and tail abnormalities (5,39,40,41), and the increased retention of cytoplasmic material, an indication of immaturity of the spermatozoa (5,40). These structural alternations and increase in neck/midpiece, and tail defects and increase of cytoplasmic material will cause higher TZI and SDI values (5,6,40). Cytoplasmic material retention, coiled tails and short tails have been indicated as of possible epididymal origin (43).

Sperm acrosomal abnormalities, especially small acrosomes, and to a certain extent also large acrosomes, are strongly related to DNA damage as determined with the CMA3 technique. CMA3 positivity is an indication of protamine deficiency and is also associated with poor fertilization rates (44). This may be due to the fact that sperm with high protamine deficiency (positivity) have lower acrosome integrity and may have a lower oocyte activating potential after ICSI. According to Nasr-Esfahani et al. (44), sperm-associated oocyte-activating factor(s) are associated with the development of the acrosome and postacrosomal sheet (or the perinuclear theca), which is completed during spermiogenesis concomitant with nuclear remodelling, where histones are replaced with protamine. As showed in the previous section, leukocytospermia is also strongly related to acrosomal abnormalities (5,6,40). Therefore, acrosome abnormalities manifested i.e., by aberrant acrosomal and postacrosme sheet anomalies and protamine deficiency may thus be regarded as leukocytospermia-induced abnormalities.

Sperm elongation is also a very distinctive abnormality in leukocytospermia as far as abnormal sperm forms are concerned. Elongated spermatozoa are regarded as a transitional stage of sperm abnormalities, according to the Düsseldorf group (45). This is due to an abnormal Sertoli cell function caused by external stress factors on the testis, in cases of leukocytospermia, possibly originating from the male urogenital tract infections. However, sperm elongation is accomplished by severe structural damage as well as severe DNA damage. The increased sperm head length results from an abnormally elongated nucleus that also presents particular membranous layers between the outer

Table 2 Effect of Leukocytospermia on Detailed Sperm Morphology Parameters as Reported in the Literature

Morphology parameter	Control group	Leukocytes (negative)	Leukocytes (positive)	*P* value
Menkveld and Kruger, 1998 (5)				
Cytological determined WBC				
Number of males per group		134	16	
Normal (%) by strict criteria		7.0(4.4)	4.3(3.5)	0.001
Elongated (%)		15.3 (13.3)	17.4 (10.4)	0.028
Tail abnormalities (%)		12.4 (9.5)	17.4 (10.4)	0.0501
Small heads (%)		10.6 (10.1)	15.2 (15.3)	(0.0643)
Neck/midpiece abnormalities (%)		26.3 (12.9)	32.1 (12.1)	(0.0930)
Germinal epithelium cells (%)		0.8 (2.1)	1.7 (2.4)	NS
Cytoplasmic residues (%)		5.7 (2.1)	7.9 (7.1)	NS
AI (% normal acrosomes)		8.3 (5.1)	6.8 (4.8)	NS
TZI value		1.5 (0.2)	1.6 (0.3)	NS
Peroxidase test determined				
Number of males per group		87	10	
Normal (%) by strict criteria		7.0 (4.4)	5.4 (3.4)	NS
Elongated (%)		14.7 (12.1)	20.7 (13.5)	NS
AI (% normal acrosomes)		7.5 (4.7)	9.5 (5.1)	NS
TZI value		1.50 (0.2)	1.54 (0.2)	NS
Sharma et al., 2001 (35)				
Number of males per group Normal (%)	28	203	25	
WHO criteria	39.79 ± 2.50	33.05 ± 0.85	28.86 ± 2.74	NS
Strict criteria	12.07 ± 0.86	9.49 ± 0.35	7.91 ± 0.96	NS
Aziz et al., 2004 (40)				
Number of males per group	13	36	20	
Normal (%) by strict criteria	10 (8–18)[a]	5 (2–12)[b]	3 (0–8)[c]	ab, ac $P < 0.05$
Acrosome damage (%)	19 (14–29)[a]	26 (20–36)	36 (30–56)[c]	ac $P < 0.05$
Nuclear abnormalities (%)	2 (1–6)[a]	7 (4–13)[b]	10 (5–12)[c]	ab, ac $P < 0.05$
Midpiece abnormalities (%)	19 (9–22)[a]	21 (15–28)[b]	26 (20–30)[c]	ab, ac $P < 0.05$
Cytoplasmic residues (%)	4 (0–7)	6 (4–11)	11 (6–19)	<0.05
Tail defects (%)	4 (2–6)	7 (4–12)	17 (7–280)	<0.05
Sperm deformity index value	1.5 (1.4–1.6)	1.7 (1.6–2.3)	1.9 (1.7–2.3)	<0.05
Menkveld et al., 2003 (6)		**NIH IIIA**	**NIH IIIB**	
Number of males per group	17	34	18	
Normal (%) by WHO criteria	34.4 (12.4)	38.9 (16.2)	36.5 (14.5)	NS
Normal (%) by Strict criteria	7.3 (5.6)	5.3 (3.1)	5.9 (4.6)	NS
AI (% normal acrosomes)	12.7 (7.3)[a]	8.7 (4.8)[b]	8.1 (3.7)[c]	ab, ac $P < 0.01$
TZI value	1.63 (0.2)	1.65 (0.3)	1.61 (0.2)	NS
Elongated spermatozoa (%)	7.2 (9.5)[a]	17.5 (15.7)	10.8 (10.7)[c]	ac $P < 0.05$

Values are means (SD), taken from Refs. 5 and 6.
Values are means ± SE, taken from Ref. 35.
Values are medians and (25th–75th) percentiles, taken from Ref 40.
NIH IIIA = prostatitis
NIH IIIB = prostatodynia

and inner leaves of the nuclear envelope. The sperm nuclear anomalies are also associated with anomalies of the neck region and persistence of cytoplasmic residual material and increased frequency of chromosomal aneuploidies rates, together with impaired chromatin compaction due to possible mechanisms such as meiotic nondisjunction or spermiogenesis anomalies (46). Low ICSI fertilization rates have also been found in men with severely elongated spermatozoa compared to other sperm morphology abnormalities (47).

It will therefore appear that leukocytospermia can have a very detrimental influence on testicular function due to the presence of proinflammatory mediators in the testis that could lead to alterations in the regulation of spermiogenesis when activated by the presence of leukocytospermia as a consequence of the male urogenital genital infection. According to Aziz et al. (40) cytokines, released by the inflammatory reaction, have been found to interfere with Sertoli cell function leading to abnormal spermiogenesis. In addition, the findings by Menkveld and

Kruger (5), Menkveld et al. (6) and Aziz et al. (40) of significantly higher proportions of sperm with cytoplasmic residues in men with leukocytospermia could also be due to defective Sertoli cell function and disorganized spermiation and due to alterations in the sperm maturation process, while the spermatozoa are transported through the epididymis.

A second potential mechanism through which leukocytospermia may induce alterations in sperm morphology is excessive ROS production. ROS (hydrogen peroxidaes, superoxide anion or hydroxyl radicals) can derive from activated granulocytes and spermatozoa, especially morphological or functional abnormal spermatozoa themselves and spermatozoa with cytoplasmic residues (48). Although ROS at low concentrations have an important physiological effect on spermatozoa (hyperactivation, capacitation, and acrosome reaction), in high concentrations they have pathologic effects, especially on the sperm membrane or sperm DNA. The damaging effect of ROS on sperm DNA is associated with poorer in vitro fertilization results and especially lower pregnancy rates. This is due to the fact that the parental genome can not be activated and development of the embryo is thus halted (49).

WHAT ARE THE EFFECTS OF ANTIBIOTIC AND ALTERNATIVE TREATMENT OF MEN WITH LEUKOCYTOSPERMIA ON SPERM MORPHOLOGY PARAMETERS?

With the successful treatment of leukocytospermia with antibiotics or alternative treatment methods, the negative relationship between leukocytospermia and sperm morphology will be confirmed when there is an improvement in sperm morphology after successful treatment of leukocytospermia. However, results of published studies are controversial. This may be due to any insufficient treatment period or alternatively due to the fact that functional and anatomical damage in the male reproductive tract, acquired as a result of the infections, are often permanent and not reversible by antibiotic treatment (50).

Successful treatment of leukocytospermia by antibiotics has been published by Branigan and Muller (51) and by Vicari et al. (52). Successful treatment with alternatives like antioxidants, immunomodulating and other natural products has been reported. Gambera et al. (41) treated leukocytospermia men with β-glucan, fermented papaya, and lactoferrin supplemented with vitamins C and E for three months. After treatment there was a reduction in leukocytes an increase in sperm motility and sperm morphology. They concluded that treatment with immunomodulating and antioxidant agents protect spermatozoa during maturation and migration through the male genital tract, resulting in a functional rescue demonstrated by improvement of semen quality. Lackner et al. (32) treated leukocytospermia men with a two-week therapy cycle regime with a specific Cox-2 inhibitor (valdecoxib, 20 mg) once daily for 12 weeks. Although the median normal sperm morphology values increased, the improvement was not of statistical significance. Oliva and Mulitgner (53) described an improvement of sperm morphology and motility in infertile males with leukocytospermia treated with ketotifen, an antihistamine-like drug, which has a stabilizing effect on mast cells. After eight weeks of treatment, a significant improvement was observed in the percentage of morphological normal spermatozoa from 35% to 44%.

CONCLUSIONS

Male urogenital tract infections can have a severe negative effect on sperm morphology (3). This negative effect does not only alter the external morphological appearance (shape) of the spermatozoa but may also alter the internal structures and the functional abilities of the sperms, like the sperm acrosome and a reduction in acrosin activity. This leads to lower in vivo and in vitro fertilization rates and especially a lower pregnancy rate due to the DNA damage caused by the increased ROS production by leukocytes and abnormal spermatozoa themselves (3). Treatment with antibiotics, for long periods, and alternative treatment methods like antioxidants and immunomodulating agents can improve sperm morphology and the functional ability of the sperms with positive outcome on fertilization rates and especially pregnancy rates (C).

REFERENCES

1. Diemer T, Ludwig M, Huwe P, et al. Influence of urogenital infections on sperm function. Curr Opin Urol 2000; 10:39–44.
2. Henkel R, Kierspel E, Stalf T, et al. Effect of reactive oxygen species produced by spermatozoa and leukocytes on sperm functions in non-leukocytospermic patients. Fertil Steril 2005; 83:635–642.
3. Weidner W, Jantos C, Schiefer HG, et al. Semen parameters in men with and without proven chronic prostatitis. Arch Androl 1991; 26:173–183.
4. Wolff H. The biologic significance of white blood cells in semen. Fertil Steril 1995; 63:1143–1157.
5. Menkveld R, Kruger TF. Sperm morphology and male urogenital infections. Andrologia 1998; 30(suppl 1):49–53.
6. Menkveld R, Huwe P, Ludwig M, et al. Morphological sperm alternations in different types of prostatitis. Andrologia 2003; 35:288–293.
7. World Health Organization. WHO Laboratory Manual for the Examination of Human Semen and Sperm-Cervical Mucus Interaction, 4th ed. Cambridge, UK: Cambridge University Press, 1999.
8. Menkveld R. The basic semen analysis. In: Oehninger S, Kruger TF, eds. Male Infertility. Diagnosis and treatment. Oxon, UK: Informa Healthcare, 2007:141–170.
9. Tomlinson MJ, White A, Barratt CLR, et al. The removal of morphologically abnormal sperm forms by phagocytes: a positive role for seminal leukocytes? Hum Reprod 1992; 10:517–522.
10. Tomlinson MJ, Barratt CLR, Cooke ID. Prospective study of leukocytes and leukocyte subpopulations in semen suggest

they are not a cause of male infertility. Fertil Steril 1993; 60:1069–1075.
11. Eggert-Kruse W, Bellmann A, Rohr G, et al. Differentiation of round cells in semen by means of monoclonal antibodies and relationship with male fertility. Fertil Steril 1992; 56:1046–1055.
12. Wolff H, Polotch JA, Martinez A, et al. Leukocytospermia is associated with poor semen quality. Fertil Steril 1990; 53:528–536.
13. Haidl G. Macrophages in semen are indicative of chronic epididymal infections. Arch Androl 1990; 25:5–11.
14. Leib Z, Bartoov B, Eltes F, et al. Reduced semen quality caused by chronic abacterial prostatitis: an enigma or reality? Fertil Steril 1994; 61:1109–1116.
15. Kiessling AA, Lamparelli N, Yin H-Z, et al. Seminal leukocytes: friends or foes? Fertil Steril 1995; 64:196–198.
16. Menkveld R, Stander FSH, Kotze TJvW, et al. The evaluation of morphological characteristics of human spermatozoa according to stricter criteria. Hum Reprod 1990; 5:586–592.
17. Menkveld R. Role of acrosome index in prediction of fertilization outcome. In: Oehninger S, Kruger TF, eds. Male Infertility. Diagnosis and treatment. Oxon, UK: Informa Healthcare, 2007; 187–194.
18. Menkveld R, Franken DR, Kruger TF, et al. Sperm selection capacity of the human zona pellucida. Mol Reprod Dev 1991; 30:346–352.
19. Menkveld R, Rhemrev JPT, Franken DR, et al. Acrosomal morphology as a novel criterion for male fertility diagnosis: relation with acrosin activity, morphology (strict criteria) and fertilization in vitro. Fertil Steril 1996; 65:637–644.
20. World Health Organization. WHO Laboratory Manual for the Examination of Human Semen and Semen-cervical Mucus Interaction, 1st ed. Cambridge, UK: Cambridge University Press, 1980.
21. World Health Organization. WHO Laboratory Manual for the Examination of Human Semen and Semen-cervical Mucus Interaction, 2nd ed. Cambridge, UK: Cambridge University Press, 1987.
22. MacLeod J, Gold RZ. The male factor in fertility and infertility. IV. Sperm morphology in fertile and infertile marriage. Fertil Steril 1951; 2:394–414.
23. Oehninger S, Acosta AA, Kruger TF, et al. Failure of fertilization in in vitro fertilization: The "occult" male factor. J In Vitro Fert Embryo Transf 1988; 5:181–187.
24. Menkveld R, Kruger TF. Advantages of strict (Tygerberg) criteria for sperm morphology evaluation. Int J Androl 1995; 18(suppl 2):36–42.
25. Menkveld R. An investigation of environmental influences on spermatogenesis and semen parameters [Ph.D., dissertation (in Afrikaans)]. South Africa: Faculty of Medicine, University of Stellenbosch, 1987.
26. Fredricsson B, Björk R. Morphology of postcoital spermatozoa in the cervical secretion and its clinical significance. Fertil Steril 1977; 28:841–845.
27. Mortimer D, Leslie EE, Kelley RW, et al. Morphological selection of human spermatozoa in vivo and in vitro. J Reprod Fertil 1982; 64;391–399.
28. World Health Organization. WHO Laboratory Manual for the Examination of Human Semen and Sperm-cervical Mucus Interaction, 3rd ed. Cambridge, UK: Cambridge University Press, 1992.
29. Menkveld R, Wong WY, Lombard CJ, et al. Semen parameters including WHO and strict criteria morphology, in a fertile and subfertile population: an effort towards standardisation of in vivo thresholds. Hum Reprod 2001; 16:1165–1171.
30. Kruger TF, Acosta AA, Simmons KF, et al. Predictive value of abnormal sperm morphology in in vitro fertilization. Fertil Steril 1988; 49:112–117.
31. Esfandiari N, Saleh RA, Abdoos M, et al. Positive bacterial culture of semen from infertile men with asymptomatic leukocytospermia. Int J Fertil 2002; 47:265–270.
32. Lackner JE, Herwig R, Schmidbauer J, et al. Correlation of leukocytospermia with clinical infection and the possible effect of anti-inflammatory treatment on semen quality. Fertil Steril 2006; 86:601–605.
33. El-Demiry MIM, Hargrave TB, Busutill A, et al. Immunocompetent cells in human testis in health and disease. Fertil Steril 1987; 48:470–479.
34. Kaleli S, Öçer F, Irez T, et al. Does leukocytospermia associate with poor semen parameters and sperm function in male fertility? The role of different seminal leukocytes concentrations. Eur J Obstet Gynecol Reprod Biol 2000; 89:185–191.
35. Sharma RK, Pasqualotto EA, Nelson DR, et al. Relationship between seminal white blood cell counts and oxidative stress in men treated at an infertility clinic. J Androl 2001; 22:575–583.
36. Arata de Bellabarba GA, Tortolero I, et al. Nonsperm cells in human semen and their relationship with semen parameters. Arch Androl 2000; 45:131–136.
37. Moskovtsev SI, Willis J, White J, et al. Leukocytospermia: relationship with sperm deoxyribonucleic acid integrity in patients evaluated for male factor infertility. Fertil Steril 2007; 88:737–740.
38. Bezold G, Politch JA, Kiviat NB, et al. Prevalence of sexually transmissible pathogens in semen from male infertility patients with and without leukocytospermia. Fertil Steril 2007; 87:1087–1097.
39. Thomas J, Fishel SB, Hall JA, et al. Increased polymorphonuclear granulocytes in seminal plasma in relation to sperm morphology. Hum Reprod 1997; 12:2418–2421.
40. Aziz N, Agarwal A, Lewis-Jones I, et al. Novel association between specific sperm morphological defects and leukocytospermia. Fertil Steril 2004; 82:621–627.

41. Gambera L, Campanella G, Piomboni P, et al. Association of antioxidants and natural immune activators in the treatment of asthenoteratospermia and abacterial leukocytosis. Minerva Ginecol 2007; 59:473–479.
42. Zalata AA, Ahmed AH, Allamaneni SSR, et al. Relationship between acrosin activity of human spermatozoa and oxidative stress. Asian J Androl 2004; 6:313–318.
43. Burrello N, Aridiacono G, Vicari E, et al. Morphologically normal spermatozoa of patients with secretory olio-astheno-teratozoospermia have an increased aneuploidy rate. Hum Reprod 2004; 19:2998–2302.
44. Nasr-Esfahani MH, Razavi S, Tavalaee M. Failed fertilization after ICSI and spermiogenic defects. Fertil Steril 2008; 89:892–898.
45. Hofmann N, Haider SG. Neue Ergebnisse morphologischer Diagnostik der Spermatogeneseströrungen. Gynäkologe 1985; 18:70–80.
46. Prisant N, Escalier D, Soufir J-C, et al. Ultrastructural nuclear defects and increased chromosome aueuploidies in spermatozoa with elongated heads. Hum Reprod 2007; 22:1052–1059.
47. Osawa Y Sueoka K, Iwata S, et al. Assessment of the dominant abnormal form is useful for predicting the outcome of intracytoplasmic sperm injection in cases of severe teratozoospermia. J Assist Reprod Genet 1999; 16:436–442.
48. Fischer MA, Willis J, Zini A. Human sperm DNA integrity: correlation with sperm cytoplasmic droplets. Urology 2003; 61:207–211.
49. Henkel R, Hajimohammad M, Stalf T, et al. Influence of deoxyribonucleic acid damage on fertilization and pregnancy. Fertil Steril 2004; 81:965–972.
50. Comhaire FH, Mahmoud AM, Depuydt CE, et al. Mechanisms and effects of male genital tract infection on sperm quality and fertilizing potential: the andrologist's viewpoint. Hum Reprod Update 1999; 5:393–398.
51. Branigan EF, Muller CH. Efficacy of treatment and recurrence rate of leukocytospermia in infertile men with prostatitis. Fertil Steril 1994; 62:580–584.
52. Vicari E. Effectiveness and limits of antimicrobial treatment on seminal leukocyte concentration and related reactive oxygen species production in patients with male accessory gland infection. Hum Reprod 2000; 15:2536–2544.
53. Oliva A, Multigner L. Ketotifen improves sperm motility and sperm morphology in male patients with leukocytospermia and unexplained infertility. Fertil Steril 2006; 85:240–243.

35 Immunological aspects of male accessory gland infection

Luciano Adorini, Mario Maggi, and Mauro Gacci

INTRODUCTION

The primary function of the immune system is to protect the host from infectious agents. Environmental pathogens threaten the host with a wide spectrum of pathologic mechanisms, and the immune response uses a complex array of protective mechanisms to control and usually eliminate infectious organisms. All of these mechanisms rely on detecting structural features of the pathogens that mark them as distinct from host cells. Such host–pathogen discrimination is essential to permit the host to eliminate the pathogen without excessive damage to its own tissues. Host mechanisms for recognition of microbial structures can be broadly distinguished in two general classes: innate immune responses encoded by genes in the host germline recognizing molecular patterns shared by many microbes but absent in the mammalian host; and adaptive immune responses encoded by gene elements that somatically rearrange to assemble antigen-binding molecules with exquisite specificity for unique microbial and environmental structures.

Because the immune system uses many different effector mechanisms to destroy the broad range of microbial cells and particles it encounters, it is critical for the immune response to avoid unleashing these destructive mechanisms against its own tissues via a series of mechanisms promoting tolerance to self, as failure of self-tolerance can lead to autoimmune diseases (1).

In this chapter, we will review the basic immunological aspects of male accessory gland infections, and in particular discuss the relationship between infections and induction of autoimmune pathology in these organs.

General Features of Innate and Adaptive Immunity

The innate immune system comprises an array of defense mechanisms encoded in the germline genes of the host, from epithelial barriers and mucociliary blankets to bioactive molecules including cytokines, chemokines, lipid mediators of inflammation, bioactive amines, antibacterial peptides, and enzymes. Importantly, the innate immune system includes cell-surface receptors that bind molecular patterns expressed by invading microbes. Innate immune responses can be induced in virtually any cell, but they are primarily mediated by specialized cell types, such as macrophages, dendritic cells (DCs), and natural killer cells. Innate immunity is characterized by rapid, local responses, largely based on the production of proinflammatory mediators, in particular cytokines, chemokines, and reactive oxygen species. This is triggered by recognition of stereotyped patterns conserved in infectious microorganisms via surface molecules able to recognize distinct structural components of pathogens (2).

Unlike the innate immune system, the adaptive immune system manifests exquisite specificity for its target antigens by virtue of the antigen-specific receptors expressed on the surfaces of T and B lymphocytes. The antigen-specific receptors of the adaptive response are assembled by somatic rearrangement of germline gene elements to form T-cell receptor (TCR) and immunoglobulin genes. The assembly of antigen receptors from a collection of a few hundred germline-encoded gene elements permits the formation of millions of different antigen receptors, each with potentially unique specificity for a different antigen (1).

Adaptive immune responses are induced by cells specialized in antigen processing and presentation, in particular DCs, are mediated by cells specialized in antigen recognition, carried out by T and B lymphocytes, and are primarily orchestrated by $CD4^+$ T lymphocytes (1). To select lymphocytes able to respond to foreign molecules while remaining tolerant to self-components, the strategy of the immune system has been to generate a vast repertoire of antigen-specific receptors, distribute it clonally in different lymphocytes, and then eliminate cells capable of recognizing self-components with high affinity, while permitting the differentiation of T cells potentially able to recognize foreign antigens. However complex the mechanisms utilized, the basis for tolerance to self-components is relatively simple. Firstly, T cells expressing high-affinity receptors for self-antigens can be physically eliminated during thymic development via clonal deletion. Although this is a primary mechanism of self-tolerance, it does not completely eliminate T cells specific for self-antigens. Self-reactive T cells that have been exported to the periphery can then be functionally inactivated upon antigen recognition in the absence of appropriate co-stimulatory signals, a process denominated clonal anergy. Finally, peripheral self-reactive T cells can be suppressed by other T cells (1).

Innate recognition of infection can lead to the induction of adaptive immune responses and activate autoreactive lymphocytes via a number of mechanisms, including molecular mimicry, bystander activation, and triggering of Toll-like receptors (TLRs).

Toll-like Receptors

Recognition of microbial infection and initiation of host defense responses is controlled by multiple mechanisms. Innate immune recognition, also known as pattern recognition, is based on the detection of molecular structures that are unique to microorganisms, and each pattern recognition receptor has a broad specificity potentially binding to a large number of microbial molecules sharing a common structural motif or pattern. There are several functionally distinct classes of pattern recognition receptors (2), but the best characterized are represented by TLRs, a family of about 10 different transmembrane receptors that recognize viral nucleic acids and several bacterial products (3). The full range of TLR functions in antimicrobial defence has not yet been determined, but TLRs are known to elicit inflammatory and antimicrobial responses after activation by their microbial ligands (2). TLRs activate multiple steps in the inflammatory reactions that help to eliminate the invading pathogens and coordinate systemic defenses. Notably, TLRs activate tissue-resident macrophages to produce proinflammatory cytokines, including tumor-necrosis factor interleukin-1β (IL-1β), IL-6, and chemokines like IL-8, which coordinate local and systemic inflammatory responses (2). In addition, TLRs control multiple DC functions, and activate signals that are critically involved in the initiation of adaptive immune responses, which can include autoimmune responses.

MALE ACCESSORY GLAND INFECTIONS

Definition

Male accessory gland infections (MAGI) is a complex syndrome caused by bacterial and immunologic agents, resulting in a chronic active infection of prostate, prostate and seminal vesicle, or prostate with seminal vesicle and epididymis (4). According to the WHO standardization, MAGI is diagnosed if the male presents abnormal spermatozoa and specific characteristics of medical history, physical examination, and laboratory parameters (see flowchart) (5).

ABNORMAL SPERMATOZOA
(OLIGO-ASTHENO-TERATO-AZOO-SPERMIA)
ASSOCIATED TO:

↓

GROUP A (Clinical Symptoms & Signs)
History: urinary tract infections (UTI), sexually-transmitted diseases
Signs: abnormal palpation (volume and thickness) of epididymis, deferent, abnormal digital rectal examination (prostate or seminal vesicle)

GROUP B (Prostatic secretion: EPS or VB3 according to Meares-Stamey test) (6)
Direct: EPS: Expressed prostatic secretions
Indirect: VB3: Urine after prostate massage
Leukocytes >10 ($400\times$)

GROUP C (Ejaculate analysis)
Elevated *white blood cell counts* with positive peroxidase ($>10^6$/mL)
Positive *bacterial culture* (Gram negative: $>10^3$ CFU/mL, Gram positive: $>10^4$ CFU/mL)
Abnormal *chemical–physical* aspect and/or *viscosity* and/or *pH* and/or *biochemical* and/or *inflammatory* markers and/or *reactive oxygen species*

↓

MAGI diagnosis if two parameters are positive:
***each* from a different group (A-B, A-C, OR B-C)**
or *both* from group C (C-C)

Source: From Ref. 5.

Epidemiology

MAGI is rising as a relevant health problem because 12% of male partners of infertile couples with abnormal semen quality present with MAGI (7). 15% of adult males could be affected by prostatitis, that is frequently associated to MAGI in infertile males (8), while the overall incidence of men with a previous or current diagnosis of prostatitis is estimated to be from 5% to 16% (9), with generally comparable rates among different populations from North America, Europe, and Asia (10).

Etiopathogenesis

At present, the etiology and pathogenesis of MAGI remains unknown but urinary tract infections (UTI) seem to be involved in the promotion of a large proportion of cases (11). E. coli, and in a minimal part non-E. coli strains such as Enterococcus, Proteus, Klebsiella, Pseudomonas, Chlamydia, Neisseria, Mycobacterium tuberculosis are the most frequently isolated microbial agents in MAGI-associated UTI.

Moreover, self-reactivity directed against the prostate by the immune system seems to be involved in the etiology of the disease, but it is still unclear if this autoreactive process could be consequent to bacterial infection of the urethra, prostate, seminal vesicle, or epididymis, which could activate an inflammatory response leading to autoimmunity (12). The induction of an autoimmune process can also induce antisperm antibodies, with a detrimental impact on male fertility (13).

Clinical Presentation and Diagnosis

Pathologic conditions such as prostatitis, vesiculitis, and epididymitis, that may facilitate the formation of antisperm antibodies can be clinically relevant or, less frequently, be totally asymptomatic. Overall, the prevalence of prostatitis-like symptoms in MAGI has been reported to be between 6% and 9% (14). According to ultrasound criteria, 42% of bacterial MAGI had prostatitis, 26% had prostatovesiculitis, and 32% had prostatovesicular epididymitis (15). Clinical history, physical examination, ultrasound, urine and ejaculate analysis, and microbiological culture are mandatory to formulate the correct diagnosis, to identify the site of infection and to plan treatment strategies.

Prostatic inflammation (prostatitis) begins as an inflammatory disease of the prostatic ducts and acini, progressing to periglandular inflammation with subsequent disruption of the ducts and glands, and spreading of the inflammatory process into the stromal tissue. Prostatitis is the most common urologic disorder in men younger than 50 years and the third most common urologic diagnosis in men older than 50 years (after BPH and prostate cancer), representing 8% of urology office visits (16).

Prostatitis is characterized by pelvic pain and no specific diagnosis accounting for the pain, while voiding symptoms may or may not be present (17). Symptoms are recorded and analyzed with the National Institutes of Health Chronic Prostatitis Symptom Index (NIH-CPSI) that has been validated by the Chronic Prostatitis Cohort study and the Chronic Prostatitis Collaborative Research Network clinical trials (18). Allergies, sinusitis, erectile dysfunction, and irritable bowel syndrome are the most frequently reported comorbidities (19). Lower urinary tract symptoms suggestive of prostatitis, such as frequency, urgency, dysuria, have a significant negative impact on the quality of life , and contribute or cause erectile dysfunction (20); moreover, prostatitis can be associated to altered semen quality parameters with severe impact on male fertility (21).

The NIH consensus definition and classification identifies four categories of prostatitis (22). Category I includes acute bacterial prostatitis and category II chronic bacterial prostatitis. Category III, also known as chronic prostatitis/chronic pelvic pain syndrome (CP/CPPS), is defined by pelvic pain in the absence of demonstrable bacterial infection, and is further subdivided into category IIIA or inflammatory, and category IIIB or noninflammatory, based on the presence of leukocytes in expressed prostatic secretion or seminal plasma, respectively. Molecular studies have documented bacterial DNA sequences in prostate tissue from CP/CPPS patients, suggesting that prostatic colonization and/or infection can occur in these patients, but further research is needed to define the role of bacteria in the etiology of CP/CPPS (23). Category IV, or asymptomatic inflammatory prostatitis, is defined by the presence of leukocytes in seminal secretions or by inflammatory infiltrates detected in histological specimens, in the absence of typical chronic pelvic pain. CP/CPPS (NIH category III) is common in medical practice and its prevalence rate in the general population ranges from 5% to 14.2% (24). Therefore, about 60% to 80% of all prostatitis could be classified as CP/CPPS.

The NIH consensus definition recognizes that pain is the main symptom in "abacterial chronic prostatitis" (with variable voiding and sexual dysfunction) and represents the optimal criterion to differentiate CP patients from control patients or patients experiencing other genitourinary problems (e.g., BPH). A prospective–descriptive study conducted in 20 Italian centers reported a 12.8% rate as prevalence of a clinical diagnosis of prostatitis (25). CP/CPPS may cause morbidity through symptoms and quality of life can be severely compromised. CP/CPPS is still poorly understood, often inadequately treated, and further studies are needed to clarify the relationship among its aspects (26). Interestingly, leukocyte counts do not necessarily correlate with symptom severity (27) and more reliable markers are needed.

AUTOIMMUNE NATURE OF CP/CPPS

CP/CPPS is still an enigmatic syndrome but immunological, neurological, and endocrine dysfunctions have been proposed to be involved in disease development (28). Evidence indicating a predominant autoimmune component in the pathogenesis of CP/CPPS is, however, emerging (29), and the autoimmune nature of CP/CPPS is also supported by experimental models of prostatitis (30). These models have been quite extensively characterized, demonstrating that immunization of rats or mice with prostate gland extracts can induce T cell and antibody responses to prostate antigens, associated with histological evidence of prostate inflammation (30).

We could demonstrate expression of all TLRs tested by human and mouse prostate cells (Fig. 1), extending previous observations documenting selected TLR expression by BPH cells (31,32). TLRs expressed by human BPH cells are functional and their triggering by viral or bacterial products, such as poly I:C and LPS, induces production of proinflammatory chemokines like IL-8 and CXCL10, and cytokines like IL-6 (33). In addition to the growth-promoting properties of IL-8 and IL-6 on prostate cells (34–36), the capacity of IL-8 and CXCL10 to recruit inflammatory cells could play a role in inducing and maintaining chronic inflammatory conditions of the prostate, such as those observed in CP/CPPS patients. Thus, prostate cells represent targets of TLR agonists, which can lead to the production of proinflammatory cytokines and chemokines that are able to mediate chronic prostate inflammation and prostatic hyperplasia.

Our data may be interpreted to infer that the association between infection and CP/CPPS could reflect the triggering by microbial products of signal transduction via TLRs expressed by prostate cells, leading to production of proinflammatory cytokines and chemokines that contribute to create the conditions for an autoimmune attack. This pathogenetic mechanism, along with genetic susceptibility and induction of adaptive immune responses, may precipitate autoimmune diseases, as recently shown in the induction of autoimmune myocarditis by a combination of TLR stimulation and CD40-mediated triggering of self-peptide–loaded DCs (37). Activation of TLRs in target tissues could also be involved in the pathogenesis of systemic autoimmune diseases, as suggested for TLR9 in systemic lupus erythematosus (38).

Clinical Evidence

Autoreactive $CD4^+$ and $CD8^+$ T cells specific for prostate antigens exist in normal individuals (39), and this T-cell repertoire could potentially become activated to mount an autoimmune response. Indeed, peripheral blood mononuclear cells and $CD4^+$ T cells from CP/CPPS patients proliferate in response to seminal plasma (12,40) and to specific prostate antigens (41,42), indicating expression of the autoreactive T-cell repertoire in

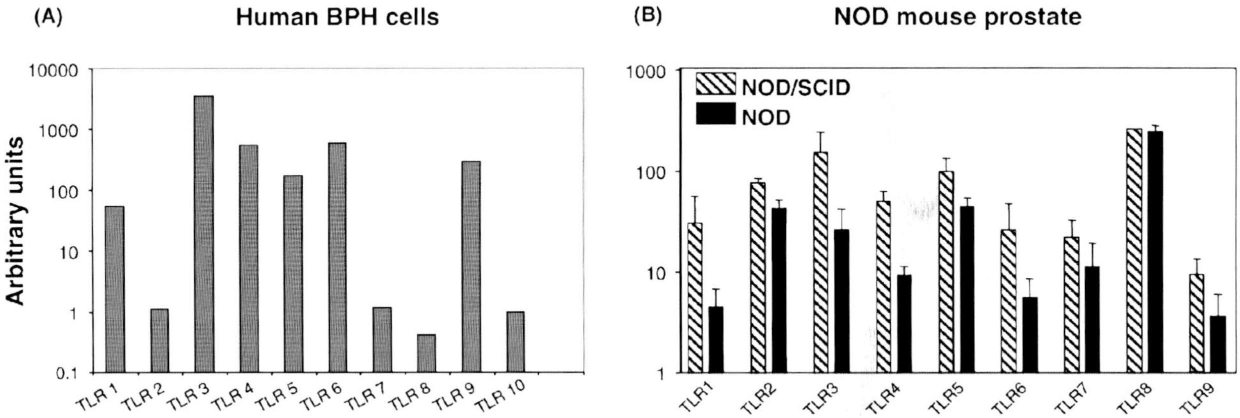

Figure 1 TLR expression by human BPH cells and NOD mouse prostate. (A) Quantification of TLR mRNA expression by real-time RT-PCR in human BPH cells. mRNA levels are shown as arbitrary units normalized to GAPDH expression. Data are from one representative experiment out of 3 performed. (B) Quantification of TLR mRNA expression by real-time RT-PCR on freshly isolated prostates from 10-week-old NOD/SCID (stippled bars) or 8-week-old NOD male mice (filled bars). The levels of mRNA are shown as arbitrary units normalized to GAPDH expression. Data are mean ± SE from three experiments. Note the similar level of TLR expression in prostates from NOD and NOD/SCID mice, which are immunodeficient and thus devoid of intraprostatic lymphomononuclear cell infiltration, demonstrating constitutive expression of TLRs by NOD prostate cells.

disease pathogenesis. High-titer IgG autoantibodies to prostate-associated proteins are found in patients with CP/CPPS (43), further indicating a T cell–dependent autoimmune process. In addition, CP/CPPS patients show higher levels in seminal plasma, compared to controls, of proinflammatory cytokines like IL-1β and TNF-α, and chemokines like IL-8 (44–49).

Increased Seminal Plasma Cytokines and Chemokines in CP/CPPS

We have examined seminal plasma levels of eight cytokines and nine chemokines in healthy controls compared to patients affected by CP/CPPS (49). Among the cytokines tested, although the effects were of low magnitude, the proinflammatory cytokines IL-1α, IL-1β, IL-6, and IL-12p70 were significantly elevated in CP/CPPS, while the anti-inflammatory cytokine IL-10 was increased in CP/CPPS IIIB patients compared to controls, as previously reported (50). The chemokines CCL3, CCL4, CCL17, CCL22, and IL-8, were also significantly increased in seminal plasma from CP/CPPS patients (49). The concomitant increase of several inflammatory cytokines and chemokines in CP/CPPS is consistent with an important chronic inflammatory component in the pathogenesis of this disease (29,51).

In addition, our data indicate that IL-8, an important mediator of inflammatory processes, is a reliable biomarker of CP/CPPS, and can discriminate between CP/CPPS IIIA and IIIB patients (49). The potential value of IL-8 as a surrogate marker of disease is further supported by the positive correlation of IL-8 levels with symptom scores and serum PSA values in CP/CPPS patients. IL-8 is an inflammatory chemokine functioning primarily as a neutrophil chemoattractant and activating factor, but can also recruit basophils and T cells, and is a potent angiogenic factor (52). IL-8 is secreted by multiple cell types and exerts its effects by binding with high affinity to two cell-surface receptors—the chemokine receptors CXCR1 and CXCR2 (52).

IL-8 plays an important role in different inflammatory diseases, like rheumatoid arthritis (53), gastritis (54), inflammatory bowel disease (55), atherosclerosis (56), and inflammatory lung disease (57). IL-8 has been found elevated in seminal plasma of patients affected by CP/CPPS IIIA (46), but in this study no IL-8 increase was observed in CP/CPPS IIIB patients. In a more recent study, IL-8 was found elevated in CP/CPPS patients, but they were not categorized further (48). Our observation of significantly increased IL-8 levels in CP/CPPS IIIB compared to controls, although still significantly lower than CP/CPPS IIIA (49), reveals an inflammatory process also in IIIB patients, in agreement with previous data (58). Interestingly, our data show, for the first time, significantly increased IL-8 levels in seminal plasma of BPH patients (49), consistent with the notion that chronic inflammation may have a prominent role also in the induction and progression of BPH (51,59). Our data show that IL-8 is expressed in situ by epithelial and stromal prostate cells, and is functional, as shown by the recruitment of CXCR1 and CXCR2-positive leukocytes, as well as $CD15^+$ neutrophils (49). Therefore, IL-8 may not only serve as a reliable biomarker applicable to diagnosis, prognosis, and assessment of treatment efficacy in CP/CPPS patients, but does actually represent an important driver of prostate inflammation and an interesting therapeutic target in itself for the treatment of this condition.

Recommendations

- MAGI is diagnosed according to the WHO standardization (5), and symptoms are recorded and analyzed with the National Institutes of Health Chronic Prostatitis Symptom Index (NIH-CPSI) (18). **[Level of evidence 1a; Grade of recommendation A]**
- Prostate cells represent targets of TLR agonists, which can lead to the production of proinflammatory cytokines and chemokines able to mediate chronic prostate inflammation and prostatic hyperplasia (31–36). **[Level of evidence 2a; Grade of recommendation B]**
- IL-8 can discriminate between CP/CPPS IIIA and IIIB patients (49), and actually represents an important driver of prostate inflammation and an interesting therapeutic target in itself for the treatment of this condition. **[Level of evidence 2b; Grade of recommendation B]**

REFERENCES

1. Paul WE. Fundamental Immunology. 6th ed. Philadelphia: Wolters Kluwer/Lippincott Williams & Wilkins, 2008.
2. Medzhitov R. Recognition of microorganisms and activation of the immune response. Nature 2007; 449(7164):819–826.
3. Akira S, Uematsu S, Takeuchi O. Pathogen recognition and innate immunity. Cell 2006; 124(4):783–801.
4. Diemer T, Ludwig M, Huwe P, et al. Influence of urogenital infection on sperm function. Curr Opin Urol 2000; 10(1):39–44.
5. Rowe P, Comhaire F, Hargreave T, et al. World Health Organization manual for the standardized investigation, diagnosis and management of the infertile male, 1st ed. Cambridge, New York, Melbourne, Madrid: Cambridge University press, 2000.
6. Meares EM Jr, Stamey TA. The diagnosis and management of bacterial prostatitis. Br J Urol 1972; 44(2):175–179.
7. Everaert K, Mahmoud A, Depuydt C, et al. Chronic prostatitis and male accessory gland infection–is there an impact on male infertility (diagnosis and therapy)? Andrologia 2003; 35(5):325–330.
8. Nickel JC, Teichman JM, Gregoire M, et al. Prevalence, diagnosis, characterization, and treatment of prostatitis, interstitial cystitis, and epididymitis in outpatient urological practice: the Canadian PIE Study. Urology 2005; 66(5):935–940.
9. Roberts RO, Lieber MM, Rhodes T, et al. Prevalence of a physician-assigned diagnosis of prostatitis: the Olmsted County Study of Urinary Symptoms and Health Status Among Men. Urology 1998; 51(4):578–584.
10. Lee SW, Cheah PY, Liong ML, et al. Demographic and clinical characteristics of chronic prostatitis: prospective comparison of the University of Sciences Malaysia Cohort with the United States National Institutes of Health Cohort. J Urol 2007; 177(1):153–157; discussion 158.
11. Lipsky BA. Urinary tract infections in men. Epidemiology, pathophysiology, diagnosis, and treatment. Ann Intern Med 1989; 110(2):138–150.
12. Alexander RB, Brady F, Ponniah S. Autoimmune prostatitis: evidence of T cell reactivity with normal prostatic proteins. Urology 1997; 50(6):893–899.
13. Weidner W, Krause W, Ludwig M. Relevance of male accessory gland infection for subsequent fertility with special focus on prostatitis. Hum Reprod Update 1999; 5(5):421–432.
14. Nickel JC, Downey J, Hunter D, et al. Prevalence of prostatitis-like symptoms in a population based study using the National Institutes of Health chronic prostatitis symptom index. J Urol 2001; 165(3):842–845.
15. Vicari E. Effectiveness and limits of antimicrobial treatment on seminal leukocyte concentration and related reactive oxygen species production in patients with male accessory gland infection. Hum Reprod 2000; 15(12):2536–2544.
16. Krieger JN. Classification, epidemiology and implications of chronic prostatitis in North America, Europe and Asia. Minerva Urol Nefrol 2004; 56(2):99–107.
17. Berger RE, Ciol MA, Rothman I, et al. Pelvic tenderness is not limited to the prostate in chronic prostatitis/chronic pelvic pain syndrome (CPPS) type IIIA and IIIB: comparison of men with and without CP/CPPS. BMC Urol 2007; 7:17.
18. Litwin MS, McNaughton-Collins M, Fowler FJ Jr, et al. The National Institutes of Health chronic prostatitis symptom index: development and validation of a new outcome measure. Chronic Prostatitis Collaborative Research Network. J Urol 1999; 162(2):369–375.
19. Clemens JQ, Brown SO, Kozloff L, et al. Predictors of symptom severity in patients with chronic prostatitis and interstitial cystitis. J Urol 2006; 175(3 Pt 1):963–966; discussion 967.
20. Marszalek M, Wehrberger C, Hochreiter W, et al. Symptoms suggestive of chronic pelvic pain syndrome in an urban population: prevalence and associations with lower urinary tract symptoms and erectile function. J Urol 2007; 177(5):1815–1819.
21. Motrich RD, Maccioni M, Molina R, et al. Reduced semen quality in chronic prostatitis patients that have cellular autoimmune response to prostate antigens. Hum Reprod 2005; 20(9):2567–2572.
22. Krieger JN, Nyberg L Jr, Nickel JC. NIH consensus definition and classification of prostatitis. JAMA 1999; 282(3):236–237.
23. Krieger JN, Ross SO, Riley DE. Chronic prostatitis: epidemiology and role of infection. Urology 2002; 60(6 suppl):8–12; discussion 13.
24. Schaeffer AJ, Landis JR, Knauss JS, et al. Demographic and clinical characteristics of men with chronic prostatitis:

the national institutes of health chronic prostatitis cohort study. J Urol 2002; 168(2):593–598.
25. Rizzo M, Marchetti F, Travaglini F, et al. Prevalence, diagnosis and treatment of prostatitis in Italy: a prospective urology outpatient practice study. BJU Int 2003; 92(9):955–959.
26. Turner JA, Hauge S, Von Korff M, et al. Primary care and urology patients with the male pelvic pain syndrome: symptoms and quality of life. J Urol 2002; 167(4):1768–1773.
27. Schaeffer AJ, Knauss JS, Landis JR, et al. Leukocyte and bacterial counts do not correlate with severity of symptoms in men with chronic prostatitis: the National Institutes of Health Chronic Prostatitis Cohort Study. J Urol 2002; 168(3):1048–1053.
28. Karlovsky ME, Pontari MA. Theories of prostatitis etiology. Curr Urol Rep 2002; 3(4):307–312.
29. Pontari MA, Ruggieri MR. Mechanisms in prostatitis/chronic pelvic pain syndrome. J Urol 2004; 172(3):839–845.
30. Vykhovanets EV, Resnick MI, Maclennan GT, et al. Experimental rodent models of prostatitis: limitations and potential. Prostate Cancer Prostatic Dis 2007; 10(1):15–29.
31. Konig JE, Senge T, Allhoff EP, et al. Analysis of the inflammatory network in benign prostate hyperplasia and prostate cancer. Prostate 2004; 58(2):121–129.
32. Gatti G, Rivero V, Motrich RD, et al. Prostate epithelial cells can act as early sensors of infection by up-regulating TLR4 expression and proinflammatory mediators upon LPS stimulation. J Leukoc Biol 2006; 79(5):989–998.
33. Penna G, Fibbi B, Amuchastegui S, et al. Human benign prostatic hyperplasia stromal cells as inducers and targets of chronic immuno-mediated inflammation. J Immunol 2009; 182(7):4056–4064.
34. Giri D, Ittmann M. Interleukin-8 is a paracrine inducer of fibroblast growth factor 2, a stromal and epithelial growth factor in benign prostatic hyperplasia. Am J Pathol 2001; 159(1):139–147.
35. Giri D, Ozen M, Ittmann M. Interleukin-6 is an autocrine growth factor in human prostate cancer. Am J Pathol 2001; 159(6):2159–2165.
36. Castro P, Xia C, Gomez L, et al. Interleukin-8 expression is increased in senescent prostatic epithelial cells and promotes the development of benign prostatic hyperplasia. Prostate 2004; 60(2):153–159.
37. Eriksson U, Ricci R, Hunziker L, et al. Dendritic cell-induced autoimmune heart failure requires cooperation between adaptive and innate immunity. Nat Med 2003; 9(12):1484–1490.
38. Anders HJ, Vielhauer V, Eis V, et al. Activation of toll-like receptor-9 induces progression of renal disease in MRL-Fas(lpr) mice. Faseb J 2004; 18(3):534–536.
39. Corman JM, Sercarz EE, Nanda NK. Recognition of prostate-specific antigenic peptide determinants by human CD4 and CD8T cells. Clin Exp Immunol 1998; 114(2):166–172.
40. Batstone GR, Doble A, Gaston JS. Autoimmune T cell responses to seminal plasma in chronic pelvic pain syndrome (CPPS). Clin Exp Immunol 2002; 128(2):302–307.
41. Ponniah S, Arah I, Alexander RB. PSA is a candidate self-antigen in autoimmune chronic prostatitis/chronic pelvic pain syndrome. Prostate 2000; 44(1):49–54.
42. Motrich RD, Maccioni M, Molina R, et al. Presence of INFgamma-secreting lymphocytes specific to prostate antigens in a group of chronic prostatitis patients. Clin Immunol 2005; 116(2):149–157.
43. Dunphy EJ, Eickhoff JC, Muller CH, et al. Identification of antigen-specific IgG in sera from patients with chronic prostatitis. J Clin Immunol 2004; 24(5):492–502.
44. Alexander RB, Ponniah S, Hasday J, et al. Elevated levels of proinflammatory cytokines in the semen of patients with chronic prostatitis/chronic pelvic pain syndrome. Urology 1998; 52(5):744–749.
45. Nadler RB, Koch AE, Calhoun EA, et al. IL-1beta and TNF-alpha in prostatic secretions are indicators in the evaluation of men with chronic prostatitis. J Urol 2000; 164(1):214–218.
46. Hochreiter WW, Nadler RB, Koch AE, et al. Evaluation of the cytokines interleukin 8 and epithelial neutrophil activating peptide 78 as indicators of inflammation in prostatic secretions. Urology 2000; 56(6):1025–1029.
47. Orhan I, Onur R, Ilhan N, et al. Seminal plasma cytokine levels in the diagnosis of chronic pelvic pain syndrome. Int J Urol 2001; 8(9):495–499.
48. Khadra A, Fletcher P, Luzzi G, et al. Interleukin-8 levels in seminal plasma in chronic prostatitis/chronic pelvic pain syndrome and nonspecific urethritis. BJU Int 2006; 97(5):1043–1046.
49. Penna G, Mondaini N, Amuchastegui S, et al. Seminal plasma cytokines and chemokines in prostate inflammation: interleukin 8 as a predictive biomarker in chronic prostatitis/chronic pelvic pain syndrome and benign prostatic hyperplasia. Eur Urol 2007; 51(2):524–533; discussion 533.
50. Miller LJ, Fischer KA, Goralnick SJ, et al. Interleukin-10 levels in seminal plasma: implications for chronic prostatitis-chronic pelvic pain syndrome. J Urol 2002; 167(2 Pt 1):753–756.
51. Kramer G, Mitteregger D, Marberger M. Is benign prostatic hyperplasia (BPH) an immune inflammatory disease? Eur Urol 2007; 51(5):1202–1216.
52. Baggiolini M, Loetscher P, Moser B. Interleukin-8 and the chemokine family. Int J Immunopharmacol 1995; 17(2):103–108.
53. De Benedetti F, Pignatti P, Bernasconi S, et al. Interleukin 8 and monocyte chemoattractant protein-1 in patients with juvenile rheumatoid arthritis. Relation to onset types, disease activity, and synovial fluid leukocytes. J Rheumatol 1999; 26(2):425–431.

54. Shimada T, Terano A. Chemokine expression in Helicobacter pylori-infected gastric mucosa. J Gastroenterol 1998; 33(5):613–617.
55. McCormack G, Moriarty D, O'Donoghue DP, et al. Tissue cytokine and chemokine expression in inflammatory bowel disease. Inflamm Res 2001; 50(10):491–495.
56. Boisvert WA, Curtiss LK, Terkeltaub RA. Interleukin-8 and its receptor CXCR2 in atherosclerosis. Immunol Res 2000; 21(2–3):129–137.
57. Pease JE, Sabroe I. The role of interleukin-8 and its receptors in inflammatory lung disease: implications for therapy. Am J Respir Med 2002; 1(1):19–25.
58. John H, Barghorn A, Funke G, et al. Noninflammatory chronic pelvic pain syndrome: immunological study in blood, ejaculate and prostate tissue. Eur Urol 2001; 39(1):72–78.
59. Lee KL, Peehl DM. Molecular and cellular pathogenesis of benign prostatic hyperplasia. J Urol 2004; 172(5 Pt 1):1784–1791.

36 ROS and DNA integrity—implications of male accessory gland infections

Ralf Henkel

INTRODUCTION

Data on the prevalence of permanent infertility, that is, the unfulfilled wish for children, vary considerably between 3% and 15% to 20% (1). Among all involuntary childless couples, male infertility is the reason for the unfulfilled wish for children in approximately 30% to 50% (2), which amounts to more than 7% of men who are affected by infertility during their reproductive lifetime. Thus, the prevalence of male infertility is even higher than for diabetes mellitus type 1 and 2, which is considered as a common disease (3).

Apart from progressively decreasing semen quality, which contributes to the remarkable decline in fertility rates worldwide (4), reasons for male infertility are manifold and include, among others, infections and inflammations of the male genital tract including the accessory glands. These infections/inflammations play a major role not only as they are causing dysfunction of these glands but also for the complex interaction between the release of infection-related or inflammation-related mediators and sperm function. Generally, the prevalence of male genital tract infection-related or inflammation-related infertility reportedly varies from 10% to 20% in nonselected subjects and amounts to up to 35% in a large study comprising of more than 4000 patients consulting for infertility (5). Specifically, epidemiologic studies revealed that for prostatitis, the prevalence is approximately 2% to 10% (6) while for epididymitis, which also often involves the adjacent testis in the form of an epididymo-orchitis, Krieger (7) reported approximately 600,000 new cases annually in the United States.

Traditionally, male genital tract infections/inflammations are diagnosed by means of clinical parameters or the presence of leukocytes in the ejaculate. The latter parameter can vary dramatically and the seminal concentration of leukocytes can even be elevated in fertile men. Moreover, approximately 80% of leukocytospermic men are microbiologically negative (8). Therefore, the observation of leukocytospermia is clinically not a reliable indicator of asymptomatic urogenital tract infections (9), and recent reports (10) question whether the WHO threshold of leukocytospermia ($> 1 \times 10^6$ leukocytes/mL) is too high. Moreover, there is also no common agreement about how leukocytes should be detected. Thus, there is an urgent need to identify other and better markers for male urogenital tract infections that can clearly identify affected patients as well as give predictive values for the determination of sperm fertilizing capacity.

Since the late 1980s, new diagnostic markers for the identification of male genital tract infection/inflammation have been described. Among these, the concept of oxidative stress caused by elevated levels of reactive oxygen species (ROS) (10) plays the most prominent role. ROS have been shown to have detrimental effects on sperm functions and thus, on male fertility.

NATURE OF OXIDATIVE STRESS AND ROS

Similar to any other living cell, in spermatozoa energy is produced in the mitochondria by an enzymatically controlled oxidation of hydrogen in the form of nicotinamide adenine dinucleotide (NADH). The chemical energy is then conserved in the form of adenosine triphosphate (ATP). In the course of this stepwise process, oxygen (O_2) is reduced by four electrons and highly reactive free radicals as intermediate products (Fig. 1) such as hydroxyl radicals ($^{\cdot}OH$), superoxide anion ($^{\cdot}O_2^-$), or hydrogen peroxide (H_2O_2) are formed. Such products as oxygen derivatives are called ROS. At the end of this reduction process of molecular oxygen, which is also a diradical, water (H_2O) is formed. In addition, in vivo reactions of these ROS are coupled via the Fenton and Haber–Weiss reactions (Fig. 2) in cycles where cofactors, particularly transition metal ions like Fe^{2+}/Fe^{3+}, accelerate the reaction in generating the most reactive hydroxyl radicals. Normally, the generation of these free radicals is regulated by scavengers like manganese superoxide dismutase (MnSOD), copper/zinc superoxide dismutase (Cu/ZnSOD), glutathione peroxidase (GPx), and catalase (CAT). However, in case production of free radicals increases or protective enzymes cannot neutralize these highly reactive molecules, this will lead to an imbalance of this system. Consequently, ROS will react with biomolecules such as DNA, proteins, and lipids causing damage.

From a chemical point of view, radicals are chemical intermediates that have one or more unpaired electrons. This, in turn, results in extreme reactivity, a high oxidative potential, and therefore, very short half-life times in the nanosecond (10^{-9} sec) ($^{\cdot}OH$; hydroxyl radicals) to millisecond range (10^{-3} sec) ($^{\cdot}O_2^-$; superoxide anion). Therefore, radicals practically react at the site of generation. On the contrary, some peroxyl and alkoxyl radicals, which can be formed in plasma membranes in the process of lipid peroxidation, show half-life times in the second range and are, therefore, relatively stable. Thus, such molecules can travel some distances and exert their action at other target sites. In addition, another oxygen species, hydrogen peroxide (H_2O_2), which is chemically not a radical as it does not have unpaired electrons but is also highly reactive, is persistent and can even penetrate plasma membranes because it is

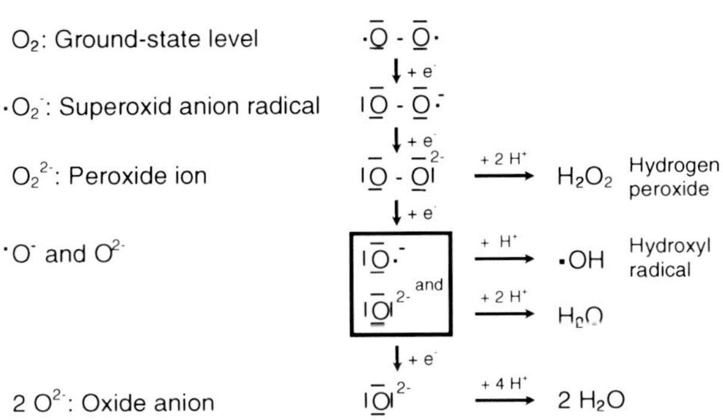

Figure 1 Oxidation forms of oxygen. If molecular oxygen, which is a diradical with two unpaired electrons, is reduced it acquires four electrons and water (H_2O) is formed. The dashes around the oxygen (O) represent paired, the points unpaired electrons.

electronically not charged. In contrast, other ROS like superoxide anion or the hydroxyl radical are nonmembrane permeable.

Considering that any living cell functions in a rather reduced state, it is of utmost importance that the equilibrium between oxidants and antioxidants is finely balanced and kept in a steady state. This reduced state is maintained, for instance, by the glutathione system. However, on the other hand, a certain limited and localized level of ROS is also essential for normal cell function (11). Thus, cells are constantly facing the interface between oxidation and reduction. In case this steady state derails for whatever reason leading to an imbalance in favor of the oxidants, which can potentially cause cellular or genetic damage, this condition is called "oxidative stress."

ORIGIN OF ROS AND OXIDATIVE STRESS

In the male genital tract and an ejaculate, sources of ROS are either leukocytes or the sperm cells themselves, whereby activated leukocytes physiologically produce up to 1000 times more ROS than spermatozoa (12). This high ROS production by leukocytes plays a major role in infections, inflammations, and cellular defence mechanisms. Basically, the cellular mechanisms for the generation of ROS in leukocytes and spermatozoa are the same. In addition, similar to leukocytes, a plasma membrane–bound NADPH oxidase system is generating superoxide radicals, which, in turn, will then dismutate under the influence of superoxide dismutase (SOD) into hydrogen peroxide as shown in the following.

$$\mathrm{NADPH} + 2\,O_2 \longrightarrow 2\,{}^{\cdot}O_2^- + \mathrm{NADP}^+ + H^+$$

$$2\,{}^{\cdot}O_2^- + 2\,H^+ \xrightarrow{\mathrm{SOD}} O_2 + H_2O_2$$

Mammalian sperm cells have an extraordinary high content of polyunsaturated fatty acids, particularly of docosahexanoic acid with six double bonds, in their plasma membrane resulting in the high membrane fluidity required for normal sperm function. On the other hand, this high amount of polyunsaturated fatty acids renders spermatozoa extremely susceptible to oxidative stress (13), impairing the membrane function and resulting in loss of fertilizing potential or even cell death. Additionally, there is evidence that ROS can seriously damage the DNA, not only in the sperm nucleus (14) but also in the mitochondria (15).

$$\left.\begin{array}{l} {}^{\cdot}O_2^- + Fe^{3+} \longrightarrow Fe^{2+} + O_2 \\ Fe^{2+} + H_2O_2 \longrightarrow Fe_{3+} + {}^{\cdot}OH + OH^- \end{array}\right\} \textbf{Fenton reaction}$$

$${}^{\cdot}O_2^- + H_2O_2 \xrightarrow{Fe^{2+}} O_2 + OH^- + {}^{\cdot}OH \qquad \textbf{Haber–Weiss reaction}$$

Figure 2 Fenton and Haber–Weiss reaction.

INFLUENCE OF LEUKOCYTE-DERIVED ROS ON SPERM NUCLEAR DNA FRAGMENTATION

Lopes et al. (14) showed that sperm nuclear DNA fragmentation can be induced by ROS, and more recently, Alvarez et al. (16) demonstrated that sperm DNA integrity was even significantly impaired in leukocytospermic semen samples. This finding is insofar of particular importance as sperm DNA fragmentation is a cause for fertilization and pregnancy failure in intrauterine insemination (IUI), in vitro fertilization (IVF), and intracytoplasmic sperm injection (ICSI), which has been confirmed in a very recent meta-analysis (17). With respect to ROS, one has to differentiate where the ROS originate, from external sources like leukocytes that are present in almost any ejaculate (8) or the spermatozoa themselves as ROS are physiologically produced in any living cell during respiration.

Although ROS have been shown to induce apoptosis in both somatic cells (18) and maturing spermatozoa, indicating an indirect way of action of oxidative stress caused by ROS leading to DNA fragmentation, there is also evidence suggesting a rather direct way of action (10). Data supporting this theory arise from studies that showed increased levels of specific forms of oxidative damage like 8-hydroxydeoxyguanosine in sperm DNA (19). Interestingly, spermatozoa from infertile men are generally more susceptible to DNA fragmentation by hydrogen peroxide (H_2O_2) than those from fertile subjects (20).

Pasqualotto et al. (21) demonstrated that infertile patients not only had elevated ROS levels but also reduced levels of antioxidant capacity. This observation supports the concept that the balance between ROS generation and antioxidant capacity in the semen plays a critical role in the pathophysiology of genital tract infection/inflammations and their impact on sperm functions and fertilization/pregnancy (22). Additionally, H_2O_2 secreted by leukocytes is persistent and can even penetrate plasma membranes, while other ROS like the superoxide anion (${}^{\cdot}O_2^-$) or the hydroxyl radical (${}^{\cdot}OH$) are nonmembrane permeable. Thus, extrinsic ROS derived from leukocytes can cause sperm nuclear DNA damage as suggested by Henkel et al. (10), and it is not only a matter of the number of leukocytes present in an ejaculate but also whether or not these leukocytes are activated. As even much lower numbers of leukocytes than 1×10^6/mL in the ejaculate and low amounts of ROS are harmful to sperm DNA integrity (10), a causality between leukocytes in the ejaculate and DNA fragmentation must not be neglected. At this point, it must also be noted that leukocyte-mediated sperm damage gains importance when spermatozoa are separated in vitro and when the seminal plasma is being eliminated.

INFLUENCE OF SPERM-DERIVED ROS

Besides the leukocyte-mediated effect of oxidants on sperm nuclear DNA fragmentation, the sperm cell's own ROS production, however, should not be neglected. Considering that normal mature spermatozoa do not contain considerable amounts of cytoplasm, sperm ROS production is extremely low. However, it is well known that as a result of a gonadal or epididymal infection or inflammation, or as Sertoli cell dysfunctions, normal sperm morphology can be decreased. Such defective sperm with poor morphology usually exhibit excess residual cytoplasm, which consequently results in a higher content of cytoplasmic enzymes (23) and then trigger sperm's own ROS production. Recent findings by Henkel et al. (10) and De Iuliis et al. (24) support the idea of Muratori et al. (25) about an involvement of ROS produced endogenously in the sperm cells as cause for sperm nuclear DNA fragmentation.

INFLUENCE OF ROS ON MITOCHONDRIAL DNA

One part of cellular DNA that has been neglected and not investigated until very recently is the DNA present in the mitochondria. Mitochondria are the powerhouse of the cell and produce most of the cell's energy during normal physiological aerobic metabolism. In the course of this process, approximately 1% to 5% of the consumed oxygen is converted into free radicals. Contrary to nuclear DNA, mitochondrial DNA (mtDNA) is not protected by histones and protamines, replicates very fast without proper proofreading, and has only a very basic repair mechanism (26); thus, mtDNA makes certain regions of the mitochondrial genome up to 100 times more susceptible to damage and mutations (27).Therefore, mtDNA is particularly prone to mutations and numerous diseases including male infertility like asthenozoospermia (28).

While earlier studies only focused on the nuclear DNA, latest research addresses mtDNA, which encodes 13 polypeptides essential for the electron transfer chain on the inner mitochondrial membrane and is, therefore, intimately involved in oxidative phosphorylation and ATP production in the mitochondria. Hence, mtDNA defects will inevitably result in a decreased mitochondrial membrane potential ($\Delta\psi_m$) and defective mitochondrial function. In turn, this is essential for sperm motility (29), and the determination of mitochondrial membrane potential has been suggested as being a highly sensitive parameter (30).

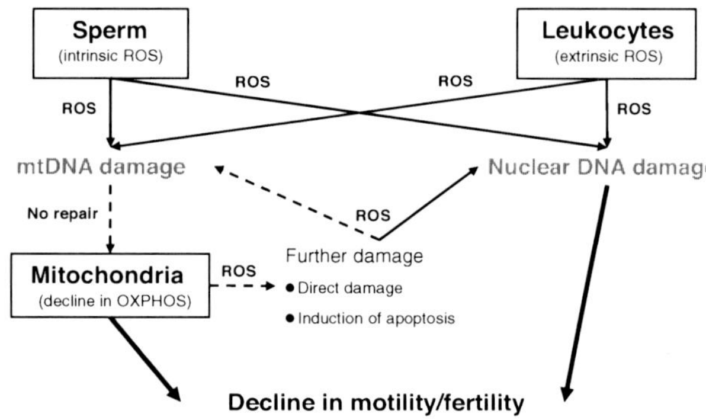

Figure 3 Putative mechanism of nuclear and mitochondrial sperm DNA damage leading to male infertility. Reactive oxygen species (ROS) derived from sperm or leukocytes can damage nuclear and mtDNA. In case of mtDNA damage, this damage can lead to a decline on oxidative phosphorylation (OXPHOS) as mtDNA encodes for proteins of the electron transport chain and there is no proper repair mechanism. This, in turn, can lead to a vicious cycle (*dashed arrows*) of further mitochondrial ROS generation, further mtDNA damage, induction of apoptosis, and nuclear DNA damage. Eventually, these processes will result in a decline in motility and the sperm fertilizing capacity.

Patients presenting with urogenital tract infections/inflammations show reduced sperm motility (31). This damage can either be triggered by direct pathogenic influences of bacteria on spermatozoa (32) or infectious mediators like ROS (33). In the light of the important role of mtDNA for the process of oxidative phosphorylation and the generation of motility and sperm function, it is conceivable that oxidative stress caused by infectious or inflammatory processes can also lead to mtDNA damage, leading to dysfunction of the mitochondrial respiratory chain with subsequent further stimulation of mitochondrial ROS production and oxidative damage. Similarly, in a vicious cycle, damage will then accelerate. Eventually, this will result in dysfunctional sperm (Fig. 3). Thus, male genital tract infections/inflammations could have underlying effects of mitochondrial diseases that could contribute to the sperms' compromised fertilizing capacity. Unfortunately, clinical studies investigating this relationship between male genital tract infection/inflammation and mitochondrial damage are not available yet.

CONSEQUENCES OF NUCLEAR DNA AND mtDNA DAMAGE FOR MALE FERTILITY AND ASSISTED REPRODUCTION

The negative impact of sperm nuclear DNA damage has repeatedly and unequivocally been shown for intrauterine insemination (34) and in vitro fertilization (35). Data obtained by Henkel et al. (35) even suggest that DNA-fragmented spermatozoa are still able to fertilize an oocyte, but at the time when the paternal genome is switched on, further development stops resulting in failed pregnancy. Even in natural conception, oxidative sperm DNA damage had a negative impact on human fertility and on the time to pregnancy (36). Although for ICSI, contradictory results have been reported in the past (14); the important contribution of sperm DNA damage to the fertilization process by any technique of assisted reproduction now appears to be beyond doubt as the number of reports confirming its importance on fertilization and the onset of pregnancy and also its detrimental effects on the health of the offspring (37) is increasing.

If there is an effect of sperm DNA damage on fertilization, it seems quite plausible that fragmented DNA is a cause for poor embryo quality, poor blastocyst development, and even early embryo death (38). In a recent report by Greco et al. (39), the authors demonstrated significantly higher percentages of nuclear DNA damage in ejaculated spermatozoa than in testicular sperm and concluded, in the light of the severe damages that can be caused for the offspring, that it is actually safer to use testicular sperm for ICSI. This might be related to the fact that testicular sperm were shown to display significantly more wild-type mtDNA than epididymal sperm (40) and could possibly be explained by the mitochondrial processes that can trigger nuclear DNA damage described earlier. Consequently, both studies (39,40) suggested the practical use of testicular sperm for ICSI rather than posttesticular sperm for ICSI as a therapeutic option in men with high levels of sperm nuclear and mtDNA damage in epididymal and ejaculated spermatozoa.

CONCLUSION

During recent years, sperm DNA fragmentation/damage has been recognized as a major contributing factor to male infertility that cannot be determined with the current semen analysis techniques according to the WHO standard (2a). As both sperm nuclear and mitochondrial DNA damage are important causes of fertilization and pregnancy failure and even a cause for early embryonic death or offspring diseases like childhood cancer, especially in males, these parameters should supplement any andrological laboratory diagnosis. This is even more important since it appears that an assault on mtDNA can not only result in poor sperm motility but also lead to nuclear DNA damage (2b). In this context, it is then imperative to investigate the cause of the DNA damage in individual patients and various hypotheses, namely *(i)* "abortive apoptosis," *(ii)* improper DNA packaging and ligation during spermatogenesis, and *(iii)* oxidative stress, which are discussed in several studies (for review see Ref. 41). For the latter hypothesis, two sources of ROS seem to be of importance, leukocytes and the spermatozoa themselves, and it appears that silent male genital tract infections/inflammations might not even lead to an increased leukocyte concentration (3). Nevertheless, significant damage to mitochondrial and nuclear DNA can be set. Therefore, in order to help patients undergoing assisted reproduction in a better way by improving pregnancy rates and preventing early childhood diseases, not only a thorough clinical andrological examination including diagnosis of male genital tract infections/inflammations should be done but also more research is necessary to investigate these important sperm parameters.

Thus, according to the current literature one can state the following:

- Sperm nuclear DNA damage is a cause of fertilization failure and pregnancy loss (B).
- A major cause for sperm DNA damage is ROS, which can be derived from male genital tract infections/inflammations (B).
- If looking at sperm DNA damage, one has to consider nuclear and mtDNA (C).

Levels of evidence (lowercase alphabets with numerals) and grade of guideline recommendations (uppercase alphabets) are in parentheses.

REFERENCES

1. Bruckert E. How frequent is unintentional childlessness in Germany? Andrologia 1991; 23:245–250.
2. Hull MG, Glazener CM, Kelly NJ, et al. Population study of causes, treatment, and outcome of infertility. Br Med J (Clin Res Ed) 1985; 291:1693–1697.
3. Nieschlag E, Behre HM. Andrology. Male reproductive health and dysfunction, 2nd ed. Berlin, Germany: Springer, 2000.
4. Skakkebaek NE, Jorgensen N, Main KM, et al. Is human fecundity declining? Int J Androl 2006; 29:2–11.
5. Henkel R, Maaß G, Jung A, et al. Age-related changes in seminal polymorphonuclear elastase in men with asymptomatic inflammation of the genital tract. Asian J Androl 2007; 9:299–304.
6. Hyeon Ku J, Woong Kim S, Paick JS. Epidemiologic risk factors for chronic prostatitis. Int J Androl 2005; 28:317–327.
7. Krieger JN. Epididymitis, orchitis, and related conditions. Sex Transm Dis 1984; 11:173–181.
8. Wolff H. The biologic significance of white blood cells in semen. Fertil Steril 1995; 63:1143–1157.
9. Barratt CL, Bolton AE, Cooke ID. Functional significance of white blood cells in the male and the female reproductive tract. Hum Reprod 1990; 5:639–648.
10. Henkel R, Kierspel E, Stalf T, et al. Effect of reactive oxygen species produced by spermatozoa and leukocytes on sperm functions in non-leukocytospermic patients. Fertil Steril 2005; 83:635–642.
11. Halliwell B. The antioxidant paradox. Lancet 2000; 355(9210):1179–1180.
12. de Lamirande E, Gagnon C. Capacitation-associated production of superoxide anion by human spermatozoa. Free Radic Biol Med 1995; 18:487–495.
13. Aitken RJ, Clarkson JS, Fishel S. Generation of reactive oxygen species, lipid peroxidation, and human sperm function. Biol Reprod 1989; 40:183–197.

14. Lopes S, Jurisicova A, Sun JG, et al. Reactive oxygen species: Potential cause for DNA fragmentation in human spermatozoa. Hum Reprod 1998; 13:896–900.
15. Lewis SEM. Importance of mitochondrial and nuclear sperm DNA in sperm quality assessment and assisted reproduction outcome. Hum Fertil 2002; 5:102–109.
16. Alvarez JG, Sharma RK, Ollero M, et al. Increased DNA damage in sperm from leukocytospermic semen samples as determined by the sperm chromatin structure assay. Fertil Steril 2002; 78:319–329.
17. Zini A, Boman JM, Belzile E, et al. Sperm DNA damage is associated with an increased risk of pregnancy loss after IVF and ICSI: Systematic review and meta-analysis. Hum Reprod 2008; 23:2663–2668.
18. Huang C, Li J, Zheng R, et al. Hydrogen peroxide-induced apoptosis in human hepatoma cells is mediated by CD95(APO-1/Fas) receptor/ligand system and may involve activation of wild-type p53. Mol Biol Rep 2000; 27:1–11.
19. Shen H, Ong C. Detection of oxidative DNA damage in human sperm and its association with sperm function and male infertility. Free Radic Biol Med 2000; 28:529–536.
20. Hughes CM, Lewis SE, McKelvey-Martin VJ, et al. A comparison of baseline and induced DNA damage in human spermatozoa from fertile and infertile men, using a modified comet assay. Mol Hum Reprod 1996; 2:613–619.
21. Pasqualotto FF, Sharma RK, Nelson DR, et al. Relationship between oxidative stress, semen characteristics, and clinical diagnosis in men undergoing infertility investigation. Fertil Steril 2000; 73:459–464.
22. Sikka SC. Relative impact of oxidative stress on male reproductive function. Curr Med Chem 2001; 8:851–862.
23. Aziz N, Saleh RA, Sharma RK, et al. Novel association between sperm reactive oxygen species production, sperm morphological defects, and the sperm deformity index. Fertil Steril 2004; 81:349–354.
24. De Iuliis GN, Wingate JK, Koppers AJ, et al. Definitive evidence for the nonmitochondrial production of superoxide anion by human spermatozoa. J Clin Endocrinol Metab 2006; 91:1968–1975.
25. Muratori M, Maggi M, Spinelli S, et al. Spontaneous DNA fragmentation in swim-up selected human spermatozoa during long term incubation. J Androl 2003; 24:253–262.
26. Croteau DL, Stierum RH, Bohr VA. Mitochondrial DNA repair pathways. Mutat Res 1999; 434:137–148.
27. Pesole G, Gissi C, De Chirico A, et al. Nucleotide substitution rate of mammalian mitochondrial genomes. J Mol Evol 1999; 48:427–434.
28. Folgero T, Bertheussen K, Lindal S, et al. Mitochondrial disease and reduced sperm motility. Hum Reprod 1993; 8:1863–1868.
29. Kasai T, Ogawa K, Mizuno K, et al. Relationship between sperm mitochondrial membrane potential, sperm motility, and fertility potential. Asian J Androl 2002; 4:97–103.
30. Marchetti C, Obert G, Deffosez A, et al. Study of mitochondrial membrane potential, reactive oxygen species, DNA fragmentation and cell viability by flow cytometry in human sperm. Hum Reprod 2002; 17:1257–1265.
31. Diemer T, Huwe P, Ludwig M, et al. Urogenital infection and sperm motility. Andrologia 2003; 35:283–287.
32. Diemer T, Huwe P, Ludwig M, et al. Influence of autogenous leucocytes and *Escherichia coli* on sperm motility parameters in vitro. Andrologia 2003; 35:100–105.
33. Fraczek M, Szumala-Kakol A, Jedrzejczak P, et al. Bacteria trigger oxygen radical release and sperm lipid peroxidation in in vitro model of semen inflammation. Fertil Steril 2007; 88(suppl 4):1076–1085.
34. Duran EH, Morshedi M, Taylor S, et al. Sperm DNA quality predicts intrauterine insemination outcome: A prospective cohort study. Hum Reprod 2002; 17:3122–3128.
35. Henkel R, Hajimohammad M, Stalf T, et al. Influence of deoxyribonucleic acid damage on fertilization and pregnancy. Fertil Steril 2004; 81:965–972.
36. Loft S, Kold-Jensen T, Hjollund NH, et al. Oxidative DNA damage in human sperm influences time to pregnancy. Hum Reprod 2003; 18:1265–1272.
37. Aitken RJ, Krausz C. Oxidative stress, DNA damage and the Y chromosome. Reproduction 2001; 122:497–506.
38. Tomsu M, Sharma V, Miller D. Embryo quality and IVF treatment outcomes may correlate with different sperm comet assay parameters. Hum Reprod 2002; 17:1856–1862.
39. Greco E, Scarselli F, Iacobelli M, et al. Efficient treatment of infertility due to sperm DNA damage by ICSI with testicular spermatozoa. Hum Reprod 2005; 20:226–230.
40. O'Connell M, McClure N, Lewis SEM. Mitochondrial DNA deletions and nuclear DNA fragmentation in testicular and epididymal human sperm. Hum Reprod 2002; 17:1565–1570.
41. Henkel R. DNA and its influence on fertilization and pregnancy. In: Kruger TF, Oehninger S, eds. Male Infertility—Diagnosis and Treatment. Oxon, United Kingdom: Informa UK Ltd., 2007:277–290.

37 Hematospermia (Hemospermia)

Nadja Engel and Hubert John

ETIOLOGY AND HISTORY

Hematospermia is defined as the macroscopic appearance of blood in semen or ejaculate. Hematospermia is considered a benign symptom, is painless that almost always resolves spontaneously, and is rarely associated with significant urological pathology and is most often considered to be idiopathic in nature. In general, hematospermia represents a trivial condition, but nevertheless, it is often alarming for the patient and his partner.

Hematospermia has been diagnosed by physicians for centuries and has been recognized by those such as Hippocrates, Galen, Paré, Morgagni, Velpeau, Guyon, and Fournier. The first comprehensive article by Hugues in 1894 was historically associated with sexual behaviur including excessive overindulgence, prolonged sexual abstinence, or interrupted coitus (1–3).

Hematospermia may manifest as a single episode or with periodic recurrences or may persist for month to years. In this chronic form is a disconcerting symptom that produces anxiety in sexually active men, who often have fear of cancer or sexually transmitted diseases (STD). Hematospermia may arise in association with pathology involving the prostate gland, seminal vesicles, vasa deferentia, ejaculatory ducts, urethra, urinary bladder, epididymis, or testes (Table 1). The most common entities that have been reported in men with hematospermia include prior prostate biopsy, prostate calculi, benign prostate hypertrophy, and inflammation or infection, such as chronic prostatitis or seminal vesiculitis, although majority of cases are thought to be idiopathic in etiology, with the most probable site of origin occurring in the seminal vesicles. Hematospermia also may be the result of neoplasm, vascular abnormalities, and systemic or iatrogenic factors. The exact incidence or prevalence of hematospermia is unknown. Persistent hematospermia can be defined as a continuous or recurrent bouts and most likely, the two forms represent similar underlying disease processes. Most men with hematospermia are young, younger than 40 years, with symptoms ranging from a few weeks to a few months in duration. Most men have an inflammatory cause or it remains idiopathic. The likelihood of recurrent hematospermia is seen in the older age group. Patients older than 40 years with persistent hematospermia associated with hematuria require urologic investigation (3–6).

It was reported that 77.5% of men had only experienced one or two episodes before visiting the urologist (4). A detailed, careful history and physical examination is the starting point in the evaluation of the man with hematospermia. It is important to obtain a detailed medical history, surgical history, such as urethral instrumentation, prostate biopsy, or injection of hem orrhoids, and drug history with regard to the use of anticoagulants and recent antithrombolytics. The amount, colour, duration, and frequency of hematospermia should be ascertained. Determination of the origin of bleeding within the ejaculation is the key, as postcoital hemorrhage from the patient's sexual partner related to vaginal microtears, menstruation, or gynecological and anorectal pathology may sometimes be mistaken for hematospermia. Also a history of prolonged and intense masturbation or sexual intercourse could lead to the congestion of genital organs and bleeding. Important is a history of a genital or perineal trauma or self-instrumentation in the urogenital region. One must ascertain the history of exposure to tuberculosis and the travel to endemic areas, where tuberculosis or schistosomiasis is found, as appropriate.

Important are also associated symptoms, such as weight loss, local or bony pain, fever, lower urinary tract symptoms, voiding complaints, and gross hematuria, that should raise the possibility of a urethral stricture or a vascular and enlarged prostate.

Sexually transmitted diseases may point to an infective cause such as urethritis, prostatitis, epididymitis, HIV, or condylomata acuminata. Other infective causes include bilharziosis, cytomegalovirus, and hydatid disease (1–14).

Inflammatory and Infection

These conditions are found to be the most common etiological factors and account for most hematospermia in the younger population and overall up to 40% of cases. Inflammatory processes cause mucosal irritation, hyperemia, and edema of the duct/gland, thus, leading to bleeding. This inflammation may be the result of traumatic, chemical, or prostate and seminal vesicle.

Infectious etiologies include viral, bacterial, mycobacterial, and parasitic infections. Seventy-five percent of the cases of hematospermia are caused by pathogens including herpes simplex virus in 42%, *Chlamydia trachomatis* in 33%, *Enterococcus faecalis* in 17%, and *Ureaplasma urealyticum* in 8% (1–14).

Obstruction

Hematospermia may also be caused by ductal obstruction and cyst formation. The mechanism involves dilatation and distention, resulting in rupture of mucosal blood vessels.

Tumors
Various benign tumors may cause hematospermia. Ectopic prostate tissue in the urethra, prostate polyps, and proliferative urethritis have been described as producing hematospermia.

Malignant tumors may be a rare cause of hematospermia, with prostate, testis, seminal vesicle tumors reported (12).

Vascular Abnormalities
Venous varicosities may also be the source of bleeding in hematospermia. In addition, vascular abnormalities associated with reproductive development in adolescence may lead to hematospermia. These conditions include arteriovenous malformation and hemangioma of the prostate, seminal vesicles and rarely, of the spermatic cord.

Trauma and Iatrogenic Causes
These are currently the most commonly seen etiologies. Transrectal prostate biopsy for prostate cancer screening is now the most common cause of hematospermia. Other causes are radiation therapy and brachytherapy for prostate cancer. There are also reports of urethral stent migration and urethral foreign bodies leading to hematospermia.

In addition, external traumas to the perineum and sex glands as well as pelvic fractures may result in hematospermia. Drugs such as warfarin and aspirin and antithrombolytic therapies are also associated.

Systemic Factors
Systemic disorders associated with hematospermia include hypertension, lymphoma, and bleeding diathesis. Risk factors for hematospermia in patients with hypertension include severe uncontrolled hypertension, increased serum creatinine, severe proteinuria, and renovascular disease. Hematological disorders may also responsible.

ANATOMY

The most frequent cause of hematospermia is inflammation or infection; the disorder may also occur because of benign or malignant neoplasm, calcification, and cysts. Pathological conditions were most frequently located in the seminal vesicles and the prostate; in the following section we have discussed about the anatomy of these structures.

The **seminal vesicles** are obliquely oriented paired accessory sex glands located superior and posterior to the prostate gland between the urinary bladder and the rectum in the extraperitoneal space and are partially covered by the parietal peritoneal lining. They are oval, rounded, or tubular in configuration; are widest in their mid-portions; and become narrow inferior medially to form the seminal vesicle excretory ducts. The normal seminal vesicles average approximately 3.1 ± 0.5 cm in length and 1.5 ± 0.4 cm in width on cross-sectional imaging. The paired vasa deferentia are continuations of the epididymis tails that ascend into the abdomen through the inguinal rings, follow the lateral pelvic wall and then curve posteriorly, medially and inferiorly to course along the superior–medial surface of the seminal vesicles, where they dilate and convolute to form the ampullary segments, usually at the level of the lateral margins of the seminal vesicles. The normal vas deferens is 30 to 45 cm in length, is of uniform calibre, and most often measures 1 mm in diameter. The normally ampullary portion of the vas deferens ranges from 3 to 7 cm in length and 2.7 to 10.0 mm in diameter and is symmetric in length bilaterally. The paired ampullae then join with the posterior medial aspects of the excretory ducts of the paired seminal vesicles to form the ejaculatory ducts at the superior surface of the prostate gland, which are symmetric and traverse the prostate gland to drain into the prostate urethra on both sides of the verumontanum. The normal ejaculatory duct is on an average 16.0 ± 3.5 mm in length and 1.5 ± 0.6 mm in width in its mid-portion, with slight tapering distally (3).

The **prostate gland** is a fibromuscular gland surrounding the prostate urethra at the bladder base within the extraperitoneal space. The prostate gland has an apex and a base, where the prostate apex is inferiorly located and the prostate base is superiorly located. The prostate gland may be separated into several zones. The peripheral zone is located posterior within the prostate gland from the base of the verumontanum to its apex, the transitional zone surrounds the proximal prostate urethra, and the central zone surrounds the transitional zone at the prostate base and the ejaculatory ducts. The surgical capsule is a band of tissue that separates the central gland from the peripheral zone and the true prostate capsule is a 2- to 3-mm fibromuscular layer that separates the peripheral zone of the prostate gland from the peri-prostate soft tissue, which is composed of fat and neurovascular bundles. The anterior fibromuscular stroma forms the entire anterior surface of the prostate gland as a thick nonglandular layer of tissue. Prostate ducts enter the base of the prostate ducts and the base of the prostate urethra and allow for the passage of prostate secretions (3).

DIAGNOSTIC PROCEDURES

Although differential diagnosis is comprehensive, the most frequent underlying causes are infections and inflammatory processes in the lower seminal passages.

History and Physical Examination

A detailed case history and medical history including surgical history is important, together with the physical examination, which is the start point in the evaluation of hematospermia. Also, one must ascertain a drug history and a history of exposure to tuberculosis and travel to endemic areas. Similar to history taking, physical examination is done in a logical and systematic manner. The physical examination besides morphological checking of the genital organs includes digital rectal examination. Rectal examination will allow assessment of the prostate gland and tenderness or induration may imply infection while a hard texture or nodule may be indicative of

Table 1 Causes of the Hematospermia

Inflammatory/infection
- Prostatitis
- Urethritis, papillary urethritis
- Epididymo–orchitis
- Seminal vesiculitis
- Genital-urinary tuberculosis (*Mycobacterium* spp.)
- Sexually transmitted disease: gonorrhoea (*Neisseria gonorrhea*), syphilis (*Treponema pallidum*), lymphogranuloma inguinale (*Chlamydia trachomatis*), herpes genitalis (herpes simplex virus), ulcus molle (*Haemophilus ducreyi*), *Ureaplasma urealyticum*, *Mycoplasma* spp., aids (HIV), condylomata acuminata (herpes virus/HPV 6, 11, 16, 18, 31, 33, 35), Morbus Bowen disease, erythroplasia Queyrat, bowenoide papulosis (herpes virus/HPV 16), cytomegalovirus
- Urinary tract infection in general: *Enterococcus faecalis*, *Streptococcus* spp., *Staphylococcus* spp., *Enterobacter* spp., *Proteus mirabilis*, *Pseudomonas* sp., *Escherichia coli*, mycosis (Candida albicans)
- Parasitic infections: bilharziosis/schistosomiasis (*Schistosoma japonicum/ haematobium/mansoni*), hydatid disease (*Echinococcus granulosus/multilocularis*), *Brucella* spp., trichomoniasis (*Trichomonas vaginalis*), *Gardnerella vaginalis*

Obstruction/congenital
- Prostate calcification
- Benign prostate hypertrophy
- Seminal vesicle calculi/dilatation/obstruction
- Ejaculatory duct calculi/dilatation/obstruction
- Seminal vesicles cysts
- Müllerian duct cysts
- Ejaculatorian duct cysts
- Utricular cyst
- Urethral stricture
- Seminal vesicle diverticula
- Prostate malakoplakia
- Seminal vesicles malakoplakia/adenomyosis

Tumors

Benign
- Condylomata acuminata of urethra or meatus urethrae
- Papillary adenoma of prostate urethra
- Leiomyoma of seminal vesicle

Malignant
- Prostate adenocarcinoma
- Prostate sarcoma
- Carcinoma of bladder or urethra
- Testicular carcinoma
- Seminal vesicle carcinoma
- Sarcoma of seminal vesicle
- Melanoma of the seminal vesicle
- Lymphoma of the seminal vesicle
- Secondary neoplasm involvement
- Distant carcinoma

Table 1 (Continued)

Vascular
- Prostate varices
- Prostate telangiectasia
- Hemangioma
- Posterior urethral veins
- Venous varicosities
- Arteriovenous malformation
- Excessive sex or masturbation

Trauma/iatrogenic
- Prostate biopsy
- Trauma of perineum, genitalia, pelvic
- Prostate injection or medication
- Seminal vesicle biopsy, injection or medication
- Postvasectomy, Postorchiectomy
- Brachytherapy, cryotherapy, thermotherapy, high-intensity focused ultrasound therapy of prostate
- Prostate or ureteral stents
- Self-instrumentation and autoerotic manipulation
- Hemorrhoidal injection or sclerotherapy
- Vaso-venous fistula or vesicle-venous fistula
- Lower ureteral extracorporeal shockwave lithotripsy

Systemic
- Hypertension
- Bleeding disorders
- Hemophilia purpurea, von Willebrand disease
- Chronic liver disease (cirrhosis of the liver)
- Leukemia, lymphoma
- Amyloidosis
- Treatment with anticoagulants, anti-fibrinolytics

Idiopathic

neoplasm especially in an older individual. On digital rectal examination, special attention should be given to the seminal vesicles and the presence of any midline masses. The groin, perineum, and external genitalia are examined with particular notice taken of the urethral meatus and needs to be done for the examination of trauma, condylomata, phimosis, or cancer. The urethral meatus should re-examined after the digital rectal examination for bloody discharge. The location of the urethra and identification of the testis with the spermatic cord is important, and the testicular and epididymis examination will also reveal the presence of infective element, including tuberculosis disease. Attention should be given to any skin lesions. The vasa deferentia should also be palpated along its course to identify any nodular induration or may show thickening. The abdomen should be palpated for any masses, in particular hepatomegaly, splenomegaly, pelvic swelling, and palpable bladder.

A full general examination including an assessment of blood pressure and temperature should be performed (1–3,6,13).

Laboratory Testing

The next step is the macroscopic analysis of the ejaculate particular for red coloration, clear hematospermia, red–yellow coloration, or hemato-pyospermia and must be enhanced by the microscopic semen analysis.

A "condom test" can be carried out where the patient is asked to collect the ejaculate in the condom, which is examined for blood. Hematospermia must also be distinguished from melanospermia, which is exceedingly rare. It is characterized by dark or black spotting in the ejaculate, which can be identified as melanin by chromatography.

Initial investigations in all cases should include full screening for sexually transmitted diseases and midstream urine with urine analysis and urine culture and will help to confirm the presence of urinary infection and hematuria. Traditionally, the incidence of positive culture is low at 6% to 29%. Urine cytology although not mentioned in the literature is a simple test to rule out the bladder pathology. If the history is suggestive of exposure to tuberculosis or schistosomiasis, urine analysis, semen and prostate secretion analysis is required for acid-fast bacilli, parasites, and fungal infections. If a sterile pyuria is noted, then further investigations are required to exclude tuberculosis as an underlying cause. Serum coagulation profile may reveal underlying bleeding disorders while the erythrocyte sedimentation rate may be raised in tuberculosis. Up to 13% of the cases of hematospermia were caused by tuberculosis. Semen analysis may be helpful for differentiating true hematospermia from other causes of ejaculate discoloration such as a malignant melanoma may also show the presence of pus cells, which then warrants further investigation in search of an infectious etiology. This includes semen culture, urethral swabs, mycobacterial culture, and viral serology. If sexually transmitted diseases are suspected, urethral cultures for *Neisseria gonorrhoeae* and *C. trachomatis* are obtained. Also should be used first void urine samples and genitourinary and serum specimens to test for *C. trachomatis, U. urealyticum,* and herpes simplex virus as well as standard bacterial cultures. In younger men, urethritis should be considered in the differential diagnosis and urethral swabs should be taken to exclude nonspecific and gonococcal urethritis.

Serum prostate antigen (PSA) level testing is performed in men $\geq$ 40 years with a family history, in patients who have a suspicious nodule on rectal examination, or men $\geq$ 50 years who are potentially at risk for prostate carcinoma. Blood should also be sent for complete blood count, urea and electrolytes, liver function tests, and clotting screen time if history and examination suggests chronic illness or bleeding diathesis (1–3,6,13).

Imaging Techniques

The next step in the diagnosis involves the noninvasive imaging techniques such as ultrasound, computed tomography (CT), magnetic resonance imaging (MRI), and transrectal ultrasonography (TRUS). With modern imaging techniques, the number of cases labelled as idiopathic has decreased dramatically. However, the dilemma lies in how far to investigate these patients. In the majority, hematospermia is a benign and self-limiting symptom, requiring only basic investigations and simple reassurance. However, it is the minority in whom hematospermia is the primary symptom of urological malignancy that must be diagnosed and treated accordingly.

Computed Tomography

CT was the first technique available for noninvasive imaging of the prostate and seminal vesicles and its limited resolution, radiation exposure, and technical complexity, and the lack of any studies on its use in hematospermia cases means that it has given way to the widespread use of TRUS (7). CT can identify calcifications, gross soft tissue masses, or cystic lesions of the prostate gland, seminal vesicles, and vasa deferentia but is less commonly used than TRUS or MRI in primary evaluation of the men with hematospermia.

Transrectal Ultrasonography

With the advent of biplane TRUS, the earlier imaging techniques are used only in specific cases. The relatively inexpensive techniques allow detailed real-time both axial and sagittal images with good resolution and without preparation or radiation. TRUS is a simple, safe, effective, and relatively noninvasive imaging technique, which can be performed as an outpatient procedure and allows objective evaluation of seminal vesicles, prostate, and ejaculatory ducts. Soft tissue masses such as polyps and tumors may be accurately delineated and measurements may be accurately obtained. Studies demonstrate that TRUS has an accurate diagnostic rate between 74% and 95% (2,12,13). Seminal vesicles were examined for the pathologies such as dilatation and calcification and space-occupying lesions such as cysts and masses. Ejaculatory ducts were examined for the presence of calculi, cysts, and dilatation. The prostate was investigated for the presence of a benign hyperplasia, calcifications, and prostatitis. The diagnosis were made according to the volume on the shape of the prostate and its internal echoes on TRUS. Especially, echoes from peripheral zone of prostate were evaluated for prostate malignancies (11). Ultrasound should be considered as the definitive primary screening modality for patients with hematospermia. The judicious use of TRUS can detect abnormalities such as calculi, obstruction, inflammation, and neoplasm of the prostate, ejaculatory duct, seminal vesicles, and ampullary portions of the vasa deferentia (7,8). Patients are placed in the left lateral decubitus position or lithotomy position. Grayscale images are obtained with a 5.0 to 9.0 MHz ultrasonography transducer in the axial and sagittal planes. Color- and power-Doppler images may also be acquired, particularly when prostate is suspected and prostate biopsy is contemplated. TRUS-guided aspiration or biopsy of the seminal vesicles or prostate gland may be performed to further elucidate the site of bleeding, to provide a definitive diagnosis if a lesion is detected, or to confirm the presence of ejaculatory duct obstruction (14). TRUS should be the imaging technique of choice in the evaluation of patients with hematospermia (7).

Magnetic Resonance Imaging

The current gold standard for imaging the accessory sex glands and their ducts is the MRI (13). The latter can detect changes in anatomical structure secondary to endocrine therapy, radiation, inflammatory disorders, or neoplasm, but the greatest advantage of MRI over TRUS is its ability to reveal hemorrhage in the seminal vesicles or prostate. Endorectal coil MRI with its excellent soft tissue contrast provide radiation-free multiplanar anatomic evaluation. It is operator independent and can be performed when TRUS is unsatisfactory or nondiagnostic. MRI may be slightly more sensitive than TRUS in detecting abnormalities (13).

Classical X-ray

The classical X-ray examinations were performed as plain film, vasography, and seminal vesiculography or vasovesical vesiculography. With help of these methods, the calcification and malignant diseases of the male genitalia can be identified. Vasovesiculography is rarely performed today and is mainly reserved for men with azoospermia with normal spermatogenesis on testicular biopsy, who are suspected to have aplasia or occlusion of the vasa deferentia and ejaculatory ducts.

The excretory urogram should be used to search for urinary tract calcification and is helpful for identifying the etiology in 6% of hematospermia cases (3,6).

Urethrocystoscopy

So far as precise diagnosis is not available using modern imaging methods, direct rigid or flexible urethrocystoscopy must be performed to observe possible condyloma, polyps, papilloma, ectopic tissues, and urethral and urinary bladder neoplasm as well as varices in the bladder neck, prostate, and urethra. Under direct vision, papillary urethritis, urethral foreign bodies, and stones can also be ascertained. Rigid urethrocystoscopy allows direct examination of the prostate urethra, bladder neck, and bladder, but it may miss intermittent bleeding sources. Flexible urethrocystoscopy allows the operator to retroflex and visualize the bladder neck and identify potential vessel varicosities (8).

Malignancies diagnosed by imaging techniques must be histologically verified by biopsies.

Table 2 shows the importance of different forms of investigations and the association for the evidence. Investigations in most cases of hematospermia are inconclusive but can be associated with serious history and examination. The diagnosis of the cases is also based on the findings of investigations (1).

IMAGING APPEARANCE OF PATHOLOGIES ASSOCIATED WITH HEMATOSPERMIA

Hemorrhage within the prostate gland, seminal vesicles, ejaculatory ducts, or vasa deferentia tends to be visualized in its subacute form in men with hematospermia; typically has increased echogenicity on TRUS, high signal intensity on T1-weighted images, and variable T2-weighted signal intensity on MRI and attenuation of > 20 Houndsfield units on CT.

Table 2 Investigation, Differential Diagnosis, and Evidence (1)

Investigation	Importance	Evidence
Medical/surgical history	+++	Differential diagnosis
Physical examination	++	Probable cause finding
Urine analysis/urine culture	++	Urinary tract infection
Culture of midstream and prostate secretion	++	Urethritis/prostatitis
Urethrocystoscopy	++	Strictures/stones/prostate varices
Transrectal ultrasonography	++	Cysts/calcification/ pathological structure
Magnetic resonance imaging	++	Morphology/pathological structure
Semen culture	++	Infection of semen
Complete blood count	+	Bleeding disease
Vasography	–	Low
Vesiculography	–	Low
Excretory urogram	–	Low

Inflammatory Disease

A chronic prostatitis is common and often associated with seminal vasculitis. On TRUS may be seen hyperechoic or hypoechoic foci, capsular irregular or thickening, and irregularity of the periurethral zone calcification from the chronic inflammatory cells. On MRI the signal intensity of the prostate gland is normal, but the T1- and T2-weighted intensity is low as contour deformation although a prostate carcinoma may also occur.

Schistosomiasis (bilharziosis) infection of the prostate and seminal vesicles is rare and should be considered when calcification of the prostate gland, seminal vesicles, or bladder wall are seen at TRUS or CT. The diagnosis can be definitively established through microscopic visualization of schistosoma eggs in the seminal fluid.

Mycobacterial infection can also lead to calcification at TRUS or CT and may be seen on MRI within the prostate gland as the watermelon sign, which is an abscess formation with calcification.

Amyloidosis is localized with amyloid deposits in the lamina propria of the seminal vesicles and in the walls of vessels or within the muscular tissue. On MRI may be seen nodular thickening. Definitive diagnosis can be made through microscopy when positive staining with Congo red and demonstration of typical green birefringence in polarized light are visualized.

Neoplasm Disease

Prostate carcinoma is the most commonly diagnosed malignancy (11). It most commonly arises from the peripheral zone of the prostate gland and occasionally from the central zone. On

TRUS, prostate carcinoma is most often hypoechoic relative to the normal peripheral zone but may sometimes be isoechoic or even hyperechoic. Asymmetry in prostate size, capsular distortion, and loss of differentiation between the central gland and the peripheral zone may also be seen. On MRI prostate cancer is typically intermediate in signal intensity on T1-weighted images and low intensity on T2-weighted images. Also may be seen extracapsular spread of tumor, pelvic lymphadenopathy, and osseous metastasis.

Prostate sarcomas are rare with variable echogenicity and signal intensity related in part to variable amounts of cystic change or necrosis.

Primary or secondary malignancies of the seminal vesicles cause irregular enlargement with focally or diffusely sometimes infiltrative growth or direct involvement of the surrounding structures. Seminal vesicle malignancies are rare.

Cysts

Cysts that may be encountered in men with hematospermia include ejaculatory duct cyst, seminal vesicle cysts, Cowper's gland cysts, utricular cysts, Müllerian duct cysts, and gland cysts. Congenital or acquired cysts of ejaculatory ducts may also lead to hematospermia. Dilatations of the ducts are usually associated with calculi.

An enlarged utricle is common in childhood and may be associated with intersex problems, cryptorchidism, hypospadias, or conditions including prune belly syndrome, Down's syndrome, and posterior urethral valves.

The Müllerian duct cyst is a congenital cystic remnant and is the homologue of the uterus and paranephric duct. On imaging, utricular and Müllerian duct cysts typically occur in the middle line of the prostate gland, whereas ejaculatory duct cysts usually occur in the paramedian location and seminal vesicles cysts occur laterally within the seminal vesicles. Müllerian duct cysts often have a teardrop shape and occur beyond the posterior–superior margin, whereas utricular cysts occur within the prostate gland. The Müllerian duct cysts do not communicate with the urethra or ejaculate duct, whereas utricular cysts communicate with the posterior urethra or ejaculatory duct. Ejaculatory duct cysts are rare, less common than Müllerian duct cyst, and are usually the result of partial distal obstruction of the ejaculatory duct. On TRUS, these appear as simple cysts and on MRI as round or oval unilocular cystic lesions in a paramedian location of the ejaculatory duct within the prostate gland.

Seminal vesicle cysts are an uncommon congenital abnormality associated with autosomal dominant polycystic kidney disease and renal anomalies such as a renal agenesis and ectopic ureteral insertion. On TRUS, these appear as round or oval anechoic lesions and on MRI or CT these are visualized as fluid-density unilocular cystic lesions. Seminal vesicle cysts contain fructose and spermatozoa. Cowper's gland duct or gland cysts usually occur in the children and rarely in adults and may be congenital or acquired. On MRI, a fluid-density unilocular cyst is typically seen to the bulbomembranous portion of the urethra.

Ejaculatory duct obstruction is a rare cause of infertility, clinically with oligozoospermia or azoospermia. TRUS, MRI, or CT may reveal absence of the vasa deferentia, dilatation of the duct, seminal vesicle with or without calculi, or another cyst formation (3,6,7,9,10).

Simple cysts are anechoic on TRUS with thin walls, round or oval in shape, and increase through transmission, whereas complex cysts may show increased echogenicity, may have internal septations, may have wall thickening, or may contain calculi (7). On MRI or CT, cysts have low signal intensity, whereas proteinaceous or hemorrhagic cysts may increase the signal intensity of < 20 Houndsfield units.

Dilatation/Calcification/Calculi

Pathologies of seminal vesicles constitute one of the most important group of pathologies that are likely to cause hematospermia. Most frequent pathological condition of seminal vesicle is dilatation. Theoretically, dilatation of seminal vesicles may be caused by inflammatory changes or an obstruction of the ejaculatory duct. Isolated dilatation of seminal vesicles may be a part of aging process. The size of seminal vesicles may vary with the frequency of sexual activities.

Calcification of seminal vesicles is another finding found in cases of hematospermia. A mechanical trauma to the prostate duct may be intraductal calcification during ejaculation, which may result in hematospermia. Another finding is calculi of ejaculatory ducts in men presenting with hematospermia. Hematospermia is the most frequent symptom in cases of calcification of seminal vesicles and calculi of the ejaculatory ducts. Especially, intermittent, spontaneously remitting hematospermia may be caused by these calculi.

When visualized, these typically appear with very low signal intensity and have a very high attenuation on CT. On TRUS appear focal regions of increased echogenicity and may occur within the prostate. More than 50% of prostate calculi are composed in part by components of urine (2,3,6,7,9,13).

Benign Prostate Hypertrophy

In patients older than 40 years, hematospermia can also be caused by a benign prostate hyperplasia.

The benign prostate hypertrophy develops in 80% from the transitional zone of the prostate gland during aging. The result is the enlargement of the central gland. On TRUS appears a hypoechoic enlargement of the gland, which may be compressed and distorted sometimes with variably echogenic nodule formation with a well-defined hypoechoic surgical capsula. This is associated with an overall increase in the prostate size and volume. Also may be seen cyst formation and calcification in the region of surgical capsule associated with clinical increased postvoid residual of the urinary bladder. On MRI appears a heterogeneous nodular enlargement of the central gland. Associated trabeculation, diverticula formation, or diffuse wall thickening of urinary bladder may also be encountered as a result of chronic outlet obstruction.

THERAPEUTIC PROCEDURES

There is no specific therapy option in the treatment of hematospermia and is based rationally on the examination results. Most patients can be treated with minimal investigations and simple reassurance (1,13). Treatment for hematospermia depends on the underlying pathological condition. The principal aim of the management is to exclude serious causes such as prostate and bladder cancer and treat any other underlying cause. If no pathology is found, then it is important to allay the anxiety and reassure the patient. The treatment of various pathogens with modalities such as systemic and local anti-inflammatory therapy, uro-oncological surgical and radiological treatment, transurethral interventions, and internal medical therapy, such as antihypertensive, anticoagulant therapy, and treatment of hematological disorders may be taken into consideration (1,2,13).

With infectious or inflammatory causes, the use of appropriate antiviral, antibiotic, or antiparasitic agents is indicated according to the sensitivity of the cultured organism. Empirical treatment may be appropriate when infection is suspected but culture is negative as it often occurs with *C. trachomatis* or *Bacteroides* spp. In these cases, treatment may be given is a full course of one of the tetracyclines or metronidazole. Individuals with recurrent hematospermia and those who are middle aged need specialist urological assessment and investigations. If infection is suspected, a course of 5-aminoquinolones such as ciproxin or trimethroprim–sulfamethoxazole and doxycycline combination would be beneficial even if the urine cultures are negative. Data suggest that with appropriate antimicrobiological treatment hematospermia should resolve in all cases. The choice for treatment of schistosomiasis is praziquantel.

Hematospermia caused by localized amyloid deposition in the seminal vesicles is intermittent and does not require any particular therapeutic intervention other than patient reassurance and long-term follow-up (1).

Cystic lesions of the seminal vesicles, prostate gland, ejaculatory ducts, or embryonal remnant may be treated with ultrasound- or CT-guided aspiration.

Transurethral unroofing of cyst or ductal obstruction as well as endourological and laparoscopic excision of seminal vesicle cysts can be done (5). Ejaculatory duct obstruction is managed by a transurethral incision at the duct opening (10). Lesions such as prostate varicosities, polyps, ectopic prostate tissues, and ejaculatory duct obstruction can be managed by transurethral resection, fulguration, dilatation, or incision (10).

Recent empirical evidence may suggest a role for antifibrinolytic drugs, especially finasteride for treating certain causes of hematospermia.

Finally, the laboratory and internal medical diagnosis pertains the types of coagulopathy and incidental revision of the anticoagulant or antihypertensive therapy.

Hematospermia is rare with 0.5% in a prostate cancer screening population (11). When a man presents with hematospermia, prostate cancer should be vigilantly performed since hematospermia is associated with an increased risk of prostate cancer (2,11). In some patients with persistent or recurrent hematospermia, it could be the only symptom of prostate cancer (2). In high-risk individuals and middle-aged individuals with a family history of prostate cancer, a follow-up with serum prostrate antigen over a period of time is desirable.

REFERENCES

1. John H, Ludwig M. Diagnostic and therapeutic procedures for hemospermia. Urologe 2003; 42:99–103.
2. Kumar P, Kapoor S, Nargund V. Haematospermia—A systemic review. Ann R Coll Surg Engl 2006; 88:339–342.
3. Torigian DA, Ramchandani P. Hematospermia: Imaging findings. Abdom Imaging 2007; 32:29–49.
4. Jones DJ. Haematospermia: A prospective study. Br J Urol 1991; 67:88–90.
5. Khan MS, Zaheer LU, Ahmed K, et al. Low-grade phyllodes tumour of the seminal vesicle treated with laparoscopic excision. Nat Clin Pract Urol 2007; 4(7).
6. Papp GK, Kopa Z, Szabo F, et al. Aetiology of haemospermia. Andrologia 2003; 35:317–320.
7. Yagci C, Kupeli S, Tok C, et al. Efficiency of transrectal ultrasonography in the evaluation of hematospermia. J Clin Imaging 2004; 28:286–290.
8. Rubinowicz DM, Soloway MS, Lief M, et al. Hemospermia and expressed tumour in the urethra: An unusual presentation of ductal carcinoma of the prostate. J Urol 2000; 163:915.
9. Furuya S, Kato H. A clinical entity of cystic dilatation of the utricle associated with hemospermia. J Urol 2005; 174:1039–1042.
10. Fuse H, Nishio R, Murakami K, et al. Transurethral incision for hematospermia caused by ejaculatory duct obstruction. Arch Androl 2003; 49:433–438.
11. Han M, Brannigam RE, Antenor JA, et al. Association of hemospermia with prostate cancer. J Urol 2004; 172:2189–2192.
12. Maheshkumar P, Otite U, Gordon S, et al. Testicular tumour presenting as hematospermia. J Urol 2001; 165:188.
13. Imran A, Nalagatla SK. Hemospermia. J Urol 2006; 177:1613–1618.
14. Wang LJ, Tsui KH, Wong YC, et al. Arterial bleeding in patients with intractable hematospermia and concomitant hematuria: A preliminary report. Urology 2006; 68:938–941.

38 Prostatic disease and male sexual dysfunction

Francesco Montorsi

CLINICAL CASE

A 54-year-old man arrives in your office for urinary symptoms. He is a heavy smoker (20 cigarettes/ day) and he is taking no medications. At physical examination, the patient is overweight (BMI = 28.4 kg/m^2.) and the external genitalia appear normal. The patient reports an increased frequency in voiding the bladder, with a small amount of urine per micturition in the last year. He does not complain nicturia. When specifically asked for, the patient reports an initial erectile dysfunction, which worsen in the last six months. He complains insufficient erections to complete a sexual intercourse in the last three months.

INTRODUCTION

Historically, lower urinary tract symptoms (LUTS) and erectile dysfunction (ED) were considered a consequence of the advancing age. In fact, large epidemiological studies demonstrated an increasing incidence of these medical conditions in the elderly. Compared to men in their 40s, men in their 50s have a 2-fold increase in their relative risk (RR) of ED. This increases to 5-fold in RR for men in their 60s (1). The Massachusetts Male Aging Study (MMAS) detailed that 52% of men from 40 to 70 years have some degree of ED, and 2/3 of these men have moderate to severe symptoms (2). Similarly, the histological presence of benign prostatic hyperplasia (BPH) steadily increases from 20% to 70% in the fourth versus the eighth decade of life (3,4). Moreover, the presence of moderate-to-severe LUTS occurs in about one-quarter of men in their 50s, one-third of men in their 60s, and about half of all men aged 80 years or older (5).

However, a variety of recent large-scale epidemiological studies analyzing very large cohorts of patients have convincingly documented an age-independent relationship between LUTS and ED, leading to a new paradigm in the fields of research, diagnosis, and treatment. In the most comprehensive study conducted to date on the association of age, LUTS, concomitant comorbidities, and male sexual dysfunction, Rosen et al. of the multinational survey of the aging male (the MSAM-7) analyzed survey results from 12,815 men aged 50 to 80 years from both the United States and Europe (6). Overall, the results of this study strongly confirmed the relationship between LUTS and sexual dysfunction in men, independent of the effects of age, other comorbidities, and lifestyle actors. In the MSAM-7, the overall prevalence of LUTS of any severity was 90%, with the prevalence of moderate-to-severe LUTS significantly related to age ($p < 0.0001$). The overall prevalence of ED (defined as difficulty achieving an erection) in the MSAM-7 was 49%, with 10% reporting complete absence of erections. The prevalence of ED was age-dependent, with rates of 31%, 55%, and 76% in men aged 50 to 59 years, 60 to 69 years, and 70 to 80 years, respectively. The multivariable analysis demonstrated that the severity of LUTS was an independent risk factors for ED, after adjusting for age, medical comorbidities, tobacco use, and alcohol consumption. Furthermore, the presence of LUTS was a stronger risk factors for ED than diabetes, hypertension, heart disease, or hyperlipidemia. This strong association between LUTS and ED was confirmed by another recent population-based study, which was conducted in Denmark. In men, the prevalence of LUTS was 39% and the prevalence of ED was 29%. In multivariate logistic regression analyses, LUTS was an independent predictor of ED (7).

Based on these epidemiological evidence, a large variety of authors investigated the possible mechanisms underlying these two common medical conditions. Several explanations have been suggested as a possible common pathway between ED and LUTS, which include (*i*) NOS/NO levels decreased or altered in the prostate and penile smooth muscle (SM), (*ii*) autonomic hyperactivity effects on LUTS, prostate growth and ED, (*iii*) increased Rho-kinase activation/endothelin activity, and (*iv*) prostate and penile ischemia.

HYPOTHESIS 1

Decreased NOS/NO Levels Theory

This theory closely adheres to the nitrergic innervation–SM cell relaxation molecular mechanism, which has a well-demonstrated role in the pathogenesis of ED. A reduced production of nitric oxide synthase (NOS)/nitric oxide (NO) in the pelvis, which includes both the penis and prostate, may represent a common link between the two diseases (Fig. 1).

The evidence of a potential single unifying concept relies on a recent observation by Bloch and colleagues, which reported that NOS/NO production of the prostate is reduced in BPH (transition zone) when compared to normal prostate tissue (8,9). It logically follows that prostate tissue levels of NO/NOS are reduced in BPH progression, which then reduces prostatic tone relaxation.

This theory is supported by some evidence in which BPH tissue NADPH-d staining and nNOS immunohistochemistry shows a qualitative decrease in the otherwise dense nitrinergic innervation of glandular epithelium, fibromuscular stroma, and blood vessels. The reduction of nNOS gene expression with increased age in adult rat prostates supports the biologic plausibility of this theory (10). A recent publication by Waldkirch and

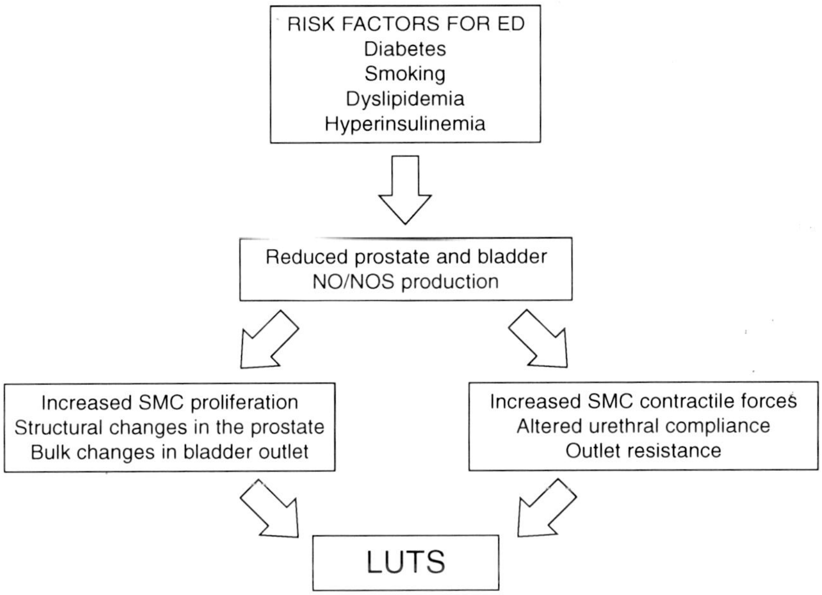

Figure 1 The NOS/NO hypothesis. Nitric oxide synthase (NOS)/nitric oxide (NO) levels decreased or altered in the prostate and penile smooth muscle.

colleagues corroborates this theory by analyzing the presence of a cGMP-dependent protein kinase-1 (cGKI), one of the downstream targets for cGMP in the process of muscle relaxation (11). The authors demonstrated the presence of cGKI isoforms alpha and beta in the transition zone of human prostate tissue. In addition, they demonstrated the co-localization of α-actin, cGMP, and cGKI isoforms, which provides further evidence for a significant role of the NO/cGMP pathway in the regulation of SM contractility in human prostate tissue. The same protein has been isolated in human penile erectile tissue, which further strengthens the NO/NOS hypothesis as a common link between ED and LUTS (12).

The physiologic role of NOS/NO is not well characterized in the prostate, the bladder, and the act of urination. In order to support the hypothesis for the reduction of NOS/NO as potential factor in LUTS, a NOS-mediated prostatic SM relaxation must occur at a critical point in the voiding reflex or as part of normal compliance. A decreased NOS activity in BPH tissue should result in altered prostatic tone and subsequently contribute to the dynamic aspect of LUTS. However, only limited data are available on the role of NOS/NO in the mechanism of voiding and controversial results have been obtained with PDE5 inhibitors in LUTS relief. The first report of an interaction between PDE5 inhibitors and LUTS improvement was published in 2002 by Sairam et al. (13) In a cohort of 112 men, the authors investigated the relationship between International Prostate Symptom Score (IPSS), International Index of Erectile Function (IIEF), and sildenafil oral medication at baseline and after three months of treatment. Sildenafil was used 'on-demand' before sexual intercourse or once daily before bedtime in case of no sexual activity. At the end of the three-month interval, all men with initially severe LUTS (6%) turned to moderate LUTS and 60% of those with initially moderate LUTS (26%) turned to mild LUTS. However, the global IPSS decreased during therapy but this was not shown to be a statistically significant improvement. Mulhall and colleagues corroborated those preliminary results by evaluating 48 men with a mean age of 62 years (14). These men had a baseline IPSS >10 and received sildenafil because of ED for three months. In this small cohort of patients, the mean reduction in the IPSS was 4.6 points ($p = 0.013$). In total, 60% of men improved their IPSS with 35% showing an at least 4-point IPSS improvement.

Recently, McVary and colleagues published the first randomized, placebo-controlled trial on the role of PDE5 inhibitors in the treatment of LUTS. A total of 369 men with a mean age of 60 years entered this trial. They investigated the effect of sildenafil for 12 weeks in participants presenting with both disorders, ED and LUTS in a 1:1 randomization ratio between sildenafil (50–100 mg/daily) and placebo.

Besides the improvement of the IIEF-EF domain, score in the sildenafil group (+9.2 vs. +1.9) under placebo ($p < 0.0001$), there was also reduction in the IPSS of −6.3 (sildenafil) versus −1.9 in the placebo group after 12 weeks ($p < 0.0001$) (15). However, a significant effect on urinary flow or any objective urodynamic parameter was not observed, suggesting a psychological improvement in general health because of PDE5 inhibitor effect on erectile function.

HYPOTHESIS 2

Autonomic Hyperactivity—Metabolic Syndrome Theory

This theory relies on the hypothesis that a dysregulation of the autonomic nervous system (ANS) provides a particular environment that may induce prostatic growth. Conversely, the

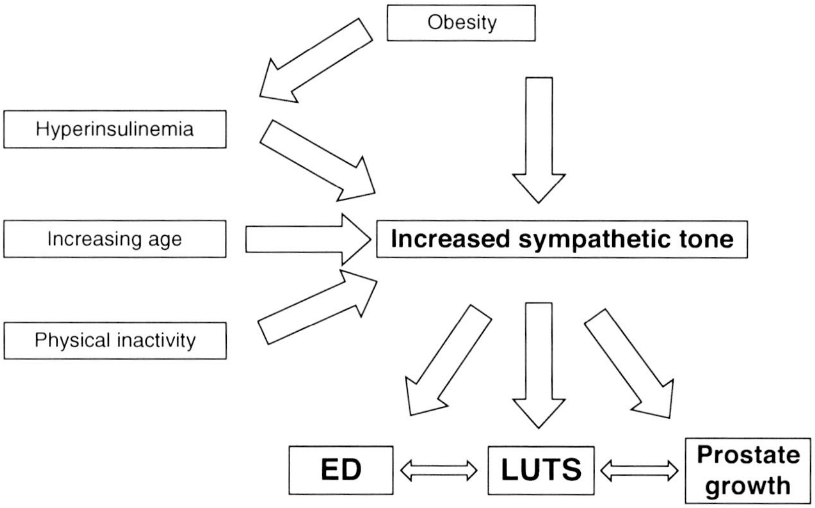

Figure 2 The autonomic hyperactivity/metabolic syndrome hypothesis.

absence of ANS stimulation should result in a regression of the gland. In this perspective, LUTS secondary to BPH is a part of the metabolic syndrome that includes glucose intolerance, insulin resistance, obesity, dyslipidemia, and hypertension, all known as risk factors for ED.

Several evidences support this theory. In 1994, McVary and colleagues demonstrated that the deafferentation of sympathetic fibers from the prostate leads to a decrease in ventral prostate weight, DNA, and protein content. Similarly, a predominance of the autonomic fibers is translated into an enlargement of the prostate gland (16). Further studies corroborated the initial findings and several investigators demonstrated an association between increased adrenergic tone in prostatic hyperplasia and ED (17–19). An experimental model purposed by Persson and colleagues observed that spontaneously hypertensive rats develop autonomic hyperactivity, prostate hyperplasia and ED, and have increased voiding frequency compared to controls (20). Similarly, in the same animals there is an altered response to cavernous nerves stimulation, which leads to SM contraction and, in turn, to ED. The acute administration of antihypertensive therapies led to an improvement in both LUTS and erectile function. The improvement in erectile function after a brief aggressive treatment may be related to improvement in structurally based vascular resistance within the penis and the decrease in responsiveness of α_1-adrenoceptor-mediated erectolytic signaling (21).

ANS hyperactivity is associated with signs and symptoms of LUTS secondary to BPH in humans also. As demonstrated by McVary and colleagues, an increased sympathetic tone (as measured by changes in blood pressure, heart rate, urinary and serum catecholamine levels) was significantly associated with the level of LUTS. After controlling all the other cofactors, (including age, BMI, abdominal obesity, C-peptide and insulin levels, physical inactivity), an increased autonomic tone was independently associated to LUTS. Moreover, autonomic hyperactivity was directly related to the severity of LUTS and to a lesser extent to the prostate total volume and transitional zone volume (22). Given that increased sympathetic activity is strongly associated with LUTS, it is highly likely that a relationship between this increased tone and ED also exists. In fact, the factors suggested as possibly affecting LUTS are all well-established risk factors for ED development and severity. It was hypothesized that noradrenaline and α1-adrenoceptors that mediate adrenergic contraction of SM in the prostate, bladder neck, urethra, and the corpus cavernosum constitute the common link. This putative explanation is attractive because it links established clinical physiologic findings of LUTS, BPH, and ED with an established basic science support (Fig. 2).

HYPOTHESIS 3

Increased Rho-Kinase Activation/Endothelin Activity

Several investigators have suggested that the alternate pathways of SM relaxation and contraction may be responsible for the relationship between ED and bladder outlet obstruction (BOO).

SM contraction has been attributed to an increase in intracellular calcium (Ca^{2+}) concentration. However, the sensitivity of muscle fibers to Ca^{2+} levels is under the regulation of several control mechanisms and proteins, which may translate into an increased SM tone, independently from an increase in intracellular Ca^{2+}. One of these regulatory systems involves the Rho-kinase pathway.

Base science studies demonstrated that Rho-kinase is activated by a G-protein, RhoA, thought to be coupled to excitatory α_1-adrenoceptors, resulting in the inhibition of SM myosin regulatory light chain (MLC) phosphatase (Fig. 3). This leads to an increase in MLC phosphorylation by basal level activity of MLC kinase and subsequent SM contraction with no changes in intracellular Ca^{2+} concentration. Rho-kinase can be regulated by levels of NO, with increases in NO altering

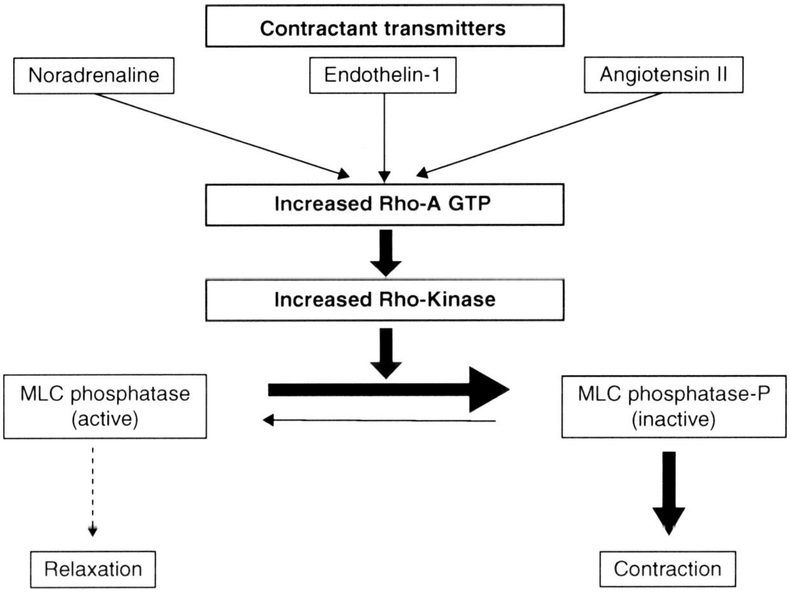

Figure 3 The increased Rho-kinase activation/endothelin activity hypothesis.

calcium concentrations (23). Rees and colleagues demonstrated that Rho-kinase is deeply involved in the regulation of SM tone, especially in condition of high basal tone (24). Using a specific inhibitor of Rho-kinase, the authors showed a decrease in human and rat prostatic SM cell proliferation and a decrease in SM contractions after adrenergic stimulation in rat prostatic tissue. An increased expression and activity of Rho-kinase is associated to an increase in calcium sensitivity of the contractile machine. A dysregulation of the Rho-kinase pathways has been demonstrated in spontaneously hypertensive rats, in the detrusor, and in the corpus cavernosum SM of rabbits with partial BOO (25,26). Chang et al. reported that corpus cavernosum SM from rabbits with partial BOO showed a broad range of molecular and functional differences versus controls. These changes include increased penile SMC contractility, reduced relaxation, and modest alterations in total SM myosin, decreased innervation, and increased SM bundle size. Interestingly enough, the same increase in calcium sensitivity has been recorded in vascular SM in hypertensive patient (27). Moreover, several factors potentially involved in the pathogenesis of both LUTS and ED (such as endothelin-1 and angiotensin II) depend on Rho-kinase activity, which acts as downstream in the regulatory pathway of SM contraction. Taken together, those observations suggest an intriguing role of Rho-kinase as a common link between the development of both ED and LUTS.

HYPOTHESIS 4

Pelvic Atherosclerosis

This theory relies on the presence of several vascular risk factors in the ageing men, which are responsible for diffuse atherosclerosis. The ubiquity of this disease suggests its possible involvement in the etiology of BPH. Risk factors such as hypertension, smoking, hypercholesterolemia, and diabetes mellitus, which are known for affecting erectile function, may be also responsible for the onset and development of LUTS (Fig. 4).

Animal models mimicking pelvic ischemia and hypercholesterolemia show a striking similarity in the SM alterations of the detrusor and corpora cavernosa. As observed by Azadzoi and colleagues, atherosclerosis-induced chronic bladder ischemia shifted the volume–pressure curve to the left and caused severe bladder fibrosis in rabbit models. At histological evaluation, the percentage of detrusor SM was severely decreased in the chronic bladder ischemia group compared with the control group. Moreover, the authors detected an increased TGF1-beta expression, as marker of ischemia-induced loss of SM fibers (28,29). Similarly, hypercholesterolemia also affects the bladder structure and compliance, albeit to a significantly lesser extent. Some years later, for prostate level, the same group detected the same structural changes highlighted in the bladder structure. In fact, using the same animal models, the authors described a significant thickening and fibrosis of the prostatic stroma as well as a cystic atrophy of the epithelium in the chronic prostate ischemia group, as compared to the control subjects. Moreover, the authors hypothesized the involvement of the impaired NO pathway in the decreased relaxation of the ischemic tissue (30). Further evidence was provided by Azadzoi et al. Using a rabbit model, they demonstrated the presence of increased prostatic tissue contraction and altered cGMP release in atherosclerotic rats. Pharmacological treatment with doxazosine and/or PDE5 inhibitors significantly reduced the SM contraction and their combined effect was more effective. The authors conclude that chronic pelvic ischemia was the underlying factor and led to both the impairment in muscle relaxation and structural changes. Moreover, they demonstrated that stimulators of NO

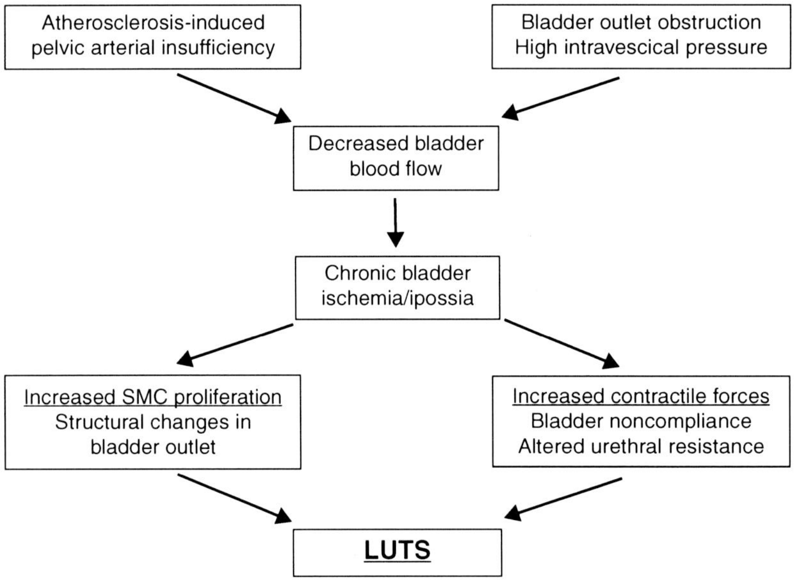

Figure 4 Atherosclerosis-induced prostate and penile ischemia hypothesis.

synthesis and cGMP production enhanced the efficacy of doxazosin in decreasing prostatic tissue contraction (31).

This hypothesis is very intriguing as it is likely to be compatible with all previous theories. Chronic ischemia may induce ANS hyperactivity, reduce NOS expression, and upregulate Rho-kinase (32).

PHOSPHODIESTERASES (PDE) IN LOWER URINARY TRACT AND PDE INHIBITORS FOR TREATMENT OF BOTH ED AND LUTS

Lower urinary tract (LUT) SMs can be relaxed by drugs that increase the intracellular concentrations of cyclic adenosine monophosphate (cAMP) and cyclic guanosine monophosphate (cGMP) (33,34). In LUT SMs, increases in cAMP seem to have a main role in bladder relaxation, whereas cGMP is important for urethral relaxation. The inactivation of both cAMP and cGMP is mediated by phosphodiesterases (PDEs), a heterogeneous group of hydrolytic enzymes. Because of their central role in SM tone regulation, PDEs have become an attractive target for drug development. The PDE5 inhibitors are nowadays routinely used for the treatment of erectile dysfunction. Therefore, it is of extreme interest to explore the role of PDEs and PDE inhibitors in the pathophysiology and treatment of LUTS.

PDEs IN THE PROSTATE

As previously described, NO/NOS synthase pathway may plays a fundamental role in the prostate. Moreover, several previous reports highlighted the presence of several precursors of the NO/cGMP system in the human prostate (35–37). Uckert and colleagues demonstrated the presence of mRNA transcripts encoding for at least 14 different isoforms of PDE in the human prostatic tissue, including transcripts encoding for PDE 1, 2, 4, 5, 7, 8, 9, and 10 in the various anatomical regions of the human prostate (38). Moreover, they investigated the effects of various PDE inhibitors on noradrenaline (NA)-mediated contractions in isolated strips of human prostatic SM. These autonomic-mediated contractions were reversed by forskolin (adenylate cyclase activator), sodium nitroprusside (NO donor), and inhibitors of PDE4 and PDE5. The authors conclude that their observation may support the use of inhibitors of PDE4 and PDE5 for treating urinary obstruction secondary to benign prostatic enlargement (39).

PDEs IN THE BLADDER

Unlike the prostate, cAMP seems to be more important than cGMP in the bladder and detrusor muscle. Truss and colleagues demonstrated the predominant presence of PDE1 and suggested that the cAMP pathway and the calcium/calmodulin-stimulated PDE1 may be involved in the detrusor physiology (40,41). Significant relaxation of human detrusor muscle in vitro, paralleled by increases in cyclic nucleotide levels, was induced by papaverine, vinpocetine (a nonselective inhibitor of PDE1), and forskolin, confirming that the cAMP pathway and PDE1 is important in regulation of detrusor SM tone (42). Similarly, PDE4 has been implicated in the control of bladder SM tone. PDE4 inhibitors reduced the in vitro contractile response in several animal models (43), and also suppressed rhythmic bladder contractions of isolated guinea pig bladder tissue (44).

PDE INHIBITORS FOR TREATING LUTS

Based on their preclinical data suggesting that PDE1 inhibitors might be beneficial in regulating detrusor SM contractility, Truss et al. presented preliminary clinical data on the use of the PDE1 inhibition. They administered vinponectine (a selective PDE1 inhibitor) to patients affected by overactive bladder and not responding to standard antimuscarinic therapy. Their findings suggested a possible role for vinpocetine in the treatment of urgency, frequency, urge incontinence, and possibly, low-compliance bladder and interstitial cystitis (45). The same group presented a larger randomized, double blind, placebo-controlled, multicenter trial with vinpocetine versus placebo in overactive bladder patients. The results showed a tendency in favor of vinponectine over placebo; however, statistical significance was reached only for a reduced micturition frequency in males ($p = 0.05$) (42).

There is abundant information available on the use of PDE5 inhibitors for the treatment of both LUTS and ED. The first report on the potential use of PDE5 inhibitors on LUTS was published in 2002 by Sairam and colleagues (13). In this open-label pilot study, they evaluated 112 men referred for ED only and treated them with sildenafil. All patients were invited to complete the IIEF and the IPSS questionnaires at baseline, at one, and at three months. They found that roughly one-third of the men had an initial IPSS ≥ 7. Their results showed no relationship between sexual function scores and urinary symptom scores before treating ED. However, they demonstrated that treatment with sildenafil appears to improve urinary symptom scores. Moreover, the authors found that a lower IPSS at baseline was a predictor of a better LUTS response to ED therapy with sildenafil (13). In 2006, Mulhall et al. published a small series of studies on 49 patients diagnosed with ED and IPSS higher or equal to 10. The patients were invited to complete a IPPS and a IIEF questionnaire after at least three months from the beginning of the therapy with sildenafil. The authors demonstrated an improvement in the IPPS score in 60% of the patients, while a significant improvement in the IPSS score (i.e., at least 4 points) was recorded in 35% of the patients (14).

In 2007, McVary and colleagues published the first randomized, placebo-controlled trial, testing the role of PDE5 inhibitors (specifically sildenafil) on LUTS (15). A total number of 369 men were randomized into two groups, the arm treated with sildenafil and the other with placebo. Patients were instructed to ingest the starting 50-mg dose of study medication once daily each night at bedtime or 30 minutes to 1 hour before sexual activity. The drug dose was titrated to 100 mg after two weeks, if tolerated. The primary study outcome was a change from baseline in EF assessed by using the EF domain of the IIEF. Secondary outcomes were changes from baseline in the other domains of the IIEF, LUTS using the IPSS, the IPSS QOL question, BPHII, Qmax, SEAR scores, and end of treatment satisfaction using EDITS. The authors concluded that sildenafil improved erectile dysfunction and LUTS in men with the two conditions. Sildenafil treatment was associated with improved quality of life and treatment satisfaction. However, the authors did not succeed in demonstrating an improvement in urinary flow rates and they concluded that this lack of evidence may mean that a new basic pathophysiology paradigm is needed to explain the etiology of LUTS.

The same group analyzed the impact of another PDE5 inhibitor, namely tadalafil, on LUTS (46). A cohort of 281 was randomized to receive either tadalafil 5 mg once a day or placebo, followed by dose escalation to 20-mg tadalafil for an additional six weeks. Primary efficacy end points were IPSS change from baseline (visit 3) to 6 and 12 weeks. Secondary efficacy end points were changed from baseline on IPSS subdomains and on urinary flow parameters. According to their results, Tadalafil significantly improved the mean change from baseline in IPSS at six and at 12 weeks. Significant improvements were also seen in the IPSS irritative and obstructive domains versus placebo. Numerical improvements were observed in the tadalafil and placebo groups at 6 and 12 weeks compared with baseline for the uroflowmetry parameters Qmax, Qave, and Vcomp. However, the differences were not significant on comparing tadalafil with placebo.

More recently, Stief and colleagues evaluated the impact of vardenafil on both ED and LUTS with a randomized, double blind, placebo-controled study, involving 222 men diagnosed with a history of BPH/LUTS for at least six months. As previously observed with the other molecules, vardenafil did improve LUTS but no significant changes in urinary flow or post void residual volume were detected (47).

COMBINED USE OF α-BLOCKERS AND PDE5 INHIBITORS FOR THE TREATMENT OF ED

The potential common link between LUTS and ED suggest that the concurrent administration of an α-blocker and a PDE5 inhibitor to patients experiencing LUTS and associated sexual dysfunction may potentiate, or improve to some extent, the beneficial effects of each drug administered alone.

Several preclinical and clinical experiences highlighted the potential role of PDE5 on LUTS, as previously discussed. Moreover, results from experimental models showed that α-blockers, especially the selective α1-blockers, have a direct relaxant effect on corpus cavernosum (48,49) and may strengthen the proerectile effect of apomorphine (50). Moreover, very recently Oger and colleagues demonstrated in vitro that the combination of alfuzosin and tadalafil is more efficient than each compound alone to relax adrenergic tone or to enhance nitrergic relaxation of the human corpus cavernosum (51).

Regarding human studies, several long-term studies highlighted an improvement in the erectile function in patients treated for BPH, potentially related to the treatment with α_1-blockers (52–54).

Kaplan and colleagues recently published the first open-label, randomized, three-arm study comparing an α1-blocker (alfuzosin) versus sildenafil versus combination of alfuzosin and sildenafil for the treatment of both ED and LUTS. In a small cohort of patients, the authors demonstrated that the effect of the combined treatment had significantly better results in both relieving LUTS and improving ED than of each drug administered alone (55). Moreover, the combination therapy was able to significantly improve the maximal flow and to significantly reduce the post void residual after micturition. The authors concluded that treatment with a combination of an α_1-blocker and a PDE5 inhibitor is safe, and in this pilot study was the most effective therapy to enhance both voiding and sexual function in men with LUTS and sexual dysfunction.

CONCLUSIONS

LUTS and sexual dysfunction are highly prevalent in aging men. Both these conditions are also significant contributors to overall quality of life. New data has been presented to indicate potential links in epidemiologic, physiologic, pathophysiologic, and treatment aspects of these two entities. There are numerous publications within the past 10 years based on sophisticated community and clinical based data suggesting a strong and consistent association between LUTS and ED. The association is supported by the consistent linear relationship of more severe LUTS with more severe ED. A significant association between LUTS, sexual satisfaction, flow rates, and prostate volume further supports this relationship. The link between ED and LUTS has biologic plausibility given the four leading theories of how these diseases interrelate, each with variable amount of supporting data. These include (*i*) NOS/NO levels decreased or altered in the prostate and penile SM; (*ii*) autonomic hyperactivity/metabolic syndrome effects on LUTS, prostate growth, and ED; (*iii*) increased Rho-kinase activation/endothelin activity; and (*iv*) pelvic atherosclerosis and subsequent prostate and penile ischemia.

A wide range of studies have attempted to evaluate the relationship between ED and LUTS by treating one symptom (i.e., ED) and measuring the impact on the other disease (i.e., LUTS). This positive effect appears to affect outcomes regardless of which disease is treated primarily, thus suggesting a common etiology or mechanism. The patient bother attributable to this affect is less clear. Large scale, placebo-controlled studies are needed to further confirm these data and elucidate the role of the combination therapy to treat these two conditions. Further studies, with rigorous methodological methods may provide an answer to the potential common biological substratum relying below LUTS and ED.

REFERENCES

1. Carson CC. Erectile dysfunction in the 21st century: whom we can treat, whom we cannot treat and patient education. Int J Impot Res 2002; 14(suppl. 1):S29–S34.
2. Feldman HA, Goldstein I, Hatzichristou DG, et al. Impotence and its medical and psychosocial correlates: results of the Massachusetts Male Aging Study. J Urol 1994; 151(1): 54–61.
3. Hermann M, Untergasser G, Rumpold H, et al. Ageing of the male reproductive system. Exp Gerontol 2000; 35:1267–1279.
4. Sampson N, Untergasser G, Plas E. The ageing male reproductive tract. J Pathol 2007; 211:206–218.
5. McVary KT. BPH: epidemiology and comorbidities. Am J Manag Care 2006; 12(5 suppl):S122–S128.
6. Rosen R, Altwein J, Boyle P, et al. Lower urinary tract symptoms and male sexual dysfunction: the multinational survey of the aging male (MSAM-7). Eur Urol 2003; 44:637–649.
7. Hansen BL. Lower urinary tract symptoms (LUTS) and sexual function in both sexes. Eur Urol 2004; 46:229–234.
8. Bloch W, Klotz T, Loch C, et al. Distribution of NOS implies a regulation of circulation, SM tone, and secretory function in the human prostate by NO. Prostate 1997; 33(1):1–8.
9. Klotz T, Bloch W, Loch C, et al. Pattern of distribution of constitutive isoforms of NO synthase in the normal prostate and obstructive prostatic hyperplasia. Urology 1997; 36:318–322. J Urol 1998; 82(suppl 1):26–33.
10. Podlasek CA, Zelner DJ, McKenna KE, et al. Morphological changes and altered NOS isoform distribution in the BB/WOR diabetic rat prostate. J Urol 2003; 169(4):285.
11. Waldkirch ES, Uckert S, Langnäse K, et al. Immunohistochemical distribution of cyclic GMP-dependent protein kinase-1 in human prostate tissue. Eur Urol. 2007; 52(2):495–501.
12. Waldkirch E, Uckert S, Sigl K, et al. Expression and distribution of cyclic GMP-dependent protein kinase-1 isoforms in human penile erectile tissue. J Sex Med 2008; 5(3):536–543.
13. Sairam K, Kulinskaya E, McNicholas TA, et al. Sildenafil improves lower urinary tract symptoms. BJU Int 2002; 90:836–839.
14. Mulhall JP, Guhring P, Parker M, et al. Assessment of the impact of sildenafil citrate on lower urinary tract symptoms in men with erectile dysfunction. J Sex Med 2006; 3:662–667.
15. McVary KT, Monnig W, Camps JL, et al. Sildenafil citrate improves erectile function and urinary symptoms in men with erectile dysfunction and lower urinary tract symptoms associated with benign prostatic hyperplasia: a randomized, double-blind trial. J Urol 2007; 177:1071–1077.
16. McVary KT, Razzaq A, Lee C, et al. Growth of the rat prostate gland is facilitated by the autonomic nervous system. Biol Reprod 1994; 51(1):99–107.
17. Golomb E, Rosenzweig N, Ellam R, et al. Spontaneous hyperplasia of the ventral lobe of the prostate in aging genetically hypertensive rats. J Androl 2000; 21:58–64.
18. Tong YC, Hung YC, Lin SN, et al. The norepinephrine tissue concentration and neuropeptide Y immunoreactivity in genitourinary organs of the spontaneously hypertensive rat. J Auton Nerv Syst 1996; 56:215–218.
19. Hale TM, Okabe H, Bushfield TL, et al. Recovery of erectile function after brief aggressive antihypertensive therapy. J Urol 2002; 168(1):348–354.
20. Persson K, Pandita RK, Spitsbergen JM, et al. Spinal and peripheral mechanisms contributing to hyperactive voiding in spontaneously hypertensive rats. Am J Physiol 1998; 275:1366–1373.

21. McVary KT, McKenna KE. The Relationship Between Erectile Dysfunction and Lower Urinary Tract Symptoms: Epidemiological, Clinical, and Basic Science Evidence. Curr Urol Rep 2004; 5(4):251–257.
22. McVary KT, Rademaker A, Lloyd GL, et al. Autonomic nervous system overactivity in men with lower urinary tract symptoms secondary to benign prostatic hyperplasia. J Urol 2005; 174:1327–1433.
23. Somlyo AP, Somlyo AV. Signal transduction by G-proteins, Rho-kinase and protein phosphatase to smooth muscle and non smooth muscle myosin II. J Physiol 2000; 522:177–185.
24. Rees RW, Foxwell NA, Ralph DJ, et al. Y-27632, A Rho-kinase inhibitor, inhibits proliferation and adrenergic contraction of prostatic smooth muscle cells. J Urol 2003; 170:2517–2522.
25. Bing W, Chang S, Hypolite JA, et al. Obstruction-induced changes in urinary bladder smooth muscle contractility: a role for Rho kinase. Am J Physiol Renal Physiol 2003; 285:F990–F997.
26. Chang S, Hypolite JA, Zderic SA, et al. Increased corpus cavernosum smooth muscle tone associated with partial bladder outlet obstruction is mediated via Rho-kinase. Am J Physiol Regul Integr Comp Physiol 2005; 289:R1124–R1130.
27. Seko T, Ito M, Kureishi Y, et al. Activation of RhoA and inhibition of myosin phosphatase as important components in hypertension in vascular smooth muscle. Circ Res 2003; 92:411–418.
28. Azadzoi KM, Tarcan T, Siroky MB, et al. Atherosclerosis-induced chronic ischemia causes bladder fibrosis and non-compliance in the rabbit. J Urol 1999; 161(5):1626–1635.
29. Azadzoi KM, Tarcan T, Kozlowski R, et al. Overactivity and structural changes in the chronically ischemic bladder. J Urol 1999; 162(5):1768–1778.
30. Kozlowski R, Kershen RT, Siroky MB, et al. Chronic ischemia alters prostate structure and reactivity in rabbits. J Urol. 2001; 165(3):1019–1026.
31. Azadzoi KM, Babayan RK, Kozlowski R, et al. Chronic ischemia increases prostatic smooth muscle contraction in the rabbit. J Urol 2003; 170(2 Pt 1):659–663.
32. Andersson K-E, Persson K. Nitric oxide synthase and nitric oxide-mediated effects in lower urinary tract smooth muscles. World J Urol 1994; 12:274–280.
33. McVary KT. Erectile dysfunction and lower urinary tract symptoms secondary to BPH. Eur Urol 2005; 47(6):838–845.
34. Wheeler MA, Ayyagari RR, Wheeler GL, et al. Regulation of cyclic nucleotides in the urinary tract. J Smooth Muscle Res 2005; 41:1–21.
35. Hedlund P, Larsson B, Alm P, et al. Nitric oxide synthase-containing nerves and ganglia in the dog prostate: A comparison with other transmitters. Histochem J 1996; 28:635–642.
36. Hedlund P, Ekstrom P, Larsson B, et al. Heme oxygenase and NO synthase in the human prostate—relation to adrenergic, cholinergic and peptide-containing nerves. J Auton Nerv Syst 1997; 63:115–126.
37. Bloch W, Klotz T, Loch C, et al. Distribution of nitric oxide synthase implies a regulation of circulation, smooth muscle tone, and secretory function in the human prostate by nitric oxide. Prostate 1997; 33:1–8.
38. Uckert S, Oelke M, Stief CG, et al. immunohistochemical distribution of cAMP- and cGMP-phosphodiesterase (PDE) isoenzymes in the human prostate. Eur Urol 2006; 49:740–745.
39. Uckert S, Kuthe A, Jonas U, et al. Characterization and functional relevance of cyclic nucleotide phosphodiesterase isoenzymes of the human prostate. J Urol 2001; 166:2484–2489.
40. Truss MC, Uckert S, Stief CG, et al. Cyclic nucleotide phosphodiesterase (PDE) isoenzymes in the human detrusor smooth muscle. II. Effect of various PDE inhibitors on smooth muscle tone and cyclic nucleotide levels in vitro. Urol Res 1996; 24:129–134.
41. Truss MC, Uckert S, Stief CG, et al. Effects of various phosphodiesterase- inhibitors, forskolin, and sodium nitroprusside on porcine detrusor smooth muscle tonic responses to muscarinergic stimulation and cyclic nucleotide levels in vitro. Neurourol Urodyn 1996; 15:59–70.
42. Truss MC, Stief CG, Uckert S, et al. Phosphodiesterase 1 inhibition in the treatment of lower urinary tract dysfunction: From bench to bedside. World J Urol 2001; 19:344–350.
43. Andersson KE, Uckert S, Stief C, et al. Phosphodiesterases (PDEs) and PDE inhibitors for treatment of LUTS. Neurourol Urodyn. 2007; 26(6 suppl):928–933.
44. Gillespie JI. Phosphodiesterase-linked inhibition of non-micturition activity in the isolated bladder. BJU Int 2004; 93:1325–1332.
45. Truss MC, Stief CG, Uckert S, et al. Initial clinical experience with the selective phosphodiesterase-I isoenzyme inhibitor vinpocetine in the treatment of urge incontinence and low compliance bladder. World J Urol 2000; 18(6):439–443.
46. McVary KT, Roehrborn CG, Kaminetsky JC, et al. Tadalafil relieves lower urinary tract symptoms secondary to benign prostatic hyperplasia. J Urol 2007; 177(4):1401–1407.
47. Stief CG, Porst H, Neuser D, et al. A randomised, placebo-controlled study to assess the efficacy of twice-daily vardenafil in the treatment of lower urinary tract symptoms secondary to benign prostatic hyperplasia. Eur Urol. 2008; 53(6):1236–1244.
48. Palea S, Barras M. Comparison of the relaxant effects of alfuzosin, phentolamine and sildenafil on rabbit isolated corpus cavernosum. BJU Int 2003; 91:873–877.
49. De Rose AF, Giglio M, Traverso P, et al. Combined oral therapy with sildenafil and doxazosin for the treatment of non-organic erectile dysfunction refractory to sildenafil monotherapy. Int J Impot Res 2002; 14:50–53.

50. Mayoux E, Ramirez JF, Pouyet T, et al. Alfuzosin improves penile erection triggered by apomorphine in spontaneous hypertensive rats. Eur Urol 2004; 45(1):110–116.
51. Oger S, Behr-Roussel D, Gorny D, et al. Combination (Palea S 2003)of alfuzosin and tadalafil exerts in vitro an additive relaxant effect on human corpus cavernosum. J Sex Med 2008; 5(4):935–945.
52. Höfner K, Claes H, De Reijke TM, et al. Tamsulosin 0.4 mg once daily: effect on sexual function in patients with lower urinary tract symptoms suggestive of benign prostatic obstruction. Eur Urol. 1999; 36(4):335–341.
53. Rosen R, Seftel A, Roehrborn CG. Effects of alfuzosin 10 mg once daily on sexual function in men treated for symptomatic benign prostatic hyperplasia. Int J Impot Res. 2007; 19(5):480.
54. Elhilali M, Emberton M, Matzkin H, et al; ALF-ONE Study Group. Long-term efficacy and safety of alfuzosin 10 mg once daily: a 2-year experience in 'real-life' practice. BJU Int. 2006; 97(3):513–519.
55. Kaplan SA, Gonzalez RR, Te AE. Combination of alfuzosin and sildenafil is superior to monotherapy in treating lower urinary tract symptoms and erectile dysfunction. Eur Urol 2007; 51(6):1717–1723.

39 Sexual dysfunction and the prostate: andrological implications of PCa, BPH, and prostatitis

Wolfgang Weidner and Richard Berges

CASE REPORT

A 62-year-old man presents in the andrological outpatient department with symptoms of dysfunctional voiding, reduced ejaculatory function, mild erectile dysfunction (ED), and pelvic pain after ejaculation. His urologist suggests a transurethral resection of the enlarged prostate as final solution of the problems. The patient and his 42-year-old spouse query about questionable side effects on the patient's sexuality, for example, retrograde ejaculation, further deterioration of erectile function, and an impairment of his postejaculatory pain.

INTRODUCTION

Sexual dysfunction in prostatic diseases has already been recognized as a side effect in the urological treatment of prostate cancer (PCa) and benign prostatic hyperplasia (BPH) for decades (1). It isagreed that erectile and ejaculatory dysfunction are predictable side effects of drug and surgical therapeutic strategies in PCa and BPH and are important topics in clinical work that are covered by standard urological teaching. In this textbook of andrology, the authors want to focus on sexual disorders addressed by patients consulting andrological specialists for therapy, for example, ED after radical prostatectomy, association between lower urinary tract symptoms (LUTS) and sexual dysfunction, and sexuality interactions with chronic prostatitis/chronic pelvic pain syndrome (CP/CPPS).

PROSTATE CANCER—RADICAL PROSTATECTOMY AND RADIOTHERAPY

Radical prostatectomy: Anatomic retropubic radical prostatectomy (RRP) has gained widespread popularity due to the provision of an excellent cancer control and low risk of urinary incontinence with a decreased risk of troublesome morbidity for the treatment of localized prostatic cancer (2). Based on neuroanatomical insights into the relationship of the neurovascular bundles with the cavernous branches of the plexus pelvicus, multiple technical surgical details improved postoperative erectile function (3). After unilateral nerve-sparing RRP, the current literature shows potency rates of about 21% to 29% (4,5). After bilateral nerve-sparing RRP, the outcome is better with postoperative erections suitable for intercourse in 70% to 86% in relevant clinical series (4–7). Multiple factors influence this positive outcome with the early age of the patient, the quality of preoperative erections, and the experience of the surgeon as most important factors. Furthermore, the outcome can be influenced by the postoperative intake of 5-phosphodiesterase (PDE5) inhibitors (8). In different comorbidities, especially, entities such as diabetes mellitus, hypertension, ischemic heart disease, and disturbances of the fat metabolism are significant negative factors for the recovery of potency after surgery (8). Montorsi et al. (9) were the first to show that by using alprostadil injections to the corpora cavernosa, the rate of recovery of spontaneous erections after nerve-sparing radical prostatectomy is higher than with observation alone. Today, pharmacological treatment with PDE5 inhibitors has acquired an established role in treating ED after prostatectomy (10). Only patients with intact erectile nerves should be expected to respond. Up to 70% of all patients treated with bilateral nerve-protective radical prostatectomy report an improvement in erectile function with any types of PDE5-I available in the market (10). In men with no tolerability (rare) or in nonresponders, intracorporal or intraurethral alprostadil administration is the next step of therapy (11). Finally the use of a vacuum device or the implantation of a penile prosthesis may be considered (Table 1).

Radiotherapy (RT): Generally, the basics of this schedule are usable also for the protection of erectile function after RT. Currently, radiological treatment options for men with localized PCa are external beam radiotherapy (EBRT) or high-dose interstitial brachytherapy in combination with temporary androgen ablation and, in case of low risk PCa, low-dose interstitial brachytherapy, which is probably the most common form of radiotherapy in these patients. Arguing a comparable long-term biochemical control and survival rates with radical prostatectomy (RP) in patients with low-risk disease, sexual function can be preserved in more than 50% after RT (12,13). Nevertheless, postradiation erectile function seems to worsen over time in about 50% of the patients who were potent before treatment (14), making an individualized counseling necessary to find out the best choice for the individual's sexual quality of life expectation. Concerning the ongoing debate, whether a postintervention PDE5 inhibitor administration has to be continous or on demand, latest data provide evidence for a paradigm shift toward on-demand therapy (15). Alprostadil injections are suggested to be started three months after surgery (11) (Table 1).

Tumor progression after RP or RT: Unfortunately, tumor progression after RRP or RT makes hormone antiandrogen therapy (ADT) necessary. ADT is indicated in locally advanced patients to improve overall survival, in lymph node positive patients to defer progression (macroscopic LNs) and overall survival (microscopic LNs), in metastatic asymptomatic patients to prevent progression to a symptomatic stage, and in symptomatic

Table 1 Andrological Counseling of Post-prostatectomy Impotence (ED) (Giessen Procedure)

Suggested	Postoperative follow-up	
Operative procedure	Direct post-op (2 wk–12 mo)	After 12 mo
Bilateral nerve sparing RRP	PDE5-inhibitor (3×/wk or on demand) failure: change to alprostadil i.c. injection (2×/wk) MUSE (2×/wk)	Penile implant (inflatable)
	Failure after 3 mo: Vacuum device	

Table 2 Items of Counseling After RRP/RT in Advanced PCa Preservation of Sexual Function

- Type of ADT (complete, intermittent, adjuvant, type of AA-drug used)
- T-serum levels, T-substitution (prudent interval after RRP)
- Drug therapy in ED (PDE5-I, prostaglandin-injection, combination of both), nonresponder: vacuum-device, penile implant

Abbreviations: ADT, antiandrogen therapy; ED, erectile dysfunction; PDE, phosphodiesterase.

patients to palliate symptoms, and to reduce the risk of fractures or urethral obstruction (16). To date, randomized prospective trials investigating ADT effects on biochemical failure after RP or EBRT do not exist. However, there is retrospective evidence in favor for early ADT. The most frequently cited study in this manner reports on 1352 patients with a PSA relapse after RP, demonstrating a significant delay of manifestation of distant metastases (17) without evidence of a better overall or cancer-specific survival, nevertheless these data are the basis for most of men to be put on ADT in this situation.

Standard surgical castration and most chemical castrations result in t-serum depletion of less than 20 ng/mL with deleterious effects on libido and erectile function (18). Of 311 men, who were sexually potent before diagnosis, 80% of those treated with ADT became impotent after one year of treatment (18). Trials with intermittent endocrine therapy demonstrated a lower incidence of side effects and a better quality of life including items of disturbed sexuality when the patients were not on treatment (19). A further possibility may be the use of antiandrogens alone (evidence from bicalutamide 150 mg/day only), which might overcome some side effects of medical castration. Although large randomized trials in patients with PSA recurrence after curative therapy are lacking, there is indirect evidence for a significant risk reduction of progression and a decrease in incidence of hot flushes, loss of libido, and ED (20). These questionable advantages have to be weighed against specific side effects of this treatment, for example, breast tenderness and gynecomastia.

In conclusion, in the absence of prospective studies, a definite recommendation for different ADT regimens after RP or RT with special reference to disturbed sexuality seems not to be possible until today. Nevertheless, the proven sexual side effects can be addressed and have not been seen as inevitable. In our experience, there is no contraindication to suggest intracavernosal injections of prostaglandins with and without oral PDE5-inhibitor intake and response rates are up to 33% to 80% with medical therapy, including 44% of those receiving PDE5-inhibitor monotherapy (21).

In PCa patients, after definitive treatment and no sign of recurrence, counseling for loss of libido may be different. As libido is most sensitive to testosterone suppression and responds to testosterone replacement therapy (TRT) very well (22), it may be valuable to rethink treatment strategies. Today it seems to be proven that TRT does not significantly increase intraprostatic androgen levels in hypogonadal men with a limited effect of TRT on PCa risk (23). Oncologically, a recent preliminary study in castration-resistant PCa demonstrated a PSA decrease under TRT. Only one case symptomatic progression occurred (24). This may underline the statement of the current EAU guideline (22) that in symptomatic hypogonadal men after a prudent interval after RRP or RT, TRT may be a thinkable alternative for the future to improve libido and sexual function. Our current approach to these patients is summarized in Table 2.

LUTS/BPH

It has been accepted for decades that in aging men with LUTS/BPH, sexual dysfunction to some extent correlates to benign prostatic obstruction and symptom severity (1). It was the merit of the Alf-One Study to demonstrate the direct interaction between severity of LUTS and sexual dysfunction (25). The key message of this study and consecutive papers such as the MSAM-7 trial (26) is that in sexually active men with LUTS/BPH and with painful ejaculation have more severe LUTS, more often ED and reduced ejaculatory volume, compared to men with LUTS only. Recently, these data have been reconfirmed in the EpiLUTS analysis of more than 11,000 men (27), demonstrating a correlation between ED measured by the IIEF and the IPSS score. Furthermore, LUTS seems to be an independent predictor of ED (28). Pathophysiologically, this interaction is highlighted in chapter 38.

Medical treatment: 5α-reductase inhibitors such as dutasteride and finasteride are acceptable treatment option for moderate/severe LUTS and enlarged prostate (30–40 mL) (29). Side effects mainly relate to sexual dysfunction with a decreased libido in 6%, ED in 8%, and decreased ejaculation in 4% (30). The EPICS Study analyzed data of a randomized double-blind trial comparing 12 months of dutasteride and finasteride therapy for drug-related adverse events to sexuality: There was no significant difference between both the drugs (31) (Table 3).

Table 3 Drug-Related Side-Effects to Sexuality

	Dutasteride (0.5 mg daily), $N = 813$	Finasteride (5 mg daily), $N = 817$
Impotence (%)	7	8
Decreased libido (%)	5	6
Ejaculatory disorder (%)	1	1
Gynecomastia (%)	1	1

Source: Modified from Ref. 31.

Concerning α_1-blockers as treatment options for patients with moderate/severe LUTS, all four α_1-blockers, for example, alfuzosin, doxazosin, tamsulosin, and terazosin seem to have similar clinical efficacy, although side effect profiles differ because of pharmacological differences with retard formulations being superior regarding tolerability, also there may be differences regarding effects on ejaculation (30,31). Nevertheless, comparative studies have failed to detect significant differences in abnormal ejaculation for tamsulosin and alfuzosin (32). If ejaculatory dysfunction is present, it rather represents a reduced ejaculatory volume. Due to the high prevalence of ED and LUTS, combination therapy with α1-blockers and PDE5 inhibitors has to be considered with caution (31): Due to the vasodilating properties of both substance groups, enhanced blood pressure reduction may occur.

BPH: TUR-P AND ALTERNATIVE TREATMENT

Surgical treatment: In this chapter, a detailed review of all side effects of standard operative procedures (TUR-P and its modifications, TUI-P, open prostatectomy) and of new techniques (both primary ablative, e.g., laser enucleation or vaporisation, or secondary ablative, e.g., microwave therapy, TUNA) is not intended. However, the typical adverse effects concerning retrograde ejaculation and ED should be known to the andrologically interested urologists and are summarized in Tables 4 and 5.

There are limited data about sexual dysfunction from alternative treatments to TUR-P mainly due to the fact that direct comparative trials are rare and definitions of side effects differ. In general it appears, that all primary ablative procedures (laser-vaporisation, laser enucleation) have similar effects on ejaculation and erectile function as with TUR-P. Due to the significant lower ability of tissue removal, secondary ablative procedures (TUMT/TUNA) tend to produce lower rates of retrograde ejaculation. A preliminary overview on alternative procedures is given in Table 5.

Table 4 Retrograde Ejaculation (RE) and ED in Standard Surgical Treatments of the Prostate (33,34)

Procedure	RE (%)	ED (%)
TUI-P	30–40	Unclear
TUR-P	50–80[a]	30[b]
Open prostatectomy	70	50

[a]Depending upon extensity of resection.
[b]Depending upon preoperative erectile function.

Table 5 Retrograde Ejaculation (RE) and ED in Alternative Ablative Procedures to TUR-P (35–42)

Procedure	RE (%)	ED (%)
Selected primary ablative alternative procedures		
Holmium laser enucleation	60–74	Not reported
KTP laser vaporisation	36–45	Not reported
Selected secondary ablative alternative procedures		
TUMT	19.8–22.2	4–8.7
TUNA	None	Not reported

PROSTATITIS AND DISTURBED SEXUALITY

The National Institutes of Health (NIH) Classification of Prostatitis Syndromes is the basis of today's scientific work in this field consented with the International Prostatitis Collaborative Network (43) (Table 6). Considering disturbed sexuality only, chronic bacterial prostatitis (NIH II) and chronic prostatitis/chronic pelvic pain syndrome (NIH III) have to be considered. Acute bacterial prostatitis (NIH I) is a severe infection with fever, inflammatory host response, and voiding disturbances, making active sexuality difficult. Type IV prostatitis is asymptomatic and not detectable by the patient. For further information see chapter on prostatitis.

SEXUAL DYSFUNCTION AND "PROSTATITIS" SYMPTOMS

Unfortunately, patients with "prostatitis" associated symptoms may exhibit a broad spectrum of sexual dysfunction such as loss of libido, ED, and ejaculatory disorders, including premature ejaculation. This general association has already been proven 30 years ago in more than 50% of men with "chronic prostatitis" sexual disorders (44). Lutz et al. (45) analyzed the interaction between pelvic pain and ED. In this study, men with significant "pelvic pain" had a higher chance to suffer from ED than

Table 6 Prostatitis NIH Classification

I. Acute bacterial (ABP)
II. Chronic bacterial (CBP)
III. Chronic prostatitis/chronic pelvic pain syndrome (CP/CPPS)
  (a) Inflammatory
  (b) Noninflammatory
IV. Asymptomatic, inflammatory

Abbreviation: NIH, National Institutes of Health.

patients without pelvic pain. Other authors stated ED in 15% (46), 23% (47) and 31% (48) of the men. In a recently published study, including 296 participants with CP/CPPS, 72% reported sexual dysfunction (49). In this study, ejaculatory dysfunction was common in most men, and in men reporting both ED and ejaculatory difficulties, worse CP/CPPS symptoms and a reduced quality of life became evident. In conclusion, symptoms of sexual dysfunction, especially ED, do occur in up to 72% of all patients searching help for "prostatitis" related symptoms, especially in case of CP/CPPS.

The second point of interest is the interaction between CP/CPPS symptoms and ejaculatory dysfunction. Two Chinese studies demonstrated the relevance of premature ejaculation (PE) in symptomatic prostatitis patients (46,49). This finding was confirmed by one study with a modern definition of PE, using the intravaginal ejaculation latency time: 77% of all men with CP/CPPS suffered from this disorder (50). Similarly, a high incidence of "inflammatory prostatitis signs" was reported in men with PE (51). Ejaculatory pain may also bother "prostatitis" patients (52). Despite lack of concrete evidence, many patients may be encouraged to refrain from ejaculation (1), although case reports have suggested the improvement of prostatitis symptoms by better drainage due to increased ejaculatory frequency (53).

Finally, therapeutic considerations have to be addressed. Concerning therapy, the 6th International Conference on New Developments in Prostate Cancer and Prostate Diseases held at Paris in 2006 summarized all types of therapy based on an evidence-based approach for all types of prostatitis and CP/CPPS (53). It was decided that only therapeutic strategies reducing symptoms, especially against pelvic pain, are interesting in this context. The use, especially, of α-blockers has to be addressed since one study (54) demonstrated a special benefit on painful ejaculation in LUTS patients. In patients with CP/CPPS, α-blockers are often prescribed as the first therapeutic choice (55). Concerning CP/CPPS, a new randomized study using alfuzosin did not demonstrate a reduction of symptoms as compared to placebo (56). This outcome contradicts with the widespread use of α-blockers in all types of prostatitis and is especially not in concordance with several trials of the last decade. In conclusion, as discussed for years among the experts, α-blocker therapy does not seem to work clearly against symptoms in CP/CPPS. Questionable men with proven subvesical obstruction and/or proven CBP (NIH II) (57) may benefit from this type of therapy, but then side effects on ejaculatory dysfunction typical for α-blockers (see text for LUTS) have to be taken into account.

CONCLUSIONS

Localized PCa can be treated by bilateral nerve-sparing RRP, with a preservation of erection in up to 70% to 80% of cases (Evidence 2, Grade A recommendation).

RT of localized PCa results in ED in about 50% of cases (Evidence 2, Grade A recommendation).

Pharmacological treatment for penile rehabilitation is standard after nerve-protective RRP (Evidence 2, Grade A recommendation).

In tumor progression of PCa after RRP or RT, different therapeutic strategies have to be discussed for preservation of sexual function with different approaches for libido and erection (Evidence 3, Grade B recommendation).

BPH/LUTS is associated with ED and ejaculatory dysfunction (Evidence 1, Grade A recommendation).

5α-Reductase inhibitors have defined side effects to libido, ED, and ejaculation (level of evidence 1, Grade A recommendation).

α_1-Blockers, used for BPH/LUTS are associated with ejaculatory dysfunction, especially with reduced ejaculatory volume (level of evidence 2, Grade A recommendation).

Common deobstructive surgery in BPH/LUTS (e.g., TUR-P) results in significant retrograde ejaculation (level of evidence 3, Grade A recommendation) and ED in 30% to 50% (level of evidence 3, Grade B recommendation).

Alternative ablative procedures (lasers) result in similar rates of retrograde ejaculation (primary ablative) and none or less ejaculatory dysfunction (secondary ablative) (level of evidence 2, Grade B recommendation)

In spite of and contrary to the widespread acceptance of disturbed sexuality in NIH II and III prostatitis, the confirmation of this interaction is not possible.

Therapy of CBP and CP/CPPS with α-blockers to improve prostatitis symptoms does not seem to be superior to placebo, if subvesical infection is excluded (level of evidence 2, Grade B recommendation).

REFERENCES

1. Burger B, Weidner W, Altwein JE. Prostate and Sexuality: An Overview. Eur Urol 1999; 35:177–184.
2. Walsh PC. Anatomic radical prostatectomy: evolution of the surgical technique. J Urol 1998; 160:2418–2424.
3. Walsh PC. Technique of vesicourethtral anastomosis may influence recovery of sexual function following radical prostatectomy. Urol Clin North Am 1994; 2:59.
4. Noldus J, Michl U, Graefen M, et al. Patient-reported sexual function after nerve-sparing retropubic prostatectomy. Eur Urol 2002; 42:118–124.
5. Rabbani F, Stapleton AMF, Kattan MW, et al. Factors predicting recovery of erections after radical prostatectomy. J Urol 2000; 164:1929–1934.
6. Walsh PC, Marschke P, Ricker D, et al. Patient reported urinary continence and sexual function after anatomic radical prostatectomy. Urology 2000; 55:58–61.
7. Catalona WJ, Carvahal GF, Mager DE, et al. Potency, continence and complication rates in 1870 consecutive radical retropubic prostatectomies. J Urol 1999; 162:433–438.
8. Meuleman EJ, Mulders PF. Erectile function after radical prostatectomy: a review. Eur Urol 2003; 43:95–101.

9. Montorsi F, Guazzoni G, Strambi LF, et al. Recovery of spontaneous erectile function after nerve-sparing radical retropubic prostatectomy with and without early intracavernous injections of alprostadil: results of a prospective randomized trial. J Urol 1997; 158:1408–1410.
10. Montorsi F, Burnett AL. Erectile dysfunction after radical prostatectomy. BJU Int 2004; 93:1–7.
11. Montorsi F, Briganti A, Salonia A, et al. Current and future strategies for preventing and managing erectile dysfunction following radical prostatectomy. Eur Urol 2004; 45:123–133.
12. Pinkawa M, Gagel B, Piroth MD, et al. Erectile dysfunction after external beam radiotherapy for prostate cancer Eur Urol 2009; 55:227–236.
13. Pinkawa M, Gontero P. The motion: Radiotherapy for prostate cancer preserves sexual function to a greater extent than nerve sparing radical prostatectomy. Eur Urol 2009; 56:212–214.
14. Zelefsky MJ, Chan H, Hunt M, et al. Longterm outcome of high dose intensity modulated radiation therapy for patients with clinically localized prostate cancer. J Urol 2006; 176:1415–1419.
15. Montorsi F, Brock G, Lee J, et al. Effect of nightly versus on-demand vardenafil on recovery of erectile function in men following bilateral nerve-sparing radical prostatectomy. Eur Urol 2008; 54:924–9313.
16. Berges R. Hormonal treatment of prostate cancer. In: Berges R, Tombal B, eds. Androgens and Prostate Cancer. Lier, Belgium: Smart Healthcare, 2009:63–92.
17. Moul JW, Wu H, Sun L, et al. Early versus delayed hormonal therapy for prostate specific antigen only recurrence of prostate cancer after radical prostatectomy. J Urol 2004; 171:1141–1147.
18. Potosky AL, Reeve BB, Clegg LX, et al. Quality of life following localized prostate cancer treated initially with androgen deprivation therapy or no therapy. J Natl Cancer Inst 2002; 94:430–437.
19. Bruchovsky N, Klotz L, Crook J, et al. Quality of life, morbidity, and mortality results of a prospective phase II study of intermittent androgen suppression for men with evidence of prostate-specific antigen relapse after radiation therapy for locally advanced prostate cancer. Clin Genitourin Cancer 2008; 6:46–52.
20. McLeod DG, Iversen P, See WA, et al. Casodex early prostate cancer trialists' group. Bicalutamide 150 mg plus standard care vs standard care alone for early prostate cancer. BJU Int 2009; 97:247–254.
21. Di Blasio CJ, Malcolm JB, Derweesh IH, et al. Patterns of sexual and erectile dysfunction and response to treatment in patients receiving androgen deprivation therapy for prostate cancer. BJU Int 2008; 102:39–43.
22. Wang C, Nieschlag E, Swerdloff R, et al. Investigation, treatment and monitoring of late-onset hypogonadism in males: ISA, ISSAM, EAU, EAA and ASA recommendations. Int J Androl 2009; 32:1–10.
23. Isbarn H, Pinthus JH, Marks LS, et al. Testosterone and prostate cancer: Revisiting old paradigms. Eur Urol 2009; 56:48–56.
24. Szmulewitz R, Mohile S, Posadas E, et al. A randomized phase 1 study of testosterone-replacement for patients with low-risk castration-resistant prostate cancer. Eur Urol 2009; 56:97–104.
25. Nickel JC, Elhilali M, Vallancien G. Benign prostatic hyperplasia (BPH) and prostatitis: prevalence of painful ejaculation in men with clinical BPH. BJU Int 2005; 95:571–574.
26. Rosen R, Altwein J, Boyle P, et al. Lower urinary tract symptoms and male sexual dysfunction: the multinational survey of the aging male (MSAM-7). Eur Urol 2003; 44:637–649.
27. Wein AJ, Coyne KS, Tubaro A, et al. The impact of lower urinary tract symptoms on male sexual health: EpiLUTS. BJU Int 2009; 103:33–41.
28. Hansen BL. Lower urinary tract symptoms (LUTS) and sexual function in both sexes. Eur Urol 2004; 46:229–234.
29. Berges R, Dreikom K, Höfner K, et al. Therapy of benign prostate syndrome (BPS): guidelines of the German Urologists (DGU). Urologe A 2009; 48:1503–1516.
30. Madersbacher S, Alivizatos G, Nordling J, et al. EAU 2004 guidelines on assessment, therapy and follow-up of men with lower urinary tract symptoms suggestive of benign prostatic obstruction. Eur Urol 2004; 46:547–554.
31. Chapple C, Artibani W, Berges R, et al. New medical developments in the management of LUTS in adult men. In: McConnel J, Abrssams P, Denis L, Khoury S, Roehrbom C, eds. Male lower urinary tract dysfunction. Paris: Evaluation and Management Health Publication, 2006:145–194.
32. Buzelin JM, Fonteyne E, Kontturi NJ, et al. Comparison of tamsulosin with Halfuzosin in the treatment of patients with lower urinary tract symptoms suggestion of bladder outlet obstruction. Br J Urol 1977; 80:597–605.
33. Rosette J de la, Baba S, et al. New minimally invasive and surgical developments in the management of BPO. In: McConnel J, Abrams P, Denis L, Khoury S, Roehrbom C, eds. Male lower urinary tract dysfunction. Paris: Evaluation and Management Health Publication, 2006:197–233.
34. Chapple CR, McConnel JD, Tubaro A, eds. Benign Prostate Hyperplasia. Malden USA: Blackwell. 2000.
35. Kuntz RM, Ahyai S, Lehrich K, et al. Transurethral holmium laser enucleation of the prostate versus transurethral electrocautery resection of the prostate: a randomized prospective trial in 200 patients. J Urol 2004; 172:1012–1016.
36. Montorsi F, Naspro R, Salonia A, et al. Holmium laser enucleation versus transurethral resection of the prostate: results from a 2-center, prospective, randomized trial in patients with obstructive benign prostatic obstruction. J Urol 2004; 172:1926–1929.

37. Te AE, Malloy TR, Stein BS, et al. Photoselective vaporization of the prostate (PVP) for the treatment of benign prostate (BPO): 12 months results from the first U.S. multicenter prospective trial [abstract]. J Urol 2003; 169:(suppl):465.
38. Reich O, Schlenker B, Gratzke C, et al. Plasma vaporisation of the prostate: initial clinical results. Eur Urol 2009; 57:693–698.
39. De la Rosette JJMCH, Laguna MP, Gravas S, et al. Transurethral Microwave Thermotherapy: The Gold Standard for Minimally Invasive Therapies or Patients with Benign Prostatic Hyperplasia? J Endourol 2003; 17:245–251.
40. Walmsley K, Kaplan S. Transurethral microwave thermotherapy for benign prostatic hyperplasia: Separating truth from marketing hype. J Urol 2004; 172:1249–1255.
41. Hoffman RM, McDonald R, Monga M, et al. Transurethral microwave thermotherapy vs transurethral resection for treating benign prostatic hyperplasia: a systematic review. BJU Int 2004; 94:1031–1036.
42. Hill B, Bel Ville W, Bruskewitz R, et al. Transurethral needle ablation versus transurethral resection of the prostate for the treatment of symptomatic benign prostatic obstruction: 5-year results of a prospective, randomized, multicenter clinical trial. J Urol 2004; 171(6, Pt 1 of 2):2336–2340.
43. Krieger JN, Nyberg L, Nickel JL. Consensus definition and classification of Prostatitis. JAMA 1999; 282:236–237.
44. Keltikangas-Jarvinen L, Jarvinen H, Lehtonen T. Psychic disturbances in patients with chronic prostatitis. Ann Clin Res 1981; 13:45–49.
45. Lutz MC, Roberts RO, Jacobson DJ, et al. Cross-sectional associations of urogenital pain and sexual function in a community based cohort of older men: Olmsted County, Minnesota. J Urol 2005; 174:624–628.
46. Anderson RU, Wise D, Sawyer T, et al. Sexual dysfunction in men with chronic prostatitis/chronic pelvic pain syndrome: improvement after trigger point release and paradoxical relaxation training. J Urol 2006; 176:1534–1538.
47. Liang CZ, Zhang XJ, Hao ZY, et al. Prevalence of sexual dysfunction in Chinese men with chronic prostatitis. BJU Int 2004; 93:568–570.
48. Trinchieri A, Magri V, Cariani L, et al. Prevalence of sexual dysfunction in men with chronic prostatitis/chronic pelvic pain syndrome. Arch Ital Urol Androl 2007; 79:67–70.
49. Lee SW, Liang ML, Yuen KH, et al. Adverse impact of sexual dysfunction in CP/CPPS. Urology 2008; 71:79–84.
50. Gonen M, Kalkan M, Cenker A, et al. Prevalence of premature ejaculation in Turkish men with chronic pelvic pain syndrome. J Androl 2005; 26:601–603.
51. Screponi E, Carosa E, Di Stasi SM,et al. Prevalence of chronic prostatitis in men with premature ejaculation. Urology 2001; 58:198–202.
52. Ilie CP, Mischinau DL, Pemberton RJ. Painful ejaculation. BJU Int 2007; 99:1335–1339.
53. Schaeffer AJ, Anderson RU, Krieger JN, et al. Statement on prostatitis. The assessment and management of male pelvic pain syndrome, including prostatitis. In: Edition MLUTD, ed. 6th International Conference on New Developments in Prostate Cancer and Prostate Diseases. Paris: Health Publications 2006:343–375.
54. Nickel JC, Elhilali M, Emberton M, et al. The beneficial effect of alfuzosin 10 mg once daily in real-life practice on lower urinary tract symptoms (LUTS), quality of life and sexual dysfunction in men with LUTS and painful ejaculation. BJU Int 2006; 97:1242–1246.
55. Wagenlehner FME, Weidner W. No benefit of alphablockers for chronic prostatitis. Nat Rev Urol 2009; 6:183–184.
56. Nickel JC, Krieger JN, McNaughton-Collins M, et al. Alfuzosin and symptoms of chronic prostatitis-chronic pelvic pain syndrome. New Engl J Med 2008; 359:2663–2673.
57. Weidner W. Treating chronic prostatitis: Antibiotics no, alpha-blockers may be. Ann Intern Med 2004; 141:639–640.

40 Psychological abnormalities of male sexual function

Emmanuele A. Jannini and Andrea Lenzi

INTRODUCTION: A *PARS DESTRUENS*

The field of sexology arose in the medical environment. Originally, there was no clear distinction between physical (sometime called "organic" or, without reason, "physiological") and psychological function. The interpretation of erectile dysfunction (ED), here used as a paradigm of all other sexual dysfunctions, as a psychogenic symptom is mainly due to psychoanalytic tradition and the founders of modern psychosexology, Masters and Johnson (1). On the basis of their assertion that over 90% of impotence is psychogenic, diagnosis and therapy have been left to the psychologist (i.e., to a medical nonexpert) for at least 15 years, condemning legions of patients with ED to learn to live with their disorder rather than cure it. However, the spread of radioimmunological measurement, echo Doppler flowmetry, and neurophysiological procedures has overturned the assumption of these two masters who, of course, did not have access to these techniques. It is now know that the etiology of ED is predominantly organic, making the sexologist's role in the diagnostic and therapeutic process of apparently secondary importance in comparison with that of the doctor (2). Thus, from one error (ED is always psychogenic, i.e., psychological reductionism) another arose: that ED is exclusively a medical issue, that is, medical reductionism. In fact, this fault may persist if a simple medical therapy—even if etiological and targeted—is considered as sufficient in itself to completely restore erectile function. In reality, anxiety and depression almost always accompany ED (3) and if unexplored and untreated can invalidate an exclusively "medical" therapy.

The etiology of ED and other sexual dysfunctions is traditionally considered as either organic or psychogenic (4,5) in a dichotomized view, which is far from reality. Every patient whose impotence is due to an organic disorder, especially if longstanding (which unfortunately is often the case), builds his own world of fear, anxiety, worry, depression, and distress around his disorder (6). Furthermore, anyone who has treated a patient with ED of any origin will know that even the most organic impotence—such as that caused by diabetes (7)—is *also* psychogenic (8). In fact, when a sexual encounter results in frustration and stress rather than gratification, it is almost impossible not to construct a vicious psychoneuroendocrine (9) circle of distress and depression, "spectator syndrome" and performance anxiety (Fig. 1). All impotence of organic origin therefore also has a psychogenic aspect [or is "mixed," as it is classified by some (10)]. **All**, not just some. Even when there is a recognizable organic cause of ED, such as diabetes, it quickly develops an emotional component, so clinicians need to recognize that in most cases there will be both organic and psychogenic elements in ED. It must also be considered that the sufferer must continue to live, or survive, despite his impotence. For this reason, this "structured" symptom, in psychological terms, can be more difficult to resolve than the underlying organic cause.

So whatever the cause, all impotence is at least partly psychogenic. This classification is thus at the very least unhelpful, and essentially redundant.

Another reason to avoid a dichotomized taxonomy is the borderline condition that has been recently named "subclinical erectile dysfunction" (SED), or the pathological condition of men experiencing a lack of erection who are unaffected by ED (11). Borderline organic and psychological causes are both present in this condition, which is characterized by a psychosomatic–somatopsychic loop, which may lead to overt ED.

How should we classify those cases where there is no physical cause or disease underlying the symptom? Are there any laboratory or psychometric tests that can distinguish patients with an undoubtedly psychogenic origin? Despite some attempts (12), the answer is unfortunately no. It is, therefore, impossible to objectively demonstrate with instrumental, psychometric, or psychological tests that a given event or existential condition is "the" cause of the ED (as the detection of *Streptococcus pneumoniae* would be for pneumonia), the definition "psychogenic," with the meaning of "generated by the psyche," is abusive and unjustifiable (13). However, this reasoning does not at all mean that psychological causes of sexual dysfunctions do not exist.

Conventional wisdom teaches that ED is diagnosed by "exclusion" (14). Unfortunately, no one can be sure that all etiologies have actually been excluded. In fact, we have no proof that we now know every technique necessary to make a diagnosis, nor that we have perfected our pathophysiological knowledge of ED. An example is the thyroidal etiology of ED: Only recently was it discovered that thyroid diseases could affect sexual desire and cause ED and ejaculatory disturbances, which are easily cured once euthyroidism is achieved (15).

The diagnosis can therefore never be of exclusion, but rather of probability. A negative medical diagnosis does not mean that the cause is psychogenic, simply because it is unknown. This is analogous to the diagnosis of one of the most common diseases as "essential" hypertension (high blood pressure with no identifiable cause), which even though no organic cause has been found is considered a psychosomatic disorder with a solid

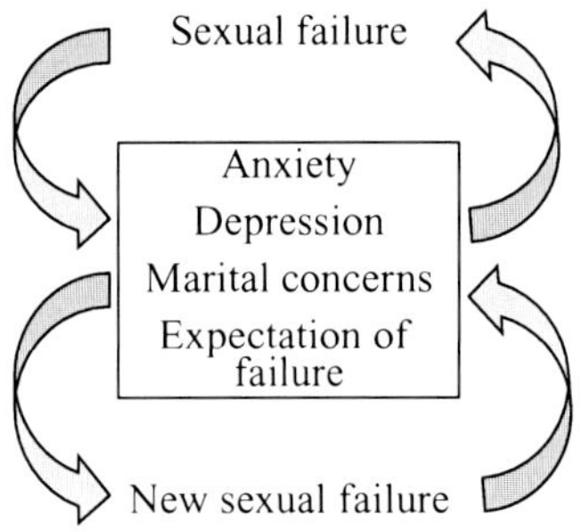

Figure 1 The loop. Irrespective of the etiology of the sexual failure (relational, intrapsychic, organic, mixed), a psychological reaction is always structured, leading to an ever-present psychological concause.

organic etiology, to be "organically" treated with weight loss, regular exercise, a low–fat and low-sodium diet, and drugs. The classification of sexual dysfunctions into organic/psychogenic should thus be abandoned in favor of organic/nonorganic or idiopathic, recognizing that whatever the cause, the psychogenic component is inseparable in the case of a symptom like impotence, so easily capable of unhinging a couple's relationship.

After this critical analysis, aimed at demolishing common dangerous myths in the psychosexological approach to male patients with sexual dysfunction, the following paragraphs (the *pars construens*) will deal with the psychological causes, concauses, and epiphenomenal effects of the most frequent sexual symptoms, such as loss of libido, hypogonadism, impotence, and ejaculatory disturbances.

HYPOACTIVE SEXUAL DESIRE

As sexual desire is apparently mainly a subjective, psychological drive, psychological factors should be prevalent in the etiology of hypoactive sexual desire disorder (HSDD). This symptom has been defined as "**Persistently or recurrently deficient (or absent) sexual fantasy and desire for sexual activity** (. . .) **[leading] to marked distress or interpersonal difficulty**" (16). The inclusion of the word "disorder" in the definition of this condition is important, as the absence of libido per se (as may also happen in the voluntarily celibate), if it does not cause distress, is not a symptom.

HSDD is far more common (or admitted to)—and therefore studied—in women than in men. This may be in part due to the common, hormone-dependent impairment of the libidinal machinery caused by menopause. Furthermore, males diagnosed with HSDD are significantly older than women diagnosed with this condition (17). As with other sexual dysfunctions, HSDD can be lifelong, and thus generalized, acquired, or both generalized and situational.

The major causes or concauses are (*i*) marital (or relational) and intrapsychic (such as depression), (*ii*) the presence of another sexual dysfunction, and (*iii*) organic etiologies, such as use of drugs affecting desire, hypogonadism, or a severe medical illness (18).

Marital factors are frequently involved. A long-term relationship is a common reason for a drop in desire (acquired, situational HSDD). This is not a true HSDD, as desire for other actual or potential partners is fully conserved.

Other relational factors can directly induce HSDD. For example, using the SIEDY structured interview and the Middlesex Hospital Questionnaire test (MHQ-test) (19), it has been demonstrated that HSDD is directly correlated with the partner's libido (20). His/her adequate libido and even climax reaction during intercourse would reinforce the patient's feeling of sexual competence and therefore desire. HSDD can also be caused by a disabling illness of the partner, due to both physical and psychological distress and reduced partner receptivity. Other features in the relationship may also significantly contribute to the symptom. For example, an overt conflict between the couple or with other household members and its associated negative feelings, such as hostility, resentment and anger, may affect the man's ability to become sexually interested.

Lack of job satisfaction can also impair male sexual desire through an intrapsychic mechanism (21).

HSDD is associated with a significant increase in numerous **intrapsychic symptoms** (depression, free-floating anxiety, and somatization) but not with hysterical traits (22). Depression typically reduces libido, either directly or as a side effect of antidepressants. General distress (whether with work or within the family) is another important cause of loss of desire. Paraphilias and sexual secrets, such as those regarding sexual orientation or gender identity, may also be a cause of intrapsychic HSDD.

HSDD can be **secondary** to another sexual dysfunction: in this frequent case, an avoidance mechanism is clearly involved. Based on the stimulus theory, this may be due to a psychoendocrine mechanism: a reduction or absence in sexual activity—perhaps caused by impotence or another sexual dysfunction in the couple—leads to a reduction in testosterone production (23), probably through an alteration in the GnRH pulse generator (9), and consequently HSDD. In other cases, the "other" sexual dysfunction (usually impotence) can be consciously or unconsciously rejected by the patient. This is of particular importance, because in some cultures men may be more comfortable with the self-diagnosis of HSDD than to admit to the more humiliating ED, even to themselves.

There is also a strong link between a man's perceptions of his own masculinity and virility and his ability to father a child. For this reason HSDD is frequently observed in male infertility (24).

Finally it should be noted that the cause–effect relationship between low libido and the described psychopathological features is often problematic: in many cases, the relational or intrapsychic symptoms are not the cause but the consequence of the loss of desire. This possibility must be always be considered during the assessment of subjects suffering from HSDD.

EFFECTS OF HYPOGONADISM ON PSYCHOSOCIAL PARAMETERS

Psychosocial impairment is not easy to define scientifically. Symptoms of this "syndrome" (depressed mood, anxiety, irritability, reduced cognitive capacity, loss of sense of wellbeing) (25) are largely unspecific. However, psychosocial impairment cannot be denied in either general hypogonadism or hypogonadism in the aging male.

A decline in testosterone can be associated with some degree of dysphoria (26). This link is so close that these symptoms can be simply attributed to the aging process (27). Furthermore, as if locked in a vicious circle, these psychosocial symptoms may be the basis of sexual symptoms (hypoactive sexual desire, erectile dysfunction, ejaculatory dysfunction) that are typical of both the elderly and, to some extent, hypogonadism. Sexual dysfunction can further exacerbate psychosocial impairment in a perverse loop pattern that should be approached therapeutically with medical counseling on possible lifestyle changes (risk factors, sport, diet), by restoring sexual function, and, when necessary, with androgen replacement therapy (ART). The social issues faced by the elderly further complicate this scenario. The loss of social power due to retirement and of body image due to aging itself are deeply linked with the attitude of a society—such as our own Western one—which is culturally unable to deal with the sexual needs of its older members. This can be considered an "antisexual syndrome" of the society against the sexuality of the elderly (28).

The majority of steroid hormones strongly affect animal and human behavior as well as social attitudes. Testosterone production in particular has been closely connected to achieving dominant positions in rank-controlled animal societies. On this basis, it has been inferred that low androgen levels may substantially affect cognitive abilities, concentration, and general mood.

ERECTILE DYSFUNCTION

A detailed, careful medical, psychological, and sexual history is essential in evaluating ED—-but, unfortunately, not sufficient in itself. Questionnaires (29) and structured interviews (30) are widely used in ED diagnosis (19). They are powerful and useful instruments, but also very dangerous if the diagnosis relies on them alone, as they will never reach a 100% predictive value. Nonetheless, sexual inventories can be considered a guide but not a substitute for an in-depth sexual history. However, their uncritical use may jeopardize diagnosis if the complexity of human sexual behavior is not taken into account or sexual function and dysfunction are oversimplified and trivialized with mere numbers, such as the score obtained from an inventory (31).

The common interpretation of ED as a disorder in itself rather than a symptom leads to diagnostic errors such as those which give particular importance to the patient's psychosexual history. The belief that the organic or psychogenic nature can be recognized through the patient's history is only apparently correct. In reality, it may be dangerous and misleading. Table 1,

Table 1 Distinguishing Features of Impotence

Erectile dysfunction	Psychogenic (nonorganic)	Organic
Onset	Acute	Insidious
Relationship with existential event	Present	Absent
Relationship with physical disease	Absent	Present
Characteristics	Selective, intermittent, transitory	Worsening, absolute
Nocturnal erections	Present/reduced	Absent
Spontaneous erections	Present/reduced/absent	Absent
Erections on masturbation	Present	Absent

which is widely reported in the literature, is undoubtedly useful in guiding the clinician, but the patient's history can lead to gross errors. For example, a history of sexual violence since childhood does not necessarily indicate a psychogenic cause, especially if the patient is diabetic. Neither is diabetes itself necessarily at the heart of the ED, given that up to 30% of male diabetics have normal erectile function (32). Along the same lines, the fact that a given patient experiences normal function within his marriage but is impotent in an extramarital relationship (or vice versa) does not necessarily indicate that the sole cause is performance anxiety in one or other situation.

The concept of the *locus minoris resistentiae* (area of least resistance) is an old one but still a valid, useful way of thinking. This must be considered in evaluating causes or concauses of ED; In the previous example, for instance, so-called situational impotence is not necessarily a psychological disturbance (33), but could be a symptom of an organic breakdown of a physiological system, which manifests only under (psychological) stress and not in subjectively nonstressful situations. No cardiologist would fail to attribute a solid organic basis to angina pectoris just because it manifested only in conditions of psychophysical stress! Chest pain in angina patients normally only manifests in more psychologically or physically demanding situations, while the heart remains completely asymptomatic in normal, nonstressful conditions. Is there any reason why ED should not be the same?

A large body of literature deals with the psychosocial etiologies of ED (34). Again, while it is clear that these causes may specifically affect the ability to obtain or maintain an erection, the presence of a psychological issue must always be considered a concause or a possible cause. It is impossible to demonstrate that it is "the" cause: psychological factors are frequently found in combination with organic causes.

In the **intrapsychic** environment, many factors may act directly on virility (Table 2) and others indirectly, throughout a sociocultural mechanism. This is the case of the frequent myths about male sexuality ("men always want and can have sex,"

Table 2 Intrapsychic Causes or Concauses of Erectile Dysfunction

- Performance anxiety
- Depression
- Negative expectations
- Professional stress
- Traumatizing experiences
- Loss of self-esteem
- Loss of autonomy
- Rigid sexual education

fixation on the standard macho model of sex, etc.). Traditional sex education is often inadequate, with its focus on reproductive biology, perpetuation of sexual myths, and inability to provide a framework for personal growth and interaction, and is, therefore, an important psychological risk factor. Furthermore, contemporary role models and media can also be unhelpful or even misleading—especially performance-orientated models, where sexuality is a matter of "success" or "failure." Anxiety, probably through an adrenergic mechanism, is one of the major psychological cofactors of ED (35,36). Shabsigh et al. reported that ED is associated with a high incidence of depressive symptoms regardless of age, marital status, or comorbidities (3). However, this is not pure ED, as it is almost always secondary to HSDD. It is also important to note that patients with ED and depression are more likely to discontinue their treatment than other patients with ED.

Finally, of the psychological abnormalities of ED, alexithymia—defined as difficulty in identifying feelings and distinguishing between feelings and the bodily sensations of emotional arousal—is a personality trait not rarely found in impotent men (37). Although easily considered a causative element, alexithymia can also be a consequence of erection-related doubts.

Erectile dysfunction can cause significant problems for the patient, his partner, and their relationship. However, relationship difficulties can also be an important concause of ED (20). For this reason, treating ED should involve the partner wherever possible. As with HSDD, **relational** factors are important in ED pathogenesis and maintenance. Risk factors for developing relational ED include the presence of chronic conflicts (firm roles of dominance and dependence), habit and the couple's routine, loss of sex appeal, disparity of income with respect to the female partner, and, obviously, jealousy following the discovery of an extramarital relationship.

Finally, ED has a substantial impact on health-related **quality of life**. Positive correlations between erectile function and self-esteem, confidence, and relationship satisfaction suggest that improved erectile quality can ameliorate the long-term psychosocial quality of life (38). Improvement of ED by effective pharmacological treatments is associated with a marked improvement in depressive symptoms, anxiety, and general quality of life (39). For this reason, sildenafil and related drugs (tadalafil and vardenafil) can be considered as "psycho-drugs," acting on mind and behavior in a somatopsychic way.

EJACULATORY DYSFUNCTIONS: PREMATURE EJACULATION

Ejaculatory disorders are classified as disorders of emission, ejaculation itself, and orgasm (40). While the list of etiological causes of impotence is large and growing, for the most frequent ejaculatory disorder—premature ejaculation (PE)—it is still quite short, with psychological causes being the most studied in past years (41). PE has been perceived as a psychological concern, either a learned behavior or a response to a meaningful event/interaction or sexual anxiety (42). For this reason, the psychophysiological model has been applied to the study of ejaculatory response for well over four decades. This approach illustrates the complex relationship emerging among cognitive, affective, and physiological components of ejaculation control. Furthermore, systematic use of psychopathological procedures is a crucial aid in differential diagnosis of various PE subtypes (43).

Premature ejaculation is a frequent male sexual complaint (44). While there are strong indications that lifelong PE is a mainly neurobiologically determined dysfunction (45), acquired PE is a symptom with numerous acquired causes (46): urological, such as prostate infection/inflammation (subclinical prostatitis) (47), neurological (48), hormonal, such as hyperthyroidism (15,49), and psychological (relational and intrapsychic) (41,50).

Psychoanalytic theories are based on the idea that distortions of belief and false convictions about sexuality are established in childhood as a consequence of adverse influences on sexual behavior. Destructive attitudes are usually exerted by parents, but also by other power figures within and outside the family (51). This, in a Freudian perspective, may lead to sexual dysfunctions such as PE. Classic psychoanalytic theories identified a sadistic or narcissistic behavior in PE (52). For other psychoanalysts, however, men who ejaculate prematurely are typically passive and masochistic in their marriage and obsessive–compulsive in character. These theories were the basis of Helen S. Kaplan's first idea that PE is the result of an unconscious hatred of women (53). By ejaculating quickly, a man symbolically and physically "steals" the woman's orgasm. However, the same researcher rejected her own theory when she found that men with PE do not have any particular neuroses or personality disorders (54).

Premature ejaculation has been considered as common, if not normal, during early sexual experiences. Masters and Johnson added other connected etiological causes to this concept, building **behavioral theories** on PE: the risk of unwanted discovery (such as copulating in a car), experiences with prostitutes, and anxiety due to poor sexual education (e.g., lack of adequate knowledge of contraceptive methods) can worsen ejaculatory control, already physiologically poor at a young age (Table 3) (1).

Table 3 Psychosocial Factors Involved in Premature Ejaculation

- GUILT (sexual activity considered sinful, e.g., premarital or extramarital sex)
- FEAR (of pregnancy, sexually transmitted diseases, being discovered)
- ANXIETY (general or related to sexual performance)

Source: From Ref. 50.

Kaplan's original etiological explanation is also connected with the role of early experiences: a man with PE has not allowed himself to receive the sensory feedback of those sensations occurring immediately before orgasm, which would enable him to bring his ejaculatory reflex under voluntary control (54). She compares this mechanism to control of enuresis, obtained when a child recognizes the sensation of a full bladder. In the same way, lack of awareness of preejaculatory sensations may lead to PE.

Finally, anxiety (over sexual performance generally, but also over other, extrasexual factors) has frequently been suggested as a cause (55). This is in accordance with Kaplan's theory: anxiety may block pre-ejaculatory sensations. It should be noted again that anxiety may also be the effect rather than the cause of sexual dysfunction.

EJACULATORY DYSFUNCTIONS: DEFICIENT EJACULATION

Even if much rarer than PE, delayed or inability to reach ejaculation and/or orgasm is a clinical symptom, which may seriously impair a couple's sexual life. A continuing problem with deficient ejaculation is usually taken personally by the partner, who begins to feel less attractive, sexy, and sexually adequate. Marital stress, sexual dissatisfaction, inhibited sexual desire, and avoidance of sexual contact may result if the symptom is not addressed and remedied.

Delayed ejaculation (DE), or ejaculatory insufficiency, is an inhibition of the ejaculatory reflex with absent or reduced seminal emission and impaired ejaculatory contractions, possibly with reduced or absent orgasm. Estimates of DE incidence range from 1% to 4% of sexually active men. Men with DE may be able to ejaculate with great effort and after prolonged intercourse (30 to 45 minutes), or be unable to ejaculate in some circumstances. The symptom can occur both during intercourse and with manual stimulation in the presence or absence of a partner (*relative* and *absolute* DE, respectively). If ejaculation is totally absent, the condition is called male anorgasmia (46).

Psychological etiologies may be the result of strict religious backgrounds (causing sex to be viewed as sinful), lack of attraction to a female partner, idiosyncratic conditioning caused by unique or atypical masturbation patterns, psychologically traumatic events (such as being discovered in masturbation or illicit sex, or learning that his partner is having an affair), and homosexual attraction. Ejaculatory overcontrol may mirror an overcontrolled personality, frequently found in these patients. Delayed ejaculation has been also recently explained as having an "autosexual" rather than heterosexual or homosexual orientation (56). Ejaculation during masturbation is in fact often normal in DE. However, even if it is considered a psychorelational symptom, DE may often be associated with medical therapy or with infection/inflammation of the prostate and seminal vesicles (46).

In conclusion, multiple psychobiological causes are associated with DE, a still obscure condition that substantially impairs the couple's psychosexual equilibrium (57).

The condition of a man who has never ejaculated through any form of stimulation, such as "wet dreams," masturbation, or coitus (primary or complete **anejaculation**, or *impotentia ejaculationis*), occurs in 0.14% of the general population, according to Kinsey et al. (58). These patients originated from differing social and intellectual levels, but a feature common to them all was a strict education. Other psychological factors underlying this condition are poorly defined. In fact, psychosexual counseling and/or psychotherapy are not as effective as in other types of nonorganic sexual dysfunction. Anejaculation, in contrast to DE, appears to be mainly caused by organic etiologies. The best way to deal with lifelong anejaculation thus far seems to be to inform the patients about the biological and psychological inhibiting factors they need to avoid, and to discourage unrealistic expectations of psychotherapy. However, psychotherapy may be useful in subgroups, particularly in the absence of effective and safe drugs (59).

CONCLUSION: THE ROLE OF COUNSELING IN ANDROLOGICAL PRACTICE

The availability of the first effective oral treatment for ED (60) has led to a significant increase in men seeking andrological diagnosis and treatment. However, the apparently easy medical approach has induced some clinicians to neglect counseling and the relational, interpersonal, and psychological impact of sexual dysfunction and its diagnosis and treatment. In fact, a brief explanation of sexual physiology in dysfunctions is no less essential than giving information on food intake to diabetic patients (61). Counseling may uncover and resolve hidden conflicts (anger and grief). The clinician, who should try to facilitate communication between partners, may explore relationship issues, uncovering a need for professional couple therapy in complicated cases.

In the last three to four decades, the only real novelty in the management of sexual diseases has been their medical treatment. In fact, behavioral therapies (62) are still used without substantial modification of the original definitions and format (63). The field of psychosexology has only recently taken the task of scientifically demonstrating the efficacy of psychosexual therapies seriously. Following this path, talking therapies will continue to play a pivotal role in sexology, not as an alternative to but probably in conjunction with medical treatments in complicated cases.

There are many men with sexual dysfunctions, and their number is expected to grow, as will awareness of the possibility of seeking help. It is clear that the best therapeutic results are obtained when the psychorelational impact of diagnosis and therapy are taken into account. For this reason, an integrated model has been proposed, with the coresponsibility of the doctor (exclusion of physical diseases and prescription of medicines) and the psychologist (taking care of psychological aspects) in the management of dysfunctional patients (64).

There are several elements in favor of, and also against, this model, making it problematic. As clarified in the introduction, any sexual dysfunction, even if due to the most organic of causes, may dramatically affect the couple's psychology, behavior, and relationship, with profound echoes in their life. Thus the presence of a psychosexologist in the diagnostic and therapeutic team is more than useful. Re-establishing erectile function or ejaculatory control and re-establishing satisfactory sexual interaction with the partner are totally different objectives, and when the latter is not achieved, men may represent with treatment failure or withdraw from treatment altogether. The risk with medical and surgical therapies alone is in fact their focus on the penis as the central dysfunctional element, failing to appreciate the couple as the real source of the problem (20). Thus a combination of both medical and psychological professional experiences seems necessary.

Against the sometimes idealistic integrated model are the problems of a lack of guarantee of its therapeutic outcome, the high cost of a talking therapy and the fact that few psychologists are really able to achieve both a good, effective relationship with their patients and a good partnership with the doctors. The Global Study of Sexual Attitudes and Behaviours [GSSAB] survey demonstrated that worldwide only 5.5% of men with a sexual dysfunction talked to a psychiatrist, psychologist, or marriage counselor about their sexual problems (65). In addition, the distinction between body and mind is obsolete, cultural and artificial, and frequently not appreciated by patients. This distinction takes inadequate account of modern physiological research and belies the axiom that all psychological processes have a somatic basis. It is in fact far more than a trivial mantra to repeat that the only right way to approach to patients with sexual dysfunction is holistically. Integrated medical and psychosexological sex therapy requires mutual understanding and respect for the different disciplines involved in sexual health. This is unfortunately not always possible due to both psychological and medical reductionisms and the original sins of the old psychosexology and new sexual medicine that this chapter has attempted to obviate.

REFERENCES

1. Masters W, Johnson,VE. Human Sexual Inadequacy. Boston: Little, Brown Co, 1970.
2. Carson C, Kirby R, Goldstein I. Textbook of Erectile Dysfunction. Oxford Isis Medical, 1999.
3. Shabsigh R, Klein LT, Seidman S, et al. Increased incidence of depressive symptoms in men with erectile dysfunction. Urology 1998; 52:848–852.
4. Jeffcoate WJ. Impotence: science and sciencibility. Br Med J (Clin Res Ed) 1986; 292:783–784.
5. Usta MF, Erdogru T, Tefekli A, et al. Honeymoon impotence: psychogenic or organic in origin? Urology 2001; 57:758–762.
6. Rosen RC. Psychogenic erectile dysfunction. Classification and management. Urol Clin North Am 2001; 28:269–278.
7. De Berardis G, Franciosi M, Belfiglio M, et al. Erectile dysfunction and quality of life in type 2 diabetic patients: a serious problem too often overlooked. Diabetes Care 2002; 25:284–291.
8. Wyllie MG. The underlying pathophysiology and causes of erectile dysfunction. Clin Cornerstone 2005; 7:19–27.
9. Carosa E, Benvenga S, Trimarchi F, et al. Sexual inactivity results in reversible reduction of LH bioavailability. Int J Impot Res 2002; 14:93–99; discussion 100.
10. Lue TF. Erectile dysfunction. N Engl J Med 2000; 342:1802–1813.
11. Jannini EA, Lenzi A, Isidori A, et al. Subclinical erectile dysfunction: proposal for a novel taxonomic category in sexual medicine. J Sex Med 2006; 3:787–793; discussion 794.
12. Speckens AE, Hengeveld MW, Lycklama à Nijeholt GA, et al. Discrimination between psychogenic and organic erectile dysfunction. J Psychosom Res 1993; 37:135–145.
13. Sachs BD. The false organic-psychogenic distinction and related problems in the classification of erectile dysfunction. Int J Impot Res 2003; 15:72–78.
14. Magee MC. Psychogenic impotence: a critical review. Urology 1980; 15:435–442.
15. Carani C, Isidori AM, Granata A, et al. Multicenter study on the prevalence of sexual symptoms in male hypo- and hyperthyroid patients. J Clin Endocrinol Metab 2005; 90:6472–6479.
16. American Psychiatric Association. Diagnostic and statistical manual of mental disorders (DSM-IV-TR), 4th ed. Washington: APA, 2000.
17. Segraves R, Balon R, Clayton A. Proposal for changes in diagnostic criteria for sexual dysfunctions. J Sex Med 2007; 4:567–580.
18. Kaplan HS. Disorders of Sexual Desire. New York, NY: Simon and Schuster, 1979.
19. Corona G, Jannini EA, Maggi M. Inventories for male and female sexual dysfunctions. Int J Impot Res 2006; 18:236–250.
20. Corona G, Petrone L, Mannucci E, et al. Assessment of the relational factor in male patients consulting for sexual dysfunction: the concept of couple sexual dysfunction. J Androl 2006; 27:795–801.
21. Corona G, Petrone L, Mannucci E, et al. The impotent couple: low desire. Int J Androl 2005; 28(suppl 2):46–52.

22. Hatzichristou D, Rosen RC, Broderick G, et al. Clinical evaluation and management strategy for sexual dysfunction in men and women. J Sex Med 2004; 1:49–57.
23. Jannini EA, Screponi E, Carosa E, et al. Lack of sexual activity from erectile dysfunction is associated with a reversible reduction in serum testosterone. Int J Androl 1999; 22:385–392.
24. Lenzi A, Lombardo F, Salacone P, et al. Stress, sexual dysfunctions, and male infertility. J Endocrinol Invest 2003; 26:72–76.
25. Sternbach H. Age-associated testosterone decline in men: clinical issues for psychiatry. Am J Psychiatry 1998; 155:1310–1318.
26. Yesavage JA, Davidson J, Widrow L, et al. Plasma testosterone levels, depression, sexuality, and age. Biol Psychiatry 1985; 20:222–225.
27. Tenover JL. Male hormone replacement therapy including "andropause". Endocrinol Metab Clin North Am 1998; 27:969–987, x.
28. Carosa E, Volpe R, Martini P, et al. Psychosocial issues of ART in aging male. J Endocrinol Invest 2005; 28:117–121.
29. Rosen RC, Riley A, Wagner G, et al. The international index of erectile function (IIEF): a multidimensional scale for assessment of erectile dysfunction. Urology 1997; 49:822–830.
30. Petrone L, Mannucci E, Corona G, et al. Structured interview on erectile dysfunction (SIEDY): a new, multidimensional instrument for quantification of pathogenetic issues on erectile dysfunction. Int J Impot Res 2003; 15:210–220.
31. Corona G, Petrone L, Mannucci E, et al. Difficulties in achieving vs maintaining erection: organic, psychogenic and relational determinants. Int J Impot Res 2005; 17:252–258.
32. Giuliano FA, Leriche A, Jaudinot EO, et al. Prevalence of erectile dysfunction among 7689 patients with diabetes or hypertension, or both. Urology 2004; 64:1196–1201.
33. Williams W. Psychogenic erectile impotence–a useful or a misleading concept? Aust N Z J Psychiatry 1985; 19:77–82.
34. Corona G, Ricca V, Bandini E, et al. Association between Psychiatric Symptoms and Erectile Dysfunction. J Sex Med 2008; 5:458–468.
35. Aversa A, Rocchietti-March M, Caprio M, et al. Anxiety-induced failure in erectile response to intracorporeal prostaglandin-E1 in non-organic male impotence: a new diagnostic approach. Int J Androl 1996; 19:307–313.
36. Corona G, Mannucci E, Petrone L, et al. Psycho-biological correlates of free-floating anxiety symptoms in male patients with sexual dysfunctions. J Androl 2006; 27:86–93.
37. Michetti PM, Rossi R, Bonanno D, et al. Male sexuality and regulation of emotions: a study on the association between alexithymia and erectile dysfunction (ED). Int J Impot Res 2006; 18:170–174.
38. Althof SE, O'Leary MP, Cappelleri JC, et al. Impact of erectile dysfunction on confidence, self-esteem and relationship satisfaction after 9 months of sildenafil citrate treatment. J Urol 2006; 176:2132–2137.
39. Seidman SN, Roose SP, Menza MA, et al. Treatment of erectile dysfunction in men with depressive symptoms: results of a placebo-controlled trial with sildenafil citrate. Am J Psychiatry 2001; 158:1623–1630.
40. Jannini EA, Lenzi A. Ejaculatory disorders: epidemiology and current approaches to definition, classification and subtyping. World J Urol 2005; 23:68–75.
41. Jannini EA, Simonelli C, Lenzi A. Sexological approach to ejaculatory dysfunction. Int J Androl 2002; 25:317–323.
42. Althof S. The psychology of premature ejaculation: therapies and consequences. J Sex Med 2006; 3(suppl 4):324–331.
43. Rowland DL, Slob AK. Understanding and diagnosing sexual dysfunction: recent progress through psychophysiological and psychophysical methods. Neurosci Biobehav Rev 1995; 19:201–209.
44. Jannini EA, Lenzi A. Epidemiology of premature ejaculation. Curr Opin Urol 2005; 15:399–403.
45. Waldinger MD. The neurobiological approach to premature ejaculation. J Urol 2002; 168:2359–2367.
46. Jannini EA, Simonelli C, Lenzi A. Disorders of ejaculation. J Endocrinol Invest 2002; 25:1006–1019.
47. Screponi E, Carosa E, Di Stasi SM, et al. Prevalence of chronic prostatitis in men with premature ejaculation. Urology 2001; 58:198–202.
48. Colpi GM, Fanciullacci F, Beretta G, et al. Evoked sacral potentials in subjects with true premature ejaculation. Andrologia 1986; 18:583–586.
49. Corona G, Petrone L, Mannucci E, et al. Psycho-biological correlates of rapid ejaculation in patients attending an andrologic unit for sexual dysfunctions. Eur Urol 2004; 46:615–622.
50. Jannini EA, Lenzi A. Couple therapy for premature ejaculation. In: Kandeel RF, Lue T, Pryor JL, Swerdloff RS, eds. Male Sexual Dysfunction: Pathophysiology and Treatment. New York, NY: Informa, 2007:351–362.
51. Bieber I. The psychoanalytic treatment of sexual disorders. J Sex Marital Ther 1974; 1:5–15.
52. Ellis H. Studies in the Psychology of Sex. New York, NY: Random House, 1936.
53. Kaplan H. The New Sex Therapy: Active Treatment of Sexual Dysfunction. New York, NY: Brunner/Mazel, 1974.
54. Kaplan HS. How to Overcome Premature Ejaculation. New York, NY: Brunner-Mazel, 1989.
55. Dunn KM, Croft PR, Hackett GI. Association of sexual problems with social, psychological, and physical problems in men and women: a cross sectional population survey. J Epidemiol Community Health 1999; 53:144–148.

56. Apfelbaum B. Retarded ejaculation. A much misunderstood syndrome. In: Leiblum SR, Rosen RC, eds. Principles and Practice of Sex Therapy, 3rd ed. New York, NY: Guilford Press, 2000:205–241.
57. Corona G, Mannucci E, Petrone L, et al. Psychobiological correlates of delayed ejaculation in male patients with sexual dysfunctions. J Androl 2006; 27:453–458.
58. Kinsey A, Pomeroy WB, Martin CE. Sexual Behavior in the Human Male. Philadelphia: W.B. Saunders, 1948.
59. Waldinger MD, Schweitzer DH. Retarded ejaculation in men: an overview of psychological and neurobiological insights. World J Urol 2005; 23:76–81.
60. Jannini EA, Lenzi A, Wagner G. New perspectives in the pharmacotherapy of erectile dysfunction. IDrugs 2003; 6:1165–1172.
61. Jannini EA, Lenzi A, Wagner G. Behavioural Therapy and Counselling. In: Schill WB, Comhaire FH, Hargreave TB, eds. Andrology for the Clinician. Berlin: Springer, 2006:598–607.
62. Barnes T. Integrated sex therapy: the interplay of behavioral, cognitive and medical approaches. In: Carson CC, Kirby ES, Goldstein I, eds. Textbook of Erectile Dysfunction. Oxford: Isis Medical Media, 1999:465–484.
63. Shover L, Leiblum S. The stagnation of sex therapy. J Psychol Human Sex 1994; 6:5–10.
64. Jannini EA, Lenzi A. Introduction to the integrated model: medical, surgical and psychological therapies for the couple. J Endocrinol Invest 2003; 26:128–131.
65. Moreira E, Glasser DB, Laumann E, et al. Help-seeking behavior for sexual problems according to gender: results from the global survey of sexual attitudes and behaviors. In: VII Latin American Congress for the Study of Impotence and Sexuality; 2003; Cartagena, Colombia.

41 Ejaculatory disorders

Nancy L. Brackett, Charles M. Lynne, Dana A. Ohl and Jens Sønksen

ANATOMY AND PHYSIOLOGY OF EJACULATION

Ejaculation is the process of allowing transport of sperm through the urethra and expulsion of semen from the urethral meatus. The organs involved in the ejaculatory process are the epididymis, vas deferens, prostate, seminal vesicles, bladder neck, external urethral sphincter, and bulbourethral glands (1). In normal ejaculation, anatomic structures are precisely coordinated via neural centers to allow normal ejaculation to take place.

Sperm are stored in the cauda epididymis prior to ejaculation. Research using an animal model has shown that fluid is first slowly expelled from the cauda epididymis into the vas deferens during sexual excitement. Sperm are then rapidly transported via peristalsis through the vas deferens and into the urethra during ejaculation. In the animal model, residual cauda fluid persisting in the urethra is transported back into the cauda epididymis where it is again stored until the next ejaculation (2). This storage function can become disordered by neurological conditions (3), or infrequent ejaculation (2,4). In such cases, distal migration down the Wolffian structures can occur leading to storage of sperm in the seminal vesicles, a condition detrimental to sperm motility (3).

The vasa run up from the testes, in the spermatic cord, entering the retroperitoneum and separating from the spermatic cord to course over the ureter, and turn medially under the prostate. There they run medial and parallel to the seminal vesicles, eventually coalescing with the (excretory ducts of the) seminal vesicles to become the ejaculatory ducts. The ejaculatory ducts course through the prostate and open into the urethra on the sides of the verumontanum.

Once seminal fluid is expelled through the ejaculatory ducts into the urethra, it is normally expelled forcibly in an antegrade direction. In sequence, first the bladder neck closes, preventing retrograde ejaculation. Then contractions of the periurethral muscles cause rhythmic forceful expulsion of semen through the urethra. Expansion of the posterior urethra has been postulated to cause the rhythmic contractions; however, contractions are observed in neurologically normal men with the absence of seminal emission, such as testis cancer patients who underwent a radical retroperitoneal lymph node dissection. This observation suggests that periurethral muscle activity is part of the central reflex, rather than a response to posterior urethral expansion.

The exact mechanisms mediating this coordinated reflex are not completely understood. Studies in men with spinal cord injury suggest that an extremely high pressure contraction of the external sphincter/periurethral muscles is the event that immediately precedes the ejaculatory reflex threshold. For example, men with high pressure contractions in response to penile vibratory stimulation always ejaculated, whereas those without such muscle contraction never ejaculated (5). This finding suggests that proprioception within the external sphincter may be important in initiating responses through the neurological pathways described below. In any event, the external urethral sphincter must relax enough to allow the pressure gradient built up in this "pressure chamber" to forcibly expel the semen outward from the urethra in an antegrade direction.

Neural Control of Ejaculation

Neural control of ejaculation consists of the ejaculatory reflex that is mediated at the thoracolumbar level and involves a coordinated interaction of the sympathetic and parasympathetic autonomic nervous systems. Higher-level control of the ejaculatory reflex is probably initiated centrally and may be inhibited centrally as well via the cortex, thalamus, hypothalamus, midbrain, and pons (6,7). Centrally, dopaminergic structures are thought to be excitatory to the ejaculatory reflex while serotonergic receptors are thought to be inhibitory (8,9). Additional somatic input directly into the reflex comes from the dorsal nerve of the penis.

A "pressure chamber" phenomenon, created by seminal emission and closure of the bladder neck, is mediated by sympathetic outflow via lumbar sympathetic ganglia and the hypogastric nerve. Secretions of the prostate gland and seminal vesicles result from parasympathetic outflow (S2–4) via the pelvic nerve. Contractions of the bulbocavernosal muscles, ischiocavernosal muscles, and pelvic floor result in forceful expulsion of the ejaculate. These functions are mediated by somatic efferents from segments S2–4 (Fig. 1).

ABNORMALITIES OF EJACULATION

Anatomic Abnormalities of Ejaculation

Ejaculatory Duct Obstruction

Obstruction of the ejaculatory ducts may be complete or partial. Complete ejaculatory duct obstruction (EDO) is generally recognized as a condition caused either by atresia of the ends of the ejaculatory ducts or by obstruction of the distal ends of the ejaculatory ducts such as by midline prostatic cysts (usually originating in the prostatic utricle). Those men with atretic distal prostatic ducts may have cystic fibrosis gene mutations as seen also in men with congenital bilateral absence of the vas deferens. The clinical findings are: azoospermia, low seminal

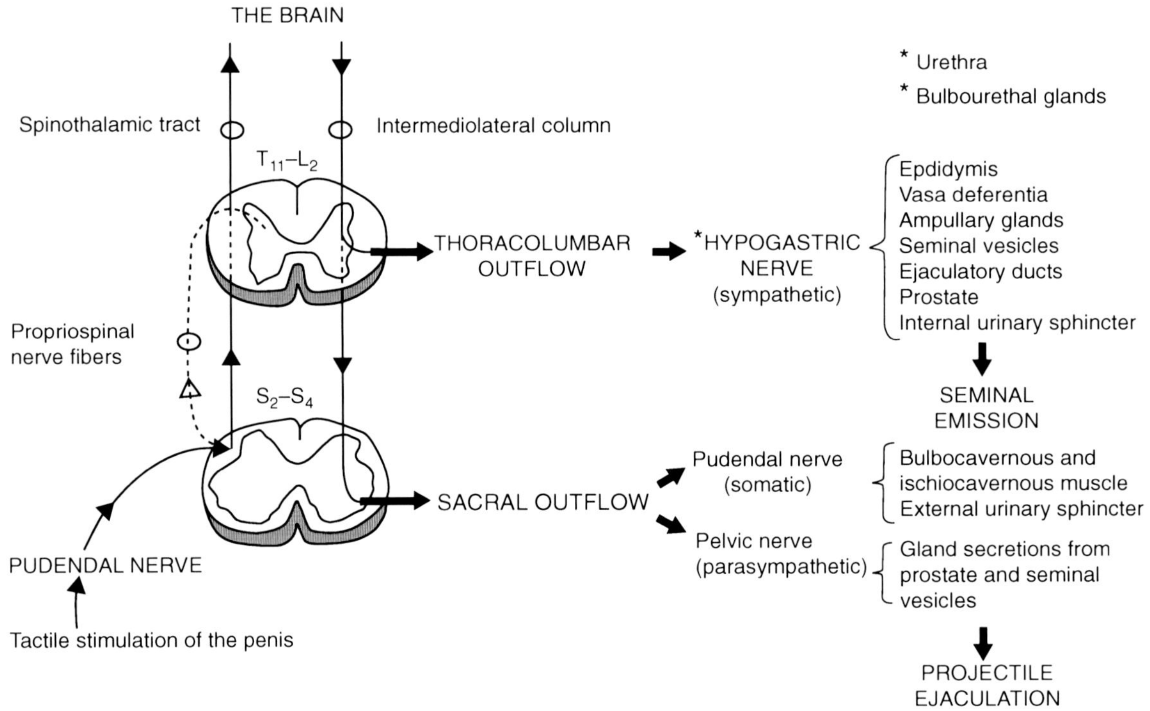

Figure 1 Spinal inervation of ejaculation.

fluid volume (<1 cc), absence of fructose in the seminal fluid, and an acidic pH of the seminal fluid. A carefully performed transrectal ultrasound of the prostate can often demonstrate dilated ejaculatory ducts as they course through the prostate or the midline cysts.

Partial EDO is a controversial diagnosis, not universally accepted by all urologists. It is thought that some problems of abnormal sperm morphology and motility previously thought to be idiopathic (and with sperm volumes > 1 cc) can be explained by partial EDO. The major argument against this belief is that the diagnosis is presumptive and that the treatment, transurethral resection of the ejaculatory ducts (TURED), may have significant morbidity, including reduced fertility (10).

TURED enjoys a high success rate resulting in increased seminal volume and reappearance of sperm in the ejaculate. Urine contamination of the ejaculate, reflux into the prostate, and scarring of the urethra, however, can lead to complications. In cases in which the ejaculatory ducts may not be dilated, such as presumed partial EDO, postoperative scarring may result in complete obstruction. Midline cysts may be aspirated or excised in some instances.

Congenital Bilateral Absence of the Vas Deferens (CBAVD)

Congenital bilateral absence of the vas deferens (CBAVD) is highly associated with mutations of the cystic fibrosis gene (the cystic fibrosis transmembrane conductance regulator gene, CFTR). More than 80% of men with CBAVD will have at least one mutation of the gene. Over 95% of men with cystic fibrosis will have an abnormality of the Wolffian duct structures, primarily absences of the vasa. Men with CBAVD will also have varying degrees of malformation of the epididymis although the caput is usually intact. The seminal vesicles likewise are commonly hypoplastic or atretic and may appear absent or abnormal on transrectal ultrasound (11).

Clinically, men with CBAVD present as do men with complete EDO; azoospermia, low ejaculate volume, absence of seminal fructose, and an acid seminal pH. The vasa are, of course, not palpable. To date, CBAVD is not reconstructible. Usually testicular function is normal and sperm retrieval coupled with IVF/ICSI is commonly employed to achieve pregnancy. Prior to commencing attempts at pregnancy, both the man and his partner should undergo testing for CFTR gene mutations and receive genetic counseling.

Bladder Neck Incompetence

As discussed in the earlier section on anatomy and physiology, the bladder neck must close in order for an orderly sequence of antegrade ejaculation to occur. All else being normal, bladder neck incompetence results in retrograde ejaculation. Occasionally, this condition may be seen as a spontaneous problem. More commonly, retrograde ejaculation, due to an incompetent internal sphincter, is a result of medication (see the section on α-adrenergic antagonists), diabetic neuropathy or other neurogenic causes, or anatomic causes.

In the past, Y-V plasty of the bladder neck had been employed to surgically treat young boys for a variety of conditions, such as vesicoureteral reflux, urinary tract infections, dysfunctional voiding, and enuresis (12). It was not effective for these conditions, and has been abandoned. However, an occasional patient will still be seen with this condition. Reversal of Y-V plasty is difficult. With the use of relatively simple sperm retrieval techniques (discussed later in this chapter), and the availability of the common assisted reproductive technologies, an attempt at surgical revision of the previously operated bladder neck is usually not necessary nor advisable.

Neuropathic Abnormalities of Ejaculation

Table 1 lists the major causes of neurogenic ejaculatory dysfunction.

Diabetes

Genital urinary (GU) dysfunction is common in Type I diabetics. Diabetic "cystopathy" and erectile dysfunction have been well described, occurring in up to 87% and 75%, respectively, of men with Type I diabetes (13). Ejaculatory dysfunction is not as well described or reported. In surveys, it may be included as a part of ED. Clinically, ejaculatory dysfunction will be recognized as an absence of ejaculate. This condition will be caused either by retrograde ejaculation (poor closure of the bladder neck) or by anejaculation (failure of emission), and is now considered part of the broader spectrum of diabetic sympathetic autonomic neuropathy. Ejaculatory dysfunction is said to be present in up to 40% of men with Type I diabetes (14).

To produce an antegrade ejaculate and/or attempt a pregnancy through normal intercourse, almost any sympathomimetic drug may be used to close or "tighten" the bladder neck (see the section on pharmacologic management), although results are variable and usually disappointing (15). For most couples, some sort of assisted conception will be necessary, and in most instances, the protocols for retrieving and using retrograde sperm will be satisfactory. Men more severely affected who are truly anejaculatory (failure of emission) will usually require electroejaculation or surgical sperm retrieval to obtain sperm for assisted conception.

Low Abdominal/Pelvic Surgery

Surgery in the retroperitoneum and pelvis in proximity to the sympathetic and parasympathetic plexi that supply the GU organs commonly leads to varying degrees of injury to those structures. The superior hypogastric plexus, rich in sympathetic fibers, lies in a midline presacral position just below the aortic bifurcation and is vulnerable to injury during classic open surgery for abdominal aortic aneurysm, aortobifemoral bypass, and some colorectal and pelvic tumors. Injury to this structure may lead to disinnervation of the bladder neck, which can result in retrograde ejaculation. The pelvic splanchnic nerve(s) in the perirectal area, rich in parasympathetic fibers, may commonly be injured during radical rectal surgery. In addition to erectile and urinary dysfunction, 36% to 60% rates of ejaculatory dysfunction have been reported after this type of surgery (16).

Table 1 Neurogenic Causes of Ejaculatory Dysfunction

Diabetes
Low abdominal/pelvic surgery
Multiple sclerosis
Myelodysplasia
Retroperitoneal lymph node dissection
Spinal cord injury
Stroke/traumatic brain injury

Multiple Sclerosis

Multiple sclerosis (MS), a demyelinating disease, affects both the brain and spinal cord. Autonomic dysfunction, often vague, may be an early sign of MS but as the disease progresses the GU system is heavily involved. Reportedly, voiding dysfunction is present in up to 97% of patients, erectile dysfunction in up to 73%, and ejaculatory and/or orgasmic dysfunction in 50%, while libido is reduced in only 40% (17). The autonomic nervous system symptoms may wax and wane along with the somatic symptoms. Men with MS who are anejaculatory respond to assisted ejaculation in much the same way as men with spinal cord injury, although certain caveats must be followed. Men with MS are generally sensate, and if electroejaculation is employed, heavy conscious sedation or general anesthesia will be necessary. Similarly, penile vibratory stimulation, if performed with the degree of intensity required to induce ejaculation, may be intolerable, due to preserved penile sensation. Additional considerations are that treatment regimens for men with MS may include steroids and/or immunosuppressive medications with accompanying effects on testicular function and spermatogenesis.

Myelodysplasia

Spinal dysraphism involves the lumbar vertebrae in over 90% of cases and the lower thoracic vertebrae in another 5% (18). Most of these patients will have urologic problems and, as they progress through puberty into adulthood, sexual problems as well. An excellent study by Decter et al., of 57 men attending a multidisciplinary spina bifida clinic, documented the sexual functioning of these men. Forty-one had erections, including 27 who ejaculated with erection. Of 11 patients who attempted to father children, 8 were successful. The patients' neurological level of dysfunction did not seem to be predictive of either erectile or ejaculatory competence. Those men with lower (and less severe) neurologic levels of dysfunction appeared to have a better chance of achieving fatherhood (19).

Retroperitoneal Lymph Node Dissection (RPLND)

The paravertebral sympathetic ganglia at the thoracolumbar levels are in close proximity to the para-aortic and paracaval lymph nodes involved in metastatic spread from testicular cancers and may be injured and/or resected during RPLND. The superior hypogastric plexus, comprised of postganglionic fibers from these ganglia, lies approximately in a midline presacral position and may also be involved to some degree in the dissection. These structures contain sympathetic fibers responsible for seminal emission and bladder neck closure. Historically, retrograde ejaculation or anejaculation has been the sequelae of most concern in this procedure since the disease being treated occurs so commonly in men of the age of planning for parenthood. The surgical templates designed to spare at least a part of these structures have reduced the risk of loss of ejaculatory function. The highest rates of success in preserving ejaculatory function have been reported with nerve sparing RPLND. When the surgical anatomy and findings are favorable, ejaculation can be preserved in up to 95% of patients undergoing this procedure (20). With the advent of laparoscopic lymph node dissection, there have been some reports of laparoscopic RPLND being successful in preserving ejaculation in all of the patients in which the procedure was successfully completed (21,22).

Spinal Cord Injury

Spinal cord injury (SCI) is a disease of young men. In men with a conus or cauda equina injury occurring below sacral cord levels responsible for ejaculation, up to 18% retain their ability to ejaculate (23). These very low lesions are uncommon and the vast majority of men with SCI cannot ejaculate without technical or medical assistance. The two most studied and reliable methods of assisted ejaculation are penile vibratory stimulation and electroejaculation that are described later in this chapter.

Stroke and Traumatic Brain Injury

In general, patients who have sustained either a stroke or traumatic brain injury (TBI) will complain of the same types of sexual disorders, which include a decline in libido, sexual satisfaction, coital frequency, erection, and orgasmic ability (16). Ejaculatory dysfunction per se is usually not reported and is implied in reports and discussions of orgasmic dysfunction. Because of the profound effects of brain injury/dysfunction on the patients' psychological, cognitive, and social functions, it is not clear what role these factors or any resultant or residual physical disability may play in the sexual dysfunctions so often reported (24). Compounding the issue of ejaculatory dysfunction are potential side effects of medications (see: Pharmacologic Abnormalities of Ejaculation). These drugs include antihypertensives, antidepressants, and other psychoactive medications. Finally, as we learn more about the role of supraspinal dopaminergic and serotonergic centers on ejaculatory function (8,9), we may be able to identify more clearly an organic basis for ejaculatory (as well as other autonomic) dysfunction seen after brain injuries.

Functional Abnormalities of Ejaculation

Functional abnormalities of ejaculation include conditions that cannot be attributed to an anatomical or neurological cause of the problem. This category includes premature ejaculation (PE) and delayed ejaculation, both of which may be thought of as abnormalities of orgasmic threshold.

Premature Ejaculation

PE is one of the most common sexual complaints, with 31% of men ages 18 to 59 reporting a problem (25). PE is characterized by a lack of voluntary control over ejaculation with concomitant distress, i.e., in which the sexual or emotional well-being of one or both partners is negatively affected. Because there is great variation in both how long it takes men to ejaculate and how long both partners want sex to last, researchers have begun to formulate a quantitative definition of PE.

An intravaginal ejaculation latency time (IELT) of less than one minute is considered "definite" PE, and an IELT of between 1 and 1.5 minutes is considered "probable" PE (26).

Delayed Ejaculation (Retarded Ejaculation, Primary Anejaculation, and Anorgasmia)

Delayed ejaculation is present when a man is unable to ejaculate, either during intercourse, or with manual stimulation in the presence of a partner. Men with delayed ejaculation may be entirely unable to ejaculate in some circumstances (e.g., during intercourse), or may be able to ejaculate only with great effort and after prolonged intercourse (e.g., 30–45 minutes).

Delayed ejaculation may be lifelong or acquired, occurring in 8% of men aged 18 to 59 (25). Evaluation should rule out neurological conditions and confirm the presence of nocturnal emissions, suggesting that the ejaculatory reflex can function normally.

Many cases of lifelong anorgasmia are thought to be due to psychological factors, such as strict religious upbringing, lack of attraction for a partner, traumatic events, or conditioning caused by unique or atypical masturbation patterns (27). Various medications may also contribute to delayed ejaculation (see below).

In cases where delayed ejaculation is interfering with procreation, extreme measures, such as electroejaculation (28) or surgical sperm retrieval, may be used to obtain sperm for assisted conception procedures.

Pharmacologic Abnormalities of Ejaculation

As discussed in the Anatomy and Physiology section above, there are central (supraspinal) areas of ejaculatory control that may be either under serotonergic control and have an inhibitory effect, or under dopaminergic control and have an excitatory effect, on ejaculation. In the autonomic nervous system, while the roles of the sympathetic and parasympathetic components are well described, pharmacologic dysfunction seems, for the most part, to be linked to medications that exhibit strong α-sympathetic blockade. In today's society, antidepressants are widely used not only for the treatment of depression but also for all forms of anxiety. α-Sympathetic blockade has become the first line choice of treatment for the symptoms of benign prostatic hyperplasia related to bladder outlet obstruction.

Antidepressants
The most common antidepressants used today are the family of selective serotonin reuptake inhibitors (SSRIs), which, as their name describes, inhibit the uptake of serotonin into the presynaptic cell, thus resulting in more serotonin available at the synapse. The older antidepressants of the tricyclic family also inhibit serotonin reuptake. The net effect is to inhibit ejaculatory and orgasmic function (29). These drugs may also inhibit dopamine activity, thereby decreasing its stimulatory effect on ejaculation.

α-adrenergic Antagonists
Sympathetic α_1-adrenergic nerves control the closure of the bladder neck and the transport of seminal fluid throughout the ejaculatory reflex. In addition, smooth muscle fibers in the blood vessels and prostate are primarily innervated by α_1-adrenergic fibers. As a result, medications designed to treat prostatism and hypertension can interfere with both closure of the bladder neck and seminal emission during ejaculation. Orgasmic sensation is usually preserved and the men so affected complain of little or no ejaculate (30). Newer blockers, more selective for the α_{1a} fibers found in the prostate, have been developed.

A study by Hellstrom and Sikka compared tamsulosin and alfuzosin on ejaculatory function. The more selective α_{1a} drug, alfuzosin, produced a decrease in ejaculatory volume in 21% of the subjects taking it while the older less selective tamsulosin had a significant decrease in ejaculatory volume in almost 90% of those subjects (35% reporting no ejaculate) (30).

MANAGEMENT OF ABNORMALITIES OF EJACULATION

For convenience, a management algorithm (Fig. 9) is provided at the end of this section.

Nonsurgical Management

Pharmacologic
The neuropharmacology of ejaculation and drug-related causes of ejaculation have been discussed in earlier sections of this chapter. With these sections in mind, it should be easy to understand the evolution of our current methods of pharmacologic management.

Anejaculation and retrograde ejaculation
α-Adrenergic neural innervation is compromised in conditions such as anemission; retrograde ejaculation not due to anatomic causes; or "nerve sparing" RPLND. In such conditions, α agonists may be useful. Often their response may be related to the severity of the problem. They will not be helpful in most cases of SCI. In situations in which some degree of innervation is preserved, especially if some sensation of orgasm is present, they may be useful. In diseases that are progressive such as diabetes or MS, the efficacy of these treatments will depend on the stage of progression and may decline as time passes (31,32).

In the case of retrograde ejaculation, as described above, the most commonly available sympathomimetic drugs may be used to try to achieve bladder neck closure in order to induce antegrade ejaculation (15). Pseudoephedrine, 60 mg four times daily, phenylpropanolamine, 75 mg twice daily, or ephedrine sulfate, 50 mg four times daily are examples of common dosage regimens (33,34). Their use should be restricted to a few days before the planned need for sperm to avoid the tachyphylaxis that may be seen with the prolonged use of sympathomimetic medications. Midodrine is an α_1-adrenergic agonist often used to support blood pressure in quadriplegic men with neurogenic orthostatic hypotension. It has been reported to be useful in increasing the success of antegrade ejaculation in men with SCI (35) but has not yet found widespread use outside of the area of SCI.

Imipramine, a tricylic antidepressant that also has α-adrenergic actions, has been used successfully to reverse retrograde into antegrade ejaculation in 10 out of 23 men with diabetes (25 mg twice daily) in a recent study (36). In the same study, there was no statistically significant difference in success rates when comparing imipramine with the use pseudoephedrine (120 mg twice daily). However, when both drugs were given together 16 out of 23 men responded with antegrade ejaculation.

Premature ejaculation
There are few published guidelines for the management of PE. The European Guidelines on Ejaculatory dysfunction (37) and The American Urological Association Guideline on the Pharmacologic Management of Premature Ejaculation (38) suggest that PE can be treated successfully with some SSRIs or with topical anesthetics. The guidelines state that medications of the SSRI class are the most effective in treating PE. These medications include the following selective inhibitors and their dosage regimens: fluoxetine, 5 to 20 mg/day; paroxetine, 10 to 40 mg/day or 20 mg three to four hours preintercourse; sertraline, 25 to 200 mg/day or 50 mg four to eight hours preintercourse. Nefazodone, citalopram, and fluvoxamine have been reported to be ineffective. The nonselective SRI clomipramine (25–50 mg/day or 25 mg 4–24 hours preintercourse) was also found to be effective (38). More recently, dapoxitine has been reported to be useful (39).

Lidocaine 2.5%/prilocaine 2.5% cream applied to the head of the penis 20 to 30 minutes before intercourse (to achieve numbing of the glans) has also been reported to be effective in treating PE (37) but has not achieved the popularity of the orally administered medicines.

Sperm Retrieval in Refractory Retrograde Ejaculation
Often, medical management of retrograde ejaculation will fail to produce an antegrade specimen and sperm retrieval procedures must be utilized to retrieve the sperm in the bladder. Depending on the level and quality of sperm production, the retrieved sperm can be processed and used for any assisted reproductive procedure (40,41). The sperm can be cryopreserved and used later for in vitro fertilization in combination with

intracytoplasmic sperm injection (ICSI) (42). The technique used in the case of men with SCI undergoing electroejaculation (EEJ) will be described in a later section. In any case, certain concepts should be followed. The healthy urine acidic pH is very hostile to sperm (43). Often the urine is infected and should be cultured and treated accordingly.

Alkalinization of the urine is desirable either by administration of oral alkalizing agents or by the instillation of 20 to 40 cc of a buffered sperm-friendly media such as used for sperm washing (44). If catheterization to instill media or retrieve the specimen is used, a nonspermicidal lubricant (serum albumin for example) should be used.

The sperm should be removed from the bladder as soon as possible after ejaculation. Since the bladder is usually emptied before ejaculation and a small amount of media (if used) is present, this removal will usually necessitate another catheterization. Catheterization and lavage with a sperm wash media is the most efficient way to obtain the most complete specimen although many patients will object to the catheterization. In those instances, one must rely on the patient's ability to completely void the bladder contents. Those contents may contain only a very small volume. If voiding is not satisfactory, the patient may be catheterized after the failed voiding, or he may return on another day for another attempt at semen retrieval by voiding postejaculatory urine.

Finally, any sperm obtained should be immediately separated from the bladder contents and processed appropriately for the selected assisted reproductive technology.

Neurostimulatory

Neurostimulatory methods may be used to induce ejaculation in men with neurogenic anejaculation. Men with SCI are the most-studied group of patients with neurogenic anejaculation (45). The most common neurostimulatory methods to induce ejaculation in men with SCI are penile vibratory stimulation (PVS) and EEJ.

Penile vibratory stimulation

The method of PVS involves placing a vibrator on the glans penis (Fig. 2). The vibration delivers mechanical stimulation to the penis with the goal of recruiting the ejaculatory reflex to induce ejaculation. PVS-induced ejaculation requires an intact ejaculatory reflex arc to provide transmission of afferent stimuli from the penis to the sacral, lumbar and lower thoracic segments of the spinal cord, and efferent stimuli from these segments to the ejaculatory organs. It has been demonstrated that intact dorsal penile nerves are necessary for PVS-induced ejaculation in men with SCI (46).

A variety of devices may be used to induce ejaculation in men with SCI (47–49). These devices are typically sold as over-the-counter massagers, and are not engineered specifically for ejaculation of neurologically impaired men. Variable success rates have been reported using these devices (50,51). In 1994, Sonksen et al. (52) reported on the importance of vibratory amplitude for achieving successful ejaculation by PVS of men with SCI. The study showed that an amplitude of 2.5 mm (versus lower amplitudes) was optimal for inducing ejaculation in men with SCI. Based on this research, a vibrator was engineered specifically for inducing ejaculation in men with SCI. This vibrator, called the FERTI CARE®, continues to be the only commercially available device developed especially for this purpose (www.Multicept.com) (Fig. 3).

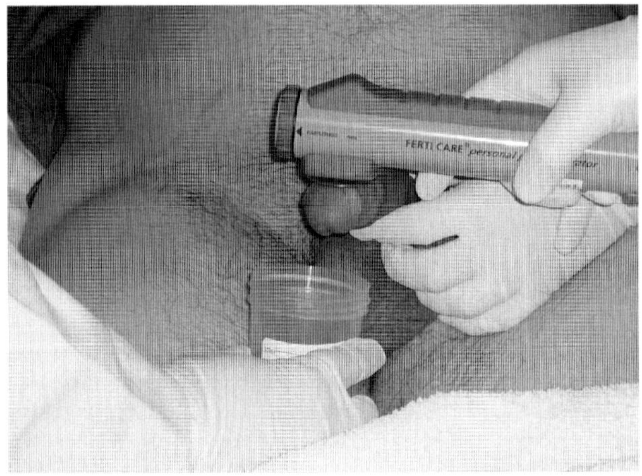

Figure 2 Penile vibratory stimulation is recommended as the first line of treatment for anejaculation in men with SCI.

The procedure of PVS has been well described in a number of publications (50,51,53).

The typical protocol involves placing a vibrator on the penis for 6 to 10 minutes, stopping every 2 minutes to inspect the penile skin for edema or abrasions. Patients with a level of injury at or rostral to neurologic level T6 are pretreated with nifedipine 20 mg sublingually, prior to administration of PVS, to manage potential autonomic dysreflexia (54–56).

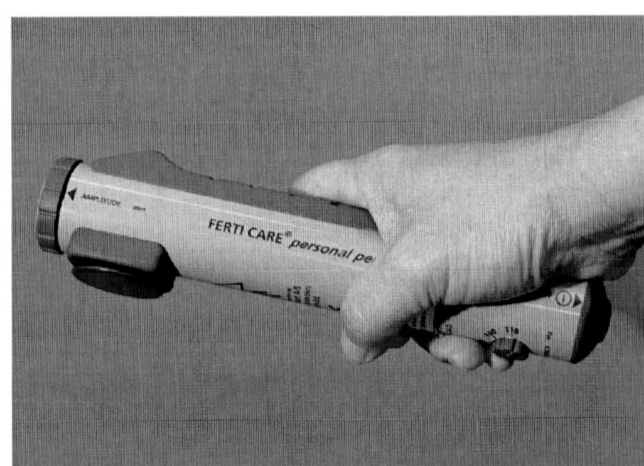

Figure 3 The Ferti Care vibrator, pictured here, was engineered specifically for ejaculation by men with SCI.

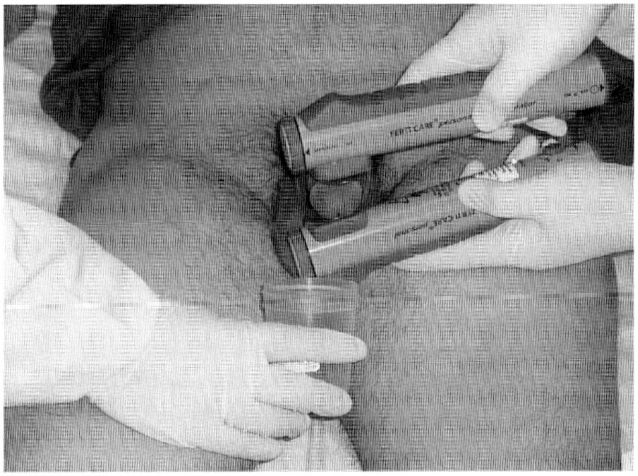

Figure 4 Individuals who cannot respond to PVS with one vibrator may respond to PVS with two vibrators.

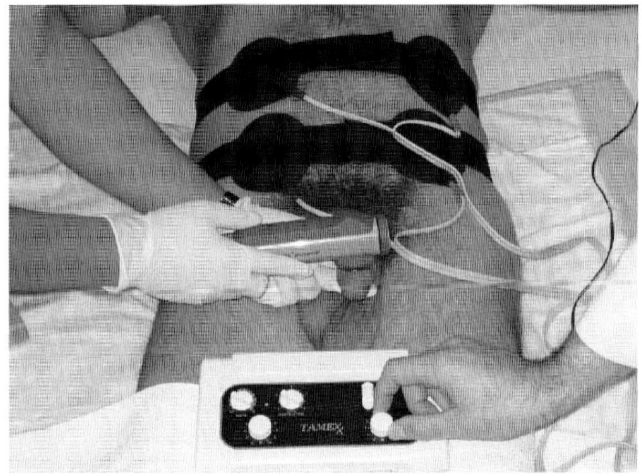

Figure 5 PVS, in combination with abdominal electrical stimulation using a commercially available device, has been shown to be successful in some men who do not respond to PVS alone.

If a patient is unable to ejaculate with a high amplitude vibrator, other methods may be employed to facilitate ejaculation with PVS, such as application of two vibrators (57) (Fig. 4), use of abdominal electrical stimulation in addition to PVS (58) (Fig. 5), or oral administration of Viagra or Midodrine prior to PVS (36,59).

Electroejaculation

Men who cannot produce an ejaculate via PVS are often referred for EEJ (Fig. 6). EEJ is a method of retrieving semen from anejaculatory men (60,61). Unlike PVS, which may be performed at home by some patients, EEJ requires administration by a

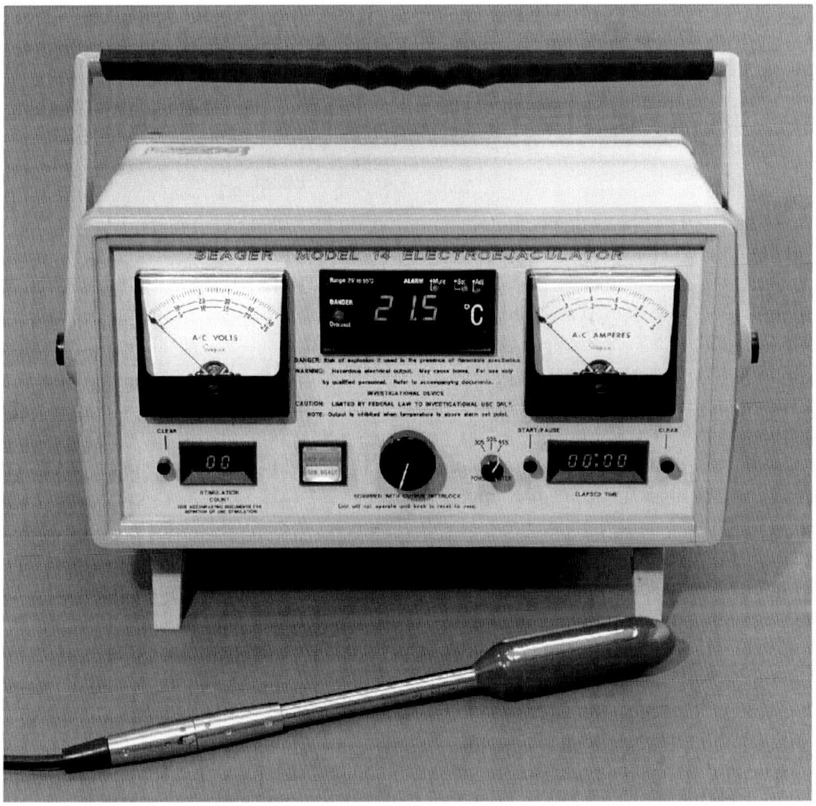

Figure 6 Electroejaculation is a method to retrieve semen when PVS fails.

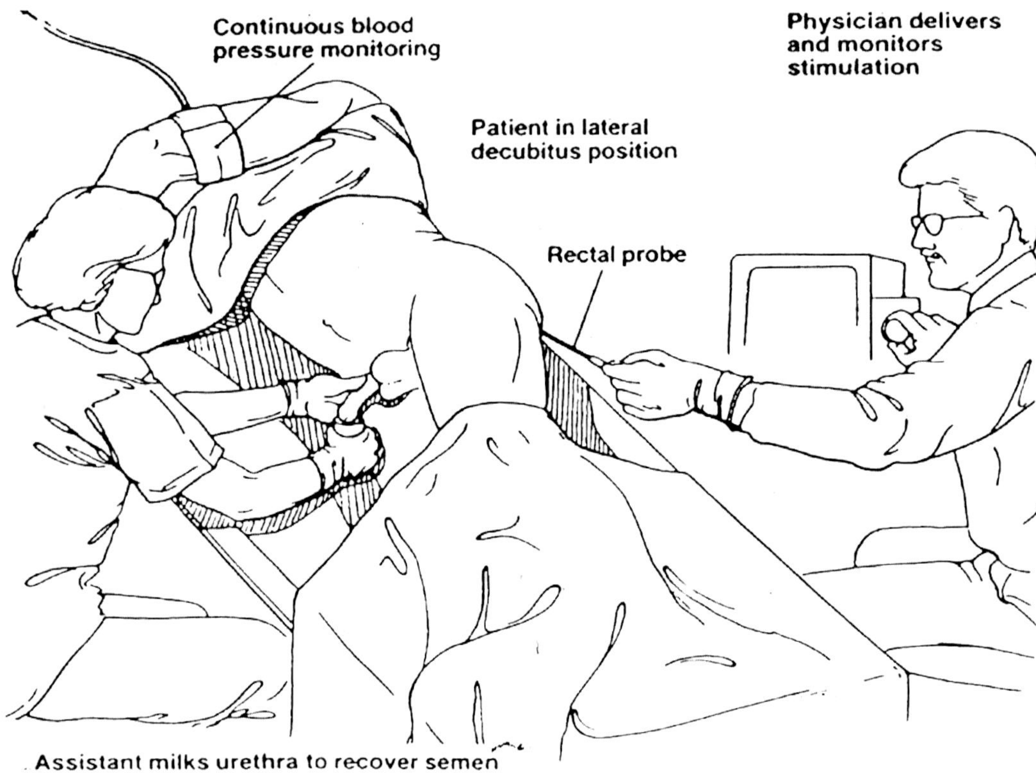

Figure 7 Electroejaculation must be performed by a specially trained physician. Electroejaculation is effective in retrieving semen in 95% of men with SCI and it is a useful alternative for semen retrieval in cases of PVS failure.

specially trained physician. To perform EEJ, the patient is placed in the lateral decubitus position (Fig. 7). A probe is placed in the rectum. The probe contains electrodes that are positioned toward the prostate and seminal vesicles. Electric current is delivered through the probe that stimulates emission of semen.

EEJ is a safe, reliable method of semen retrieval in men with SCI. The technique of EEJ has been described in numerous publications (62–65). Practitioners generally employ the following protocol: Patients with a level of injury at or rostral to T6 are pretreated with nifedipine to manage possible autonomic dysreflexia. Immediately prior to EEJ, the bladder is catheterized to reduce the potential contact of sperm with urine in cases of retrograde ejaculation. To further optimize the bladder environment, 10 to 20 mL of a buffering medium (such as sperm wash medium) may be instilled into the bladder. Rectoscopy is performed prior to initiation of EEJ to assure there are no preexisting lesions or colitis, which are relative contraindications for the procedure.

The EEJ stimulation is delivered in a wave-like pattern with voltage progressively increasing in 1 to 5 V increments until ejaculation occurs. Historically, the recommended administration of EEJ in humans was to maintain delivery of electric current until ejaculation occurred (60,66). This method of current delivery typically resulted in a higher proportion of sperm in retrograde versus antegrade fractions (67,68). Recent evidence, however, suggests that complete cessation of electrical activity between voltage peaks may be optimal for maximum antegrade ejaculation (5,65).

During EEJ, antegrade ejaculate will be released intermittently, often dribbling in nature. The urethra may have to be milked. The voltages and currents reported to successfully produce ejaculation range from 5 to 25 V and 100 to 600 mA, respectively. To completely empty the system, 10 to 20 stimulations may be required. After the procedure, the bladder is catheterized again to obtain the retrograde fraction, which may be substantial in some patients. Rectoscopy is performed after the procedure to exclude injury to the rectum.

Patients with complete spinal injuries can undergo EEJ without anesthesia. Those with significant sensory sparing or normal sensation will require general anesthesia for EEJ. The EEJ procedure can be painful in men with partly preserved sensation, and they may require either general anesthesia or conscious sedation before treatment (69,70).

PVS and EEJ continue to be the most widely used methods of semen collection in men with SCI. Both methods are safe, reliable and effective (45,71,72). PVS, however, offers advantages over EEJ. For example, PVS equipment is approximately 1/20 the cost of EEJ equipment (i.e., approximately $800 vs. $16,000 in the year 2008). Compared to EEJ, PVS is preferred more by patients and results in a higher yield of sperm in the antegrade fraction (67,68). Unlike EEJ, which requires administration by a physician, PVS may be performed at home by selected couples. The advantage of EEJ is its effectiveness with PVS failures (65,73,74).

A review of ejaculatory success rates in a large series of patients with SCI (75) showed that 88% responded to PVS if their level of injury was at or rostral to T10, versus 15% who responded if their level of injury was at or caudal to T11. EEJ was performed on PVS failures, 95% of whom ejaculated. The 5% of men who did not ejaculate with EEJ were all patients with retained pelvic sensation who experienced pain at low voltages (1–4 V) on their first trial of EEJ, and did not want to continue with further trials of EEJ under sedation or general anesthesia.

Prostate Massage

The name, prostate massage, is a misnomer for the mechanical expression of the contents of the reproductive tract. Prostate massage has been used to collect semen from men with neurogenic anejaculation (76). The use of prostate massage in the algorithm of semen retrieval methods is unclear. For example, PVS and EEJ result in a greater chance of obtaining sperm and result in a higher yield of total motile sperm compared to prostate massage (77). In cases where practitioners lack training or equipment for PVS or EEJ, prostate massage may be a useful alternative for semen retrieval in men with SCI.

Surgical Sperm Retrieval

Surgical sperm retrieval (SSR) is a method of retrieving sperm from reproductive tissue. A variety of techniques may be used including testicular sperm extraction (TESE), testicular sperm aspiration (TESA) (Fig. 8), microsurgical epididymal sperm aspiration (MESA), percutaneous epididymal sperm aspiration (PESA), and aspiration of sperm from the vas deferens (78–84). Unlike PVS and EEJ, SSR was not developed to treat anejaculation. Instead, SSR was originally developed to retrieve sperm from men without SCI, who were azoospermic, i.e., men who had no sperm in their ejaculate.

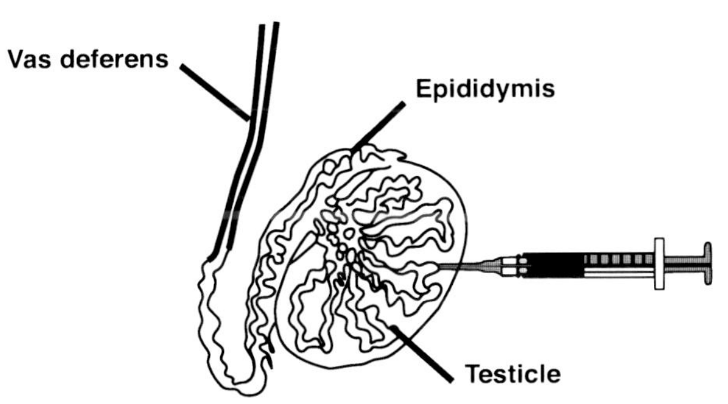

Figure 8 Testicular sperm aspiration (TESA). Use of surgical sperm retrieval in men with SCI is controversial.

In the algorithm of sperm retrieval methods in men with SCI, SSR should be performed only if PVS or EEJ fail or are not possible. Relative to PVS and EEJ, SSR is an expensive and invasive method that results in a lower yield of total motile sperm. The low yield of sperm from SSR commits the couple to the most invasive and expensive of the assisted conception methods, namely ICSI. The higher sperm yields possible with PVS and EEJ widen the options for assisted conception in couples with an SCI male partner, potentially significantly reducing the cost and invasiveness to the couple.

The application of SSR to men with SCI is controversial. A recent survey (75) indicated that some practitioners are using SSR as the first line of treatment for anejaculation in men with SCI. The primary reasons given by these practitioners for not offering PVS or EEJ were a lack of equipment and/or lack of training in these techniques (75). Ejaculation success rates, however, indicate that PVS and EEJ warrant consideration in centers not currently offering these options for couples with SCI male partners (75).

Special Concerns for Male Partners with Spinal Cord Injury

Semen Quality in Men with Spinal Cord Injury

The majority of men with SCI have a distinct semen profile characterized by normal total sperm numbers but abnormally low sperm motility (85–88). The cause of this condition is unknown, but does not seem to be related to simple lifestyle factors such as elevated scrotal temperature from sitting in a wheelchair, infrequency of ejaculation, methods of bladder management, or methods of assisted ejaculation (67,68,89–93). Evidence suggests that abnormal transport of sperm into the seminal vesicles (3) and/or toxic factors in the seminal plasma (94–98) may contribute to the problem.

Reproductive Options for Couples with SCI Male Partners

With improvements in rehabilitation law and medicine, men with SCI have become increasingly integrated into society. Marriage and children are important to these men. The majority of men with SCI cannot ejaculate during sexual intercourse, and require some form of technical or medical assistance to father a child. The same assisted conception methods used for the general male factor infertility population may be used for the SCI population. These methods include intravaginal insemination (sometimes called "at home" insemination), intrauterine insemination, and in vitro fertilization, with or without ICSI. The choice of method depends on a number of factors including the method of sperm retrieval, the total motile sperm count, any possible female factors, and the financial capabilities of the couple. Although definitive studies have not yet been performed, pregnancy outcomes using sperm from men with SCI seem to

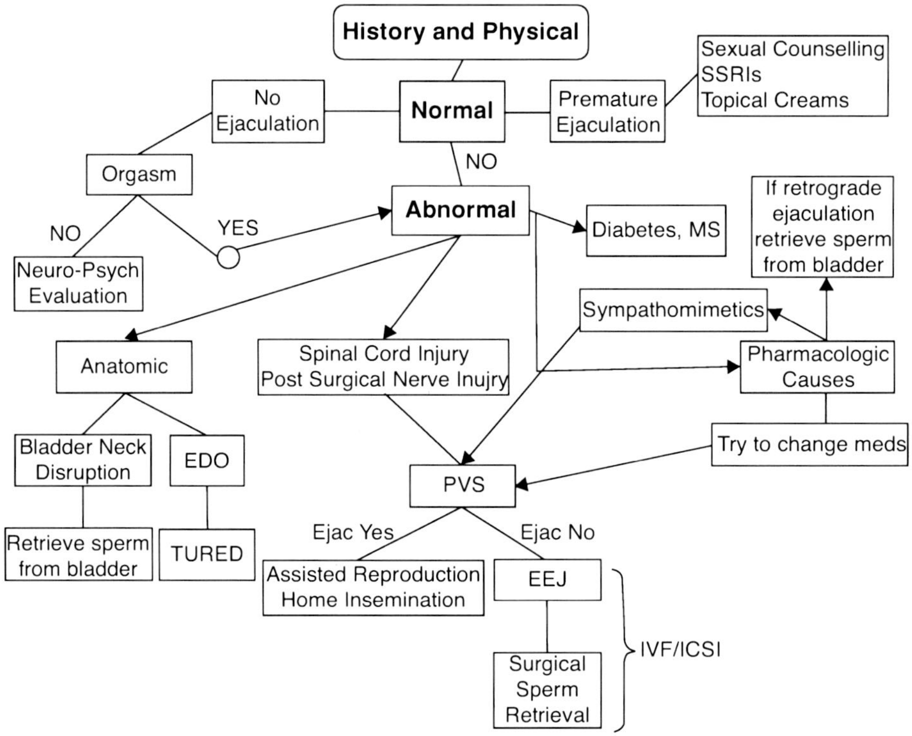

Figure 9 Schematic for Evaluation and Management of Ejaculatory Dysfunction.

be similar to those using sperm from non-SCI patients with male factor infertility (75).

REFERENCES

1. Thomas AJ. Ejaculatory dysfunction. Fertil Steril 1983; 39:445–453.
2. Prins GS, Zaneveld LJ. Radiographic study of fluid transport in the rabbit vas deferens during sexual rest and after sexual activity. J Reprod Fertil 1980; 58:311–319.
3. Ohl DA, Menge A, Jarow J. Seminal vesicle aspiration in spinal cord injured men: insight into poor semen quality. J Urol 1999; 162:2048–2051.
4. Jarow JP. Seminal vesicle aspiration of fertile men. J Urol 1996; 156:1005–1007.
5. Sonksen J, Ohl DA, Wedemeyer G. Sphincteric effects during penile vibratory ejaculation and electroejaculation in men with spinal cord injuries. J Urol 2001; 165:426–429.
6. Giuliano F, Clement P. Neuroanatomy and physiology of ejaculation. Annu Rev Sex Res 2005; 16:190–216.
7. Coolen LM, Allard J, Truitt WA, et al. Central regulation of ejaculation. Physiol Behav 2004; 83:203–215.
8. Wolters JP, Hellstrom WJ. Current concepts in ejaculatory dysfunction. Rev Urol 2006; 8(suppl 4):S18–S25.
9. Giuliano F, Clement P. Physiology of ejaculation: emphasis on serotonergic control. Eur Urol 2005; 48:408–417.
10. Fisch H, Lambert SM, Goluboff ET. Management of ejaculatory duct obstruction: etiology, diagnosis, and treatment. World J Urol 2006; 24:604–610.
11. Samli H, Samli MM, Yilmaz E, et al. Clinical, andrological and genetic characteristics of patients with congenital bilateral absence of vas deferens (CBAVD). Arch Androl 2006; 52:471–477.
12. Ochsner MG, Burns E, Henry HH. Incidence of retrograde ejaculation following bladder neck revision as a child. J Urol 1970; 104:596–597.
13. Vinik AI, Maser RE, Mitchell BD, et al. Diabetic autonomic neuropathy. Diabetes Care 2003; 26:1553–1579.
14. Dunsmuir WD, Holmes SA. The aetiology and management of erectile, ejaculatory, and fertility problems in men with diabetes mellitus. Diabet Med 1996; 13:700–708.
15. Lue TF, Giuliano F, Montorsi F, et al. Summary of the recommendations on sexual dysfunctions in men. J Sex Med 2004; 1:6–23.
16. Rees PM, Fowler CJ, Maas CP. Sexual function in men and women with neurological disorders. Lancet 2007; 369:512–525.
17. Haensch CA, Jorg J. Autonomic dysfunction in multiple sclerosis. J Neurol 2006; 253(suppl 1):I3–I9.
18. Bauer S, Koff S, Jayanthi V. Voiding dysfunction in children: neurogenic and non-neurogenic. In: Walsh P, Retik

A, Vaughn E, et al., eds. Campbell's Urology. Philadelphia, PA: Elsevier Science, 2002: 2231–2261.
19. Decter RM, Furness PD, III, Nguyen TA, et al. Reproductive understanding, sexual functioning and testosterone levels in men with spina bifida. J Urol 1997; 157:1466–1468.
20. Walsh PC, Retik AB, Vaughan ED Jr, et al., eds. Campbell's Urology. Philadelphia, PA: Saunders, 2002.
21. Holman E, Kovacs G, Flasko T, et al. Hand-assisted laparoscopic retroperitoneal lymph node dissection for nonseminomatous testicular cancer. J Laparoendosc Adv Surg Tech A 2007; 17:16–20.
22. Neyer M, Peschel R, Akkad T, et al. Long-term results of laparoscopic retroperitoneal lymph-node dissection for clinical stage I nonseminomatous germ-cell testicular cancer. J Endourol 2007; 21:180–183.
23. Bors E, Comarr AE. Neurological disturbances of sexual function with special reference to 529 patients with spinal cord injury. Urol Surv 1960; 10:191–222.
24. Korpelainen JT, Nieminen P, Myllyla VV. Sexual functioning among stroke patients and their spouses. Stroke 1999; 30:715–719.
25. Laumann EO, Paik A, Rosen RC. Sexual dysfunction in the United States: prevalence and predictors. JAMA 1999; 281:537–544.
26. Waldinger MD, Zwinderman AH, Olivier B, et al. Proposal for a definition of lifelong premature ejaculation based on epidemiological stopwatch data. J Sex Med 2005; 2:498–507.
27. Perelman MA, Rowland DL. Retarded ejaculation. World J Urol 2006; 24:645–652.
28. Stewart DE, Ohl DA. Idiopathic anejaculation treated by electroejaculation. Int J Psychiatry Med 1989; 19:263–268.
29. Seidman S. Ejaculatory dysfunction and depression: pharmacological and psychobiological interactions. Int J Impot Res 2006; 18(suppl 1):S33–S38.
30. Hellstrom WJ, Sikka SC. Effects of acute treatment with tamsulosin versus alfuzosin on ejaculatory function in normal volunteers. J Urol 2006; 176:1529–1533.
31. Kamischke A, Nieschlag E. Update on medical treatment of ejaculatory disorders. Int J Androl 2002; 25:333–344.
32. Gilja I, Parazajder J, Radej M, et al. Retrograde ejaculation and loss of emission: possibilities of conservative treatment. Eur Urol 1994; 25:226–228.
33. Proctor KG, Howards SS. The effect of sympathomimetic drugs on post-lymphadenectomy aspermia. J Urol 1983; 129:837–838.
34. Thiagarajah S, Vaughan ED Jr, Kitchin JD, III. Retrograde ejaculation: successful pregnancy following combined sympathomimetic medication and insemination. Fertil Steril 1978; 30:96–97.
35. Soler JM, Previnaire JG, Plante P, et al. Midodrine improves ejaculation in spinal cord injured men. J Urol 2007; 178:2082–2086.
36. Arafa M, El Tabie O. Medical treatment of retrograde ejaculation in diabetic patients: a hope for spontaneous pregnancy. J Sex Med 2008; 5:194–198.
37. Colpi G, Weidner W, Jungwirth A, et al.; EAU Working Party on Male Infertility. EAU guidelines on ejaculatory dysfunction. Eur Urol 2004; 46:555–558.
38. Montague DK, Jarow J, Broderick GA, et al. AUA guideline on the pharmacologic management of premature ejaculation. J Urol 2004; 172:290–294.
39. Pryor JL, Althof SE, Steidle C, et al. Efficacy and tolerability of dapoxetine in treatment of premature ejaculation: an integrated analysis of two double-blind, randomised controlled trials. Lancet 2006; 368:929–937.
40. Braude PR, Ross LD, Bolton VN, et al. Retrograde ejaculation: a systematic approach to non-invasive recovery of spermatozoa from post-ejaculatory urine for artificial insemination. Br J Obstet Gynaecol 1987; 94:76–83.
41. Shangold GA, Cantor B, Schreiber JR. Treatment of infertility due to retrograde ejaculation: a simple, cost-effective method. Fertil Steril 1990; 54:175–177.
42. Okada H, Goda K, Koshida M, et al. Pregnancy by insemination of cryopreserved spermatozoa from a man with retrograde ejaculation: a case report. J Reprod Med 2004; 49:389–391.
43. Crich JP, Jequier AM. Infertility in men with retrograde ejaculation: the action of urine on sperm motility, and a simple method for achieving antegrade ejaculation. Fertil Steril 1978; 30:572–576.
44. Suominen JJ, Kilkku PP, Taina EJ, et al. Successful treatment of infertility due to retrograde ejaculation by instillation of serum-containing medium into the bladder. A case report. Int J Androl 1991; 14:87–90.
45. Brown DJ, Hill ST, Baker HW, et al. Male fertility and sexual function after spinal cord injury. Prog Brain Res 2006; 152:427–439.
46. Wieder JA, Lynne CM, Ferrell SM, et al. Brown-colored semen in men with spinal cord injury. J Androl 1999; 20:594–600.
47. Szasz G, Carpenter C. Clinical observations in vibratory stimulation of the penis of men with spinal cord injury. Arch Sex Behav 1989; 18:461–474.
48. Beretta G, Zanollo A, Colpi GM, et al. Vibration massage in genito-sexual rehabilitation of spinal cord injuries. Our experience. [Italian]. Minerva Urol Nefrol 1985; 37:203–206.
49. Bennett CJ, Seager SW, Vasher EA, et al. Sexual dysfunction and electroejaculation in men with spinal cord injury: review. J Urol 1988; 139:453–457.
50. Brackett NL. Semen retrieval by penile vibratory stimulation in men with spinal cord injury. Hum Reprod Update 1999; 5:216–222.
51. Sonksen J, Ohl DA. Penile vibratory stimulation and electroejaculation in the treatment of ejaculatory dysfunction. Int J Androl 2002; 25:324–332.

52. Sonksen J, Biering-Sorensen F, Kristensen JK. Ejaculation induced by penile vibratory stimulation in men with spinal cord injuries. The importance of the vibratory amplitude. Paraplegia 1994; 32:651–660.
53. Elliott S. Sexual dysfunction and infertility in men with spinal cord disorders. In: Lin V, ed. Spinal Cord Medicine: Principles and Practice. New York: Demos Medical Publishing, 2003:349–365.
54. Elliott S, Krassioukov A. Malignant autonomic dysreflexia in spinal cord injured men. Spinal Cord 2006; 44:386–392.
55. Sheel AW, Krassioukov AV, Inglis JT, et al. Autonomic dysreflexia during sperm retrieval in spinal cord injury: influence of lesion level and sildenafil citrate. J Appl Physiol 2005; 99:53–58.
56. Steinberger RE, Ohl DA, Bennett CJ, et al. Nifedipine pretreatment for autonomic dysreflexia during electroejaculation. Urology 1990; 36:228–231.
57. Brackett NL, Kafetsoulis A, Ibrahim E, et al. Application of 2 vibrators salvages ejaculatory failures to 1 vibrator during penile vibratory stimulation in men with spinal cord injuries. J Urol 2007; 177:660–663.
58. Kafetsoulis A, Ibrahim E, Aballa TC, et al. Abdominal electrical stimulation rescues failures to penile vibratory stimulation in men with spinal cord injury: a report of two cases. Urology 2006; 68:204–211.
59. Giuliano F, Rubio-Aurioles E, Kennelly M, et al. Efficacy and safety of vardenafil in men with erectile dysfunction caused by spinal cord injury. Neurology 2006; 66:210–216.
60. Ohl DA. The use of electroejaculation for ejaculatory abnormalities. In: Whitehead ED, Nagler HM, eds. Management of Impotence and Infertility. Philadelphia, PA: Lippincott, 1994:294–313.
61. Ohl DA, Wolf LJ, Menge AC, et al. Electroejaculation and assisted reproductive technologies in the treatment of anejaculatory infertility. Fertil Steril 2001; 76:1249–1255.
62. Ohl DA. Electroejaculation. Urol Clin North Am 1993; 20:181–188.
63. Seager SW, Halstead LS. Fertility options and success after spinal cord injury. [Review]. Urol Clin North Am 1993; 20:543–548.
64. Sonksen J, Ohl DA, Momose H, et al. Treatment of infertility. Spinal Cord 1999; 37:89–95.
65. Brackett NL, Ead DN, Aballa TC, et al. Semen retrieval in men with spinal cord injury is improved by interrupting current delivery during electroejaculation. J Urol 2002; 167:201–203.
66. Shaban SF, Seager SW, Lipshultz LI. Clinical electroejaculation. Med Instrum 1988; 22:77–81.
67. Brackett NL, Padron OF, Lynne CM. Semen quality of spinal cord injured men is better when obtained by vibratory stimulation versus electroejaculation. J Urol 1997; 157:151–157.
68. Ohl DA, Sonksen J, Menge AC, et al. Electroejaculation versus vibratory stimulation in spinal cord injured men: sperm quality and patient preference. J Urol 1997; 157:2147–2149.
69. Perkash I, Martin DE, Warner H, et al. Reproductive biology of paraplegics: results of semen collection, testicular biopsy and serum hormone evaluation. J Urol 1985; 134:284–288.
70. Sarkarati M, Rossier AB, Fam BA. Experience in vibratory and electro-ejaculation techniques in spinal cord injury patients: a preliminary report. J Urol 1987; 138:59–62.
71. Kolettis PN, Lambert MC, Hammond KR, et al. Fertility outcomes after electroejaculation in men with spinal cord injury. Fertil Steril 2002; 78:429–431.
72. Utida C, Truzzi JC, Bruschini H, et al. Male infertility in spinal cord trauma. Int Braz J Urol 2005; 31:375–383.
73. Nehra A, Werner M, Bastuba, et al. Vibratory stimulation and rectal probe electroejaculation as therapy for patients with spinal cord injury: semen parameters and pregnancy rates. J Urol 1996; 155:554–559.
74. DeForge D, Blackmer J, Garritty C, et al. Fertility following spinal cord injury: a systematic review. Spinal Cord 2005; 43:693–703.
75. Kafetsoulis A, Brackett NL, Ibrahim E, et al. Current trends in the treatment of infertility in men with spinal cord injury. Fertil Steril 2006; 86:781–789.
76. Engin-Uml SY, Korkmaz C, Duru NK, et al. Comparison of three sperm retrieval techniques in spinal cord-injured men: pregnancy outcome. Gynecol Endocrinol 2006; 22:252–255.
77. Momen MN, Fahmy I, Amer M, et al. Semen parameters in men with spinal cord injury: changes and aetiology. Asian J Androl 2007; 9:684–689.
78. Craft I, Tsirigotis M. Simplified recovery, preparation and cryopreservation of testicular spermatozoa. Hum Reprod 1995; 10:1623–1626.
79. Tsirigotis M, Pelekanos M, Beski S, et al. Cumulative experience of percutaneous epididymal sperm aspiration (PESA) with intracytoplasmic sperm injection. J Assist Reprod Genet 1996; 13:315–319.
80. Haberle M, Scheurer P, Muhlebach P, et al. Intracytoplasmic sperm injection (ICSI) with testicular sperm extraction (TESE) in non-obstructive azoospermia—two case reports. Andrologia 1996; 28(suppl 1):87–88.
81. Kahraman S, Ozgur S, Alatas C, et al. High implantation and pregnancy rates with testicular sperm extraction and intracytoplasmic sperm injection in obstructive and non-obstructive azoospermia. Hum Reprod 1996; 11:673–676.
82. Craft I, Tsirigotis M, Courtauld E, et al. Testicular needle aspiration as an alternative to biopsy for the assessment of spermatogenesis. Hum Reprod 1997; 12:1483–1487.
83. Westlander G, Hamberger L, Hanson C, et al. Diagnostic epididymal and testicular sperm recovery and genetic aspects in azoospermic men. Hum Reprod 1999; 14:118–122.

84. Chiang H, Liu C, Tzeng C, et al. No-scalpel vasal sperm aspiration and in vitro fertilization for the treatment of anejaculation. Urology 2000; 55:918–921.
85. Linsenmeyer TA. Male infertility following spinal cord injury. J Am Paraplegia Soc 1991; 14:116–121.
86. Denil J, Ohl DA, Menge AC, et al. Functional characteristics of sperm obtained by electroejaculation. J Urol 1992; 147:69–72.
87. Brackett NL, Nash MS, Lynne CM. Male fertility following spinal cord injury: facts and fiction. Phys Ther 1996; 76:1221–1231.
88. Sonksen J, Ohl DA. Penile vibratory stimulation and electroejaculation in the treatment of ejaculatory dysfunction. Int J Androl 2002; 25:324–332.
89. Brackett NL, Lynne CM, Weizman MS, et al. Scrotal and oral temperatures are not related to semen quality or serum gonadotropin levels in spinal cord-injured men. J Androl 1994; 15:614–619.
90. Laessoe L, Sonksen J, Bagi P, et al. Effects of ejaculation by penile vibratory stimulation on bladder reflex activity in a spinal cord injured man. J Urol 2001; 166:627.
91. Das S, Dodd S, Soni BM, et al. Does repeated electroejaculation improve sperm quality in spinal cord injured men? Spinal Cord 2006; 44:753–756.
92. Ohl DA, Denil J, Fitzgerald-Shelton K, et al. Fertility of spinal cord injured males: effect of genitourinary infection and bladder management on results of electroejaculation. J Am Paraplegic Soc 1992; 15:53–59.
93. Sønksen J, Ohl DA, Giwercman A, et al. Effect of repeated ejaculation on semen quality in spinal cord injured men. J Urol 1999; 161:1163–1165.
94. Brackett NL, Davi RC, Padron OF, et al. Seminal plasma of spinal cord injured men inhibits sperm motility of normal men. J Urol 1996; 155:1632–1635.
95. Brackett NL, Lynne CM,Aballa TC, et al. Sperm motility from the vas deferens of spinal cord injured men is higher than from the ejaculate. J Urol 2000; 164:712–715.
96. Cohen DR, Basu S, Randall JM, et al. Sperm motility in men with spinal cord injuries is enhanced by inactivating cytokines in the seminal plasma. J Androl 2004; 25:922–925.
97. Basu S, Aballa TC, Ferrell SM, et al. Inflammatory cytokine concentrations are elevated in seminal plasma of men with spinal cord injuries. J Androl 2004; 25:250–254.
98. Brackett NL, Cohen DR, Ibrahim E, et al. Neutralization of cytokine activity at the receptor level improves sperm motility in men with spinal cord injuries. J Androl 2007; 28:717–721.

42 Diagnostic management of erectile function—clinical andrology

Chi-Ying Li, Giulio Garaffa, and David J. Ralph

INTRODUCTION

Erectile dysfunction (ED) is defined as the consistent or recurrent inability to achieve or maintain an erection sufficient for sexual activity (1). Transient ED and inadequate erection affects as many as 52% of men between the ages of 40 and 70, whilst chronic ED affects about 5% of men in their 40s and 15% to 25% of men by the age of 65, as reported by the first large epidemiological study on ED (2). The incidence of ED increases with age, however, it is important to remember that it is not an inevitable consequence of ageing and that advancing age does not preclude sexual interest. With increasing life expectancy, it is anticipated that both the incidence and prevalence of ED will rise.

Recent studies have demonstrated associations between ED and other cardiovascular diseases; consequently the management of ED now concentrates on screening for and prevention of cardiovascular diseases as well as treating the ED itself (3).

Simple, effective treatments are available for ED with good response rates (see chapter on conservative treatment of ED). The rate of response is improved by effective communication and patient education (4,5). Patients should have the available treatment options explained, including the benefits, limitations, and the potential complications of each modality. Patients should have all three phosphodiesterase (PDE5) inhibitors explained and be given the opportunity to try all three. They can choose their preferred option. This has been demonstrated to improve response rates (6).

A directed medical and detailed sexual history enables the physician to make an accurate diagnosis of ED. This in combination with identifying patients' ideas, concerns, and expectations and allows the formulation of a treatment plan that can be tailored to the needs and lifestyle of each individual patient.

The treatment plan is thus formulated jointly between the physician and patient. Where possible, the patients' partner should be involved, taking into consideration the patients' and partners' preferences and aspirations (7,8).

In order to successfully manage ED, the diagnostic pathway remains the most important component as it allows the physician to make an accurate diagnosis, detect and prevent other sinister underlying cardiovascular conditions, and administer the most effective and suitable treatment modality according to the patients' requirements.

SEXUAL AND MEDICAL HISTORY

Key points

- Ascertain the correct diagnosis of ED.
- Establish the likely pathophysiology of ED, organic versus psychogenic or mixed ED.
- Identify risk factors of ED.
- Identify contraindications to subsequent ED treatment.
- Ascertain patient's sexual practice so that the treatment may be tailored to the individual needs of the patient.

Ascertain the Correct Diagnosis of ED

Obtaining a detailed sexual history is essential to the accurate diagnosis and successful treatment of ED. Whilst style and approach may vary between physicians and indeed from patient to patient, it is important to establish an open and trusting doctor–patient relationship to create an atmosphere that facilitates the taking of a detailed sexual history. The correct diagnosis of ED should be established from other causes of sexual dysfunction, e.g., secondary to ejaculatory disorders. The Brief Sexual Symptom Checklist (BSSC) (9) has been developed to initiate this process. This is shown in Table 1. Once a rapport has been established, greater detail can be entered into regarding the sexual history.

The next step is to ascertain further information on "the when, the how, and the why." Below are some questions that can help to initiate this process.

The when:

How long have you had difficulty with erection?
Did it happen suddenly or gradually?

The how:

With sexual stimulation, are you able to achieve an erection?
If partial erection—if your best ever performance was 10 out of 10, how would you rate yourself now?
With an erection, are you able to penetrate?
Are you able to maintain the erection once penetration has occurred?
Are you able to maintain the erection until completion?
Do you achieve orgasm?
Do you ejaculate with orgasm?

And the why:

Are you in a long-term relationship?
Are you looking forward to sex?

Table 1 The Brief Sexual Symptom Checklist

1. Are you satisfied with your sexual function? Yes/No. If No, please continue.
2. How long have you been dissatisfied with your sexual function?
3.
   a. The problem(s) with your sexual function is: (mark one or more)
      - problems with little or no interest in sex
      - problems with erection
      - problems with ejaculation too early during sexual activity
      - problems taking too long, or not being able to ejaculate or have orgasm
      - problems with pain during sex
      - problems with penile curvature during erection
      - others

   b. Which problem is most bothersome?
4. Would you like to talk about it with your doctor?

Do you wake up in the morning with an erection?
Do you masturbate?
Is the erection quality/sexual experience improved with masturbation? Or with a different partner?

Establish the Likely Pathophysiology of ED, Organic Versus Psychogenic or Mixed ED

Once the diagnosis of ED has been established, the next step is to ascertain the underlying cause for ED and distinguish between organic versus psychogenic ED.

Some features of organic versus psychogenic ED are summarized in Table 2.

An important factor to bear in mind is that most patients with ED have complex pathophysiology and frequently an underlying mixed etiology.

Identify Risk Factors of ED

ED may be the manifestation of an underlying medical condition. It is equally important to take a directed medical history as a well-structured sexual history. This may also help in differentiating between organic versus psychogenic causes of ED.

Conditions associated with ED can be broadly divided into vasculogenic, neurogenic, endocrine, anatomical, drugs, and psychogenic causes. A list of these are summarized in Table 3.

As part of identifying risk factors to ED, it is advisable that recommendations to modify risk factors are also given, including stop smoking (19), regular exercise, and maintaining healthy weight, might prevent ED (20,21).

In many cases, the etiology of ED is multifactorial. Overall 75% to 80% of ED is caused by vascular or neural disorders, or combination of both.

Table 2 Features of Organic versus Psychogenic ED

Organic	Psychogenic
Older population	Younger patients
Gradual onset	Sudden onset
No morning tumescence	Good morning tumescence
Normal ejaculation and libido	PE/inability to ejaculate
Risk factors in previous medical history	Recent life events/relationship problems
Drugs/smoking	Psychological problems

[a]Except secondary to trauma or surgery.
Abbreviations: PE, premature ejaculation.

Table 3 Conditions That Are Associated with ED

Categories	Risk factors
Vasculogenic	Endothelial dysfunction (10), risk factors include hypertension, smoking (11,12), hypercholesterolemia (13) and diabetes mellitus (DM) (14) Veno-occlusive ("venous leak")
Neurogenic	Parkinson's, Alzheimer's disease, cerebral vascular accident, multiple sclerosis, head injury, tumor, temporal lobe epilepsy and peripheral neuropathy, for instance DM autonomic neuropathy and vitamin B deficiency in chronic alcoholism (15)
Endocrine	Hypogonadism, affecting 17% of men with ED (16), hyperprolactinemia, hyper- or hypothyroidism. Hyperprolactinemia that can occur in association with DM, chronic renal failure, and cirrhosis of the liver
Anatomical	Postradical prostatectomy, ED occurs in approximately 60% (17) and approximately 10–28% post-TURP (Trans-Urethral Resection of Prostate) (18). Other abdominal or pelvic surgery including abdominoperineal resection, aortoiliac bypass, and pelvic radiotherapy. Other causes include spinal cord injury or trauma
Drugs	Thiazide diuretics (spironolactone), α-methyldolpa, reserpine that depletes central dopamine store, all dopamine receptor blockers (chlorpromazine, haloperidol) and agents that block the effect of endogenous dopamine (cimetidine, verapamil) Others include cocaine, which can cause ED through effects on central dopamine, increases peripheral α-adrenergic activity, and endothelial dysfunction
Psychogenic	Stress, anxiety, and depression

Identify Contraindications to Subsequent ED Treatment (see also chapter on treatment of ED)

Prior to commencing treatment of ED, it is prudent to establish if the patient has any medical condition or concomitant therapy that would be contraindicated in subsequent ED treatment. The commonest oral pharmacotherapy, PDE5 inhibitors, is contraindicated in patients receiving nitrates or those with recent stroke, unstable angina or, myocardial infarction (<6 weeks), and those with hereditary degenerative retinal disorders.

Other important drug interactions include patients taking antifungal (intraconazole and ketaconazole) and protease inhibitors (Indinavir and Ritonavir); where the dosage of the PDE5 inhibitor treatment should be reduced (22). Caution should also be exercised in patients taking α-blockers (22). The use of an intracavernosal or intraurethral route is contraindicated and the use of PDE5 inhibitors is cautioned, in patients predisposed to prolonged erection, such as sickle cell anemia, multiple myeloma, leukemia, and patients with penile implants (23).

Ascertain Patients' Sexual Practice and Tailor the Treatment Plan

This is the opportunity to dive deeper into the psychosocial aspects of sexual dysfunction. It is important to explore past and present relationships and enquire about other aspects of the patients' life including interpersonal relationships, family life, and support. In order to formulate a successful treatment plan, the patients' ideas, concerns, and expectations should be elicited. This is achieved through detailed questioning of patients' sexual practice and preferences and adjusting the treatment plan accordingly.

OBJECTIVE ASSESSMENT OF SEVERITY OF ED

Key points

- Various tools available to objectively assess ED.
- These must not replace detailed medical and sexual history.

Over the past decade, outcome measure tools have been developed to objectively assess ED in the form of self-administered questionnaires. They were originally intended for outcome assessment in clinical trials but can also be applied to the clinical setting.

While it is not mandatory to use these questionnaires for the diagnosis of ED, physicians may find these helpful in assessing the severity of ED or as a tool for assessing progress pre- and posttreatment.

Several instruments have been designed to measure the level of sexual function, some of which are still emerging from their validation process; however, they have overall demonstrated reliability and validity.

These include the following:

1. Changes in sexual functioning questionnaire (CSFQ) (24).
2. International Index of Erectile Function (IIEF) (25).
3. Sexual Health Inventory for Men (SHIM / IIEF-5) (26).
4. Male Sexual Health Questionnaire (MSHQ) (27).

The commonest employed questionnaire, which also demonstrates the highest internal consistency and reliability (9) as is recommended in many ED management guidelines (7,28,29), is the IIEF and more recently the development of a simplified IIEF-5, which is shorter and quicker to administer than the original.

Although these tools are helpful in providing an objective assessment of the severity of ED, an important concept to bear in mind is that no questionnaire should be used as a substitute for a detailed medical and sexual history.

PHYSICAL EXAMINATIONS

Key points

- Screening for cardiovascular diseases.
- Secondary sexual characteristics including external genitalia.
- Assessment of general health status.

In most cases of ED, physical examination is unlikely to point to the underlying pathophysiological process; nonetheless, it constitutes an important part of the management of ED.

In recent studies, various risk factors have been shown to be associated with ED (30–32). It is thought that ED is the first clinical symptom of a generalized vascular endothelial dysfunction, thus presenting before other sinister cardiovascular diseases. This lead time in clinical presentation is thought to be useful in detecting underlying cardiovascular conditions (3,33–36). Consequently, the management of ED now centers not only in treatment of ED but also in prevention of other cardiovascular diseases.

All patients should have a full physical examination.

This should include the following:

1. Cardiovascular system: Measurement of heart rate, blood pressure, heart sounds and examining for peripheral pulses.
2. Abdominal examination including external genitalia with particular focus on secondary sexual characteristics or the presence of gynecomastia. Assess testicular size, the penile shaft for fibrosis that may suggest Peyronie's disease and phimosis.

Digital rectal examination is not mandatory in the assessment of ED (29), but should be included in those with genitourinary or prolonged history of ejaculatory symptoms and in the elderly population, particularly if there is also a history of urinary symptoms.

Neurological examination should be carried out to assess possible underlying neurological conditions that may contribute to the underlying etiology of ED.

This is also an opportunity to assess patients' general fitness.

It is important to consider that sexual intercourse is a form of physical activity requiring a degree of exercise tolerance. In the majority of patients with coronary artery disease, it is safe to resume sexual activities (37). However, if it was thought that sexual activities were medically inadvisable, e.g., in patients with a history of severe ischemic heart disease, unstable angina, recent myocardial infarction or, severe heart failure; caution should be exercised.

The underlying cause for the impaired exercise tolerance must be sought and patient referred for treatment of the underlying condition accordingly, before commencing therapy for ED.

In the United States, the Princeton Consensus Panel, consisting of urologists, cardiologists, pharmacologists, and psychologists, devised a guideline for the management of patients presenting with ED (38) and concomitant cardiovascular conditions.

Patients are divided into three groups: low, intermediate, and high risk. Those in the low-risk group can have their ED treatment initiated; while those in the intermediate and high-risk groups should be referred for specialist investigations. The guideline can be summarized in Figure 1.

It is advisable for the physical examination to be completed in the presence of a chaperone.

LABORATORY TESTS

Key points

- Screening for cardiovascular risk factors.
- Serum blood tests for ED.

Screening for Cardiovascular Risk Factors

Screening for other cardiovascular diseases is an integral part of the management of ED; the same applies for baseline laboratory testing.

ED may be part of a generalized vascular endothelial dysfunction. Since its symptoms manifest before other cardiovascular diseases, this lead time is useful in detecting otherwise asymptomatic and more sinister underlying cardiovascular conditions (33,34).

Therefore, all patients presenting with ED who have no previous diagnosis of diabetes or hypercholesterolemia should have a baseline fasting blood glucose and lipid levels measured.

Serum Blood Tests for ED

Routine measurement of morning (08:00–11:00) testosterone, follicle stimulating hormone (FSH)/leutinizing hormone (LH), and prolactin is currently controversial. However, in the second international consultation on sexual dysfunction, the committees recommended that men with ED should have a morning testosterone level checked (9). This is supported by a recent comprehensive review article, which concludes that testosterone replacement improves libido and the response to PDE5 inhibitors (39). In addition, ED secondary to hypogonadism is potentially reversible with supplementary testosterone (40).

If the first morning testosterone sample is borderline or low, it should be repeated together with second line investigations. These should include LH/FSH, sexual hormone-binding globulin, prolactin, and thyroid function test.

Prostatic-specific antigen (PSA) should be measured if clinically indicated or dependent on the local guidance for PSA screening programs, as these may differ (7,28,29), but certainly before commencement of testosterone therapy.

Recent evidence has demonstrated a significant incidence of hypogonadism with the ageing process (41). Furthermore, it is proposed that the process of ageing is the primary etiology of hypogonadism in the elderly population. It is also known as the male andropause or androgen deficiency of the aging male (ADAM).

Although the evidence supporting an association between ageing and ED, and between ageing and hypogonadism is convincing, there is no consistent evidence to support a direct link between testosterone levels and erectile status (16,42,43). However, various studies have demonstrated that testosterone replacement therapy improves sexual desire and response to ED treatments (44). This forms the basis for the current rationale of checking testosterone levels in those presenting with ED, as testosterone replacement therapy may be considered in those failing initial ED treatment.

In ED patients where initial treatment with PDE5 inhibitors has failed; the diagnosis, and hence consideration of initiating testosterone therapy should be based on the clinical history of loss of libido, supported by laboratory evidence of low serum testosterone.

Controversy arises over the level that defines low testosterone and at which replacement therapy should be initiated. The current recommendation prepared by the International Society of Andrology and the International Society for the Study of the Ageing Male as part of EAU guideline suggests substitution for total testosterone <231 ng/dL or free testosterone <52 pg/mL (45).

SPECIAL INVESTIGATION TECHNIQUES

Most patients presenting with ED do not require special investigation, though these may be indicated as follows (28,29):

- Young patients with lifelong history of ED.
- ED as a result of trauma where surgical intervention is being considered.
- Abnormalities of penis or testes found on examination/assessment for penile deformities.
- Prior to surgical intervention having failed conservative treatment options.
- History of complex psychiatric/psychosexual disorders.
- At patients' requests/medicolegal indications.

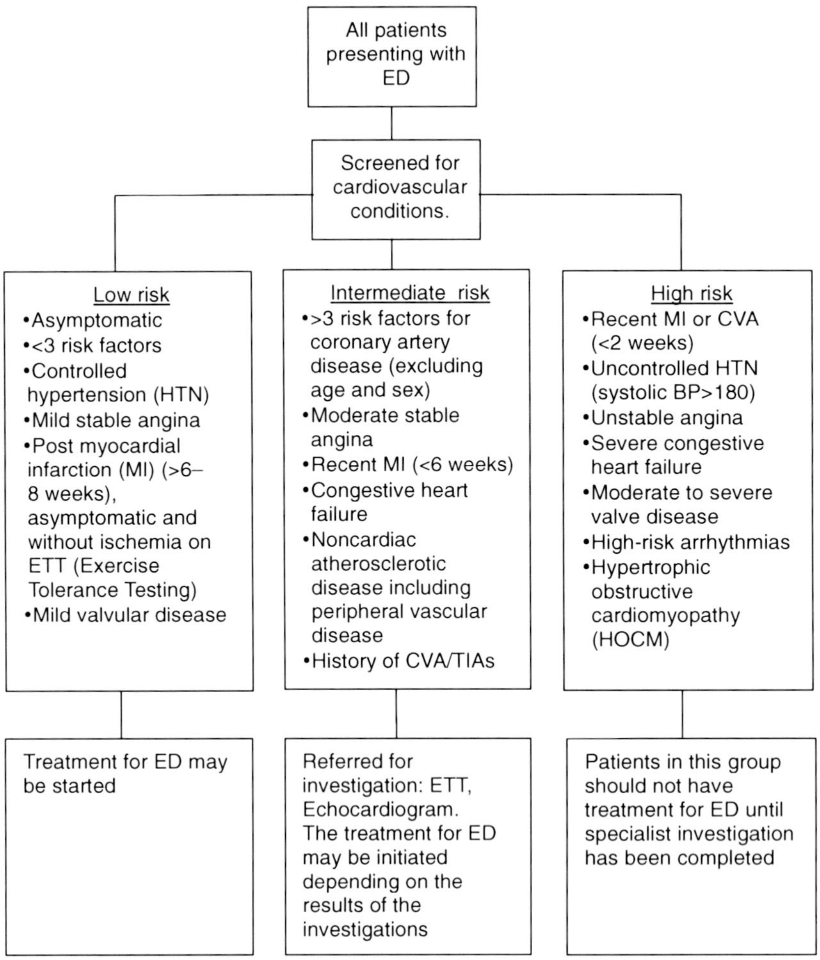

Figure 1 Summary flow chart of the Princeton Consensus Panel recommendations.

Nocturnal Penile Tumescence and Rigidity (NPTR)

Indication
NPTR is used in differentiating between organic and psychological causes of ED. NPT is associated with cycles of REM (rapid eye movement) sleep and is consequently largely unaffected by psychological aspects of ED.

Most men have four to six episodes of NPT in an eight-hour sleep cycle.

Procedure
Ideally, the NPTR should be carried out in a sleep center using either an Erectiometer® or a Rigiscan® that measures penile rigidity by recording at 20 seconds intervals via transducers placed at the base and the coronal sulcus of the penis.

Interpretation
Normal values: >70% rigidity per event lasting 10 minutes. In the presence of a good quality erection, the cause of ED is likely to be psychogenic.

Intracavernosal Vasoactive Drug Injection

Indication
This is mainly used for assessment of penile curvature, e.g., Peyronie's disease and congenital penile curvature.

Duplex Doppler ultrasound may also be used in conjunction to assess penile blood flow and further identify plaques or fibrosis.

Procedure
Using aseptic technique, intracavernosal injection of vasoactive substance, Alprostadil (PGE1), Papaverine or Phentolamine, is made on one side of the penis.

Doppler ultrasound assessment can be introduced once erection has developed.

Interpretation
A pharmacologically induced erection will reveal potential cavernous deformity. A normal response does not exclude arterial insufficiency and many patients may have borderline arterial insufficiency.

Penile Duplex Doppler—Vascular Assessment

Indication
Assessment of the vascular status—arterial blood supply and veno-occlusive mechanism of the penis (46).

Procedure
Doppler studies can be used, after intracavernosal injection of PGE1 pharmacotherapy to induce an artificial erection, to identify: cavernous arterial diameter, cavernous artery acceleration time, peak systolic arterial velocity (PSV), systolic rise time, end diastolic arterial velocity (EDV), and index of vascular resistance (RI).

Interpretation
A PSV >35 cm/sec indicates normal cavernous arterial flow. PSV <25 cm/sec indicates cavernous arterial insufficiency (sensitivity 100%, specificity 95%). PSV 25 to 35 cm/sec indicates borderline penile arterial flow. EDV >5 cm/sec (RI <0.8 with normal PSV) signifies pure veno-occlusive dysfunction (VOD). EDV >5 cm/sec with PSV <25 cm/sec signifies mixed etiologies.

Cavernosogram/DICC (29)

Indication
Primary ED (lifelong history) in young men to confirm VOD. It is used to identify isolated venous leakage that may respond surgical ligation. Also may identify site-specific leaks at sites of trauma and Peyronie's plaques.

Procedure
Using aseptic technique, 20 μg PGE1 is injected intracavernosally. A butterfly needle is inserted vertically into the penis and used to infuse saline. The infusion is started and the flow rate necessary to maintain erection with cavernous pressure >100 mm Hg is recorded. Fifty to hundred milliliters of radiographic contrast is instilled and radiographs taken to demonstrate the corpora cavernosa. Detumescence is achieved by intracavernosal injection of phenylephrine, if needed.

Interpretation
Normal intracavernosal pressure is >90 mm Hg.

Normal infusion rate required to maintain erection is <20 mL/min. If >20 mL/min flow is required to maintain erection, a VOD is diagnosed. False positive may occur if the penis is not fully erected as one may be observing venous drainage and not leakage.

Internal Pudendal Arteriography

Indication
Only for selected cases where revascularization procedures are considered, usually to locate an arterial lesion demonstrated on Doppler Ultrasound Scan (USS), e.g., ED in young men as a result of pelvic trauma.

Penile angiography may also be used in high flow priapism prior to embolization.

Procedure
Selective internal pudendal angiography.

Interpretation
Isolated arterial occlusion may be demonstrated for preoperative planning of revascularization procedure.

In the case of priapism, an arteriovenous fistula may be demonstrated.

CONCLUSION

With the increasing incidence and prevalence of ED, it is important to remember that a detailed, patient-centered sexual and medical history, supported by simple baseline evaluation tools, allows accurate diagnosis of ED and identification of the underlying cause, while the process of diagnosing or preventing other cardiovascular diseases can be initiated.

With the wide variety of ED therapeutic options available, effective patient communication, informing patients of the characteristics of different treatment modalities, giving patients adequate opportunity to trial different options, and addressing the specific needs of individual patients are the key elements in improving success rates in the management of ED.

KEY MESSAGES

1. Detailed sexual history is paramount to the accurate diagnosis and successful treatment of ED (Level 4, grade C).
2. ED is associated with other cardiovascular diseases, thus management of ED should include screening for and prevention of cardiovascular diseases as well as treating the ED itself (Level 2a, grade B).
3. Most patients with ED do not require special investigations; however, these may be indicated in some (Level 2a, grade B).

REFERENCES

1. NIH Consensus Conference. Impotence. NIH Consensus Development Panel on Impotence. JAMA 1993; 270(1):83–90.
2. Feldman HA, Goldstein I, Hatzichristou DG, et al. Impotence and its medical and psychosocial correlates: results of the Massachusetts Male Aging Study. J Urol 1994; 151(1):54–61.
3. Ponholzer A, Temml C, Obermayr R, et al. Is erectile dysfunction an indicator for increased risk of coronary heart disease and stroke? Eur Urol 2005; 48(3):512–518.
4. Gruenwald I, Shenfeld O, Chen J, et al. Positive effect of counseling and dose adjustment in patients with erectile dysfunction who failed treatment with sildenafil. Eur Urol 2006; 50(1):134–140.
5. Hatzichristou D, Moysidis K, Apostolidis A, et al. Sildenafil failures may be due to inadequate patient instructions and

follow-up: a study on 100 non-responders. Eur Urol 2005; 47(4):518–522.

6. Stroberg P, Hedelin H, Ljunggren C. Prescribing all phosphodiesterase 5 inhibitors to a patient with erectile dysfunction—a realistic and feasible option in everyday clinical practice—outcomes of a simple treatment regime. Eur Urol 2006; 49(5):900–907.
7. Montague DK, Jarow JP, Broderick GA, et al. Chapter 1: the management of erectile dysfunction: an AUA update. J Urol 2005; 174(1):230–239.
8. Hatzimouratidis K, Hatzichristou DG. A comparative review of the options for treatment of erectile dysfunction: which treatment for which patient? Drugs 2005; 65(12):1621–1650.
9. Rosen RC, Hatzichristou D, Broderick G, et al. Clinical evaluation and symptom scales: sexual dysfunction assessment in men. In: Lue TF, Basson R, Rosen RC, et al., eds. Sexual Medicine; Sexual Dysfunctions in Men & Women. Second International Consultation on Sexual Dysfunctions. 2nd ed. Paris: Health Publications, Editions 21, Chapter 7, 2004:173–206.
10. Solomon H, Man JW, Jackson G. Erectile dysfunction and the cardiovascular patient: endothelial dysfunction is the common denominator. Heart 2003; 89(3):251–253.
11. Bacon CG, Mittleman MA, Kawachi I, et al. A prospective study of risk factors for erectile dysfunction. J Urol 2006; 176(1):217–221.
12. Austoni E, Mirone V, Parazzini F, et al. Smoking as a risk factor for erectile dysfunction: data from the Andrology Prevention Weeks 2001–2002 a study of the Italian Society of Andrology (s.I.a.). Eur Urol 2005; 48(5):810–817.
13. Roumeguère T, Wespes E, Carpentier Y, et al. Erectile dysfunction is associated with a high prevalence of hyperlipidemia and coronary heart disease risk. Eur Urol 2003; 44(3):355–359.
14. Bacon CG, Hu FB, Giovannucci E, et al. Association of type and duration of diabetes with erectile dysfunction in a large cohort of men. Diabetes Care 2002; 25(8):1458–1463.
15. Saenz dT I, Angulo J, Cellek S, et al. Pathophysiology of erectile dysfunction. J Sex Med 2005; 2(1):26–39.
16. Martinez-Jabaloyas JM, Queipo-Zaragoza A, Pastor-Hernandez F, et al. Testosterone levels in men with erectile dysfunction. BJU Int 2006; 97(6):1278–1283.
17. Stanford JL, Feng Z, Hamilton AS, et al. Urinary and sexual function after radical prostatectomy for clinically localized prostate cancer: the Prostate Cancer Outcomes Study. JAMA 2000; 283(3):354–360.
18. Hanbury DC, Sethia KK. Erectile function following transurethral prostatectomy. Br J Urol 1995; 75(1): 12–13.
19. Pourmand G, Alidaee MR, Rasuli S, et al. Do cigarette smokers with erectile dysfunction benefit from stopping?: a prospective study. BJU Int 2004; 94(9):1310–1313.
20. Rosen RC, Friedman M, Kostis JB. Lifestyle management of erectile dysfunction: the role of cardiovascular and concomitant risk factors. Am J Cardiol 2005; 96(12B):76M–79M.
21. Esposito K, Giugliano F, Di PC, et al. Effect of lifestyle changes on erectile dysfunction in obese men: a randomized controlled trial. JAMA 2004; 291(24):2978–2984.
22. British National Formulary 61, 54 ed. London: RPS Publishing, 2007.
23. British National Formulary 59, 54 ed. London: RPS Publishing, 2007.
24. Clayton AH, McGarvey EL, Clavet GJ. The Changes in Sexual Functioning Questionnaire (CSFQ): development, reliability, and validity. Psychopharmacol Bull 1997; 33(4):731–745.
25. Rosen RC, Cappelleri JC, Gendrano N III. The International Index of Erectile Function (IIEF): a state-of-the-science review. Int J Impot Res 2002; 14(4):226–244.
26. Rosen RC, Cappelleri JC, Smith MD, et al. Development and evaluation of an abridged, 5-item version of the International Index of Erectile Function (IIEF-5) as a diagnostic tool for erectile dysfunction. Int J Impot Res 1999; 11(6):319–326.
27. Rosen RC, Catania J, Pollack L, et al. Male Sexual Health Questionnaire (MSHQ): scale development and psychometric validation. Urology 2004; 64(4):777–782.
28. Wespes E, Amar E, Hatzichristou D, et al. EAU Guidelines on erectile dysfunction: an update. Eur Urol 2006; 49(5):806–815.
29. Hackett G, Dean J, Kell P, et al. British Society for Sexual Medicine—Guidelines on the Management of Erectile Dysfunction. J Sex Med. 2008; 5(8): 1841–1865.
30. Chiurlia E, D'Amico R, Ratti C, et al. Subclinical coronary artery atherosclerosis in patients with erectile dysfunction. J Am Coll Cardiol 2005; 46(8):1503–1506.
31. Ponholzer A, Temml C, Mock K, et al. Prevalence and risk factors for erectile dysfunction in 2869 men using a validated questionnaire. Eur Urol 2005; 47(1):80–85.
32. Vlachopoulos C, Rokkas K, Ioakeimidis N, et al. Prevalence of asymptomatic coronary artery disease in men with vasculogenic erectile dysfunction: a prospective angiographic study. Eur Urol 2005; 48(6):996–1002.
33. Montorsi F, Briganti A, Salonia A, et al. Erectile dysfunction prevalence, time of onset and association with risk factors in 300 consecutive patients with acute chest pain and angiographically documented coronary artery disease. Eur Urol 2003; 44(3):360–364.
34. Montorsi P, Ravagnani PM, Galli S, et al. Association between erectile dysfunction and coronary artery disease. Role of coronary clinical presentation and extent of coronary vessels involvement: the COBRA trial. Eur Heart J 2006; 27(22):2632–2639.

35. Seftel AD, Sun P, Swindle R. The prevalence of hypertension, hyperlipidemia, diabetes mellitus and depression in men with erectile dysfunction. J Urol 2004; 171(6, pt 1):2341–2345.
36. Sun P, Swindle R. Are men with erectile dysfunction more likely to have hypertension than men without erectile dysfunction? A naturalistic national cohort study. J Urol 2005; 174(1):244–248.
37. Jackson G, Betteridge J, Dean J, et al. A systematic approach to erectile dysfunction in the cardiovascular patient: a Consensus Statement—update 2002. 2002; 56(9):663–671.
38. Jackson G, Rosen RC, Kloner RA, et al. The second Princeton consensus on sexual dysfunction and cardiac risk: new guidelines for sexual medicine. J Sex Med 2006; 3(1): 28–36.
39. Mikhail N. Does testosterone have a role in erectile function? Am J Med 2006; 119(5):373–382.
40. Lue TF, Giuliano F, Montorsi F, et al. Summary of the recommendations on sexual dysfunctions in men. J Sex Med 2004; 1(1):6–23.
41. Harman SM, Metter EJ, Tobin JD, et al. Longitudinal effects of aging on serum total and free testosterone levels in healthy men. Baltimore Longitudinal Study of Aging. J Clin Endocrinol Metab 2001; 86(2):724–731.
42. Kupelian V, Shabsigh R, Travison TG, et al. Is there a relationship between sex hormones and erectile dysfunction? Results from the Massachusetts Male Aging Study. J Urol 2006; 176(6, pt 1):2584–2588.
43. El-Sakka AI, Hassoba HM. Age related testosterone depletion in patients with erectile dysfunction. J Urol 2006; 176(6, pt 1):2589–2593.
44. Greenstein A, Mabjeesh NJ, Sofer M, et al. Does sildenafil combined with testosterone gel improve erectile dysfunction in hypogonadal men in whom testosterone supplement therapy alone failed? J Urol 2005; 173(2):530–532.
45. Nieschlag E, Swerdloff R, Behre HM, et al. Investigation, treatment and monitoring of late-onset hypogonadism in males. ISA, ISSAM, and EAU recommendations. Eur Urol 2005; 48(1):1–4.
46. Aversa A, Sarteschi LM. The role of penile color-duplex ultrasound for the evaluation of erectile dysfunction. J Sex Med 2007; 4(5):1437–1447.

43 Conservative treatment of erectile dysfunction

Thomas C. Stadler, Uwe Hartmann, Armin J. Becker, and Christian G. Stief

INTRODUCTION

Erectile dysfunction (ED) has been defined as the consistent or recurrent inability of a man to attain and/or maintain a penile erection sufficient for satisfying sexual performance. Consistency is an important aspect of the definition of ED. Erectile difficulties must be reported to occur on a consistent or recurrent basis in order to qualify for the diagnosis of ED. A three-month minimum duration is generally accepted for establishment of the diagnosis. In some instances of trauma or surgically induced ED (e.g., postprostatovesiculectomy or postcystectomy), the diagnosis may be confirmed prior to three months. Although ED is a benign disorder, it is closely related to physical and psychosocial health, and has an essential influence on the quality of life of both patients and their partners. Clinically, the diagnosis of ED is primarily based on patient's self-report. The diagnosis may be supported by objective testing (or partner's report), nevertheless these measures cannot displace the patient's self-report in classifying the disorder. The necessary reliance on patient's reports implies that cultural factors and patient–physician communication and relation will be important determinants in defining and diagnosing the disorder.

A recent review of the current epidemiological data shows a high incidence and prevalence of moderate to severe ED worldwide. In large-scale studies, the prevalence of ED ranges from 19.2% to 52% (1,2). ED shares common risk factors with cardiovascular disease, such as lack of exercise, obesity, smoking, hypercholesteremia, and metabolic syndrome. Modification or elimination of risk factors (predominantly initiation of exercise and weight loss) may reduce the risk of ED and may even to some extent rehabilitate erectile function.

Only psychogenic ED, posttraumatic arteriogenic ED in young patients and ED deriving from hormonal disorders can be potentially cured with specific treatment modalities. The vast majority of men with ED will be treated symptomatically with no cause-specific treatment options. This fact leads to a structured treatment strategy that depends on efficacy, safety, degree of invasiveness, and costs as well as patient and partner satisfaction. Pharmacological therapies can act centrally or peripherally on the end organ (the corpus cavernosum penis) or both. These drugs act via various pathways inducing smooth muscle relaxation and promoting erection.

FIRST-LINE THERAPY—PHARMACOLOGICAL OPTIONS

Erection depends on the relaxation of the penile cavernosal smooth muscle. Although the control mechanism is complex, nitric oxide (NO) is the most important chemical mediator of smooth muscle relaxation. NO is released directly from parasympathetic nerve endings and from vascular endothelium in response to sexual stimulation. NO acts on smooth muscle cells by stimulation of the enzyme guanylate cyclase to convert guanosine triphosphate (GTP) into the active second messenger cyclic guanosine monophosphate (cGMP) that induces smooth muscle relaxation. cGMP is broken down by the enzyme phosphodiesterase (PDE) into inactive GMP.

There are various types of PDE in the human body, of which PDE5 is the most important subtype for penile smooth muscle activity. The cGMP concentration in the smooth muscle cell is the result of a balance between the intensity of the NO stimulus and the rate of cGMP breakdown by PDE5, which is why PDE5 plays an important role in the regulation of penile erectile activity and offers an important starting point in the treatment of ED. Drugs that inhibit PDE5 therefore increase the action of cGMP and with that enhance penile cavernous and vascular smooth muscle relaxation and erection in response to sexual stimulation. Table 1 provides recent pharmacological options.

PDE5 inhibitors are the reference class in oral ED therapy. Three potent selective PDE5 inhibitors are currently available for clinical use with European Medicines Agency (EMEA) approval and with proven efficacy and safety for the treatment of ED: sildenafil, vardenafil, and tadalafil. They are not initiators of erection, but they require sexual stimulation in order to facilitate and to prolongate an erection. PDE5 inhibitors are highly effective and well tolerated, as demonstrated by controlled clinical trials and clinical practice experience. The class is registered for on-demand use. The clinical action of PDE5 inhibitors may be detected after the first intake; however, a concluding treatment success evaluation should not be performed after several times of application (at least four to six times). Patients must be taught how to optimally use the drug, particularly regarding the need for sexual stimulation and adequate dosing. The treatment results are therefore improved by sufficient patient education. There is a variability of onset of action for the three substances (which may be at least 15–30 minutes). The duration of action is about 6 to 12 hours for sildenafil and vardenafil and up to 24 to 36 hours for tadalafil.

Sildenafil (Viagra™) was the first PDE5 inhibitor for clinical use in ED, meanwhile with millions of men treated. It is effective (erection with more rigidity sufficient for vaginal penetration) after 30 to 60 minutes from administration. A heavy fatty meal may reduce or prolongate absorption. It is available in 25, 50, and 100 mg doses. The recommended starting dose is 50 mg and

Table 1 Pharmacological Treatment of Erectile Dysfunction

Substance	Mechanism of action	Indication	Contraindications	Dosage/application
Prostaglandin E1 (alprostadil) Intracavernous	Rise of intracellular cAMP, smooth muscle relaxation	All forms of ED	Coagulation disorders and anticoagulation therapy; Peyronie's disease	5–40 μg via intracavernous injection
Intraurethral		Mild to moderate organogenic ED	Peyronie's disease, urethral anomalies	250–1000 μg intraurethral
Yohimbine	α_2-adrenergic antagonist	Psychogenic and marginal organogenic ED	None	3 × 10 mg for at least 6 wk
Sildenafil	Selective PDE5 inhibitor, cavernous smooth muscle relaxation	All forms of ED	Concomitant medication with NO Donors, retinitis pigmentosa	25–100 mg approx. 60 min prior to sexual performance
Tadalafil	Selective PDE5 inhibitor, cavernous smooth muscle relaxation	All forms of ED	Concomitant medication with NO Donors, retinitis pigmentosa	5–20 mg approx. 30 min prior to sexual performance
Vardenafil	Selective PDE5 inhibitor, cavernous smooth muscle relaxation	All forms of ED	Concomitant medication with NO Donors, retinitis pigmentosa	5–20 mg approx. 25–60 min prior to sexual performance

this should be adapted according to the response and side effects. Efficacy may be maintained for up to 12 hours. In premarketing studies, after 24 weeks of treatment in a dose–response study, improved erections were reported by 56%, 77%, and 84% of the men taking 25, 50, and 100 mg of sildenafil, respectively, compared to 25% of those taking placebo (3). The efficacy of sildenafil in almost every subgroup of patients with ED is more than established (4). *Tadalafil* (Cialis™) is administered in 10 and 20 mg doses. It is effective from 30 minutes after administration, but its highest efficacy is expected after about 2 hours. Efficacy is maintained for up to 36 hours and not influenced by food. The recommended starting dose is 10 mg; this should be adapted according to response and side effects. Improved erections were reported by 67% and 81% of the men taking 10 and 20 mg of tadalafil compared to 35% in the control placebo group (5). Tadalafil also improved erections in difficult-to-treat subgroups (6, 7). Vardenafil (Levitra™) displays its effect about 30 minutes after administration. Its effect may be influenced by a fatty meal. It can be administered in 5, 10, and 20 mg doses. The recommended starting dose is 10 mg, adapted to the response and side effects (8). In vitro, it is 10-fold more potent than sildenafil. However, this does not necessarily imply greater clinical efficacy (9). After 12 weeks of treatment and in a dose–response study, improved erections were reported by 66%, 76%, and 80% of the men taking 5, 10, and 20 mg of vardenafil respectively, compared to 30% in the control placebo group (10). Vardenafil also improved erections in difficult-to-treat subgroups.

Safety Issues for PDE 5 Inhibitors

All three PDE5 inhibitors are associated with class-related side effects including headache, dizziness, dyspepsia, facial flushing, and nasal congestion, which are highly variable and may be declining with continued application or substance switches. Other side effects such as visual abnormalities under sildenafil and vardenafil (due to additional PDE6 inhibition) or myalgia and back pain under Tadalafil may vary according to the specific compound used. However, adverse events are generally mild in nature and self-limited by continuous use; the drop-out rate due to adverse events is similar to placebo (11). PDE5 inhibitors are strictly contraindicated in patients receiving organic nitrates and NO donors. In patients receiving concomitantly an α-blocker, recommendations may vary from caution to contraindication depending on the PDE5 inhibitor and the α-blocker being used. Physicians must carefully follow the label instructions of these drugs.

PDE5 inhibitors undergo hepatic metabolism via cytochrome P450 CYP3A4. CYP3A4 inhibitors, such as erythromycin, ketoconazole, and protease inhibitors, can increase the levels of PDE5 inhibitors. In patients taking these drugs, administration of PDE5 inhibitors at the lowest available dosage must be considered.

Cardiovascular Safety

Clinical trials and postmarketing data of all PDE 5 inhibitors demonstrated no increase in myocardial infarction rates. None of the PDE5 inhibitors adversely affects total exercise time or time to ischemia during exercise testing in men with stable angina pectoris. In fact they may actually improve exercise tests (12–14). Nitrates are totally contraindicated with all PDE5 inhibitors due to unpredictable hypotension. The duration of interaction between organic nitrates and PDE5 inhibitors is dependent on the PDE5 inhibitor and nitrate under study. If a patient develops angina while on a PDE5 inhibitor, other agents may be administered instead of nitroglycerine or until the appropriate time has passed (24 hours for sildenafil/vardenafil and 48 hours for tadalafil). In general, the adverse event profile of the PDE5 inhibitor will not worsen even when the patient is on multiple antihypertensive agents.

α-Blocker Interactions

All PDE5 inhibitors appear to have some interaction with α-blockers, which under some condition may result in orthostatic hypotension. Sildenafil labeling currently describes a precaution advising that 50 or 100 mg (not 25 mg) dosages should not be taken within a four-hour window of an α-blocker. The concomitant use of vardenafil with α-blockers is not recommended. However, coadministration of vardenafil with tamsulosin is not associated with clinically significant hypotension. Tadalafil is contraindicated in patients taking α-blockers with the exception of tamsulosin (15).

Dose Adjustments

Lower doses of PDE5 inhibitors may be required in patients taking ketoconazole, itraconazole, erythromycin, clarythromycin, and HIV protease inhibitors (ritonavir, saquinavir). Higher doses of the PDE5 inhibitors may be required in patients taking rifampicin, phenobarbital, phenytoin, and carbamazepine. Renal or hepatic dysfunction may require dose adjustments or warnings. In patients with hypogonadism, medication with PDE5 inhibitors under androgen supplementation improves erectile responses and provokes arterial cavernous dilatation (4).

Yohimbine is an α_2-adrenergic blocker that acts both centrally and peripherally. There is a low level of evidence for the efficacy of yohimbine in ED. The usual dosage is 15 to 30 mg per day in divided doses. Side effects include palpitations, urinary frequency, nausea, indigestion, headache, and transient hypertension.

Although its efficacy underlies that of PDE5 inhibitors, the benefit of yohimbine medication for ED seems to outweigh its risks. Therefore, some authors believe yohimbine to be a reasonable therapeutic option for ED that should be considered as initial pharmacological intervention. Particularly in ED with psychogenic components, this substance may be useful (16–18).

Androgen Replacement Therapy

Adult-onset hypogonadism is a clinical and biochemical syndrome frequently associated with advancing age and characterized by a deficiency in serum androgen levels, with or without changes in receptor sensitivity to androgens. It may affect the function of multiple organ systems and result in significant impairment of quality of life, including major alterations of sexual functions.

In patients with sexual dysfunction and at risk of developing or already suspected to suffer from hypogonadism (decreased sexual interest, changes in secondary sexual features), a testosterone (T) determination with the blood sample taken between 8:00 and 10:00 a.m. is recommended. The most accessible and reliable assays to establish the presence of hypogonadism are the measurement of bioavailable T or calculated free T (cFT). Assays for total testosterone, particularly in the elderly, may not reflect the man's true androgen status. If testosterone levels are below normal or at the lower limit of the accepted normal values, it is wise to confirm the results with a second determination together with the assessment of luteinizing hormone (LH), follicle stimulating hormone (FSH), and prolactin.

In men with ED and/or diminished sexual interest, a clear indication (a clinical picture together with biochemical evidence of hypogonadism) should exist prior to initiation of androgen substitution therapy. Contraindications should also be ruled out (prostatic or breast cancer, severe bladder neck obstruction). Testosterone can be given transdermally (with patch or gel) or intramuscularly (by injection). Since androgen replacement therapy is typically chronic or lifelong, it is essential that all patients receiving androgen therapy be followed on a regular basis. The treating physician must be familiar with the diagnostic, therapeutic, and monitoring aspects of androgen therapy. The patient should be monitored closely for possible side effects or contraindications, such as abnormal liver function, hyperlipidemia, polycythemia, prostate abnormalities (prostate cancer or severe bladder neck obstruction), hyperactivity or aggressive behavior, and sleep apnea. Inadequate therapeutic response or the appearance of significant adverse effects call for reassessment of treatment indications (19).

PSYCHOSEXUAL THERAPY

For patients with a significant psychological cause for their erectile disorder, psychosexual therapy may be helpful either alone or in combination with another therapeutic approach. In addition, clinical experience suggests that, irrespective of the exact causation of the individual ED, many patients can profit from sex counseling or sex therapy. Recently, several studies have shown that a pharmacological treatment augmented by a brief standardized educational and counseling program (either in a couple or group setting) addressing psychological or partner-related issues is superior to pharmacotherapy alone.

Modern sex therapy is a brief, structured, and direct treatment method based on the groundbreaking work of Masters & Johnson in the 1960s and 1970s. It is focused not so much on underlying or deep-rooted intrapsychic or interpersonal conflicts, but rather on the here-and-now factors interfering with an adequate sexual functioning. The most prominent of these factors is the vicious cycle of performance anxiety and avoidance behavior that can be identified in virtually every chronic ED. Any ED can only be successfully treated if this vicious cycle—either by sex therapy or by pharmacotherapy or (preferably) by a combination of both—can be dissolved. Sex therapy normally entails between 8 and 20 treatment sessions over three to six months. The treatment concept consists of two essential components: (1) Homework assignments carried out by the patient and/or the couple at home aimed at inducing new and corrective sexual and emotional experiences. (2) Therapeutic sessions in which the individual experiences including conflicts and obstacles surfacing in the course of the treatment are analyzed and the next steps planned. The most famous assignment is the sensate focus exercise intended to detach the couple from performance pressure or inhibition, thereby opening up new ways for a relaxed and sensuous eroticism. In subsequent phases, the genitals are involved in these exercises that are slowly but continuously expanded until successful coitus is eventually possible. For predominantly psychogenic ED, the outcome of sex therapy is satisfactory with approximately two-thirds of patients reporting a full or considerable improvement that tends to be relatively stable over time. As sex counseling and sex therapy can be easily combined with pharmacotherapy, these options should be given careful consideration in the treatment of ED.

CONCLUSIONS ON ORAL DRUGS

The introduction of oral therapy for ED has been a revolution in the management of this disorder. The advantages of oral drug therapies include broad patient acceptance, ease of administration, and relative efficacy. The disadvantages include specific contraindications such as the concomitant use of nitrates with respect to PDE5 inhibitors and the relative costs. Discontinuation rates in clinical trials are low. In clinical practice, discontinuation rates may be higher for a number of reasons, including inadequate patient education and follow-up, cost, and possibly psychological factors. Good patient information about the optimal ways of applying treatment (dosage, need for sexual stimulation, etc.) is important for the success of treatment and patient satisfaction. ED nevertheless remains a multifaceted process and introduction of a rapid and easy pharmacological solution does not eliminate the need for management of the associated psychological issues.

SECOND-LINE THERAPY—LOCAL VASOACTIVE AGENT APPLICATION

The introduction of intracavernosal injection therapy in the early 1980s was a milestone in the treatment of ED. It was the first time that a safe and highly effective pharmacologic treatment option was available for men with ED. Alprostadil (Caverject®, Edex/Viridal®) is the most frequently used single agent approved for ED treatment with intracavernous injection (Table 1). It is the most efficient monotherapy for intracavernous treatment in 5 to 40 μg doses. Drug combinations (mainly alprostadil/papaverine/phentolamine, "Trimix") may increase efficacy in appropriate settings. The erection appears after 5 to 15 minutes and lasts according to the dose injected (20,21). An office training programme (one or two visits) is required for the patients to learn the correct injection process and location.

Alprostadil (prostaglandin E1) acts primarily via specific receptors on the surface of the smooth muscle cell to stimulate the enzyme adenylate cyclase. This enzyme converts adenosine triphosphate (ATP) into cyclic adenosine monophosphate (cAMP). Injection of PGE1 therefore causes a rise in intracellular cAMP, causing a decrease in intracellular calcium, thereby inducing smooth muscle relaxation. PGE1 therapy is associated with good efficacy and tolerability in most forms of ED, the clinical effect is less dependent from sexual stimulation than that of PDE5 inhibitors.

Efficacy rates for intracavernous alprostadil of more than 70% are presented with sexual activity reported after 94% of the injections and satisfaction rates of 87% to 93.5% in patients and 86% to 90.3% in partners. Complications of intracavernous alprostadil include penile pain (up to 50% of patients, after 11% of injections), prolonged erections (5%) up to priapism (1%), and cavernous body fibrosis (2%) (22). After four hours of erection, patients are advised to consult the doctor to avoid any damage to the intracavernous muscles, which would provoke permanent and irreversible impotence. A 19-gauge needle is used to aspirate blood and therefore to decrease the intracavernous pressure. This simple method is usually sufficient to make the penis flaccid. However, if the penis regains its rigidity after this, phenylephrine intracavernous injection is required at a dose starting at 200 μg every five minutes, increasing to 500 μg if necessary. If this is an ever-occurring problem, the dose is usually reduced for the next injections.

Papaverine was the first drug to be used in this indication. It is now rarely used as a single agent, but mainly in combination with PGE1 and/or phentolamine in patients refractory to both oral and single-agent injection therapy. Papaverine is a nonselective inhibitor of the enzyme PDE in the penis, thereby inhibiting the breakdown of both cyclic GMP and cyclic AMP resulting in a fall in the cytoplasmatic calcium concentration leading to smooth muscle relaxation.

Phentolamine, when injected alone, has a modest therapeutic effect. However, it has a synergistic action when combined with drugs such as papaverine or combinations of papaverine and PGE1 (as for example used in the Trimix). It acts as an inhibitor of both α_1 and α_2-adrenoceptors antagonizing the action of noradrenaline on the cell. When injected into the corpus cavernosum, it promotes erections by blocking the tonic sympathetic neuronal activity that normally produces smooth muscle contraction (23).

Although the technique of intracavernosal injection is simple and relatively painless, patients must be taught to inject themselves in the right way, first under professional supervision and later at home. The solution is to be injected slowly with a fine needle into the side of the penis shaft with the syringe held perpendicular to the skin. The needle is removed and pressure is applied to the injection site. The drug is massaged gently throughout the shaft of the penis for approximately 30 seconds to 1 minute. Erection normally occurs within 5 to 10 minutes. Some patients may have difficulties performing self-injections because of poor manual dexterity or poor visual acuity. Obesity can make it difficult for the patient to see his penis, in which case the use of a mirror or injection by the partner may be helpful. Autoinjectors can also be beneficial. These autoinjectors are similar to those used to apply insulin.

The dose for initial injections must be estimated depending on the probable etiology of the ED. Patients with neurogenic or psychogenic ED can respond to small PGE1 doses of 2.5 to 5 μg. Patients with severe vasculogenic ED may fail to respond even to high doses of single agents. It is usually not worth increasing the dose of PGE1 to more than 40 μg, but it is preferable to try a substance combination with papaverine or phentolamine or both (Trimix). Twenty-five percent of the patients who fail to respond to PGE1 alone will respond to a combination (24).

The duration of response of intracavernous injection may be between 50 minutes and 2 to 3 hours. The patient must be advised that if his erection lasts for more than about four hours he should promptly seek medical attention. Treatment with 5 to 10 μg of terbutaline orally may abort prolonged erection with out the need for further treatment. The risk of prolonged erections is greater with papaverine and mixtures containing papaverine than with PGE1 as a single agent.

In patients with an increased risk of developing priapism, injection therapy is contraindicated. The use of anticoagulants is not an absolute contraindication, but extra care must be taken to avoid excessive bruising. In patients with Peyronie's disease, an aggravation of penile deviation must be expected.

Since the introduction of PDE5 inhibitors, intracorporeal injection has mainly been used for patients failing to respond to oral therapy. The success rate is about 70% for PGE1 and 80% for Trimix (20, 24). With time, a large proportion of patients will drop out and stop treatment. There are a number of reasons for this high drop-out rate including ineffective therapy, patient dissatisfaction, partner dissatisfaction, and serious concomitant illness. Only one out of three or four patients continues treatment three to four years after starting.

Intraurethral Therapy

As the urethral mucosa is permeable to drugs, alprostadil (PGE1), in the form of a semisolid pellet, can be administered into the urethra via an application system called MUSE (medicated urethral system for erection). The transfer of active substances to the corpora cavernosa occurs primarily via venous channels that communicate between the corpus spongiosum and the corpora cavernosa. MUSE is available in a range of doses of PGE1 from 250 to 1000 μg. Erection starts within 15 to 30 minutes and lasts 30 to 60 minutes (21, 25). Efficacy (45% of cases) is inferior to that obtained with PDE5 inhibitors or intracavernosal injection. The strength of erection can be improved by application of constriction ring in order to reduce proximal absorption. Although 80% of the drug is absorbed from the urethra within 10 minutes of application, the level of PGE1 in the ejaculate could be harmful in pregnant women, in which case, a condom should be used.

The MUSE applicator is inserted up to the collar into the meatus. The injector button is pushed down to release the pellet containing PGE1 into the urethra. The patient then massages the penis to help the distribution of the medication pellet. Side effects include penile pain, urethral burning, and hypotension, and the clinical success rate is lower than that achieved by intracavernosal therapy.

Topical (intrameatal) application of the combination of alprostadil and a dermal permeation enhancer is associated with a certain efficacy and tolerability that need to be confirmed by further studies (26).

VACUUM TUMESCENCE DEVICE

In case of contraindications or intolerabilities of pharmacological treatment, a vacuum tumescence device (VTD) can be an adequate alternative noninvasive treatment option that is effective for all etiologies of ED (27, 28). It consists of a plastic cylinder, a vacuum pump to induce erection and constriction ring to maintain erection. The erection that is induced by the vacuum device is different from normal erection, as there is no relaxation of the trabecular smooth muscle. The cylinder is placed over the penis and held firmly against the mons pubis to obtain an air-tight seal. This should be supported by the use of contact-gel. Suction then is applied to the vacuum pump (manual or electric) to produce a negative pressure leading to engorgement of the penis by increased blood influx into the corpora cavernosa. After the erect state is achieved, a constriction ring is slipped from the cylinder onto the base of the penis to inhibit venous drainage and with that to maintain erection. The vacuum then is released via a valve and the cylinder can be removed. The constriction rings may have various shapes and sizes, some feature a notch that fits over the urethra to make ejaculation easier. Usually the time taken to attain erection is 2 to 3 minutes. The ring should not be left on the penis for more than 30 minutes.

Contraindications to the use of VTDs include pathologic and iatrogenic bleeding conditions and often Peyronie's disease. The penis may appear rather cyanotic and cold and may become painful with time. Numbness and delayed ejaculations were reported. VTDs are effective to allow intercourse in 70% to 80% of users and the drop-out rate at one year is about 60% that is similar to the drop-out rate for injection treatment. In one study, average use of VTD was 3.5 times per month. A vacuum device could be used in patients in stable relationships in whom the mechanism of ED is easily understood and accepted. It is also better accepted in older patients (29,30).

THIRD-LINE THERAPY—PENILE PROSTHESIS

Penile prostheses represent the ultima ratio in ED treatment when all other modalities have failed or are contraindicated (31). Generally, there are two sorts of cavernous body implants: malleable devices and inflatable, hydraulic devices. Malleable prostheses consist of a pair of flexible silicone rods. They are available in various sizes, but can also be trimmed to fit patients individually. They provide an adequate rigidity for vaginal penetration and can be bent down when they are not in use. However, in times of inflatable devices being widely available and being more convenient for the patients, they are becoming less important and should be reserved for special indications.

Modern inflatable three-piece penile prostheses are composed of a pair or cylinders, a pump, and a reservoir. They are more complex to implant, but show more satisfactory results. The two inflatable cylinders are inserted in the corpora cavernosa and connected to a pump valve that is placed in the scrotum and inflates or deflates the cylinders. The fluid is provided by a reservoir placed beneath the rectus abdominis muscle. In most cases, excellent erect and flaccid states with good cosmetic results and a high patient satisfaction can be achieved. Complications and adverse events include pain, infections, and mechanical failures. Higher infection rates are observed in patients with diabetes, autoimmune diseases, and in patients undergoing prosthesis revisions, though, infection rates may be reduced with new and effective antibiotic-coated implants (32). Generally, infection requires prosthesis explantation.

Satisfaction rates range from 66% to 92% for patients and from 60% to 80% for their partners. Still, as the implantation of a penile prosthesis results in the irreversible destruction of the cavernous bodies, this intervention remains the last choice in ED treatment. The indication and the actual intervention should be left to the accounted specialists.

CONCLUSIONS

The worldwide availability of PDE5 inhibitors for oral use associated with high efficacy and safety rates even in difficult-to-treat populations (e.g., patients with diabetes mellitus, after radical prostatectomy) has revolutionized ED treatment. Treatment options for patients not responding to oral drugs (or with contraindications) include intracavernous injections, intraurethral alprostadil, VTDs, and implantation of penile prostheses. Generally, with all these treatment options, any form of ED can be treated, though, not in all patients full rehabilitation can be achieved.

Besides specific diagnostic approaches, physicians should assess the cardiac fitness of patients as well as their sexual, medical, and psychosocial history prior to treating ED. Any successful pharmacological treatment for ED demands a degree of integrity of the penile mechanisms of erection. The search for the ideal pharmacological therapy for erectile failure aims at fulfilling the following characteristics: good efficacy, easy administration, freedom from toxicity and side effects, a rapid onset and a possible long-acting effect. The intention of therapy should be viewed as restoration of a satisfactory sexual life, not only a rigid erection.

CASE REPORT

A 64-year-old man reports increasing episodes of erectile disorders for over nine months on first presentation. The patient describes frequent matutinal and nocturnal erections; however, his erection in most cases is not sufficient for vaginal penetration.

A prostatic hyperplasia is well-known, though, miction has not yet been heavily affected (nycturia 2×). Due to a hypertensive condition he has been taking ß-blockers for over four years. The patient used to smoke one pack of cigarettes until a few years ago. By now he had reduced smoking to a very low level that he believes to be responsible for his increasing weight; he has gained over 20 pounds over the last four years. Two years ago, diabetes was diagnosed that does not require medical treatment yet.

Now the psychological strain has aggravated, so that the patient and his younger wife require further evaluation of the ED.

The auscultation of heath and lungs shows no pathological findings. Palpations of genitalia and abdomen as well as digital rectal examination are inconspicuous. IIEF-Score: 17, BMI 28.2. There is a slight elevation of cholesterol levels; PSA is 1.7 ng/mL. The hormone status is normal. His blood pressure is fluctuating between 130/90 mm Hg and 160/90 mm Hg.

The intracavernosal injection of prostanglandin E1 provoked an E4–E5 erection under a blood flow of 20 cm/sec in the profound penile arteries. Taken together these findings reveal an almost normal cavernous body function, although a reduction in the arterial peak flow is already observable.

After the discussion of all possible treatment options, the patient prefers a medicamentous attempt with PDE5 inhibitors, the financial aspects were well considered. By now, the standard dose enables the patient to have a satisfying sex life with weekly sexual intercourse with fully rigid erections. Moreover, a concomitant diet modification and increased sportive activities were recommended. With that, a weight reduction of 20 pounds is to be achieved over one year. Even though the antihypertensive medication is still indicated, efforts to change the substance class might be helpful.

CONCLUSIVE MESSAGES

- PDE5 inhibitors are recommended as the first-line treatment of ED of any organic origin (Grade of evidence B).
- Cavernous body injection with alprostadil has shown high efficacy in second-line treatment of ED (Grade of evidence B).

REFERENCES

1. Feldman HA, Goldstein I, Hatzichristou DG, et al. Impotence and its medical and psychosocial correlates: results of the Massachusetts Male Aging Study. J Urol 1994; 151(1):54–61.
2. Braun M, Wassmer G, Klotz T, et al Epidemiology of erectile dysfunction: results of the 'Cologne Male Survey'. Int J Impot Res 2000; 12(6):305–311.
3. Goldstein I, Lue TF, Padma-Nathan H, et al.; Sildenafil Study Group. Oral sildenafil in the treatment of erectile dysfunction. 1998. J Urol 2007; 167(2, pt 2):1197–1203.
4. Guay AT, Perez JB, Jacobson J, et al. Efficacy and safety of sildenafil citrate for treatment of erectile dysfunction in a population with associated organic risk factors. J Androl 2001; 22:793–797.

5. Brock GB, McMahon CG, Chen KK, et al. Efficacy and safety of tadalafil for the treatment of erectile dysfunction: results of integrated analyses. J Urol 2002; 168(4, pt 1):1332–1336.
6. Frajese GV, Pozzi F, Frajese G. Tadalafil in the treatment of erectile dysfunction; an overview of the clinical evidence. Clin Interv Aging 2006; 1(4):439–449.
7. Porst H. IC351 (tadalafil, cialis): update on clinical experience. Int J Impot Res 2002; 14(suppl 1):57–64.
8. Pryor JP. Vardenafil: update on clinical experience. Int J Impot Res 2002; 14(suppl 1):65–69.
9. Saenz de Tejada I, Angulo J, Cuevas P, et al. The phosphodiesterase inhibitory selectivity and the in vitro and in vivo potency of the new PDE5 inhibitor vardenafil. Int J Impot Res 2001; 13(5):282–290.
10. Hellstrom WJ. Current safety and tolerability issues in men with erectile dysfunction receiving PDE5 inhibitors [published online ahead of print July 26, 2007]. Int J Clin Pract 2007; 61(9):1547–1554.
11. Arruda-Olson AM, Mahoney DW, Nehra A, et al. Cardiovascular effects of sildenafil during exercise in men with known or probable coronary artery disease. JAMA 2002; 287:719–725.
12. Porst H, Rosen R, Padma-Nathan H, et al. The efficacy and tolerability of vardenafil, a new, oral, selective phosphodiesterase type 5 inhibitor, in patients with erectile dysfunction: the first at-home clinical trial. Int J Impot Res 2001; 13(4):192–199.
13. Montorsi F, Deho F, Salonia A, et al. Pharmacological management of erectile dysfunction. BJU Int 2003; 91:446–454.
14. Shakir SAW, Wilton LV, Bshier A, et al. Cardiovascular events in users of sildenafil: result from first phase of prescription event monitoring in England. BMJ 2001; 322:651–652.
15. Guillaume M, Lonsdale F, Darstein C, et al. Hemodynamic interaction between a daily dosed phosphodiesterase 5 inhibitor, tadalafil, and the alpha-adrenergic blockers, doxazosin and tamsulosin, in middle-aged healthy male subjects. J Clin Pharmacol 2007; 47(10):1303–1310.
16. Galitzky J, Riviere D, Tran MA, et al. Pharmacodynamic effects of chronic yohimbine treatment in healthy volunteers. Eur J Clin Pharmacol 1990; 39:447–451.
17. Ernst E, Pittler MH. Yohimbine for erectile dysfunction: a systematic review and meta-analysis of randomised clinical trials. J Urol 1998; 159:433–436.
18. Hatzimouratidis K, Hatzichristou DG. A comparative review of the options for treatment of erectile dysfunction: which treatment for which patient? Drugs 2005; 65(12):1621–1650.
19. Nieschlag E, Swerdloff R, Behre HM, et al.; International Society of Andrology (ISA); International Society for the Study of the Aging Male (ISSAM); European Association of Urology (EAU). Investigation, treatment and monitoring of late-onset hypogonadism in males. ISA, ISSAM, and EAU recommendations. Eur Urol 2005; 48(1):1–4.
20. Kunelius P, Lukkarinen O. Intracavernous self-injection of prostaglandin E1 in the treatment of erectile dysfunction. Int J Impot Res 1999; 11(1):21–24.
21. McVary KT. Clinical practice. Erectile dysfunction. N Engl J Med 2007; 357(24):2472–2481.
22. Alexandre B, Lemaire A, Desvaux P, et al. Intracavernous injections of prostaglandin E1 for erectile dysfunction: patient satisfaction and quality of sex life on long-term treatment. J Sex Med 2007; 4(2):426–431.
23. Goldstein I. Oral phentolamine: an alpha-1, alpha-2 adrenergic antagonist for the treatment of erectile dysfunction. Int J Impot Res 2000; 12(S1):75–80.
24. Seyam R, Mohamed K, Akhras AA, et al. Prospective randomized study to optimize the dosage of trimix ingredients and compare its efficacy and safety with prostaglandin E1. Int J Impot Res 2005; 17(4):346–353.
25. Spivack AP, Peterson CA, Cowley C, et al. Long-term safety profile of transurethral alprostadil for the treatment of erectile dysfunction. J Urol 1997; 157:A792.
26. Goldstein I, Payton TR, Schechter P. A double blind, placebo-controlled, efficacy and safety study of topical gel formulation of 1% alprostadil (Topiglan) for the in-office treatment of erectile dysfunction. Urology 2001; 57:301–305.
27. Earle CM, Seah M, Coulden SE, et al. The use of the vacuum erection device in the management of erectile impotence. Int J Impot Res 1996; 8(4):237–240.
28. Opsomer RJ, Wese FX, De Groote P, et al. The external vacuum device in the management of erectile dysfunction. Acta Urol Belg 1997; 65(4):13–16.
29. Soderdahl DW, Thrasher JB, Hansberry KL. Intracavernosal drug-induced erection therapy versus external vacuum devices in the treatment of erectile dysfunction. Br J Urol 1997; 79(6):952–957.
30. Köhler TS, Pedro R, Hendlin K, et al. A pilot study on the early use of the vacuum erection device after radical retropubic prostatectomy. BJU Int 2007; 100(4):858–862.
31. Sexton WJ, Benedict JF, Jarow JP. Comparison of long-term outcomes of penile prostheses and intracavernosal injection therapy. J Urol 1998; 159(3):811–815.
32. Wilson SK, Zumbe J, Henry GD, et al. Infection reduction using antibiotic-coated inflatable penile prosthesis. Urology 2007; 70(2):337–340.

44 Surgery for erectile dysfunction

Levent Gurkan, Mathew C. Raynor, and Wayne J. G. Hellstrom

Erectile dysfunction (ED) affects 152 million people worldwide—a number estimated to reach 322 million by 2025 (1). ED results in significant reduction in self esteem and overall quality of life (2). Today, generally accepted first-line treatment options include oral therapies and vacuum erection devices. Second-line options are intraurethral suppositories and intracavernosal injection therapy. Surgery is reserved as the final approach for treatment failures. This chapter focuses on the surgical management of ED, including implantation of penile prosthesis and penile vascular surgery.

PENILE IMPLANT SURGERY

The history of penile prosthetic surgery dates back to the late 1930s when rib cartilage was placed subcutaneously to provide sufficient penile rigidity for sexual intercourse. This was followed by acrylic splints, polyethylene rods, and pure silicone implants (3). A milestone in penile implant surgery was the concept of placing cylinders intracavernosally introduced by the Egyptian surgeon Beheri in 1966 (4). His idea was subsequently incorporated with success with inflatable (5) and malleable prostheses (6). These devices have continued to improve over the past few decades and implant surgery is currently associated with high patient-satisfaction rates, increased mechanical reliability, and fewer overall complications. This section will focus on patient selection, available penile prosthesis devices, basic surgical procedures, and the management of complications.

Patient Selection

Candidates for implantation of penile prosthesis surgery include those who have failed medical therapy or for whom medical therapy is contraindicated. Patients are encouraged to use the vacuum erection device; unfortunately patient satisfaction and long term compliance is lower with this device (7). The potential implant patient must be informed about possible postoperative loss in penile length, sensory issues, and the small chance of infection to avoid any unrealistic expectations. The patient should realize that an implant will provide penile rigidity; however, it will not improve desire or cure any existing orgasmic or ejaculatory dysfunctions (8). The type of penile prosthesis and surgical technique employed for implantation depends on both patient factors and physician preference.

Penile Implants

There are two classes of penile implants: inflatable and semirigid. American Medical Systems (AMS) (Minnetonka, Minnesota) and Coloplast (Humlebaek, Denmark) (formerly Mentor) are the two major companies producing both inflatable and malleable prosthesis types. In the United States, inflatable devices outsell semirigid devices by a ratio of 4:1 (9). Although inflatable devices are superior in terms of providing full rigidity when erect and nearly complete flaccidity when detumesced, they require some manual dexterity; therefore, semirigid devices are more suitable for patients with diminished manual capabilities. Also, mechanical reliability is generally higher in semirigid devices with few failures reported in the literature (10). Current semirigid devices include the Genesis (Coloplast), AMS 650, and Duraform (AMS) (Fig. 1).

Inflatable penile prostheses can be subdivided into two-piece and three-piece devices. In two-piece devices, the reservoir is incorporated into the scrotal pump (Coloplast Excel) or into the base of the cavernosal cylinders (AMS Ambicor). Thus, intra-abdominal placement of the reservoir is circumvented. These devices can be especially useful in patients with previous complicated pelvic or abdominal surgeries, such as kidney transplant patients, or when adhesions or synthetic mesh may preclude easy placement of the reservoir (11). Two-piece prostheses are preconnected and generally placed through a penoscrotal approach.

Three-piece devices are composed of paired cylinders, a scrotal pump, and a reservoir. Paired cylinders are sized according to intraoperative measured lengths and placed within the corpora cavernosa. The scrotal pump includes an inflation pump and a deflation activator and is positioned in the scrotum in a dependent location. The reservoir is customarily placed into the extraperitoneal space of Retzius alongside the bladder (Fig. 2). Currently available three-piece devices differ in cylinder width and expansion properties. Standard cylinders expand in width and are available in the AMS CX and Coloplast Titan devices. Placement of these prostheses requires a standard dilatation of the corpora cavernosa to at least 12 to 14 mm. AMS LGX, which also requires a standard dilatation, expands in both width and length. Narrow-base implants are available for complex situations where dilatation is not easily accomplished (Coloplast Titan NB, AMS CXM, and AMS CXR). Both companies produce implants that appear similar; however, they differ greatly in cylinder construction and structure. Coloplast cylinders are made of Bioflex, a synthetic material similar to polyurethane under trademark protection, which is more durable than silicone. Early AMS devices used only silicone, which resulted in occasional aneurysm of the cylinders. Therefore, a three-layer construct consisting of inner and outer layers of silicone and an

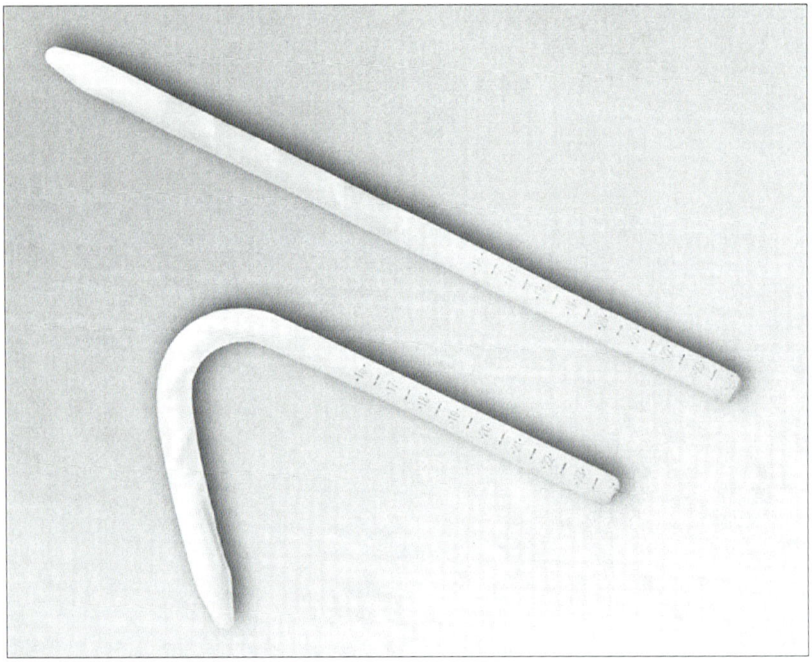

Figure 1 An example of a semirigid device. (Coloplast-Genesis).

intervening layer of polypropylene was developed to improve cylinder reliability. With the addition of paralyne in 2001, a micropolymer to enhance lubricity between these layers, three-year mechanical survival rates for cylinders have improved from 88.4% to 97.9% (12). In order to decrease the incidence of infection, both implant companies have developed different surface coating methodologies. AMS introduced InhibiZone in 2000, a combination of minocycline and rifampin impregnated into the external surfaces of all components of the three-piece prosthesis, except the rear tip extenders (Fig. 3). This antibiotic coating has significantly reduced infection rates by half in first-time implants without any risk factors, in diabetic patients, and in revision surgeries (13). Mentor (now Coloplast) introduced a hydrophilic coating in 2002 that reduces bacterial adherence and absorbs antibiotics when the implant is soaked intraoperatively. A countrywide comparison after its introduction to the market showed that the hydrophilic coating decreased infection rates from 2.07% to 1.06% (14). This new coating allows the surgeon to choose his/her preferred antibiotic solution. However, no head–to-head studies have been conducted to compare the efficacies of these different methodologies in reducing infection rates.

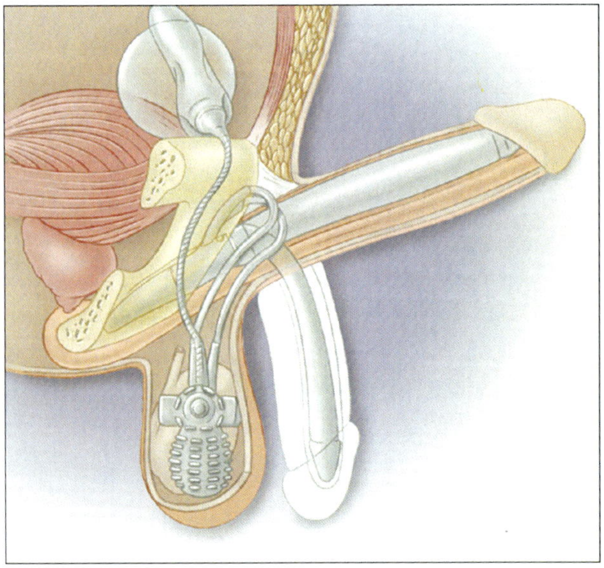

Figure 2 Schematic view of implanted three-piece penile prosthesis.

Refinements in design of the scrotal pump have also taken place. Recently, AMS introduced the "Momentary Squeeze (MS™)" pump (Fig. 3), which is designed as a one-touch button to allow complete cylinder deflation and simplify patient education. A similar pump design (OTC™) was introduced by Coloplast recently in Europe, Canada, and the United States (Fig. 4). Another longstanding problem is autoinflation, the involuntary inflation of cylinders, usually initiated by increased intra-abdominal pressure and a tight neo-capsule that has formed around the reservoir. This led to the development of a lock-out valve in the reservoir by Coloplast, which prevents back-flow of fluid from the reservoir. This valve system has decreased autoinflation rates from 11% to 1.3% (15). AMS recently introduced an integrated lock-out mechanism located in the scrotal pump.

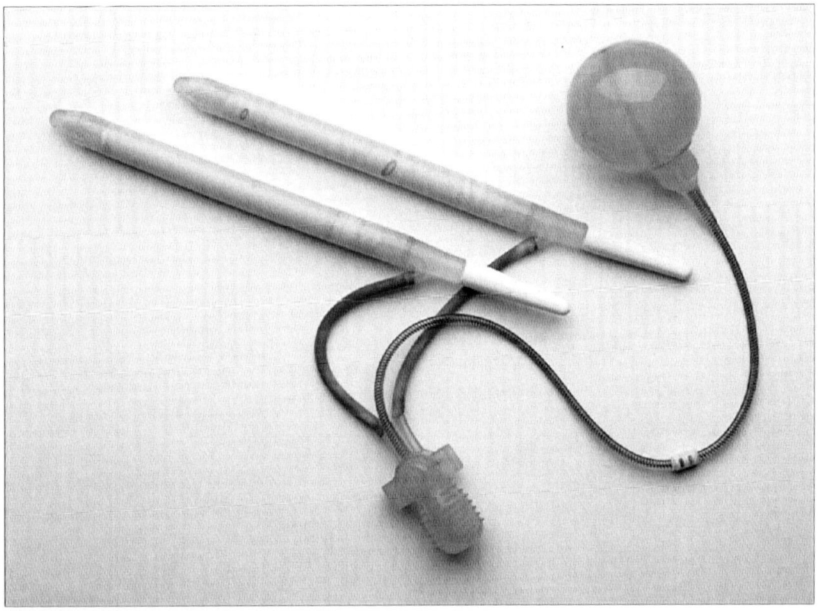

Figure 3 AMS three-piece penile prosthesis (700CX) with InhibiZone coating and "MS" pump design.

Surgical Technique

An important step in penile implant surgery is preoperative preparation. Understandably, surgeons have their particular preferences, but in general patients are instructed to scrub the surgical site three days preoperatively with antiseptic solution. Broad-spectrum antibiotics are administered preoperatively in order to attain sufficient tissue levels at the time of surgery. The patients are shaved immediately before scrubbing. Most surgeons prep with iodopovidone for at least 10 minutes. Currently, some implanting surgeons have begun using alcohol-based skin preparation products on the basis of promising reports from the orthopedic implant literature. Unfortunately, to date, there is no evidence-based published data on use of any of these products for penile implant surgery. Surgical gloves provide less than an optimal barrier; some authorities recommend iodopovidone on their fingertips or double gloving (9) to minimize potential contamination.

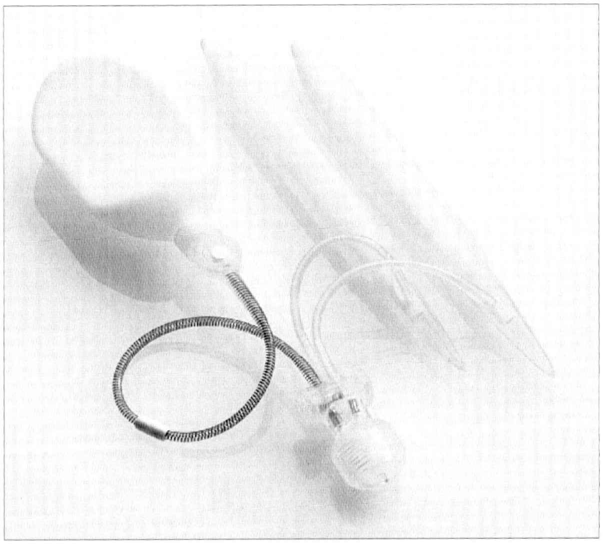

Figure 4 Coloplast three-piece penile prosthesis (Titan) with hydrophilic coating and new pump design.

Placement of an implant can be performed through a variety of approaches depending on the surgeon's comfort and training. The subcoronal approach is ideal for semirigid implants and is less time consuming and easier to perform. Two-piece devices are usually placed through a penoscrotal incision, whereas three-piece devices can be implanted via a penoscrotal or infrapubic approach (16). Until recently, the majority of protheses in the United States were placed through an infrapubic approach. However, many implanting surgeons have concerns about potential injury to the dorsal sensory nerves of the penis, which is circumvented with the penoscrotal approach. For many surgeons, the blind placement of the reservoir is a major disadvantage of this approach compared to an infrapubic incision. Traditionally, during the penoscrotal approach, sharp dissection exposes both corpora cavernosa and care should be taken to avoid injury to the corpus spongiosum. Placing stay sutures prior to corporotomy and prosthesis implantation avoids any inadvertent cylinder puncture. Ideally, the corporotomy should be made as proximal along the corpora as possible in order to decrease patient discomfort postoperatively in palpating the tubing under the scrotal skin. Dilatation of the cavernosal space can be a source of iatrogenic complications. In first-time surgeries, dilatation is usually straightforward. Conversely, after infection or cases of priapism, corporal fibrosis can severely limit dilatation. Dilatation of scarred corporal bodies is usually possible with care to avoid tunical perforation. In cases where routine dilatation of fibrosed corpora cavernosal tissue is not easily accomplished, other techniques have been suggested, including the use of cavernotomes, open corporeal excavation (17), ultrasound-guided cavernotomy (18), and optical corporotomy (19). The use of cavernotomes in these complex cases is associated with a higher complication rate (20).

Placement of the reservoir is performed under direct visualization during the infrapubic approach, while in the penoscrotal approach, the reservoir is placed by palpation. The transversalis fascia is punctured at the medial aspect of the inguinal ring, medial to the testicular cord structures, and a space is created for the reservoir alongside the bladder, in the space of Retzius. Both Coloplast and AMS produce reservoirs of different volumes. Typically, the larger reservoirs are used for cylinders longer than 18 cm. In cases where previous surgery has obliterated the space of Retzius, the surgeon may consider placement of a two-piece device or, if needed, can place the reservoir in an ectopic location, usually anterior to the transversalis fascia and posterior to the rectus muscle. As noted, the newer prosthesis models incorporate a lock-out valve mechanism that reduces the incidence of autoinflation. Partial inflation of the implant for 1 to 2 days after the surgery will prevent any bleeding from the corporotomy sites. A pressure dressing is also applied to the scrotum to prevent hematoma formation. The urinary catheter and pressure dressings can be removed the following morning and the implant deflated at the same time. This should be performed by the surgeon or someone with knowledge of the workings of these devices as the most uncomfortable reports of the prosthesis surgery recounted by patients is dressing removal and device deflation (21).

Complications

Infection associated with penile implant surgery is considered a catastrophic event. Although the incidence is very low in first-time implants (1% to 3%), revision surgeries report a higher risk of infection (7–18%) (22). The most common microorganism responsible for infection is *Staphylococcus epidermidis*, an opportunistic skin microorganism with low toxicity. Infection associated with this microorganism usually presents later in the clinical course with most patients complaining of persistent pain or drainage. Early infections, on the other hand, are associated with more virulent microorganisms, such as *Staphylococcus aureus, Pseudomonas, Escherichia coli, or Enterococcus*. These infections are usually accompanied by systemic symptoms such as fever and chills with purulent drainage and erythema. Historically, standard of care was removal of the implant, long-term antibiotics and reimplantation of a new device in 3 to 6 months. However, this approach resulted in significant corporal scarring and loss of penile length, making subsequent implantation procedures significantly more difficult. Mulcahy et al. introduced the salvage procedure in order to preserve penile length and avoid subsequent delayed implantation. The procedure involves removing all components of the device, copious irrigation of the wound with a structured order of antibacterial agents (Table 1) and immediate reimplantation of a new antibiotic-coated implant. This procedure carries a success rate of greater than 84% (23). New evidence suggests that patients undergoing revision surgery for mechanical malfunction should also undergo a salvage procedure as up to 66% of patients with clinically uninfected prostheses had positive identification of microorganisms on the explanted components at the time of revision (24). Culture of clinically uninfected implants explanted for mechanical failure showed that 43% were positive for organisms and 80% were positive for biofilm formation (25). Clinically, a decrease in infection rate has been reported for revision surgeries using a salvage protocol (26).

Table 1 Salvage Procedure

- Remove all parts of the implant
- Irrigate all compartments with seven antibiotic solutions
- Antibiotics (Kanamycin, bacitracin)
- Half-strength hydrogen peroxide
- Half-strength povidone-iodine
- Pressure irrigation with 1-g vancomycin and 80-mg gentamycin in 5 L irrigating solution
- Half-strength povidone-iodine
- Half-strength hydrogen peroxide
- Antibiotics (Kanamycin, bacitracin)
- Change gown, gloves, surgical drapes, and instruments
- Insert new prosthesis
- Close wound without using any drains
- Prolonged antibiotic treatment after surgery

For those patients experiencing length loss and corporal scarring after removal of an infected prosthesis, placement of a narrow-base device is recommended as this can act as a tissue expander and, if deemed necessary, replaced with a standard prosthesis at a later date. This technique can regain penile length and increase patient satisfaction (20). Tunical perforation can be identified intraoperatively during corporal dilatation or postoperatively by a malpositioned cylinder. Distal tunical perforation is typically identified during dilatation by crossover of the dilators. Correction involves placement of a dilator within the unaffected cavernosal body and redilating the contralateral side. If distal perforation results in a urethral injury, it is recommended to leave a urethral catheter and postpone placement of the prosthesis. Proximal tunical perforation during dilatation was treated historically with a "wind sock" repair, first described by Mulcahy in 1987 (27). A cup of a synthetic material is anchored to the cavernotomy in order to create an artificial crus and prevent proximal migration of the implant (27). This technique has reported infection rates as high as 30%, mainly because the space created between the synthetic materials was suitable for bacterial growth (28). A simpler method of repair involves placement of a single nonabsorbable suture through the corporotomy and the rear-tip extender in order to stabilize the cylinder until a fibrous capsule is formed around the cylinder. Patients are then instructed to cycle the prosthesis daily and to avoid any axial pressure for at least three months that might, in turn, dislocate the prosthesis (29). Late erosion of the implant through the distal tunica is recognized as the tip of the penile prosthesis becomes palpable just beneath the penile skin, the so called "impending erosion." Repair should be performed promptly as any delay may result in erosion through the skin causing contamination and infection. Historically it was corrected using synthetic (30) or autologous materials (31). However, the natural tissue repair technique as described by Mulcahy can be performed—the fibrous capsule around the cylinder is used to buttress the tunica. It appears that natural tissue repair with rerouting of the malpositioned cylinder and repair of the tunical defect achieves superior results with a shorter operative time, less postoperative pain, lower infection rates, and lower rates of cylinder erosion (30). Mechanical failure rates have improved dramatically since introduction of the inflatable prostheses. With various design alterations by both Coloplast and AMS, long-term mechanical survival rates over 10 years are ≥90% (12).

Conclusion

Although penile implants are an invasive treatment option, they offer the highest reliability for patients unresponsive to conservative therapies with excellent patient and partner satisfaction rates.

PENILE REVASCULARIZATION

Indications

Penile revascularization procedures are indicated only in select patients with ED. These patients include young, well-motivated men with documented arteriogenic ED, usually resulting from pelvic trauma. The hallmark of arteriogenic ED is difficulty in achieving erections, whereas the ability to maintain an erection is usually preserved. Patients with risk factors for endothelial dysfunction such as diabetes mellitus, hypertension, coronary artery disease, hypercholesterolemia, or continued tobacco abuse are usually excluded from this surgical intervention.

Diagnosis

Evaluation of men being considered for penile revascularization begins with a complete history and physical exam. The patient is questioned about previous erectile function, including the ability to achieve and maintain erections, libido, and penile sensation. Ejaculatory and orgasmic disorders should be elucidated. Questions regarding the mechanism of injury are explored as there should be a definable correlation between the injury and the onset of ED. Risk factors for vascular disease are identified. Physical examination focuses on penile pathology such as the presence of Peyronie's plaques or corporeal fibrosis. Patients should have attempted and failed a trial of nonsurgical therapies. Some men with arteriogenic ED may respond well to phosphodiesterase type 5 inhibitors (PDE5 inhibitors) or intracavernosal injection therapy. Since these men typically have an intact veno-occlusive mechanism, improving arterial inflow with pharmacotherapy should improve erectile function. Further evaluation consists of cavernous injection of a vasoactive agent and penile duplex Doppler ultrasound assessment. Doppler evaluation measures peak systolic velocities, end-diastolic velocities, and resistive indices. Reduced peak systolic velocities correlate highly with the presence of arterial insufficiency. Peak systolic velocities below 25cm/s are diagnostic of arterial insufficiency (32). Corroboration with pelvic arteriography is needed in patients with isolated arterial insufficiency. Pelvic and selective internal pudendal arteriography identifies the site of arterial injury and documents the presence of patency of the inferior epigastric vessels that are used for revascularization procedures. Arteriography is performed after administration of vasoactive agents such as papaverine, phentolamine, or alprostadil in order to allow for maximum vasodilatation and visualization of penile vasculature. Arteriography is often complicated by congenital variations in penile vascular anatomy and can make diagnoses difficult. Young healthy patients with a discrete arterial injury or obstruction are obvious candidates for penile revascularization procedures.

Surgery

Isolation of the inferior epigastric artery can be performed through a variety of approaches. Typically, a midline incision extending from the umbilicus to the pubis was necessary to harvest the vessels. Some advocate the use of semilunar lower-abdominal incisions or a paramedian incision. More recent reports describe epigastric vessel harvesting through minimally invasive techniques such as laparoscopically (33), robotically, and even using a video-assisted endoscopic vessel dissector (34). These minimally invasive procedures reduce surgical morbidity and recovery time. The inferior epigastric artery is isolated with the surrounding veins and fat in order to preserve adventitial blood supply. The vessels are transposed to the pelvis for microsurgical revascularization. The epigastric artery is dissected down to the level of its origin at the external iliac artery with care taken to avoid kinking of the vessel during transposition to the pelvis. During laparoscopic or robotic vessel harvesting, the vessels can be transposed through a separate port placed in the suprapubic area. Revascularization can be undertaken by a variety of microscopic anastomotic techniques. Anastomosis to the dorsal penile artery can be performed in an end-to-end or end-to-side manner. Arterialization of the deep dorsal vein as described by Virag is another approach. This technique has undergone many subsequent variations with similar success rates. In cases where the inferior epigastric vessels are not adequate, a saphenous vein graft from the superficial femoral artery can be performed (35). In cases of deep dorsal vein arterialization, including distal subcoronal plexus, ligation limits the possibility of subsequent glans hyperemia.

Results

Early methods of penile revascularization were complicated mainly by thrombosis and occlusion of the anastomosis. Patency rates have improved with modifications of the anastomotic techniques. Several studies have examined the long-term outcomes of penile revascularization procedures with varying results. Jarow et al. followed 11 patients for an average of 50 months after undergoing revascularization. They found a 91% improvement in these patients after strict patient-selection criteria were employed. Two-thirds of these patients were able to achieve spontaneous erections with another 27%, responding to intracavernosal injections (36). Manning et al. examined 62 men after revascularization with a mean follow-up of 41 months. Spontaneous erections were seen in 34% of patients with an additional 20% responding to vasoactive injections. They noted a 69% success rate in younger patients (37). Vardi et al. studied 52 patients over a mean period of 70.8 months. The overall success rate was 48%. Patients younger than 28 years had a 73% success rate versus 23% for those older than 28 years. Also, nonsmokers were found to have a much higher success rate versus smokers (57% vs. 29%) (38). Recent evidence, however, disputes the claim that only younger patients respond well to revascularization. Kayigil et al. examined healthy elderly males without other risk factors undergoing dorsal vein arterialization. After a mean follow-up of 22 months, there was a 60.5% success rate. In this series there was no significant difference between men less than 60 or those older than 60 years of age (39).

Complications

The most common complications from penile revascularization procedures are penile edema and ecchymoses. These are typically self-limited and not clinically significant. A more concerning complication is penile numbness due to surgically induced neuropraxia or direct injury to the dorsal nerves. Also, penile shortening can occur due to scar formation. Anastomotic leaks have been reported usually due to trauma involved with early intercourse. Injuries can range from mild, self-limited hematoma to a complete disruption of the anastomosis. A more common, but avoidable, complication is glans hyperemia. This complication is more likely to occur with dorsal vein arterialization procedures and its risk can be reduced by ligating the subcoronal plexus of veins just proximal to the glans.

VENOUS SURGERY

Indications

As with penile revascularization procedures, an even greater controversy exists regarding the use of penile venous ligation surgery for treatment of ED. Questions continue to surround the long-term outcomes of venous surgery for veno-occlusive dysfunction as well as which patients are best suited. Ideally, ED patients with documented venous leak from an isolated site and normal arterial function or men with congenital tunical malformations or aberrant venous tributaries are best suited for this type of surgery. Patients with veno-occlusive dysfunction typically complain of difficulty obtaining or maintaining erections, even with sexual stimulation. These patients should not be considered for surgical therapy before failing all conservative therapies, including oral PDE5 inhibitors and intracavernosal injections. Risk factors for vascular disease, such as hypertension, diabetes, and tobacco use must be elucidated. Patients should be thoroughly counseled on the risks of venous surgery as well as the long-term outcomes, which are generally not superlative. They also need to be informed of the prosthetic options available.

Diagnosis

Evaluation begins with a thorough history and physical examination. Patients are questioned about the duration of ED to determine whether this is a primary or secondary condition. Primary ED in the setting of veno-occlusive dysfunction may point to a congenital cause. Questions regarding the ability to obtain and maintain erections with sexual stimulation with or without pharmacologic assistance are also important. Physical examination ensures normal penile anatomy without Peyronie's plaques or other physical findings that may alter treatment. Further evaluation involves the use of penile duplex Doppler ultrasound assessment. After intracorporeal injection of vasoactive agents, peak systolic and end-diastolic velocities are measured. Venous leak can be diagnosed with high sensitivity when the end-diastolic velocity is greater than 5cm/s (40). Resistive indices less than 0.75 are also another accurate and noninvasive method of determining veno-occlusive dysfunction. Confirmatory diagnostic techniques recommended by most authorities include pharmacologic cavernosometry and cavernosography. Dynamic infusion cavernosometry involves the infusion of saline intracorporeally while simultaneously measuring intracorporeal pressure. The test is performed after administering an intracorporeal vasoactive agent. Veno-occlusive dysfunction is diagnosed by an inability to maintain intracorporeal pressure at a level equal to systolic blood pressure or by rapid detumescence following cessation of saline infusion. Concomitantly, cavernosography is performed with instillation of contrast material intracorporeally. Radiographs are used to localize the exact site of venous leak. Typically, multiple sites of venous leak are identified. Generalized glandular leak portends a poor prognosis for this type of surgery.

Surgery

Once a patient is deemed a candidate for penile venous surgery and has been counseled regarding other treatment options and long-term outcomes, surgical treatment involves dissection of the superficial and deep dorsal veins. Communicating veins between the deep and superficial systems are individually ligated. Buck's fascia is incised to expose the deep dorsal vein and is ligated. Dissection is carried proximally and distally to ligate perforating vessels from the deep dorsal vein system. Communicating circumflex veins are identified laterally between the corpora cavernosa and the corpus spongiosum and ligated. Caution must be exercised when dissecting the deep dorsal vein to avoid lateral dissection and the risk of injury to dorsal penile arteries and nerves. If cavernosography/cavernosometry demonstrates isolated crural leakage, then ligation of the proximal crura may be considered.

Results

Short-term results for penile venous surgery are generally good; however, long-term results are somewhat disappointing. This fact leads many to question the utility of venous surgery for ED. In fact, the AUA guidelines recommend placement of a penile prosthesis as the only surgical option for treatment of ED (41). Many patients undergoing venous ligation do experience an improvement in erection quality following surgery and additional patients may now respond to intracavernosal injection therapy. This early response is short-lived in majority of the patients. However, a surgery that allows one to not resort to a penile prosthesis is considered a benefit by many younger men. One of the largest series of patients undergoing deep dorsal vein resection with long-term follow-up showed a success rate of only 11.2% (42). Berardinucci et al. followed 100 men undergoing deep dorsal vein ligation and after three months, success was reported in 62% of patients. However, this success declined to 31% after 45 months (43). One subgroup of patients who may benefit includes those with primary ED due to congenital malformations of venous drainage or isolated crural leak. These patients typically exhibit a sustained and durable improvement in their erection quality (44).

Complications

Common complications following venous surgery include penile edema and ecchymoses, which are usually self-limited.

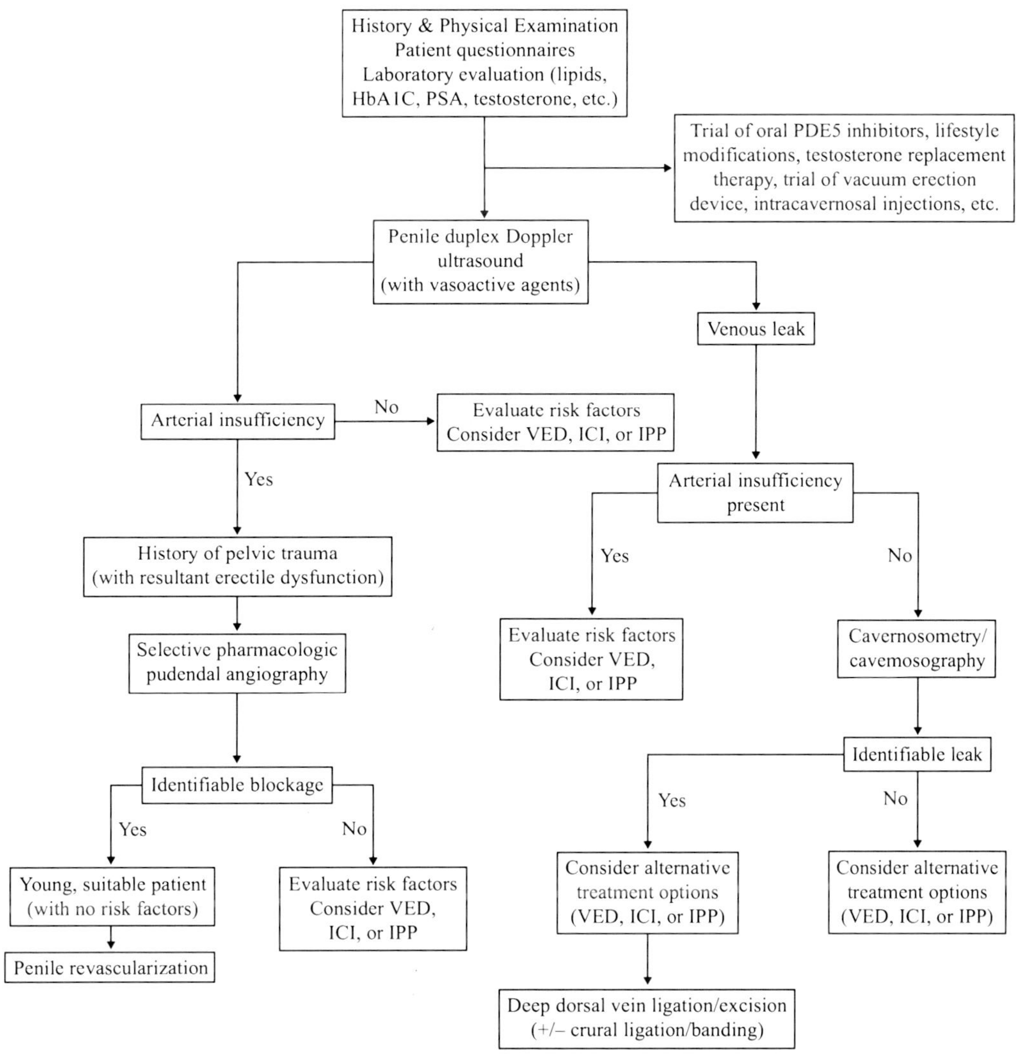

Figure 5 Flow-chart for diagnosis and treatment of vasculogenic erectile dysfunction.

Penile numbness, in varying degrees, can occur in a significant percentage of patients and may last for one year or more. Also, penile shortening has been shown to occur in up to 40% of patients (45).

Conclusions

Vascular surgery for ED has varying degrees of success. Higher success rates and longer duration of improvement can be seen with rigorous selection criteria. Patients that are young, healthy, and have documented arterial insufficiency after pelvic trauma can have long-term durable outcomes from penile revascularization procedures, whether this includes arterial bypass or deep dorsal vein arterialization. Patients with documented venous leak from an identifiable site, especially those with primary ED or young patients with a short duration of ED, may benefit from penile venous surgery. Any patient under consideration for vascular surgery for ED should be thoroughly counseled regarding the risks, complications, and long-term outcomes and must have failed a course of conservative therapy prior to proceeding with surgical therapy.

The evaluation and treatment of the ED patient requires a multidisciplinary approach including psychological, hormonal, and vascular assessment. The majority of patients today are treated medically, while surgery remains an option for nonresponders and for those who are not suitable for medical therapy. Among the surgical procedures, penile implantation is the only procedure recommended by most authorities, while penile venous surgery and penile arterialization might be an option only in selected cases (46). A simplified flowchart is provided for the treatment of ED (Fig. 5).

KEY MESSAGES:

- Candidates for penile prosthesis surgery include nonresponders to medical therapy and those for whom medical therapy is contraindicated. (grade C recommendation)
- Advances in penile prosthesis technology, including a lock-out valve mechanism and antibiotic coating, significantly improve long-term success rates of surgery. (level 2b evidence)
- Revision surgeries have higher infection and complication rates (level 2a), especially if special tools such as cavernotomes are required during the operation. (level 2a evidence)
- A single step surgery using a "salvage procedure" for revision of an infected prosthesis has a higher success rate while it diminishes potential fibrosis and scarring seen during the classical two-step revision. (level 2b evidence)
- A "washout procedure" is recommended during all revision surgeries as it has been shown to decrease capsule tissue culture positivity. (level 2a evidence)
- Due to inconsistent and low long-term success rates reported for penile venous surgery and penile arterialization, placement of a penile prosthesis remains as the only "recommended" surgical option in the treatment of ED. (grade B recommendation)

REFERENCES

1. Ayta IA, McKinlay JB, Krane RJ. The likely worldwide increase in erectile dysfunction between 1995 and 2025 and some possible policy consequences. BJU Int 1999; 84(1): 50–56.
2. O'Leary MP, Althof SE, Cappelleri JC, et al., and The United States Self-Esteem and Relationship Questionnaire Study Group. Self-esteem, confidence and relationship satisfaction of men with erectile dysfunction treated with sildenafil citrate: a multicenter, randomized, parallel group, double-blind, placebo controlled study in the United States. J Urol 2006; 175(3 Pt 1): 1058–1062.
3. Sadeghi-Nejad H. Penile prosthesis surgery: a review of prosthetic devices and associated complications. J Sex Med 2007; 4(2):296–309.
4. Beheri, GE. Surgical treatment of impotence. Plast Reconstr Surg 1966; 38(2):92–97.
5. Scott FB, Bradley WE, Timm GW. Management of erectile impotence. Use of implantable inflatable prosthesis. Urology 1973; 2(1):80–82.
6. Small MP, Carrion HM, Gordon JA. Small-Carrion penile prosthesis. New implant for management of impotence. Urology 1975; 5(4):479–486.
7. Gontero P, Fontana F, Zitella A, et al. A prospective evaluation of efficacy and compliance with a multistep treatment approach for erectile dysfunction in patients after non-nerve sparing radical prostatectomy. BJU Int 2005; 95(3):359–365.
8. Mulcahy JJ, Austoni E, Barada JH, et al. The penile implant for erectile dysfunction. J Sex Med 2004; 1(1):98–109.
9. Henry GD, Wilson SK. Updates in inflatable penile prostheses. Urol Clin North Am 2007; 34(4):535–547.
10. Akand M, Ozayar A, Yaman O, et al. Mechanical failure with malleable penile prosthesis. Urology 2007; 70(5):1007.e11–e12.
11. Cuellar DC, Sklar GN. Penile prosthesis in the organ transplant recipient. Urology 2001; 57(1):138–141.
12. Wilson SK, Delk JR, Salem EA, et al. Long-term survival of inflatable penile prostheses: single surgical group experience with 2,384 first-time implants spanning two decades. J Sex Med 2007a; 4(4 Pt 1):1074–1079.
13. Wilson SK, Zumbe J, Henry GD, et al. Infection reduction using antibiotic-coated inflatable penile prosthesis. Urology 2007b; 70(2):337–340.
14. Wolter CE, Hellstrom WJ. The hydrophilic-coated inflatable penile prosthesis: 1-year experience. J Sex Med 2004; 1(2):221–224.
15. Wilson SK, Henry GD, Delk JR Jr, et al. The Mentor Alpha-1 prosthesis with reservoir lock-out valve: effective prevention of auto-inflation with improved capability for ectopic reservoir placement. J Urol 2002; 178:1475–1478.

16. Montague DK, Angermeir KW. Surgical approaches for penile prosthesis implantation: penoscrotal vs infrapubic. Int J Impot Res 2003; 15(suppl 5):s134–s135.
17. Montague DK, Angermeier KW. Corporeal excavation: new technique for penile prosthesis implantation in men with severe corporeal fibrosis. Urology 2006; 67(5):1072–1075.
18. Shaeer, O. Penile prosthesis implantation in cases of fibrosis: ultrasound-guided cavernotomy and sheathed trochar excavation. J Sex Med 2007; 4(3):809–814.
19. Shaeer, O. Penoscopy optical corporotomy and resection for prosthesis implantation in cases of penile fibrosis, Shaeer's technique. J Sex Med 2007; 4(5):1214–1217.
20. Wilson SK, Delk JR 2nd, Mulcahy JJ, et al. Upsizing of inflatable penile implant cylinders in patients with corporal fibrosis. J Sex Med 2006; 3(4):736–742.
21. Brinkman MJ, Henry GD, Wilson SK, et al. A survey of patients with inflatable penile prostheses for satisfaction. J Urol 2005; 174(1):253–257.
22. Jarow, JP. Risk factors for penile prosthetic infection. J Urol 1996; 156(2 Pt 1):402–404.
23. Mulcahy, JJ. Long-term experience with salvage of infected penile implants. J Urol 2000; 163(2):481–482.
24. Henry GD, Carson CC, Wilson SK, et al. Revision washout decreases implant capsule tissue culture positivity: a multicenter study. J Urol 2008; 179(1):186–190.
25. Silverstein AD, Henry GD, Evans B, et al. Biofilm formation on clinically noninfected penile prostheses. J Urol 2006; 176(3):1008–1011.
26. Henry GD, Wilson SK, Delk JR 2nd, et al. Revision washout decreases penile prosthesis infection in revision surgery: a multicenter study. J Urol 2005; 173(1):89–92.
27. Mulcahy JJ. A technique of maintaining penile prosthesis position to prevent proximal migration. J Urol 1987; 137(2):294–296.
28. Knoll LD, Furlow WL. Corporeal reconstruction and prosthetic implantation for impotence associated with non-dilatable corporeal cavernosal fibrosis. Acta Urol Belg 1992; 60(1):15–25.
29. Mulcahy JJ. Crural perforation during penile prosthetic surgery. J Sex Med 2006; 3(1):177–180.
30. Carson CC, Noh CH. Distal penile prosthesis extrusion: treatment with distal corporoplasty or Gortex windsock reinforcement. Int J Impot Res 2002; 14(2):81–84.
31. Alter GJ, Greisman J, Werthman PE, et al. Use of prefabricated tunica vaginalis fascia flap to reconstruct the tunica albuginea after recurrent penile prosthesis extrusion. J Urol 1998; 159:128–132.
32. Benson CB, Aruny JE, Vickers MA Jr. Correlation of duplex sonography with arteriography in patients with erectile dysfunction. AJR 1993; 160(1):71–73.
33. Lund GO, Winfield HN, Donovan JF. Laparoscopically assisted penile revascularization for vasculogenic impotence. J Urology 1995; 153(6):1923–1926.
34. Kawanishi Y, Kimura K, Nakanishi R, et al. A minimally invasive method for harvesting the epigastric artery for penile revascularization. BJU Int 2004; 94(9):1391–1396.
35. Rao DS, Donatucci CF. Vasculogenic impotence. Arterial and venous surgery. Urol Clin North Am 2001; 28(2):309–319.
36. Jarow JP, DeFranzo AJ. Long-term results of arterial bypass surgery for impotence secondary to segmental vascular disease. J Urol 1996; 156(3):982–985.
37. Manning M, Kunemann KP, Scheepe JR, et al. Long-term followup and selection criteria for penile revascularization in erectile failure. J Urol 1998; 160(5):1680–1684.
38. Vardi Y, Gruenwald I, Gedalia U, et al. Evaluation of penile revascularization for erectile dysfunction: a 10-year follow-up. Int J Impot Res 2004; 16(2):181–186.
39. Kayigil O, Agras K, Okulu E. Is deep dorsal vein arterialization effective in elderly patients? [Published online ahead of print Nov 21, 2007]. Int Urol Nephrol 2008; 40(1):125–131.
40. Quam JP, King BF, James EM, et al. Duplex and color Doppler sonographic evaluation of vasculogenic impotence. AJR 1989; 153(6):1141–1147.
41. Montague DK, Jarow JP, Broderick GA, et al. Chapter 1: The management of erectile dysfunction: an AUA update. J Urol 2005; 174(1):230–239.
42. Schultheiss D, Truss MC, Becker AJ, et al. Long-term results following dorsal penile vein ligation in 126 patients with veno-occlusive dysfunction. Int J Impot Res 1997; 9(4):205–209.
43. Berardinucci D, Morales A, Heaton JP, et al. Surgical treatment of penile veno-occlusive dysfunction: is it justified? Urology 1996; 47(1):88–92.
44. Rahman NU, Dean RC, Carrion R, et al. Crural ligation for primary erectile dysfunction: a case series. J Urol 2005; 173(6):2064–2066.
45. Kim ED, McVary KT. Long-term results with penile vein ligation for venogenic impotence. J Urol 1995; 153(3 pt 1):655–658.
46. Sharaby JS, Benet AE, Melman A. Penile revascularization. Urol Clin North Am 1995; 22(4):821–832.

45 Peyronie's disease and penile curvature

Ekkehard W. Hauck, Thorsten Diemer, and Wolfgang Weidner

CASE REPORT

A 61-year-old man presented with a 19-months history of dorsal penile curvature. After an initial phase of penile pain during erection and progressive upward curvature, the symptoms stabilized after 7 months. The patient identified himself a palpable induration at the penile dorsum. The dorsal curvature of 70° remained unchanged for 12 months. Sexual intercourse was severely hampered due to the curvature despite sufficient rigidity of the penis. Drug treatment with potassium para-aminobenzoate, initiated 8 months after the onset of the disorder did not improve the penile malformation. The patient's history and physical status was apparently normal besides Dupuytren's contracture on both hands. He remembered a penile trauma during sexual intercourse 6 months before the onset of symptoms.

The clinical examination revealed a 35-mm long and 20-mm wide dorsal penile plaque with signs of calcification as indicated by ultrasound. Three-dimensional autophotography demonstrated the dorsal curvature of 70° during full erection. Colour-encoded duplex sonography performed during an intracavernosal pharmacon erection test with 20-μg alprostadil revealed normal arterial blood flow in the deep cavernosal arteries. Dynamic infusion pharmacocavernosometry and cavernosography provided no hints of a venous leakage. However, besides the curvature of 70°, a slight hourglass-like deformity at the site of the plaque became evident.

Due to the degree of curvature of about more than 60°, a double incision of the plaque and subsequent covering of the defects with grafts of bovine lyophilized pericard was performed. After this procedure, the penis was totally straightened and sexual intercourse has been facilitated to the satisfaction of the couple.

CLINICAL SYMPTOMS

Peyronie's disease is characterized by the clinical findings of penile pain, a plaque of the tunica albuginea, and penile curvature predominantly directed dorsally. 30% to 50% of the patients complain of erectile dysfunction and penile shortening. Penile curvature alone or a combination of these symptoms can severely hamper the performance of sexual intercourse. Additional psychological problems may occur (1–3).

EPIDEMIOLOGY AND NATURAL HISTORY

Usually middle-aged men with a peak between the age of 50 to 60 years are affected. However, the onset of the disease has been also reported in a wide range of age from 15 to 80 years. The prevalence of Peyronie's disease in men of that age appears to be up to 3.2% (1,2,4).

The natural course of Peyronie's disease is unpredictable ranging from spontaneous resolution of all clinical symptoms in up to 13% of the cases to severe penile curvature, erectile dysfunction, and the complete inability to perform cohabitation (5). It is not possible to predict the individual prognosis at the beginning of the disease. Penile pain seems to resolve spontaneously in the majority of patients within 12 to 18 months (1,5). The majority of patients achieve a stable stage without further alterations of symptoms by time (1). Peyronie's disease is supposed to be in a stable stage if it has lasted for at least 12 months and the patient does not suffer from pain or progression of symptoms for at least 6 months (1,6,7).

PATHOLOGICAL FINDINGS AND ETIOPATHOLOGY

Peyronie's disease is a connective tissue disorder with plaque formation in the tunica albuginea and the adjacent tissue of the corpora cavernosa (8). The plaque is predominantly located unifocally in the penile dorsum, causing a typical dorsal deviation with pain in the initial, acute phase of the disease (9). Morphologically, an inflammatory reaction with thickening of the tunica albuginea is detectable in the beginning. Later on, a fibrotic and frequently calcified plaque is typical (1,8).

The etiopathogenesis still remains unclear. Repetitive penile microtraumatization during sexual intercourse with the induction of a complex cascade of wound healing is discussed as potentially being one of the main causes. Fibrin deposition followed by an inflammatory reaction and subsequent scar formation should lead to plaque formation in the tunica albuginea (10). Genetic predisposition with certain HLA alleles and autoimmune processes in connection with infectious aspects have been under debate (1,11,12), but have been ruled out over the last years (13,14).

Since up to 30% of patients with the Peyronie's disease suffer also from Dupuytren's contracture, a so far unknown genetic predisposition seems debatable. Especially the TGF-β signal transduction system has been the focus of interest during the last few years (15,16,17). Besides this, many studies on possible associations to certain diseases, drugs, and other aspects have been published. However, a definitive explanation of the etiopathological pathway cannot be provided until now.

DIAGNOSTIC WORK-UP

The diagnostic work-up is simple. The patients' history will reveal data on penile pain, curvature, hampered sexual

Table 1 Efficacy of Oral Drug Therapy

Oral drug therapy Substance	Mode of study	Effect
Potassium para-aminobenzoate (Potaba®)	Placebo-controlled double blind study	**Yes** (on plaque size, on progression of curvature)
Vitamin E	Placebo-controlled double blind study	**No**
Propoleum	Placebo-controlled double blind study	**Yes** (on all symptoms, (not clinically relevant, since only available in Cuba)
Tamoxifen	Placebo-controlled double blind study	**No**
Colchicine	Placebo-controlled double blind study	**No**
Acetyl-L-Carnitine	Tamoxifen-controlled double blind study	**Yes** (on pain, on progression of curvature)

Source: From Refs. 2, 3, and 19.

intercourse, and concomitant erectile dysfunction. The plaque can be identified by palpation. The extension can be measured by the use of a ruler or by ultrasound. Calcifications as sign of chronification can be easily visualized by high-resolution ultrasound. The degree of curvature can be documented by auto-photography by the patient himself during erection from three different angles as suggested by Kelâmi (18). However, the photodocumentation can also be performed during a pharmacon erection test that should be performed in every case before surgery. During this test color coded duplexsonography allows assessment of the penile arterial flow. Dynamic infusion cavernosography can provide information on hourglass deformity, a pathological venous network, and intracorporal plaques. Cavernous leakages can be detected or excluded by cavernosometry.

TREATMENT

Different conservative treatment options of uncertain efficacy are available. The majority of patients initially prefer conservative treatment. However, the patients' high expectations frequently cannot be fulfilled (19). The indication for conservative therapy appears to be the early painful and progressive stage of the disease. Surgery should only be performed in the stable stage (1). That means, Peyronie's disease should have lasted for at least 12 months and the patient should not have suffered from pain or progression of symptoms for at least 6 months (1,7,19).

Conservative Treatment

Since the natural course of the disorder is not homogenous, it is not possible to predict the individual prognosis at the beginning of the disease. Only penile pain seems to resolve spontaneously in the majority of patients within 12 to 18 months (5). The different individual unpredictable natural courses are the reason why it is so difficult to assess the efficacy of a conservative treatment modality (19). The outcome referred to a conservative approach may be just in the range of the natural history. For this reason, the efficacy of conservative therapy of Peyronie's disease can only be proven in randomized, placebo-controlled studies that comprise a representative number of patients. However, many studies published so far have not fulfilled these criteria. Herein, data of the recently published studies are in the focus since the study design of the older approaches is usually considered inappropriate.

Oral Drug Therapy

During the last years studies on the use of potassium para-aminobenzoate (Potaba™), vitamin E, colchicine, tamoxifen, propoleum, acetyl-L-carnitine, and propionyl-L-carnitine have been published (Table 1) (2,3,19). A recent survey regarding drug therapy demonstrated that the majority of patients (76%) are treated by the use of potassium para-aminobenzoate (46%) or vitamin E (29%) (20). Other substances play a minor role.

Potassium para-aminobenzoate (Potaba) seems to be useful to stabilize the disorder and prevent progression of penile curvature in patients during the early stage of the disease. Moreover, it can reduce plaque size significantly. No significant effect on reduction of pain has been observed (21). Thus the administration of potassium para-aminobenzoate can be an option, if the prevention of progression of the disease is intended (19,21).

The use of **vitamin E** is widely performed. However, there is no evidence that vitamin E has a significant effect on the symptoms of Peyronie's disease (22). The data on **tamoxifen** and on **colchicine** indicate alterations or 'improvements' of the disorder only in the range of the natural history (19). Studies on the effect of **propoleum** have been published several times by the same group of authors (23). This substance is patented in Cuba and availability is restricted to this country. The scientific value is limited although significant effects on the symptoms such as pain, diminution of curvature, and plaque size have been described in a prospective, placebo-controlled, double blind trial. In recent studies **acetyl-L-carnitine** and **propionyl-L-carnitine** have been investigated with interesting results, however, these studies combined the administration of these substances with other drugs or did not establish a placebo-controlled group (24,25).

Table 2 Efficacy of Intralesional Drug Therapy

Intralesional drug therapy Substance	Mode of study	Effect
Verapamil	Placebo-controlled double blind study	**No**
Interferon alfa	Placebo-controlled single blind study	**Yes** (on decrease of curvature, on improvement of sexual function)
Collagenase	Placebo-controlled double blind study	**Yes** (only on mild curvature)
Betametasone	Placebo-controlled single blind study	**No**
Hyaluronidase	Placebo-controlled double blind study	**No**

Source: From Refs. 2, 3, and 19.

Intralesional Drug Therapy

The direct injection of a substance into the plaque should provide the advantage of a high local concentration of the drug. Systemic side effects can be reduced. The intralesional injection can be painful for the patient. Frequent injections require a high degree of compliance. The indication for intralesional drug therapy seems to be the same as for oral drug therapy (19).

Several substances have been applied for intralesional drug therapy of Peyronie's disease: verapamil, interferon alfa-2a and interferon alfa-2b, collagenase, cortisone, and hyaluronidase [Table 2 modified after (2,3,19)].

Following the demand for a significant effect in prospective, randomized, controlled trials a significant effect could be only revealed for collagenase in cases of mild curvature (26). For **interferon alfa** and **verapamil** a positive effect could only be demonstrated in patients with short-case history in single blinded studies (27–29) while the only double blind approach resulted in insignificant effects of verapamil (30). **Corticosteroids** are a traditional option in intralesional therapy. However, only one randomized, single-blinded, placebo-controlled study on the use of corticosteroid has been published so far, revealing that betamethasone is not effective (31).

Iontophoresis

Iontophoresis is the use of electrokinetic transport of charged molecules for improvement of transdermal drug transport into diseased tissue (32). The combination therapy of verapamil and dexamethasone was significantly effective compared to placebo on reduction of plaque size, curvature, and pain, respectively (33). Furthermore, iontophoresis appears to be a cost-effective method because the patient can perform this therapy by himself at home using a machine on loan from a company and not only as in-office therapy. The drugs applied are commonly available, and they are cheap (19).

Extracorporeal Shock Wave Therapy

Extracorporeal shock wave therapy (ESWT) was on the rise during the last decade. However, its therapeutic mechanism is unclear. An improvement of vascularization with consecutive resorption of calcification has been discussed in this connection. Concerning its pain-relieving effect, a direct disturbance of pain receptors or "hyperstimulation analgesia" could be the mode of action (34). In Peyronie's patients, ESWT seems to reduce packing and clumping of collagen fibers in the plaque (35). The first noncontrolled studies reported enthusiastically on good results (34). However, the studies with exact documentation of the symptoms before and after the intervention could not reveal significant effects on the most important symptoms, penile curvature and plaque size (36–38). The exploratory meta-analysis of the studies published so far in peer-reviewed journals could not demonstrate a significant effect of ESWT on penile curvature or plaque size (34). ESWT seems to have an effect on penile pain during erection and, consecutively, on the improvement of sexual function. Pain seems to resolve faster after ESWT treatment than during the course of the natural history (34): The data of the only single blinded approach confirm this tendency (39). ESWT may be only beneficial to achieve freedom from pain within short time (19,34).

Radiation Therapy

Radiation therapy has been used for the treatment of Peyronie's disease for long time. However, this is not an evidence-based mode of treatment concerning Peyronie's disease (19). No prospective, randomized, placebo-controlled studies have been published. The majority of recently published studies are retrospective analyses often lacking clear parameters how the effect of the therapy was defined and measured (40). So far, radiation therapy cannot be recommended as a standard procedure (19).

Surgical Therapy

Surgery for Peyronie's disease seems to be the ideal mode of treatment to correct penile curvature. For the majority of cases, good results of penile straightening can be achieved by plication procedures or by incision and grafting procedures. However, some aspects have to be considered during the process of decision for the individual therapy (41,42).

The different surgical procedures should be carefully discussed with the patient. The intention of surgery is to straighten the penis for improving the ability to perform sexual intercourse. There is no indication and proven benefit for resection of the plaque in a straight penis.

Progressive stage →	Stable stage →		→Combination with erectile dysfunction
Pain (no calfication)	Curvature <60°	Severe curvature >60°, short penis	Erectile dysfunction (ineffective conservative therapy)
↓	↓	↓	↓
Potassium para-minobenzoate (Potaba®)	Plication (Essed-Schroeder, or Nesbit procedure)	Incision graft	Penile implant with or without graft
Intention: Stop of progression	Intention: penile straightening, simple procedure	Intention: penile straightening, avoid loss of length	Intention: penile straightening ED-therapy

Figure 1 Giessen flow chart of treatment-scheme of Peyronie's disease. *Source:* From Refs. 3 and 47.

Surgery should only be performed in the stable stage of the disease (1,6,7,41,42). That means, Peyronie's disease should have lasted for at least 12 months and the patient does not suffer from pain or progression of symptoms for at least 6 months. If a patient does not fit with these criteria, a progression of symptoms may occur, especially a recurrence of penile curvature rapidly after surgery (7,41). The second important aspect is the degree of penile curvature (41,42). If sexual intercourse is hampered severely, it should be elucidated if this restriction is really related to the penile angulation. The problem could be mainly caused by erectile dysfunction that can be treated by PDE5 inhibitors. If the patient is fully potent and asks for a penile straightening procedure in cases of minor curvature as less than 30°, the indication for surgery should be discussed very carefully (41,42). These curvatures do not really cause a restriction of sexual intercourse. This fact should be well explained to the patient.

TECHNICAL PROCEDURES

The indication for the right surgical technique should be discussed with the patient according to the flow-sheet (Fig. 1). In cases of a curvature less than 60°, a contralateral plication procedure with or without excision of ellipses as described by Nesbit or Essed and Schroeder, respectively, seems to be the ideal approach (43–45). These procedures are surgically easier to perform than other elaborated techniques. After a preferable circumcision the penis is denuded in the sleeve technique for the optimal approach. An artificial erection is performed by the injection of saline solution with high pressure into the corpora cavernosa to visualize the degree of curvature and the localization of the *punctum maximum*. Then, contralaterally to the curvature, plication sutures using an inverting stitch technique are placed (46). In case of the Nesbit procedure, the small ellipsoid pieces of tunica are excised before. Usually these sutures are placed parallel to the urethra in case of upward direction of the curvature. If there is an additional lateral component of the curvature, the sutures have to be placed transversely. The result is proved by another artificial erection. If necessary, additional sutures can be placed to modify the result.

The plication procedure always causes a shortening of the penis due to the technique itself, depending on the degree of curvature that has to be corrected. If curvature is severe (>60°) or if the penis is relatively short, the placation is not the ideal approach (1,3,6,7,42). In these cases, an incision and grafting procedure as inaugurated by T. Lue is recommended (48,49). In these cases the neurovascular bundle has to be dissected completely after degloving the penile shaft. This should be carefully performed to avoid disturbance of penile sensation especially of the glans penis. Then, the plaque is incised once or twice with I- to H-shaped incisions. This leads to penile straightening by relaxation of the dorsal penis. The defects are covered by a graft, i.e., vein, bovine lyophilized pericard, or others (50). Besides the problem of lost sensitivity, erectile function also deteriorates in up to 20% of the patients. Thus, this technique is especially provided for patients with full erectile capacity. Otherwise, there is a high risk of postoperative erectile dysfunction.

If a patient suffers from severe erectile dysfunction preoperatively that does not respond to PDE5 inhibitors, the insertion of a penile implant is the therapy of choice. This can be combined with straightening procedures by penile cracking as recommend by Wilson (51) or with relaxation incisions (52). These incisions do not have to be covered with a graft since fibrosis will develop around the implant by itself, however, graft coverage might help to stabilize the penile implant.

CONCLUSIONS

Therapy of Peyronie's disease depends of the stage of the disorder. It should be conservative in the early, inflammatory stage. However, an ideal mode of conservative treatment is not available. Surgery should only be performed in the stable stage. The choice of the procedure depends on the degree of curvature, penile length, and the occurrence of concomitant erectile dysfunction (3,19,37,42,50). A therapeutical algorithm is provided in Figure 1.

KEY MESSAGES

- Peyronie's disease indicates a prevalence of up to 3.2%. in the male population. After an initial inflammatory phase, the disease enters into a stable phase typified by the cessation of pain and the lack of progression of the penile curvature (Level 1b).
- Medical treatment may be useful in the inflammatory phase of the disease although the use of most drugs is not evidence-based (Level 1a). Potassium para-aminobenzoate may be useful to stop the progression of the disease and ease pain (Level 1b, Grade A).
- Surgical correction of the curvature should only be performed in the stable phase of the disease, since early surgery leads to more complications and recurrences of the disease (Level 2b, Grade B).
- Surgical procedures to correct the penile curvature are well established. Good results are yielded with either plication procedures or incision techniques combined with penile grafting (Level 2a, Grade A).
- Severe ED associated with PD requires penile correction combined with the implantation of penile prosthesis (Grade A).

PENILE CURVATURE

About 0.4% to 0.6% of men suffer from congenital penile curvature. In these cases the penile angulation is usually directed to the ventral side. The reason is a different growth of the corpora cavernosa with a lack of the ventral corporal length. This deficiency of length causes the ventral curvature during erection sometimes accompanied by a lateral or torsion component. Usually young men present during adolescence (53). Besides Peyronie's disease--as a disorder not characteristic for these young patients--a chorda without hypospadia is the only differential diagnosis. Lacking differentiation of the corpus spongiosum, Buck' s fascia, and Colle's fascia with fibrosis in the area of the urethra is the reason for the ventral curvature. The fibrotic material should be excised.

Diagnosis of congenital penile curvature comprises the characteristic history of the congenital disorder, penile palpation and ultrasound, supplemented by three-dimensional self-photography in the Kelâmi-technique (18).

The only therapeutical option is a plication procedure in the Nesbit or Essed-Schroeder technique, achieving a high degree of patient's satisfaction (43–45).

REFERENCES

1. Gholami SS, Gonzalez-Cadavid NF, Lin CS, et al. Peyronie's disease: a review. J Urol 2003; 169:1234–1241.
2. Hauck EW, Heitz M, Schreiter F, et al. Induratio penis plastica. Aktuel Urol 1999; 30:386–404.
3. Hauck EW, Diemer T, Weidner W. Peyronie's disease – Conservative and surgical therapy. Urologe A 2006; 45:243–259.
4. Schwarzer U, Sommer F, Klotz T, et al. The prevalence of Peyronie's disease: results of a large survey. BJU Int 2001; 88:722–730.
5. Gelbard MK, Dorey F, James K. The natural history of Peyronie's disease. J Urol 1990; 144:1376–1379.
6. Lue TF, Gelbard MK, Gueglio G, et al. Peyronie's disease. In: Jardin A, Wagner G, Khoury S, Giuliano F, Padma-Nathan H, Rosen R, eds. Erectile Dysfunction. 1st International Consultation on Erectile Dysfunction. Plymouth: Plymbridge Distributors Ltd, 2000:439–476.
7. Kadioglu A, Akman T, Sanli O, et al. Surgical treatment of Peyronie's disease: a critical analysis. Eur Urol 2006; 50:235–248.
8. Davis CJ Jr. The microscopic pathology of Peyronie's disease. J Urol 1997; 157:282–284.
9. Weidner W, Schroeder-Printzen I, Weiske WH, et al. Sexual dysfunction in Peyronie's disease: an analysis of 222 patients without previous local plaque therapy. J Urol 1997; 157:325–328.
10. Devine CJ Jr, Somers KD, Jordan GH, et al. Proposal: Trauma as the cause of the Peyronie's lesion. J Urol 1997; 157:285–290.
11. Ralph DJ, Mirakian R, Pryor JP, et al. The immunological features of Peyronie's disease. J Urol 1996; 155:159–162.
12. Ralph DJ, Schwartz G, Moore W, et al. The genetic and bacteriological aspects of Peyronie's disease. J Urol 1997; 157:291–294.
13. Hauck EW, Hauptmann A, Weidner W, et al. Prospective analysis of HLA classes I and II antigen frequency in patients with Peyronie's disease. J Urol 2003; 170:1443–1446.

14. Hauck EW, Domann E, Hauptmann A, et al. Prospective analysis of 16S rDNA as a highly sensitive marker for bacterial presence in Peyronie's disease plaques. J Urol 2003; 170:2053–2056.
15. El-Sakka AI, Hassoba HW, Pillarisetty RJ, et al. Peyronie's disease is associated with an increase in transforming growth factor-beta protein expression. J Urol 1997; 158:1391–1394.
16. Hauck EW, Hauptmann A, Schmelz HU, et al. Prospective analysis of single nucleotide polymorphisms of the transforming growth factor β-1 gene in Peyronie's disease. J Urol 2003; 169:369–372.
17. Haag SM, Hauck EW, Szardening-Kirchner C, et al. Alterations in the transforming growth factor (TGF)-β pathway as potential factor in the pathogenesis of Peyronie's disease. Eur Urol 2007; 51:255–261.
18. Kelâmi A. Autophotography in evaluation of functional penile disorders. Urology 1983; 21:628–629.
19. Hauck EW, Diemer T, Schmelz HU, et al. A critical analysis of nonsurgical treatment of Peyronie's disease. Eur Urol 2006; 49:987–997.
20. Hauck EW, Bschleipfer T, Haag SM, et al. Assessment among German urologists of various conservative treatment modalities for Peyronie's disease. Results of a survey. Urologe A 2005; 44:1189–1196.
21. Weidner W, Hauck EW, Schnitker J. Potassium paraaminobenzoate (POTABA™) in the treatment of Peyronie's disease: A prospective, placebo-controlled, randomized study. Eur Urol 2005; 47:530—536.
22. Pryor JP, Farell CR. Controlled clinical trial of vitamin E in Peyronie's disease. Prog Reprod Biol Med 1983; 9: 41–45.
23. Lemourt Oliva M, Rodriguez Barroso A, Puente Guillen M, et al. Propóleo y enfermedad de Peyronie. Arch Esp Urol 2003; 56:805–813.
24. Biagotti G, Cavallini G. Acetyl-L-carnitine vs tamoxifen in the oral therapy of Peyronie's disease: a preliminary report. BJU Int 2001; 88:63–67.
25. Cavallini G, Biagotti G, Koverech A, et al. Oral propionyl-L-carnitine and intraplaque verapamil in the therapy of advanced and resistant Peyronie's disease. BJU Int 2002; 89:895–900.
26. Gelbard MK, James K, Riach P, et al. Collagenase versus placebo in the treatment of Peyronie's disease: a double-blind study. J Urol 1993; 149:56–58.
27. Hellstrom W, Eichelberg C, Pryor JL, et al. A single-blind, multi-center, placebo-controlled study to assess the safety and efficacy of intralesional interferon alpha-2b in the non-surgical treatment of Peyronie's disease [abstract 1065]. J Urol 2003; 169(suppl):274.
28. Rehman J, Benet A, Melman A. Use of intralesional verapamil to dissolve Peyronie's disease plaque: a long-term single-blind study. Urology 1998; 51:620–626.
29. Nicolai M, Cipollone G, Iantorno R, et al. Intralesional verapamil injection versus placebo in Peyronie's disease [abstract 450]. J Urol 1998; 159 (suppl 5):117.
30. Steiger M, Ohlig W, Ludwig G. Verapamil versus Placebo als Injektionstherapie der Induratio penis plastica: Langzeitergebnisse einer Doppel-blind-Studie [abstract V7.6]. Urologe A 1999; 38(suppl 1):S58.
31. Cipollone G, Nicolai M, Mastroprimiano G, et al. Betametasone versus placebo nella malattia di la Peyronie. Arch Ital Urol Androl 1998; 70:165–168.
32. Singh J, Maibach HI. Topical iontophoretic drug delivery in vivo: historical development, devices and future perspectives. Dermatology 1993; 187:235–238.
33. Di Stasi S, Giannantoni A, Stephen RL, et al. A prospective, randomized study using transdermal electromotive administration of verapamil and dexamethasone for Peyronie's disease. J Urol 2004; 171:1605–1608.
34. Hauck EW, Mueller UO, Bschleipfer T, et al. Extracorporeal shock wave therapy for Peyronie's disease: exploratory meta-analysis of clinical trials. J Urol 2004; 171:740–745.
35. Mirone V, Imbimbo C, Palmieri A, et al. A new biopsy technique to investigate Peyronie's disease associated histologic alterations: results with two different forms of therapy. Eur Urol 2002; 42:239–244.
36. Michel MS, Ptaschnyk T, Musial A, et al. Objective and subjective changes in patients with Peyronie's disease after management with shock wave therapy. J Endourol 2003; 17:41–44.
37. Strebel RT, Suter S, Sautter T, et al. Extracorporeal shock wave therapy for Peyronie's disease does not correct penile deformity. Int J Impot Res 2004; 16:448–451.
38. Hauck EW, Hauptmann A, Bschleipfer T, et al. Questionable efficacy of extracorporeal shock wave therapy in Peyronie's disease: results of a prospective approach. J Urol 2004; 171:269–299.
39. Hauck EW, Hatzichristodoulou G, Lahme S. ESWT in peyronie's disease. In: Chaussy C, Haupt G, Jocham D, Köhrmann KU, Wilbert D, eds. Therapeutic Energy Applications in Urology. Stuttgart, New York: Georg Thieme Verlag, 2005:137–143.
40. Paulsen F, Schneiderbauer J, Plasswilm L, et al. Significance of radiotherapy for the treatment of Peyronie's disease. In: Lahme S, ed. Peyronie's disease. Bremen: Uni-Med Verlag AG, 2005:85–93.
41. Hauck EW. Against the motion: surgery is the best choice for Peyronie's disease. Eur Urol 2006; 49:1128–1129.
42. Levine LA, Lenting EL. A surgical algorithm for the treatment of Peyronie's disease. J Urol 1997; 158:2149–2152.
43. Nesbit RM. Congenital curvature of the phallus: report of three cases with description of corrective operation. J Urol 1965; 93:230–232.
44. Nesbit RM. The surgical treatment of congenital chordee without hypospadia. J Urol 1954; 72:1178–1180.
45. Essed E, Schroeder FH. New surgical treatment for Peyronie's disease. Urology 1985; 25:582–587.

46. Knispel HH, Gonnermann D, Huland H. Modified surgical technique to correct congenital and acquired penile curvature. Eur Urol 1991; 20:107–112.
47. Hauck EW, Weidner W. François de la Peyronie and the disease named after him. Lancet 2001; 357:2049–2051.
48. Lue TF, El-Sakka AI. Venous patch graft for Peyronie's disease. Part I: Technique. J Urol 1998; 160:2047–2049.
49. El-Sakka AI, Rashwan HM, Lue TF. Venous patch graft for Peyronie's disease. Part II: Outcome analysis. J Urol 1998; 160:2050–2053.
50. Hellstrom WJG, Reddy S. Application of pericardial graft in the surgical management of Peyronie's disease. J Urol 2000; 163:1445–1447.
51. Wilson SK, Delk JR II. A new treatment for Peyronie's disease: modeling the penis over an inflatable penile prosthesis. J Urol 1994; 152:1121–1123.
52. Montorsi F, Salonia A, Maga T, et al. Reconfiguration of the severely fibrotic penis with a penile implant. J Urol 2001; 166:1782–1786.
53. Ebbehoj J, Metz P. Congenital penile angulation. Br J Urol 1987; 60:264–266.

46A Female-to-male transsexualism

Carlo Bettocchi, Fabrizio Palumbo, and David J. Ralph

INTRODUCTION

Of all gender identity disorders (GID), transsexualism is perhaps the most extreme. It can often involve drastic measures taken by the sufferer, which include procedures such as gender reassignment surgery (GRS) (1). The origin of the term transsexualism first appeared without a difference between transvestitism, effeminate homosexuality, and transsexualism. Beginning only in the forties, the term was used in the modern sense that is to denote individuals who desired to live or actually lived permanently in the social role of the opposite gender and who wanted to undergo sex reassignment (2). Homosexuality is now considered not as an identity or a sexual disorder; it refers to an individual's sexual preference for members of the same sex. Transvestitism represents instead just a preference for cross-dressing but have no desire to change their biological sex. A patient may choose to undergo GRS because of an overriding sense of having been assigned the wrong gender at birth.

In the recent version of the psychiatric classifications systems *DSM-IV* (*Diagnostic and Statistical Manual of Mental Disorders*, Fourth Edition), the term transsexualism was abandoned for the term *gender identity disorders* (GID), which was used for individuals who show a strong and persistent cross-gender identification and a persistent discomfort with their anatomical sex, or a sense of inappropriateness in the gender role of that sex as manifested by a preoccupation with getting rid of one's sex characteristics or the belief of being born in the wrong sex (3). In 1973, Fisk proposed the term *gender dysphoria syndrome* (GDS), and this term is actually used as a synonym for GID (4). In conclusion, a transsexual is a person with the external genitalia and secondary sexual characteristics of one sex but whose personal identification and psychosocial configuration is that of the opposite sex.

From an epidemiological point of view, it would seem to be a ubiquitous condition despite being difficult to quantify. According to the *DSM-IV*, there is an average prevalence of 1 in 100,000 biological women. Data collected in Sweden, England, and Wales show that there are more men than women among sex-change applicants, with an average ratio of 1:3 (women to men). The exception in this trend is represented by Polish prevalence rates: in this case, in fact, there are more women than men among sex change applicants (5). The reported prevalence of transsexualism has been also found to vary all around the world. The percentage in The Netherlands has been reported to be 1:30,400 [female-to-male transsexuals (FTM)] (6) and 1:8300 FTM patients in Singapore (7). However, less evidence is available concerning the number of patients who go on to request surgery. A Swedish study suggested that the number of individuals requesting gender reassignment is 0.17 per 100,000 (8).

DIAGNOSIS AND HORMONAL THERAPY

At present, in many countries, transsexuals are treated according to the Standards of Care of the Harry Benjamin International Gender Dysphoria Association (HBIGDA), which established the criteria for the treatment of transsexuals. These standards are based on the cooperation between psychiatrists, endocrinologists, and surgeons (9).

The process by which a person comes to receive GRS is complex and consists of different stages. The initial diagnosis is based on formal psychiatric (*DSM*) classification criteria. A transsexual is generally seen by a psychologist or psychiatrist who diagnoses GID. In this phase, it's important to make a differential diagnosis because in some patients, the basic problem could be a psychopathological disorder such as schizophrenia, transvestitism, or homosexuality or an anatomical–biological disorder such as intersexuality (where there's not a correspondence between genital organs and karyotype). In a second moment, a medical consultant, subsequently, may go on to prescribe the patient with hormones. In the FTM transsexual patients, the treatment consists of a hormonal therapy based on testosterone for a period of two years before the surgery. The endocrinologist's role will be first to detect unknown intersexual diseases through medical history, clinical examinations, and basal hormonal check-up. When the diagnosis of transsexualism is ascertained, the endocrinologist must control the absence of contraindications and then start the hormonal treatment. The first step in this phase is represented by the suppression of the original sex characteristics, using LHRH super agonists and norethisterone acetate. The second step consists of the induction of the designed sex characteristics, using norethisterone acetate or testosterone undecanoate (transitional phase). These two phases take a time period of two years and after that there is the third phase of the therapy (maintenance phase), which is actuated after the castration for the rest of the life of the patient and is based on the use of norethisterone acetate, testosterone undecanoate, or transdermal androgens. It is really important that the patient knows the possible undesirable side effects of this treatment, both psychological and anatomobiological. In the FTM transsexual patients are possible psychological aggression, abnormal increased libido, or psychosis on the psychological side and diabetes and liver problems on the bioanatomic side.

The "real life" test is crucial in the preoperative stages of GRS. This consists of a given period of time in which the patient lives in the role of their desired gender by dressing accordingly and even going so far as choosing a new name. The importance of this phase is to make sure the patients appear in the form of the desired sex and also because the sex change applicant in that way inform people who live in their social context about the future change of sex and live currently in their new gender role. The real-life test lasts also for 18 months and represent a middle path to evaluate the conviction of the patient and the reactions with difficulties in the social environment and toward hostile situations (10). After successful completion of this stage, the transsexual is examined by a second professional to confirm the diagnosis, and only then can they be assigned for genital surgery.

SURGICAL TREATMENT

The majority of studies produced in the literature report good satisfactory outcomes with few complications for each of the individual procedures. Many of the outcomes for these procedures relate mainly to the aesthetical appearance, the ability to void while standing, and also the capacity to perform penetrative sexual intercourse. Slightly less requested are the possibility to achieve orgasm and the scar condition. The assessment limit is the lack of controlled evidence and the unclear outcome measures.

A review of the following surgical procedures for FTM transsexuals were undertaken: hysterectomy and salpingo-oophorectomy, mastectomy, vaginectomy, metoidoplasty, phalloplasty, urethroplasty, scrotoplasty and placement of testicular prostheses, implant of penile prosthesis.

Hysterectomy and Salpingo-oophorectomy

The first step in the demolition surgery is represented by hysterectomy and consists of the surgical removal of the entire uterus and the cervix. Several studies have been led to find the better technique to use in those kind of patients. Ergenelli et al. (11) reported the use of vaginectomy, laparoscopically assisted vaginal hysterectomy, and bilateral salpingo-oophorectomy in FTM transsexuals. The importance of this technique lies in the preservation of important structure such as inferior epigastric vessels and the rectus abdominis muscle, which will be used in a second moment during the phalloplasty. The only risk is represented by the bladder perforation, which can be repaired immediately without complications. The importance of simultaneus salpingo-oophorectomy is represented by the possibility of ovarian epithelial cancer in those patients who are exposed to high levels of androgens, both endogenous and exogenous. For this reason, Hage et al. (12) also suggest this additional demolition in the treatment.

Mastectomy

Concerning the mastectomy, actually the most-used technique consists of a circumareolar approach for subcutaneus mastectomy. The second step is represented by the nipple implantation on a de-epithelialized dermal pedicle, and finally, numerous fine sutures are used for the closure to limit wrinkling. The result reported by Colic et al. (13) in the 12 patients traited consists of a naturally flat masculine breasts and a sufficient nipple and areolar vascularization. The problems that can occur depend on the size of the breasts and in case of considerable dimension, skin excision is executed, laterally and medially to the nipple–areolar complex, and in some of those circumstances, it is necessary to use a free trasplantation of nipple–areolar complex graft in combination with fusiform skin excision, resulting in a scar passing under the grafted areola.

Vaginectomy

This procedure consists of the removal of all or part of the vagina. The first step consists of a circumferential incision followed by the entering of the vesicovaginal space and the isolation of the bladder pillar. In the second step, the lower portion of the uterosacral ligament is clamped and divided and the same procedure is performed on the opposite side. Then, the bladder pillars are dissected and the mobilized vaginal cuff is extracted together with the parametrium on both sides through the vagina. After this, the posterior vaginal cuff is closed with a running locking suture; the peritoneum from the under surface of the bladder is then sewn to the anterior edge. The last step of the procedure is represented by the closure of the posterior portion of the vagina in a vertical fashion and to allow an easier follow-up cytology (14).

Phalloplasty

There is a general agreement that the ideal technique should be a one-stage procedure, cosmetically acceptable by both patient and partner. It has to permit standing to void through a competent neourethra, penetrative vaginal sexual intercourse, tactile and erogenous sensitivity, and leave minimal scarring in the donor area. There are different techniques to build a neopenis in a FTM transsexual and the most used are the forearm free flap phalloplasty, the metatoidoplasty, and the pedicled pubic phalloplasty. All these different approaches guarantee some kind of advantages or disadvantages, and then, the choice is usually performed on the patient requests, such as a satisfying aesthetic result, the ability to urinate, or a sufficient penetration for sexual function. Usually, in patients who require a certain level of erection, a second kind of surgery is requested in order to implant a penile prosthesis. At last, it will be possible to recreate a glans for an even better aesthetic result.

Metatoidoplasty

Metatoidoplasty uses the clitoris, hypertrophic after the hormonal treatment, to construct a micro phallus. The advantage of this technique, when compared to the others, is that it does not leave any scars outside the genital area; the main disadvantage is that the metatoidoplasty does not allow the creation of a neophallum with a satisfying size (Fig. 1). In a first surgical

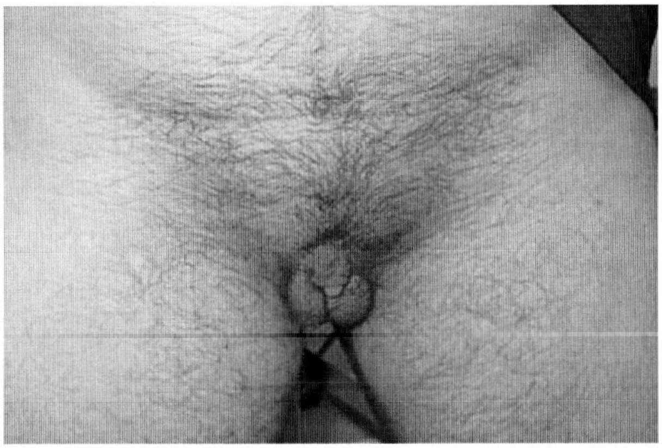

Figure 1 Metatoidoplasty.

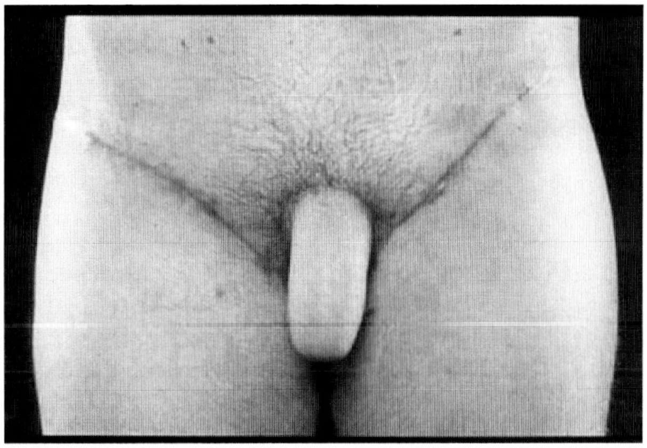

Figure 2 Forearm flap phalloplasty.

step, a caudally based pedicled flap is raised from the anterior vaginal wall and the length of this flap is devised in such a way that the flap will reach beyond the base of the clitoris. Its length varies from 5 to 7.5 cm; its width is 2 to 3 cm. The base of its pedicle envelops the dorsal half of the urethral orifice. The flap contains the muscularis layer of the ventral vaginal wall but no part of the urethral wall or bladder sphincter muscle. This vaginal flap will serve as the lining of the pars fixa of the neourethra. After the flap is raised, the donor area is sutured, thereby narrowing the vagina. In order to release the clitoral shaft by resection of the chordae, the vestibular skin between meatus and glans clitoridis is incised in a W-like fashion. The vestibular skin incisions have to be continuous with the parallel incisions on the anterior aspect of the vaginal wall. One limb of this W is extended toward the future urethral meatus at the tip of the glans clitoridis while the other limb is extended laterally and upward to include the medial surface of the right minor labium. The medial and lateral surfaces of this labium are separated. In this way, a medially pedicled vestibular–labial skin flap is fashioned at least 3 cm wide. To allow the clitoris to be transposed abdominally, the dorsal edge of the left minor labium is released. The midline vestibular skin is undermined toward the glans, hence exposing the chordae, which are resected, baring the ventral aspect of both corpora cavernosa well down in between both crura, but without severing the corpora and their neurovascular supply. Once the phallus is stretched, the vaginal mucosa and vestibular skin flaps may be sutured in a watertight fashion and rolled onto the catheter. Both flaps are anastomosed in a bevelled or even interdigitating fashion to avoid stricture. To cover and strengthen the neourethra thus created, the medial aspect of the left minor labium is de-epithelialized and sutured to cover the pendulous part of the neourethra. In this way, this external labial flap suture line does not overlie the internal urethral suture line. The lateral surface of the right labium is used to cover the perineal, fixed part of the neourethra. Extra attention is given to dorsally suture the labial flap to the inferior margin of vaginal mucosa to prevent secondary fistulas of the otherwise exposed part of the posterior urethral wall. The ventral edge of this labial skin flap is sutured to the dorsal edge of the left labial skin flap covering the pars pendula urethrae (15).

Forearm Flap Phalloplasty

The phallic reconstruction using the forearm flap was introduced since 1984 by Chang and Hwang (16) and still today represent the most common technique used in this kind of surgery (Fig. 2). The forearm flap is a fasciocutaneous flap vascularized by the radial artery and the ulnar artery; the cephalic, basilica, and medial antebrachial veins would drain the flap. Preoperatively, the Allen test is used to screen patients carefully for arterial insufficiency and if there is any doubt about the radial and ulnar arteries integrity, an angiography is performed. Then, the forearm flap is harvested from the nondominant forearm. According to the first described technique, the shaft is covered with the radial aspect of the skin paddle; a second skin island, de-epithelialized on the ulnar aspect of the skin paddle, is tubed to create the urethra. The urethral tube is then rolled within the tube of skin to form a tube-within-tube design. The deep inferior epigastric vessels are the recipient vasculature for flap transfer while the micro neurosurgical anastomosis is realized between the flap cutaneous nerve and the dorsal nerve of clitoris.

There are several modifications of this technique, but they represent just modifications in the design of the skin island and the position of the urethral paddle in relation to the skin that will eventually become shaft coverage; anyway, in all of them there are not differences in the technique of flap elevation. In the "cricket bat" modification proposed by Farrow and Boyd (17), the urethral tube extends distally, closely overlying either the radial or the ulnar artery while proximal to the urethral strip, a portion of the skin paddle provides coverage of the shaft. In a second stage, the urethral portion is tubed and transposed into the centre of the shaft portion of the skin paddle. In the Biemer's (18) modification, the urethral portion of the flap is over the artery as in the previous case and separated by two lateral paddles by a de-epithelialized strip. The lateral paddles are tabularized, and in the centre will lye the tabularised urethral paddle. Santanelli and Scuderi (19) reported the use of the island tensor fasciae latae flap procedure in FTM transsexuals, which appears to provide a safe and sensate flap for phalloplastic procedure and results in a less visible donor scar. They consider microsurgical free tissue transfer the most suitable method of choice for penile reconstruction although it does not always provide all patient goals, such as penile rigidity and donor-site disfigurement. Zielinski (20) reported a one-stage procedure for neophallus construction using a lateral groin flap in 127 FTM transsexuals, with good results in 96 patients (75.6%) and stiffness of the phallus without the use of prostheses in 47 patients. Hage et al. (21) reported on 28 patients, who underwent phalloplasties, a comparison of rectus abdominis myocutaneous pedicled flap and radial forearm free flap: they found that, in terms of functional and cosmetic outcomes, the microsurgical free flap phalloplasty techniques lead to the best results, with also regain of tactile sensitivity in the neophallus. Same study was performed by Santi et al. (22) who described a method for constructing a neopenis using the transposition of a rectus abdominis island muscle flap with resurfacing, using a radial forearm free flap. The authors, however, reported this method to be more effective than the free flap one.

All these techniques have as disadvantage the scar and the deformity of the donor site and the possibility of the development of cold intolerance in the hand of the donor side (Fig. 3). A possible solution to solve the former problem is the use of a skin-free flap harvested from other sites, such as the gluteus, to cover the forearm donor-site defect.

Pedicled Pubic Flap Phalloplasty

The phallus in this technique is fashioned from a flap of anterior abdominal wall skin, 11 cm wide and 12 cm long, measured from the base of the clitoris, incorporating the superficial external pudendal vessels (Fig. 4). After mobilizing the flap, any excess of subcutaneous tissue is excised to give a better cosmetic appearance and to facilitate the phallus tabularization. The anterior abdominal wall skin is completely mobilized up to the costal margins to enable primary closure of the abdominal wall skin. A second step is the construction of the neourethra inside the phallus by tubing a 3-cm wide strip of skin from the clitoris and labia major. During this phase, the clitoris is incorporated into the neourethra to maintain erogenous sensation. The flap that has been tubed over an 18 F silicone catheter is laid, using absorbable sutures, into the suprapubic skin flap, which is tubed to form the phallus. The perineal neourethra is built similarly from the skin of the opposite labia and toward the end of the series, the suture line is covered with a Martius fat pad in an attempt to lessen the risk of fistula formation. At the end, a suprapubic catheter is inserted to drain the bladder: this also allowed a urethrogram to be taken three weeks after surgery to exclude the presence of a urethral urinary leak. The fistula formation is eventually secondary to a stenosis in the anastomotic sites: neobulbar-native urethra or penile-neobulbar urethra. Voiding complications are the most frequently reported causes of surgical complications. For this reason, several surgeons tend to discourage their patients to request the penile urethra creation (23).

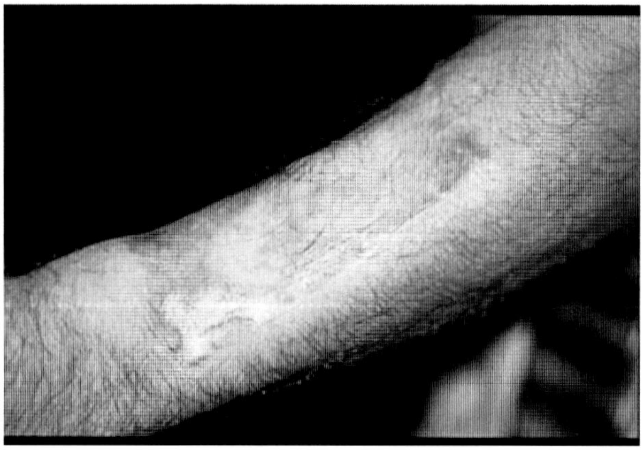

Figure 3 Arm donor site scar.

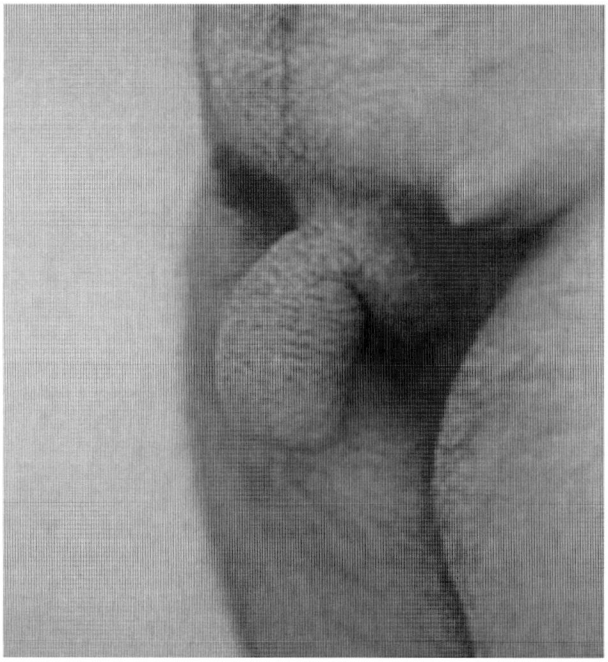

Figure 4 Pedicled pubic flap phalloplasty.

Akoz and Kargi (24) reported a single case of phalloplasty in a 21-year-old FTM transsexual using a double-pedicle composite groin flap technique. The procedure used both deep and superficial circumflex iliac vessels in the pedicle to provide greater-vascularized extended skin and bone in the flap. Two stages were used to prefabricate a neourethra before transfer of the flap. The reconstruction of the penis in an appropriate size and stiffness

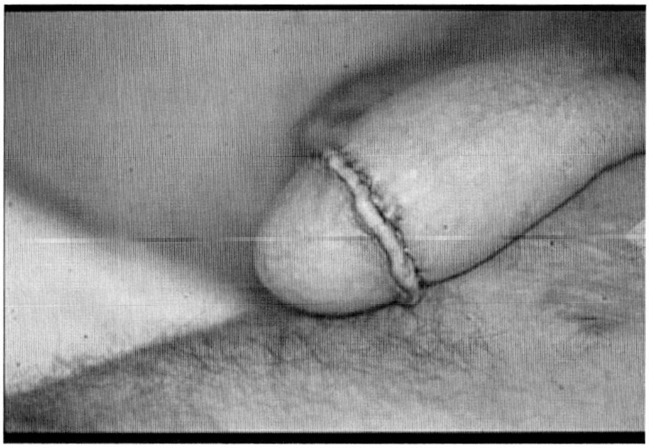

Figure 5 Glanduloplasty.

without vascular compromise was successfully obtained. Overall, it was concluded that good operative results were produced.

Glanduloplasty

The possible final step in the costruction of the penis is represented by the creation of the glans. The glansplasty is a surgical procedure that allows a neophallus to have a glans-like tip after total phalloplasty (Fig. 5). Several techniques were described but with controversial results in terms of cosmetical outcome and complications. At the moment, the most commonly used procedure is the Norfolk modification of the Munawar technique: after circumcising the tip of the neophallus, a skin flap is created and modeled to create a coronal ring, more distinct at the dorsal aspect. The donor area is than covered by a split-thickness skin graft obtained by the genito–perineal area to prevent traction on the coronal skin and to gain extra constriction by the shrinkage of the skin graft. The glansplasty can be performed simultaneously to the different phalloplasty techniques or as a separate procedure. Glansplasty has revealed to be an easy and quick to perform procedure with acceptable results and no complications.

Scrotoplasty

This technique consists of the creation of a scotal sac fashioned using the labia majora. Actually, it is accomplished by hollowing out the labia majora and attaching them to recreate a scotum-like appearance by inserting silicon implants (25). Generally, this procedure is actuated consensually with lengthening of the pars fixa of the urethra. A bifid scrotum can be constructed using a V–Y advancement of the labial skin. The advantages of this technique are represented by the small scar, which is located in the inner part of the scrotum and is covered by hairs, while the complications consist of the possibility, even if unusual, of infection, dislocation, or expulsion of the prosthesis. The rupture of the envelope of silicone gel–filled testicular prostheses is believed to be rare and possibly caused by acute or chronic pressure (26).

Penile and Testicular Prosthesis Implantation

In FTM transsexuals, another surgical challenge is represented by the request to create a certain level of rigidity in the neo phallum to allow a penetrative sexual intercourse. For decades, rib cartilage and bone transplants were the most popular entities. These techniques have been reported with high rates of failure. Rib cartilage has variable rigidity and there are no reports of patient satisfaction. Bone with periosteum tends to reabsorb with time. Implantation of a penile prosthesis instead can provide to the rigidity of the neophallus and guarantee satisfying sexual intercourse. At the moment, the prosthesis usually implanted is the hydraulic three-component type, composed of two cylinders, a scrotal pump, and a paravescical reservoir. Sometime is aesthetically preferable to implant a single cylinder because the positioning of both cylinders can sometimes distort the phallic appearance (27). The reservoir contains saline solution that is drift into the cylinders located inside the phallum, using the pomp positioned into the neoscrotum. For this kind of implant, the main problem is the absence of corpora cavernosa, which normally contains the prosthesis and avoid the erosion of tissues by the cylinders that constitute the prosthesis. In order to overcome this hurdle, in the modern technique are used vascular prosthesis of Dacron to cover the cylinder, ensure optimal encapsulation, provide collagen growth, and then remedy the erosion. This kind of Dacron socks, containing the cylinders are then anchorated to the pubes'periosteum to produce a sufficient adhesion to the inner structure and avoid prosthesis component dislocation. There is still a considerable number of prostheses removed due to infection and tissue necrosis, although the presence of external antibiotic biofilm on the prosthesis surface and also antibiotical prophylaxis are commonly used.

Once the prosthesis is implanted, the pump can simulate the presence of one testicle inside the scrotum. A second testicular prosthesis can be positioned in the controlateral emiscrotum to complete the aestethic result.

CONCLUSIONS

Majority of studies reviewed a large number of transsexual people experiencing a successful outcome in terms of subjective well-being, cosmesis, and sexual function. But the magnitude of benefit and harm cannot be reliably estimated accurately using the current available evidence. It has been recognised in other previous reviews of GRS that many studies do not use or report the rigorous treatment pathway, which a patient would have to go through in the United Kingdom. It is important to consider that these patients request a new different phenotypic appearance from both endocrinologists and surgeons and a great psychological stability from psychologists/psychiatrics. To do so, it is fundamental for a team-working group of specialists to achieve the ambitious target of a newborn person.

ACKNOWLEDGMENT

The authors give special thanks to Mr. D.J. Ralph and the UCLH Andrology Unit for kindly giving some of the figures.

REFERENCES

1. Cohen-Kettenis PT, Gooren LJG. Transsexualism: A review of etiology, diagnosis and treatment. J Psychosom Res 1999; 46:315–333.
2. Cauldwell DC. Psychopathia transexualis. Sexology 1949; 16:274–280.
3. Fauman MA. Diagnostic and Statistical Manual of Mental Disorders, 4th ed. Washington, DC: American Psychiatric Association, 1995.
4. Fisk NM. Gender dysphoria syndrome (the how, what and why of a disease). In: Laub DR. Gandy P, eds. Proceedings of the Second Interdisciplinary Symposium on Gender Dysphoria syndrome. Stanford, CA: Division of Reconstructive and Rehabilitation Surgery, Stanford University Medical Center, 1973.
5. Godlewski J. Transsexualism and anatomic sex ratio reversal in Poland. Arch Sex Behav 1988; 17:547–548.
6. Van Kesteren PJ, Gooren LJ, Megans JA. An epidemiological and demographic study of transsexuals in the Netherlands. Arch Sex Behav 1996; 25:589–600.
7. Tsoi WF. The prevalence of transsexualism in Singapore. Acta Psychiatr Scand 1988; 78:501–504.
8. Landen M, Walinder J, Lundstrom B. Incidence and sex ratio of transsexualism in Sweden. Acta Psychiatr Scand 1996; 93:261–263.
9. Walker PA, Berger JC, Green R, et al. Standards of care: The hormonal and surgical sex reassignment of gender dysphoric persons. Arch Sex Behav 1985; 14:79–90.
10. Michel A, Mormontl C, Legros JJ. A psycho-endocrinological overview of transsexualism. Eur J Endocrinol 2001; 145:365–376.
11. Ergeneli HM, Duran EH, Ozcan G, et al. Vaginectomy and laparoscopically assisted vaginal hysterectomy as adjunctive surgery in female to male transsexual reassignment: Preliminary report. Eur J Obstet Gynecol Reprod Biol 1999; 87:35–37.
12. Hage JJ, Dekker JJ, Karim RB, et al. Ovarian cancer in female to male transsexuals: Report of two cases. Gynecol Oncol 2000; 76:413–415.
13. Colic MM, Colic MM. Circumareolar mastectomy in female to male transsexuals and large gynecomastias: A personal approach. Aesthetic Plast Surg 2000; 24:450–454.
14. Markus CF, Hatch KD. Laparoscopic assisted parametrectomy/upper vaginectomy (LPUV)—Technique, applications and results. Gynecol Oncol 2005; 98:420–426.
15. Hage JJ. Metaidoioplasty: An alternative phalloplasty technique in transsexuals. Plast Reconstr Surg 1996; 97(1):161–167.
16. Chang TS, Hwang WY. Forearm flap in one-stage reconstruction of the penis. Plast Reconstr Surg 1984; 74:251–258.
17. Farrow GA, Boyd JB, Semple JL. Total reconstruction of the penis employing the "cricket bat flap" single stage forearm free graft. AUA Today 1990; 3:7.
18. Biemer E. Penile construction by the radial arm flap. Clin Plast Surg 1988; 15:425–430.
19. Santanelli F, Scuderi N. Neophalloplasty in female-to-male transsexuals with the island tensor fasciae latae flap. Plast Reconstr Surg 2000; 105:1990–1996.
20. Zielinski T. Phalloplasty using a lateral groin flap in female-to-male transsexuals. Acta Chir Plast 1999; 41:15–19.
21. Hage JJ, Bouman FG, de Graaf FH, et al. Construction of the neophallus in female-to-male transsexuals: The Amsterdam experience. J Urol 1993; 149(6):463–468.
22. Santi P, Adami M, Berrino P, et al. Neophalloplasty using a rectus abdominis muscle flap and a radial forearm free flap. Eur J Plast Surg 1992; 15:94–97.
23. Bettocchi C, Ralph DJ, Pryor JP. Pedicled pubic phalloplasty in females with gender dysphoria. BJU Int 2005; 95 (1):120–124.
24. Akoz T, Kargi E. Phalloplasty in a female-to-male transsexual using a double-pedicle composite groin flap. Ann Plast Surg 2002; 48:423–427.
25. Hage JJ, Bouman FG, Bloem JJ. Constructing a scrotum in female-to-male transsexuals. Plast Reconstr Surg 1993; 91:914-921.
26. Hage JJ, Taets van Amerongen AH, van Diest PJ. Rupture of silicone gel filled testicular prosthesis: Causes, diagnostic modalities and treatment of a rare event. J Urol 1999; 161:467–471.
27. Hoebeke P, de Cuypere G, Ceuleman S, et al. Obtaining rigidity in total phalloplasty: Experience with 35 patients. J Urol 2003; 169(1):221–223.

46B Male-to-female transsexualism

Vincenzo G. Mirone, Ciro Imbimbo, Paolo Verze, and Davide Arcaniolo

INTRODUCTION

The term "transsexual" appeared initially in the 1950s and identified an individual who aspired to or actually lived in the gender role opposite to their birth sex, whether or not hormones had been administered or surgery had been performed. Later, in the 1960s and 1970s, a variety of clinicians used the term "true transsexual." The *Diagnostic and Statistical Manual* (*DSM-III*) in 1980 recommended the term "transsexualism" as a diagnosis for anyone who expressed at least two years of continuous interest in a physiological and social gender transformation. Others with gender dysphoria could receive the diagnosis: gender identity disorder (GID) of adolescence or adulthood, nontranssexual type, or gender identity disorder not otherwise specified (GID-NOS). The *DSM-IV*, introduced in 1994, replaced the term "transsexualism" with "gender identity disorder." Individuals with a strong and persistent cross-gender identification and a persistent discomfort with their sex or a sense of inappropriateness in the gender role of that sex would be considered to have a GID of childhood, adolescence, or adulthood. For people who did not meet the specific criteria, "gender identity disorder not otherwise specified" was to be used. The latter category included a broad range of individuals, including those who wished various levels of social and physiological gender transition but did not want genital surgery. The current edition of the *Diagnostic and Statistical Manual of Mental Disorders* has five criteria that must be met before a diagnosis of GID can be given (1):

1. There must be evidence of a strong and persistent cross-gender identification.
2. This cross-gender identification must not merely be a desire for any perceived cultural advantages of being the other sex.
3. There must also be evidence of persistent discomfort about one's assigned sex or a sense of inappropriateness in the gender role of that sex.
4. The individual must not have a concurrent physical intersex condition (e.g., androgen insensitivity syndrome or congenital adrenal hyperplasia).
5. There must be evidence of clinically significant distress or impairment in social, occupational, or other important areas of functioning.

EPIDEMIOLOGY

The prevalence of transsexualism is particularly difficult to evaluate. Most centres involved in treating GIDs estimate that they treat the majority of the transsexuals of their country and therefore, only refer to data based on their clinical practice to determine transsexual prevalence rates. However, not all transsexuals contact specialised services. Some are treated by their psychiatrists and independent surgeons and others through illegal channels. Prevalence rates vary depending on the country and the era. A recent large epidemiological study conducted at major plastic surgery and gender team centers in Belgium proved an overall prevalence of 1:12,900 for male-to-female gender transpositions and 1:33,800 for female-to-male transpositions, with a male/female sex ratio of 2.43. This data is comparable to that of other Western European countries.

DIAGNOSIS

Transsexualism is not a homogeneous phenomenon. Diagnosing transsexualism is quite difficult because the results of psychological testing are not conclusive. Standards of care of the Harry Benjamin International Gender Dysphoria Association have established a diagnostic process divided into two phases for patients seeking sex-reassignment surgery (SRS) treatment (2). In the first phase, a formal diagnosis is made using DSM or International Classification of Diseases (ICD) criteria. Risk factors are estimated to ensure that the individual can tolerate the life changes that SRS will bring. In the second diagnostic phase, the patient has to live permanently in the role of the desired sex. The clinicians have to inform the family members and the patient must choose a new first name. In this phase, the patient can start hormonal therapy with different times and modalities depending upon the treatment center. A certain number of psychotherapy sessions are also required by some clinicians; however, psychotherapy is not mandatory (3).

The differential diagnosis should include nonconformity to stereotypical sex role behavior, transvestic fetishism, GID not otherwise specified (with a concurrent congenital intersex condition), and schizophrenia.

TREATMENT

Once the diagnosis of GID has been made, the therapeutic approach usually includes three stages known as triadic therapy: a real life experience in the desired gender role, hormone therapy that will induce the characteristics of the desired gender, and finally, surgery to convert the genitalia and other sex characteristics (SRS). While the patient is undergoing this triadic therapy, clinicians who are following the three therapeutic stages must take into consideration the possibility that some carefully diagnosed patients can suddenly change their minds

Table 1 Absolute and Relative Contraindications for Hormone Therapy in M-to-F Transsexuals

Absolute Contraindications	Severe diastolic hypertension Thrombophlebitis or thromboembolic disease Severe hepatic dysfunction Cerebrovascular disease
Relative Contraindications	Heavy cigarette consumption Family history of breast cancer Hyperprolactinemia Marked obesity (WHR.0.95)

Abbreviations: M-T-F, male-to-female; WHR, waist-hip ratio.

and others might choose to make only partial changes to their gender identities and forego the surgical route while still others may give up their desire to complete the triadic sequence in its entirety. Clinicians are increasingly becoming aware that not all people diagnosed with GID necessarily need or want all three elements of triadic therapy (4).

Psychotherapy

Psychotherapy is a series of highly refined interactive communications between a professional who is knowledgeable about how people suffer emotionally and how the suffering may be alleviated and one who is experiencing gender distress. The psychotherapeutic sessions initiate a developmental process by enabling a person's history to be appreciated, current dilemmas understood, and unrealistic expectations and self-destructive behavior identified. The usual objectives of psychotherapy is the enabling of a long-term, stable lifestyle with realistic chances for success in relationships, education, work, and healthy gender and role identification. Benefits from psychotherapy may be attained at every stage of gender evolution. This includes the post–surgical period when the anatomic obstacles to gender comfort have been removed and the transsexual continues to feel a lack of genuine comfort and skill in living in the new gender role (5).

Hormonal Therapy

Before administering hormonal therapy, the endocrinologist should perform a careful anamnesis, a complete clinical examination, and a basal hormonal check-up to detect possible contraindications. Relative and absolute contraindications for hormone therapy are summarized in Table 1. The desired effects of hormonal treatment are decrease in blood testosterone, increase in blood oestradiol, mammary gland hyperplasia, a decrease in erections, reduction of facial hair, modification of speech, and gynoid fat deposit. Patients must be carefully advised about possible undesirable side effects of hormonal treatment such as thrombo-embolic disorders, depression, decreased libido, hyperprolactinemia, and an increase in the bilirubin blood levels, which are most prevalent. Guidelines on hormonal treatment are summarized in Table 2 (5).

Table 2 Guidelines on Hormone Therapy

Phase	
Presurgical A.1.: suppression of the original sex characteristics (optional)	LHRH superagonists (IM monthly?) and/or spironolactone (100 ± 200 mg/day) or cyproterone acetate (50 ± 100 mg/day)
Presurgical A.2.: induction of designated sex characteristics	Ethinylestradiol (50 ± 100 mg/day) or conjugated oestrogen (1.25 ± 2.50 mg/day) or estradiol benzoate, oestradiol phenylpropionate (25 mg/2 wk) *Optional* Spironolactone (100 ± 200 mg/day) or cyproterone acetate (50 ± 100 mg/day)
Postsurgical B.: postcastration	Oestrogens (see A.2.) or transdermal form (50 ± 100 mg/day) *Optional* Progesterone (100 mg/day for 2 wk/mo) or classic post menopausal hormone therapy

Abbreviations: LHRH, luteinizing hormone–releasing hormone; IM, intramuscular.

Real-Life Experience

The objective of the real-life test is to make sure that the patient takes on the appearance of the desired sex in everyday activities, both social and professional. Also, sex change applicants must choose a new first name, dress in accordance with their new gender, inform their different social partners of his future sexual reassignment, and live correctly in their new gender role. During this period, the sex change candidates must supply proof of their social life and integration. This allows an evaluation of the degree of conviction. Indeed, everyday confrontation with reactions from the social milieu represents one of the major difficulties in sexual conversion. When clinicians assess the quality of a person's real-life experience in the new gender role, the following abilities are estimated:

1. the ability to maintain full or part-time employment;
2. the ability to thrive as a student;
3. the ability to function in community-based volunteer activities;
4. the ability to undertake any combination of items 1–3;
5. the ability to acquire a new (legal) first or last name;
6. the ability to provide documentation that people other than the therapist can predict that the patient will function in the new gender role.

Surgery

Surgical treatment for a person with a GID is not merely another elective procedure. Typical elective procedures traditionally involve only a private mutually consenting contract between a suffering person and a technically competent surgeon. Surgeries for GID can be undertaken only after a comprehensive evaluation by a qualified mental health professional has been conducted. Surgery may then be performed once written documentation testifies that a comprehensive evaluation has been made and that the person has met the eligibility and readiness criteria. Surgical procedures may include orchiectomy, penectomy, vaginoplasty, and augmenting mammaplasty. Vaginoplasty requires both skilled surgical procedure and competent postoperative treatment. Additive mastoplasty may be performed prior to vaginoplasty if the physician prescribing hormones and the surgeon have both attested that breast enlargement after undergoing hormonal treatment for two years is not sufficient for comfort in the social gender role. Other surgeries that may be performed to assist in feminization include reduction thyroid chondroplasty, suction-assisted lipoplasty of the waist, rhinoplasty, facial bone reduction, facelift, and blepharoplasty.

VAGINOPLASTY

A male-to-female gender surgical reconversion can be performed using several different techniques; however, all of them share a few basic common surgical steps:

1. Bilateral orchidectomy
2. Penile disassembling, leading to separation of urethral corpus spongiosum, corpora cavernosa, glands, and dorsal neurovascular bundle
3. Excision of corpora cavernosa and distal urethra
4. Preparation of a urethral stump and urethrocutaneous anastomosis
5. Creation of a prostatorectal space, which allows to allocate the neovagina
6. Vulvoplasty

At present, the most widely used surgical techniques are:

1. Simple penile skin inversion
2. Peno-scrotal flap
3. Onlay urethral flap (Perovic's technique)
4. Enterovaginoplasty

SIMPLE PENILE SKIN INVERSION

After anesthesia is induced, the patient is placed in the lithotomy position. A vertical perineal incision is made from the base of the penis to the midline of the scrotum to a point situated 1 cm above the anal verge. The incision is extended through the subcutaneous tissue to expose the urethral corpus spongiosus and corpora cavernosa bilaterally. A bilateral orchidectomy is performed by dissecting and suturing both spermatic cords at the level of external inguinal rings. Once this is done, the proximal ends of these structures will then retract into the inguinal canal. Then the external inguinal ring is closed bilaterally so as to avoid future weakness that can lead to inguinal hernia. The next step is the penile degloving where the penis is stretched and two circumferential incisions through the penile skin are made; one at the base of the penis and the other distally immediately under the glans. The penile skin with the glans penis is severed from the corpus spongiosum and the corpora cavernosa. The glans remains with the penile skin tube. Through sharp dissection, the penile skin is then isolated from the shaft and then reverted and placed around a silicone vaginal mold. At the tip of the mold, the penile skin is closed with a running absorbable suture. This sutured end will become the apex of neovagina. Following this step the corpus spongiosum is separated from the corpora cavernosa. The corpora cavernosa are cut in the midline and hemostatic sutures are placed through the proximal base under the pubic ramus. Section of each corpus cavernosum should be made as proximal as possible and a limited amount of tissue should remain. A running absorbable suture is routinely performed on the residual erectile tissue in order to avoid painful erection during sexual arousal. The bulbospongiosum muscle is then severed and the corpus spongiosum is mobilized. The central tendon of the perineum is incised and a careful, blunt dissection is performed to create a wide space between the rectum and prostate, where the neovagina will be placed. The Denonvilliers' fascia is then identified and the blunt dissection continues through this avascular plane, transecting the medial fibers of the levator ani muscles to obtain an optimal depth. The inverted penile skin tube distended with the vaginal mold is placed in the perineal neocavity. When the patient wishes to have external sensitivity with the creation of a neoclitoris, only a quarter of the glans is left uncovered to form the clitoris while three-quarters are de-epithelialized and placed subcutaneously to ensure a deep internal sensitivity. The base of the penile cylinder is fixed to the periosteum of the pubis by heavy nonabsorbable traction sutures. An elliptical 1.5-cm incision is then performed on the anterior wall of the neovagina by passing the adequately shortened urethra through this incision and suturing it with 4–0 absorbable sutures to the skin. The most posterior aspects of the skin tube is sutured to the posterior aspect of the initial incision. The sutures are continued laterally and frontally to form the labia majora. Finally, if necessary, cosmetic refinements can be made such as the reduction of excessive skin of the labia majora and the creation of a labia minora. At the conclusion of the procedure, a Foley catheter is inserted and a compressive dressing applied. The Foley catheter is removed after five to seven days (6).

PENO-SCROTAL FLAP

The penoscrotal flap is the most widely used vaginoplasty technique in male-to-female transsexualism. This technique is particularly advisable when a penis of a small dimension does not permit the penile skin inversion technique. With the patient under general anesthesia placed in a lithotomic position, an inverted U-shaped incision on the posterior aspect of the scrotum is performed. A pedicle scrotal flap is then created taking care to carefully preserve the subcutaneous vascularization. An ensuing penile degloving is conducted by both distal and proximal dissection. The penile and scrotal flap will constitute the anterior and posterior wall of the neovagina, respectively. The corpus spongiosum is then isolated starting from the crura up to the penile glans. Through a bilateral incision of the Buck's fascia, a plane is created between the tunica albuginea and the dorsal neurovascular bundle whose connection to the glans is carefully preserved. The plane is initially developed at the level of the distal part of the penis. The glans can now be safely detached from the corpora cavernosa, and neurovascular bundle isolation can be carried out in a retrograde fashion. At this point, all the anatomical components involved are now disassembled. A double hemostatic stitch is passed through the crura of each corpus cavernosum. The corpora are then excised as proximally as possible, erectile tissue is cauterised, and residual bleeding controlled with a running suture. Before proceeding with the steps that follow, a bilateral orchidectomy is performed. A V-shaped incision is performed on the glans and a cuneus of glandular tissue is used for neoclitoris reconstruction. In order to prevent inhestetism and uncomfortable bulging in the anterior vaginal wall, a reduction of the urethral bulb is performed with a nonabsorbable suture, taking care not to cause bladder outlet obstruction. After incision of the central tendon of the perineum, a plane is developed between the prostate and the rectum to expose the Denonvillier's fascia. The penile skin is then detubularized to obtain a pedicle flap, taking care to preserve vascularization. The penile and scrotal flaps are assembled together through an interrupted absorbable suture to constitute the neovagina. The fixation of the cul-de-sac in the retroprostatic space is crucial to prevent the neovagina from prolapsing. A prolene stitch is passed through the Denonvillier's fascia, and both the ends of the suture are passed through the penoscrotal flap at the level of the cul-de-sac. The suture is then tied while a vaginal valve keeps the neovagina in position, obtaining optimal fixation. A small incision on the anterior vaginal wall is performed to allocate the neoclitoris. The urethra is conveniently reduced and then is passed through a second incision, which is performed more ventrally. The urethra is then spatulated. Possible bleedings can be controlled with a Liga-Sure device. The urethrocutaneous anastomosis is then carried out with interrupted absorbable sutures. A hemostatic sponge is wrapped around the neomeatus to control residual bleeding. After reconstruction of the labia from the scrotal skin, a vaginal tutor is left in position. The catheter is removed five days after surgery, and the patient is discharged after seven days (7).

PEDICLED PENILE SKIN WITH A COMPOSITE URETHRAL FLAP VAGINOPLASTY--PEROVIC'S TECHNIQUE

In the Perovic's vaginoplasty technique, the neovagina is created from an inverted pedicled island penile skin flap and a vascularized urethral flap (8). After a bilateral orchidectomy, as has been described for other techniques, the penis is disassembled into its anatomical components (corpora cavernosa, the glans cap with the urethra and its neurovascular bundle, and the vascularized penile skin). The corpora cavernosa are excised as proximally as possible, the erectile tissue is destroyed, and the tunica albuginea is sutured with 2/0 absorbable sutures. The glans is divided into two parts, ventral and dorsal, as the dorsal part of the glans will form the neoclitoris. To achieve this, the glans is reduced by severing the central ventral tissue and leaving the sides of the glans intact to avoid possible injuries to the neurovascular bundle. The sides of the dorsal half of the gland are then de-epithelialized and sutured to obtain a conical shape, which is necessary for the construction of the neoclitoris. The ventral part of the glans, which is still connected to the urethra, will become the neocervix at the base of the neovagina. The bulbospongiosus muscle must be carefully separated from the bulbar urethra to preserve the fascial sheath. The urethra is then spatulated and used to create the mucosal part of the neovagina. Any bleeding in the bulbar urethra during this phase can be controlled with hemostatic sutures without using electrocautery so as to preserve the vascularization of the urethral flap. The urethra is then shortened and the neoclitoris is placed above the new urethral meatus. When reconstructing the neovagina, a vascularized island tube flap is molded from the skin of the penile body and prepuce. The incision is performed circa 2 cm above the base of the mobilized penile skin to obtain an extended vascularized pedicle for the tube. A hole is then made at the base of the pedicle to transpose the urethral flap. On the dorsal side of the skin tube flap, only the skin is incised, whereas the vascularized subcutaneous tissue remains intact. The urethral flap, which is transposed through the pedicle hole, is embedded into the skin tube and sutured. The bottom of the tube is closed with the distal part of the urethra and/or the remaining ventral half of the glans cap after the de-epithelialization of its inner side, as previously described. The tube, consisting of skin and urethral flap, is then inverted thereby forming the neovagina. If there is insufficient penile skin, the short skin tube and long urethral flap will not be in proportion. The vagina can then be formed in two ways. The proximal part at the base of the vagina is formed only by the urethral flap, which initiates secondary epithelialization. If the tube pedicle is too short to place the tube into the perineal cavity, the neovagina is created using the vascularized urethral flap and free penile skin grafts. In this case, the vascularized urethral flap plays a key role in creating the new vagina. The space for the allocation of the neovagina is created in the perineum as has been described for the other techniques. The modified Stamey procedure is used to fix the neovagina within the perineal cavity. Two 15-degree angled Stamey needles penetrate through the rectus to the left and right of the midline at the upper border of the pubic symphysis. The needles then enter laterally into the neocavity from the bladder neck. In the empty bladder, the Foley catheter balloon, which is easily palpable, enables the determination of the exact location of the bladder neck. A polypropylene U suture (0–0) in the middle lateral part of the neovagina is threaded through the eye of the needle and the needle is withdrawn suprapubically.

Table 3 Complications of Vaginoplasty

Intraoperative complications	Rectal injuries Neurovascular bundle injuries
Short term postoperative complications	Urethral perimeatal bleeding
	Neovagina-rectal fistula
	Penile or scrotal cutaneous cylinder necrosis
	Neoclitoris necrosis
	Vaginal abscess
	Wound infection
Long term postoperative complications	Neovaginal stenosis
	Adhitus
	Deep
	Neovaginal prolapse
	Urethral meatus stenosis
	Type 3 stress incontinence
Inhestetisms	Scrotaliform aspect of main labia
	Neoclitoris hypertrophy
	Persistence of an exuberant fragment of corpus cavernosum
	Maintenance of bulbar urethra
	Superior or posterior neolabial commissural inhestetisms

Both ends of the suture are pulled out of the skin of the prepubic area and knotted over bolsters under mild tension, so as to avoid necrosis of the penile flap where the sutures penetrate its wall. At this point, the neovagina is placed deep in the perineal cavity. The next step consists of a vulvoplasty. The labia minora are formed by the remaining parts of the base of the penile skin that are sutured to the de-epithelialized area of the neoclitoris. The labia majora are created by the refinement of the original scrotal skin. A peri-vaginal Jackson–Pratt drain is left for three days. The urethral catheter and vaginal packing (a condom filled with soft material) are removed seven days after surgery.

ENTEROVAGINOPLASTY

Enterovaginoplasty is a widely used technique in patients affected with vaginal aplasia caused by Mayer–Rokitansky–Kuster–Hauser syndrome but which can also be used in transsexual patients. The advantages of using this technique is the possibility of creating a neovagina of sufficient length and appearance that is similar to a natural vagina. Additionally, it is the only method that provides a vaginal lining with natural lubrication. This technique is the best choice for transsexual patients who had previously undergone a penectomy and orchidectomy as well as for patients with dissatisfactory vaginoplasty results (9).

NEOVAGINAL EXPANDING DEVICES

The neocavity, which is created in the perineal space among the rectum, the membranous urethra, and the anterior section of the prostate, should be dilated and sustained by the introduction of an expanding device that often remains in place for many months after the operation. Usually these devices are constituted of a polyurethane foam body wrapped with an expanding silicone cylinder that may expand under atmospheric pressure. A cylindrical shape with round edges is needed to avoid excessive compression in specific points and to ensure an uniform distribution of the forces. The volume of the device is regulated by an opening valve that ensures enough constant pressure to avoid contractions or stenosis. It is possible to drain eventual secretions and conduct washings through the central tube with sterile solutions in the postoperative care. The size of the device can vary from 3 to 5 cm in diameter and from 9.5 to 16 cm in length. The choice of a suitable size of the expanding device is crucial in allowing easy insertion and avoiding difficult removal (10).

COMPLICATIONS

Vaginosplasty surgical complications are common in all the techniques described earlier. All potential complications can be divided into intraoperative complications, short-term postoperative complications, long-term postoperative complications, and inesthetism (Table 3) (10).

REFERENCES

1. Diagnostic and Statistical Manual of Mental Disorders, 4th ed. American Psychiatric Association, 2000. Retrieved on September 16, 2008.
2. Meyer WIII, Bockting W, Cohen-Kettenis PT, et al. The standards of care for gender identity disorders—Sixth version, 2001. http://www.symposion.com/ijt/soc_2001/index.htm.
3. Ravenna, Anna R. Gender Identity Disorder (DSM IV 302.85) Ratified by the "Osservatorio Nazionale sull'Identità di Genere—ONIG" in June 1998. IJT 2,4. http://www.symposion.com/ijt/ijtc0602.htm.
4. Cohen-Kettenis PT, Gooren LJG. Transsexualism: A review of etiology, diagnosis and treatment. J Psychosom Res 1999; 46(4):315–333.
5. Michel A, Mormont C, Legros JJ. A psycho-endocrinological overview of transsexualism. Eur J Endocrinol 2001; 145:365–376.
6. Glenn JF. One stage operation for male transsexuals. J Urol 1980; 123:396–398.
7. Small MP. Penile and scrotal inversion vaginoplasty for male to female transsexuals. Urology 1987; 22(6):593–597.
8. Perovic SV, Stanojevic DS, Djordjevic MLJ. Vaginoplasty in male transsexuals using penile skin and a urethral flap. BJU Int 2000; 86:843–850.
9. Trombetta C, Liguoria G, Siracusano S, et al. Transverse retubularized ileal vaginoplasty: A new application of The Monti Principle—Preliminary report. Eur Urol 2005; 48:1018—1024.
10. Belgrano E, Fabris B, Trombetta C. Il Transessualismo. Identificazione di un percorso diagnostico e terapeutico. Milano, Italy: Editrice Kurtis, 1999.

47 Priapism

Emre Akkus

A 43-year-old man had been admitted to the hospital with a six hours of prolonged painful erection. His history was a very usual one. He had been tested with an intracavernosal injection test because of erectile dysfunction (ED) and right after the test, his hard erection due to the injection did not resolve, and in two hours he had severe penile pain. His blood gas results revealed ischemic low-flow priapism. Initial ice pack compression to the penis to resolve the erection did not work. Then intracavernous phenylephrine injection had been tried and luckily it worked and the erection had been resolved and penile pain diminished. The follow-up of the patient was without any complication. He experienced spontaneous morning erections, proving that no permanent pathology remained because of the priapism he had.

If this case had been admitted two to three days after the intracavernous injection test, his corpora would probably go to irreversible histopathological changes such as corporal fibrosis and he would remain with ED. If phenylephrine injection did not work, he would probably undergo a surgical intervention to save his penis and his futural sexual life. This is atypical case of a urological emergency with priapism.

The word priapism was modified from the mythological Greek God Priapus who was the symbol of bountiful agriculture and was also defined as the God of prosperity. In Greek mythology, Priapus was a minor rustic fertility god, who was the protector of livestock, fruit plants, gardens, and male genitalia. He was best noted for his huge, permanently erect penis, which gave rise to the medical term priapism. Priapos was the son of Aphrodite and Dionysos. According to legend, Hera cursed him with impotence, ugliness, and foulmindedness while he was still in Aphrodite's womb, in revenge for the hero Paris having the temerity to judge Aphrodite more beautiful than Hera. The other Gods refused to allow him to live on Mount Olympus and threw him down to Earth to Western Anatolia, where he was brought up by shepherds. Priapus joined Pan and the satyrs as a spirit of fertility and growth, though he was perennially frustrated by his impotence. Another speculation was that he had been condemned by Zeus and turned to a dwarf with a long, erect penis.

Priapus has always been shown as the god with his penis at the erect state, which was almost at his height. This mythological word has been transposed to the urology as the prolonged painful penile erection that fails to subside despite ejaculation or orgasm. Current definition of priapism is "persistent unwanted (involuntary and nonpysiological) penile erection that is not associated with sexual desire or sexual stimulation (1)." It may also be called as the pathological erection provoked by hemodynamic abnormalities. Thus, priapism is considered to be the failure of the detumescence mechanism, which may be due to excess release of contractile neurotransmitters, obstruction of draining venules, malfunction of the intrinsic detumescence mechanism, or prolonged relaxation of intracavernosal smooth muscle (2).

Even though they are not completely separate entities, there are three different types of priapism:

1. Low-flow, ischemic, or anoxic (venous) priapism
2. High-flow, nonischemic (arterial) priapism
3. Stuttering or recurrent priapism

LOW-FLOW PRIAPISM

Low-flow priapism is the most common form of priapism and also the most serious and dangerous because of the acute ischemia of the corpora cavernosa. The seriousness is directly related to severity of the obstruction and the duration of the blockage of the drainage of the corpora cavernosa. It is associated with a decrease in venous outflow and vascular stasis, which in turn cause tissue hypoxia, anoxia, and acidosis. It must be considered as a urological emergency. Cavernous hypoxia and acidosis begin after 4 hours and increase to peak levels in 24 hours. Po_2 and pH of the trapped blood decrease to the levels of anoxia and acidosis in this time frame. Penile pain occurs with significant tissue hypoxia. Hypoxia and acidosis lead to loss of contractility of the cavernous smooth muscle, impairing the venous stasis. Histological changes start with edema of the cavernous tissue, then anoxia and necrosis of the cavernous smooth muscle cells, leading to irreversible fibrosis and may be replaced by collagen, which will result in ED. Transforming Growth Factor (TGF)-beta may also play a major role in the final process.

Since the first report of priapism, which was published in 1824 by Callaway (3), there have been several causes that relate to low-flow priapism: hematological disorders, drugs, metastatic lesions, neurological, idiopathic.

Hematological disorders: Any pathological condition, which may induce blood hyperviscosity, may result in provoking venoocclusive system and hence low-flow priapism. Most common of the hematological disorders is the sickle cell disease, where clotted sickled red blood cells block or impede the venous outflow of the penile blood. Almost 23% of adult cases and approximately 635 of pediatric cases are results of sickle cell disease (4). Hematological malignancies such as leukemia, thalassemia, and thrombocythemia or hyperlipidemic parenteral nutrition that contains 20% fat emulsion may also cause priapism by the same clotting and blockage mechanism (5). Most of the cases with leukemia are chronic granulocytic type, and patients with this type of leukemia have almost 50% chance of having priapism.

Drugs: Drug use would account for most of the incidents of priapism cases. The most frequently known drugs that may cause priapism are erectogenic drugs, antidepressants (trazadone), antipsychotics (chlorpromazine), antihypertensives (especially α-adrenergic blockers), and recreational drugs (cocaine, marijuana, or alcoholism) by central and/or peripheral action. Anticoagulants (heparin), commonly used to maintain shunts especially in dialysis, may also interfere with priapism. Erectogenic drugs particularly when administered intracavernously may result with low-flow priapism. Most common of these drugs are papaverine, prostaglandin E1 (PGE1), phentolamine, and moxisylate. In most of these cases, priapism result from an over dosage of these drugs. The incidence of priapism is less with PGE1 or combinations than papaverine alone. This may be explained by the presence of some enzymes that metabolize PGE1 in the penile tissue. Also patients with neurogenic or psychogenic ED are at greater risk of pharmacologically induced priapism than vascular cases.

Metastasis: Some cancers that can metastasize to the penis and result in priapism are as follows: bladder (30%), prostate (30%), rectosigmoid (16%), and renal (11%) (6). This is most probably due to the obstruction of the venous outflow by metastatic tumor cells.

Neurological: Neurological conditions as lumbar spinal stenosis, spinal cord injuries, or disc hernias are prone to priapism, which may enhance the release of erection inducing transmitters from paraympathetic nerves or interfere with tonic discharge from the sypathetic nervous system.

Idiopathic: Some cases of priapism are known to be idiopathic. There are case reports that show that asplenic patients may experience priapism (7). Also mycoplasma penumonia may be associated with priapism that was hypothesized to be due to hypercoagulation by infection (8).

Assessment: History taking and physical examination is usually sufficient to make the proper diagnosis of low-flow priapism. Any information of a causative factor and the duration of priapism will almost be enough to understand the case. Pysical examination reveals the rigidity of the penis, which will help in the differential diagnosis of low-flow and high-flow priapism. Low-flow priapism causes rigid erections in the corpora cavernosa but a normal corpus spongiosum keeping the glans penis soft. Tenderness, severe pain (especially after four hours), and loss of elasticity of the penis also helps to identify low-flow priapism. Aspiration of cavernosal blood for blood gas analysis is also very helpful in both identifying the type of priapism and in the follow-up of the emergent treatment. Dark color (almost black) of hypoxic blood where $Po_2 < 30$ mm Hg, $CO_2 > 70$ mm Hg, and $pH < 7.2$ suggest low-flow priapism. Analysis of the blood sample may also help to exclude sickle cell disease, thalassemia, and leukemia.

Management: Low-flow priapism is a urological emergency. Since many of the cases with delayed treatment of more than 24 hours or untreated low-flow priapism will end up with ED, for medicolegal reasons prior to any type of treatment for priapism a written informed consent, which points out the fact that priapism may result in ED regardless of the treatment, is required.

Management of priapism depends upon its type (Table 1). Once low-flow priapism has been confirmed on clinical basis, it is necessary to decompress the corpora cavernosa as soon as possible. Initial approach may be to apply ice packs or a cold shower, which probably act by inducing reflex vasoconstriction. Micturition may occasionally relive priapism. Active exercise (mounting stairs) may also help in some cases perhaps by introducing a pelvic steal–type of action. It is important to be cautious not to exaggerate the physical activity to prevent overstress the cardiac coronary arteries especially in older patients. Aspiration of the cavernosal blood by a 19-gauge Butterfly needle is the next step to achieve detumescence. This may help in immediate pain relief and detumescence. If pain persists, a penile ring block by a local penile anesthesia may be considered. Depending

Table 1 Management of Priapism

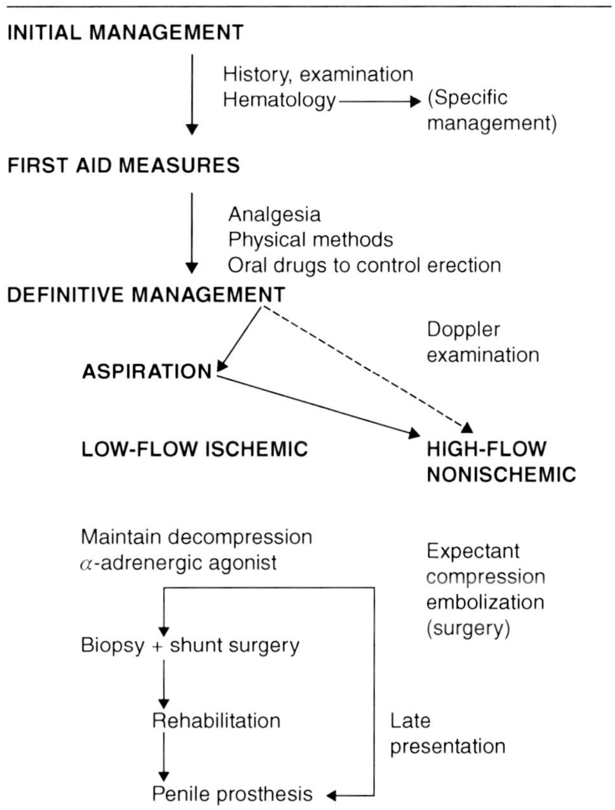

Table 2 Etiology of High-Flow Priapism

Etiology
Perineal/penile trauma
Sickle cell disease
Iatrogenic
Genitourinary disorder
Psychotropics
Metastatic tumor
Fabry's disease

on the response rate or recurrence, maintenance of slow reaspiration of blood may be helpful for persistence detumescence. Color change in the aspirated blood from black to bright red is indicative of oxygenation of the corpora. This process may take up to an hour, and blood pressure and pulse rate should be monitored accordingly. An α-adrenergic agent should be diluted accordingly if aspiration of the cavernosal blood is ineffective. Several agents may used for such purpose. Phenylefrin, etilenefrine, or norepinefrine are the drugs of choice for intracavernosal injections (Table 2). Relative contraindications for such injections are heart block and bradycardia. Hypertensive crisis and pulmonary edema may be observed with such treatments.

Even though they have limitations, it may be worthy to try oral drugs such as terbutaline and pseudoefedrin, especially in pharmacologically induced (intracavernous) priapism. But their effect remains uncertain. Similarly, intravenous injections of procyclidine or clonidine were sometimes helpful especially in idiopathic priapism, but they no longer have a major role in current treatments.

Surgical approach: Surgical therapy should be considered when conservative therapies or pharmacotherapy have failed in low-flow or ischemic priapism. The goal of the surgical treatment is to provide shunting between corpora cavernosa and corpus spongiosum via glans or vein to bypass the obstructed venoocclusive system. In low-flow priapism cases, surgery should be performed as soon as possible to avoid irreversible ultrastructural damage to the cavernous endothelium and smooth muscle. Otherwise the result will be ED. Timing of the surgery should not be longer than 24 to 36 hours (9,10). It is highly recommended to take cavernosal biopsies during shunting procedures to document the onset of irreversible muscle damage and future severe ED.

A shunt between corpora cavernosa and corpus spongiosum was first described by Ebbehoj (11) and Winter (12). Basic principle in these methods is to insert a narrow blade scalpel or Trucut biopsy needle through the glans into the corpora cavernosa to create fistula between them with multiple rotational incisions so that venous drainage is achieved. (Fig. 1). Another similar shunt technique is Al Ghorab procedure (13). The glans is incised semicircularly on the dorsum at the corona level and a circular core of tissue 5 mm in diameter is excised from each corpora to create a corpora–glandular shunt. If such shunts are not successful, then a corpora-spongiosum shunt at

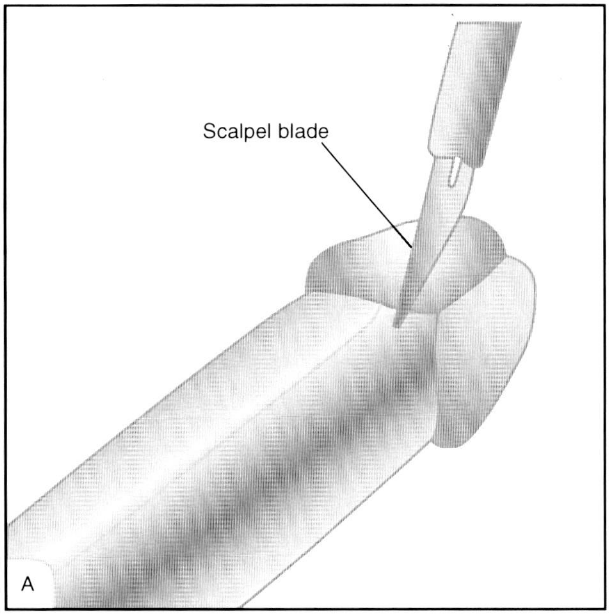

Figure 1 Shunting with scalpel blade.

the proximal part of the penis. This is done via penoscrotal, transverse scrotal, or perineal incision (13). Another surgical option is the saphenous vein–corpus cavernosum shunt, which was described by Grayhack (14). In all procedures, the aim is to obtain and observe bright red blood from the corpora to be sure that corporal tissue is oxygenized properly. After shunting procedures, dorsal veins and corpus spongiosum become the main venous drainage routes. Therefore, compressive dressings after such procedures should be avoided. Otherwise, dressings may disturb venous drainage, may cause recurrence, or may even result in necrosis of the glans or skin. Whatever the surgical method performed, recurrence of priapism after intervention should not be surprising. If intracorporeal pressure rises above 40 mm Hg recurrence is likely and larger shunts may be necessary. Severe edema and induration after several days of the surgery may mimic recurrence of priapism. Differential diagnosis can be made by measuring intracavernous blood pressure. Early complications of surgery are recurrence, bleeding, infection, skin necrosis, urethral damage, or abscess formation. Late complications are fibrosis of lacunar spaces and failure of the venous shunt. If low-flow priapism is untreated urgently or unsuccessfully, it results in necrosis of the cavernous muscle and subsequent fibrosis and hence irreversible ED. Final treatment in such patients would be penile prosthesis. Timing of the prosthesis surgery is also a dilemma. It is risky to insert penile prosthesis during shunt procedures for both infection and also for erosions. On the other hand, fibrosis may be progressive if we wait a longer period of time and thus, it will be very difficult or sometimes impossible to insert penile prosthesis even in an experienced surgeon's hands.

HIGH-FLOW PRIAPISM

The first case of high-flow priapism was published by Burt et al. in 1960 (15). Since then around 200 cases have been reported, most of them as case reports.

A pathologically increased arterial influx to the cavernous bodies leads to a "high-flow priapism" (16). High-flow priapism, also called as arterial priapism, usually occurs as a result of blunt penile and more frequently, perineal traumas and injuries leading to a laceration of the branches of the internal pudendal artery. Most common type of perineal trauma is the straddle trauma usually in bicycle accidents. It may also occur following penile revascularization surgeries or may be idiopathic, congenital, or due to neoplastic infiltration (Table 2). High-flow priapism may rarely coexist with other pathophysiological changes associated with blunt perineal trauma such as arteriogenic ED due to unilateral arterial occlusion or venoocclusive dysfunction due to site specific fibrosis of the corpus cavernosum (17). Drug abuse and intracavernous injections (PGE1) are known to be associated with low-flow priapism and contribute to only 2.5% of all the cases of high-flow priapism (18). In 16.7%, the etiology remained unclear.

The age of onset of high-flow priapism is usually during childhood because of trauma. In older men, the main reason is the malignant invasion.

The pathophysiology of high-flow priapism is when a laceration or defect in the integrity of the artery leads to high inflow and outflow case because of the unregulation of lacerated arterial blood, leaking directly into the corporal lacunar spaces. This may be called as an arterio-cavernosal or lacunar fistula. Blood from the lacerated cavernosal artery flows directly into the sinusoids and bypasses the regulatory helicine arterioles. Excess amount of arterial inflow leads to stretching of the corporal sinuses and result in penile erection. Depending on the size of the fistula, the degree of persistent erection may vary. The onset of high-flow priapism may present with delayed onset. The reason for the delay may be hypothesized that during episodes of nocturnal erections or sexual stimulation, the unorganized clot that is formed earlier in the injured artery may be disturbed by dilatation and stretching of the arterial wall triggering the high-flow priapism (19). Because of the continuous high inflow release of NO and cGMP, leading to both dilatation of the lacerated cavernosal artery and inhibition of platelet aggregation, the permanent high-flow priapism enhances. Most of the high-flow priapism cases originate from the internal pudendal artery and its branches; cavernous artery being the most common (18). The typical feature of high-flow priapism is the painless partial erection of the cavernous bodies while the corpus spongiosum and glans remain flaccid. Compression of the subalbugineal veins are incomplete because of the absence of neurological stimulus. Therefore, there is no problem with the venous outflow draining the cavernous bodies, and no ischemia within the tissues of the corpora cavernosa is seen. Oxygen saturation in the cavernous tissues may be elevated up to the arterial levels and therefore, risk of ischemic pathology is none; however, long-term changes such as intracavernous pseudoaneurysm with secondary fibrosis may cause ED. On the other hand, currently we still lack detailed information of the long-term deleterious effects of high-flow priapism on the erectile tissue ultrastructure and function, which still needs to be clarified.

Diagnosis

Several diagnostic procedures have been established for the diagnosis of high-flow priapism. Clinical presentation of high-flow priapism usually starts with the medical history of the patient. Description of a perineal or penile trauma followed by prolonged, consistent semierection is usually sufficient for the initial opinion for this entity. Adequate objective physical examination of the penis, revealing erect cavernous bodies but flaccid spongiosum and glans will support the initial diagnosis of high-flow priapism. Physical examination may also include perineal compression with the thumb. It may result with immediate tumescence, particularly in children with relapse after withdrawal of the finger imposed (piesis sign). Positive results of this maneuver in children was reported by Hatzichristou et al. (20). Although complete detumescence was not observed in the adults, partial resolution was achieved in their series.

Corporeal blood gas analysis of blood samples taken from the cavernous bodies demonstrating high oxygen saturations approaching those of arterial blood is another indicative for the diagnosis of high-flow priapism.

Perineal and penile color Doppler ultrasonography (CDU) of the penile arteries usually confirm the diagnosis of high-flow priapism (21). Since CDU is a noninvasive method and its role and effectiveness in the diagnosis is very specific, we may consider this method as the gold standard diagnostic tool for high-flow priapism. Typical features of high-flow priapism are hypoechogenic cavernosal bodies in the early state and a pseudoaneurysm with a hyperechogenic capsula within the cavernosal body in cases with long-term disease (22). Atypical arterial flow at the lacerated artery and reverse diastolic flow from the cavernous body reveal the diagnosis. CDU is also used to establish and confirm the result of the treatment in the follow-up examinations. By using CDU, the radiation exposure to the genitourinary tract can be reduced significantly. This has primary importance especially in children.

Transfemoral arteriography of the penile arteries will show the precise description of the localization of the arteriocavernous fistula. The first arteriography examination in a patient with high-flow priapism was reported in 1973 by Wheeler and Simmons (23). They have shown the fistula deriving from the branches of the internal pudendal artery. Recently, the arterial angiography and the CDU were combined during an interventional approach to reduce radiation exposure especially in children (22,24). Nuclear medicine may prove to differentiate a stagnant from a nonstagnant type of priapism. Pharmacocavernosography has only very limited value in the diagnosis of high-flow priapism.

Treatment

Successful treatment of high-flow priapism may be defined as the permanent disappearance of priapism by closing the arterial fistula while preserving erectile function. Treatment modalities for high-flow priapism were initially the same as low-flow priapism. Blood aspiration from the cavernous bodies; intracavernosal injection of α-adrenergic agonists; mechanical compression with ice packs, methylene blue; and caudal anesthesia were administered in the era when pathophysiology of high-flow priapism was unclear. Therefore, these methods have all failed. Shunt operations, which in some cases needed more than one operation, had limited value in the treatment of high-flow priapism with overall success rate of 20% (18). Open surgical ligation was another procedure performed either by ligating cavernous artery at the outlet from Alcock's canal (25) or by exploratory corporotomy followed by microsurgical closure of the fistula. Open surgical ligation resolved priapism by retrograde revascularization through the contralateral cavernous artery; however, it showed high morbidity and resulted in permanent ED. Microsurgical ligature of the fistula is a more complex procedure and can only provide satisfactory results when conducted within the first 24 hours after the onset of high-flow priapism (24). Since it is a painless disease, most patients are admitted to a hospital after several days or weeks making microsurgery impossible. Also when performing exploratory corporotomy, it may result with scarring of the tunica albuginea or cicatrical lesions of the erectile tissue, which may result in ED. Nevertheless, if angiographic embolizations fail and a well-defined capsule around the fistula can be ascertained by ultrasonography, corporotomy may still be an option (26).

Some authors suggested conservative management of watchful waiting for high-flow priapism (20,27). This may be of value especially in children. An observation period before any intervention is suggested since several cases of spontaneous resolution have been described (27). Observational period of three weeks can be useful for small arterial fistulas (26). We still lack the long-term deleterious effects of arterial priapism on erectile tissue ultrastructure and function. For large fistulas, a long observational period may jeopardize erectile tissue leading to ED. Therefore, option of watchful waiting may be hazardous because when fibrosis with subsequent ED occurs, it is irreversible. Perineal compression through a specifically designed, saddle shaped dressing held in place with a tension dressing is another conservative approach (20).

Highly selective embolization of the arterial fistula is the modern approach and first-line therapy in the treatment of high-flow priapism. Transcatheter selective embolization of the artery by autologous clots was first performed by Wear et al. in 1997 (28). This method allows temporary occlusion of the cavernous artery, permitting cicatrical closure of the arterial fistula and subsequent rechanneling of the embolized artery. Since the first embolization of the lacerated artery, different materials and techniques have been developed to perform supraselective embolizations. Transcatheter embolization with resorbable autologous clots or nonresorbable microcoils, microballoons, and gelatin sponges of the lacerated artery are widely accepted to be the most effective therapies with optimal long-term results regarding erectile function (18,29). In using such particles, there is a risk of their peripheral spread and unintentional peripheral embolization with necrosis. Autologous clots decrease temporarily the arterial inflow, thus healing of the arterial lesion occurs spontaneously (30). Dissolution of the embolic substance by endothelial-mediated lytic mechanisms enables reestablishment of arterial flow and potency is preserved (31). However, retarded clot lysis may present with ED (32). Thrombolysis and recurrent priapism may occur occasionally with autologous clot. The site of the embolizations may also vary. Embolization of cavernous, internal pudendal, common penile, and dorsal arteries may be the sites for embolizations (18).

ED following high-flow priapism treatment has been reported in 15% to 20% of the cases (33). Patients (7%) who had reported a decrease in their quality of erections needed pharmacotherapy for satisfactory sexual intercourse (26).

Transfemoral access is usually chosen to perform arteriography of the internal iliac and pudendal arteries and subsequent embolization (22,24,29). Supraselective catheterization of the lacerated arterial branch was attempted with an online control by perineal ultrasonography. Saline or diluted contrast media is injected through the catheter to control the correct placement of the catheter. The flow may be visible from the site of the fistula to cavernosa. This different flow pattern allows to distinguish the fistula from the intact penile arteries by pulsatile arterial flow, thus helping the preservation of unaffected arteries. By using this technique, arteriocavernosal fistula and other arteries that were occluded by the catheter are visualized (Fig. 2). Then transcatheter embolization is performed. Depending on the number of the fistulas, this procedure may be repeated. The success of the procedure is controlled by the disappearance of the transfistular flow in CDU while embolized material (microcoil) is visible by ultrasonography. Or, angiographic control may be performed to check the success of the procedure (Fig. 3). Control angiography may reveal another fistula, which may not be recognized before. It is important to perform thorough bilateral control angiography. Embolization should be restricted to one side to diminish the risk of permanent ED, penile gangrene, or gluteal ischemia. Transient gluteal pain is a clinical sign indicating ischemia caused by embolization procedure (34). Recently combined interventional approach of supraselective embolization with angiography and CDU has become the modern approach for high-flow priapism (22,24). This approach reduces the exposure to radiation and contrast media, which is very important especially in children who have high risk of multiple fistula requiring several embolization sessions. It also prevents an occlusion of intact arteries that effect penile perfusion. Techniques that avoid all radiation exposure, such as ultrasonography-guided compression of the fistula, have been reported (35). However, other investigators have failed to

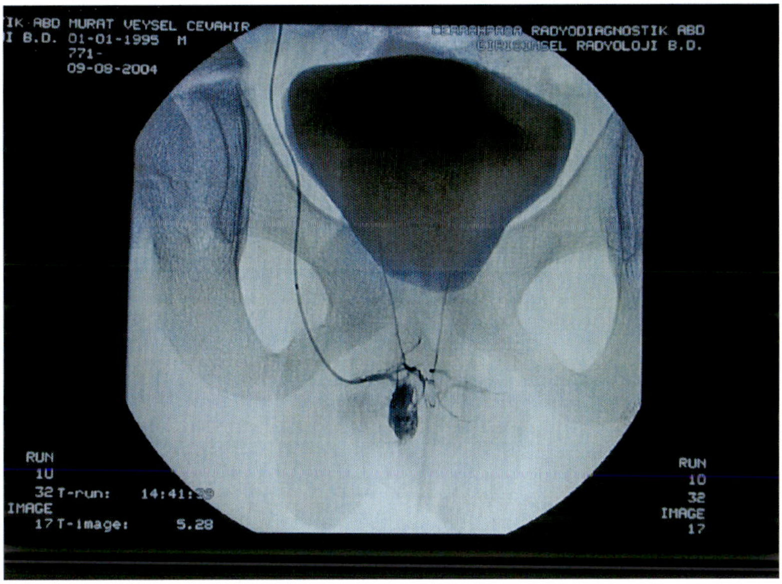

Figure 2 Arteriocavernous fistula in a high-flow priapism case.

reproduce this technique even in small fistulas (24). Although embolization of the cavernous artery is the treatment of choice, abscess formation in the corpus cavernosum because of the infected emboli and complications of the angiography technique must not be underestimated (36).

In conclusion, in patients with posttraumatic high-flow priapism, embolization of the arteriocavernosal fistula is the first-line therapy and is superior to surgical or conservative medical procedures. Supraselective embolization, with combined interventional approach with angiography and CDU, is the current modern approach in the treatment of high-flow priapism.

RECURRENT OR STUTTERING PRIAPISM

Recurrent or stuttering priapism is very uncommon and poorly understood. It is defined as multiple, brief (less than three hours) episodes several times a week for four weeks or more (3). The onset is usually during sleep with abnormal pattens of erection and detumescence does not occur upon waking. Depending upon the duration, these erections may be painful. Dysfunction of spinal or central mechanisms or abnormalities in corpora cavernosa may partially be responsible for stuttering priapism. It may present usually with high flow but rarely with low-flow ischemic episodes requiring urgent intervention. Even though

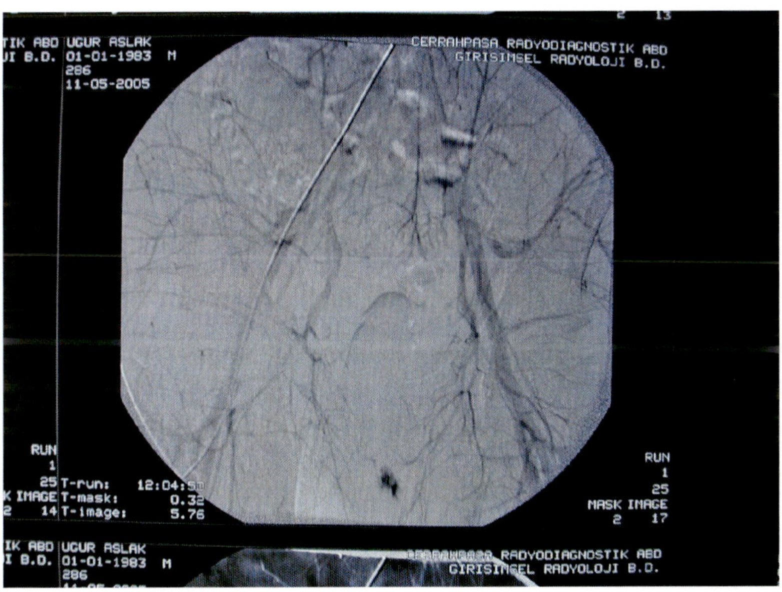

Figure 3 Transfemoral catheter guided postembolization of a case.

sickle cell disease had been taken responsible for recurrent priapism im many cases, we cannot conclude that it is confined only to sickle cell disease.

Treatment

Many men perform physical exercise routinely right after recurrent priapism, especially in the morning after waking up to bring back the detumescence. If sickle cell disease is responsible, then hematological management is necessary for the treatment. Hydration, analgesics, oxygenation, and bicarbonate and blood transfusion (if necessary) may be appropriate treatment of recurrent priapism due to sickle cell disease. The goal of hydration with intravenous fluid is to inhibit sickling by decreasing tonicity and improving circulation. Intracavernous phenylefrin (37), oral phenylpropanolamine (38), or antisickling agents such as diltiazem, calcium channel blockers, and pentoxyphylline (39,40) may be preventive or therapeutic in the management of sickle cell disease–induced recurrent priapism. Pharmacological agents such as procyclidine, terbutaline, etilefrine, stilbestrol, luteinizing hormone–releasing hormone (LHRH) agonists, and baclofen may help controlling the problem but none of them are entirely successful (1).

CONCLUSION

Priapism may be one of the urological emergencies regarding the type of the priapism. It is very important to establish the proper diagnosis as early as possible. The diagnosis and the treatment have a basic algorithm that enables the physician to approach each case appropriately (1). It is crucial to treat low-flow priapism as soon as possible. High-flow and stuttering priapism are not emergency cases. However, the proper treatment will possibly avoid possible erectile problems and the patients' future sexual lives. Whenever necessary, education of general practitioners and physicians of other related close disciplines must be done accordingly to raise the physicians' awareness to this uncommon urological entity.

ACKNOWLEDGMENT

I acknowledge Professor Firuzan Numan and Professor Civan Islak from the Department of Interventional Radiology, Cerrahpasa School of Medicine, Istanbul University, for providing me two of their slides of high-flow priapism cases.

REFERENCES

1. Pryor J, Akkus E, Alter G, et al. Priapism, Peyronie's disease, penile reconstructive surgery. In: Lue TF, Basson R, Rosen R, et al., eds. Sexual Medicine: Sexual Dysfunctions in Men and Women, 2nd International Consultation on Sexual Dysfunction. Paris, France: Montorsi Health publications, 2004:383–408.
2. Serels S, Melman A. Priapism. In: Carson C, Kirby R, Goldstein I, eds. Textbook of Erectile Dysfunction. Oxford, United Kingdom: Goldstein ISIS medical Media Ltd., 1999:529–539.
3. Stackl W, Bondil P, Cartmill R, et al. Priapism. In: Jardin A, Wagner G, Khoury S, Giuliano F, Padma-Nathan H, Rosen R, eds. Erectile Dysfunction. In: First International Consultation on Erectile Dysfunction. Paris, France: Health Publications, 2000:559–572.
4. Nelson JH, Winter CC. Priapism: Evolution of management in 48 patients in a 22 year series. J Urol 1977; 117:455–458.
5. Ekström B, Olsson AM. Priapism in patients treated with total parenteral nutrition. Br J Urol 1987; 59:170–171.
6. Powell BL, Craig JB, Muss HB. Secondary malignancies of the penis and epydidimis: A case report and review of the literature. J Clin Oncol 1985; 3:110–115.
7. Thuret I, Bardakjian J, Badens C. Priapism following splenectomy in an unstable hemoglobin. Am J Hematol 1996; 51:133–136.
8. Hirsbergh SJ, Charles RS, Ettinger JB. Pediatric priapism associated with mycoplasma pneumonia. Urology 1996; 47:745–746.
9. Winter CC, Mc Dowell G. Experience with 105 patients with priapism: Update reviews of all aspects. J Urol1988; 140:980–983.
10. Pryor JP. Priapism. In: Whittfield HN, Hendry WF, Kirby RS, Duckett JW, eds. Textbook of Genitourinary Surgery, 2nd ed. Oxford, United Kingdom: Blackwell, 1998:1384–1389.
11. Ebbehoj J. A new operation for priapism. Cand J Plast Reconstr Surg 1975; 8:241–242.
12. Winter CC. Priapism cured by creation of fistulas between glans penis and corpora cavernosa. J Urol 1978; 119:227–228.
13. Quackles R. Cure d2un cas de priapism paranastomose cavernosospongiose. Acta Urol Belg 1964; 32:5–13.
14. Grayhack JT, Mc Cullogh W, O'Connor VJ, et al. Venous by-pass to control priapism. Invest Urol 1964; 1:509–513.
15. Burt FB, Schrimer HK, Scott WW. A new concept in the management of priapism. J Urol 1960; 83:60–63.
16. Hauri D, Spycher M, Bruehlmann W. Erection and priapism: A new physiopathological concept. Urol Int 1983; 38:138–145.
17. Munarriz RM, Yan QR, Nehra A, et al. Blunt Trauma: The pathophysiology of hemodynamic injury leading to erectile dysfunction. J Urol 1995; 153:1831.
18. Kuefer R, Bartsch G Jr, Herkommer K, et al. Changing diagnostic and therapeutic concepts in high flow priapism. Int J Impot Res 2005; 17:109–113.
19. Witt MA, Goldstein I, Saenz de Tejada I, et al. Traumatic lacerations of intracavernosal arteries: The pathophysiology of nonischemic high flow arterial priapism. J Urol 1990; 143:980–983.
20. Hatzichristou D, Salpiggidis G, Hatzimouratidis K, et al. Management strategy for arterial priapism: Therapeutic dilemmas. J Urol 2002; 168:2074–2077.

21. Feldstein VA. Posttraumatic high flow priapism evaluation with color Doppler sonography. J Ultrasound Med 1993; 12:589.
22. Volkmer BG, Nesslauer T, Kuefer R, et al. High flow priapism: A combined interventional approach with angiography and color Doppler. Ultrasound Med Biol 2002; 28:165–169.
23. Wheeler GW, Simmons CR. Angiography in post-traumatic priapism. A case report. Am J Roentgenol Radium Ther Nucl Med 1973; 119:619–620.
24. Bartsch G Jr, Kuefer R, Engel O, et al. High flow priapism: Color Doppler ultrasound-guided supraselective embolization therapy. World J Urol 2004; 22(5):368–370.
25. Shapiro RH, Berger R. Post-traumatic priapism treated with selective cavernosal artery ligation. Urology 1997; 49:638–643.
26. Savoca G, Pietropaolo F, Scieri F, et al. Sexual function after highly selective embolization of cavernous artery in patients with high flow priapism: Long term followup. J Urol 2004; 172:644–647.
27. Moscovici J, Barret E, Galinier P, et al. Posttraumatic arterial priapism in the children: A study of four cases. Eur J Pediatr.Surg 2000; 10:72.
28. Wear JB Jr, Crummy AB, Munson BO. A new approach to the treatment of priapism. J Urol 1997; 117:252.
29. Kress O, Heidenreich A, Klose KJ, et al. Superselective embolization with coils in high flow priapism. Cardiovasc Intervent Radiol 2002; 25:326–329.
30. Miller SF, Chait PG, Burrows PE, et al. Posttraumatic arterial priapism in children: Management with embolization. Radiology 1995; 196:59–62.
31. Warren BA. Fibrolytic activity of vascular endothelium. Br Med Bull 1964; 20:210.
32. Bastuba MD, Saenz de Tejada I, Dinlenc CZ, et al. Arterial priapism: Diagnosis, treatment and long term follow up. J Urol 1994; 151:1231–1237.
33. Ciampalini S, Savoca G, Buttazzi L, et al. High-flow priapism: Treatment and long term followup. Urology 2002; 59:110.
34. Steers WD, Selby JB. Use of methylene blue and selective embolization of the pudendal artery for high flow priapism refractory to medical and surgical treatments. J Urol 1991; 146:1361–1363.
35. Sancak T, Conkbayır I. Post-traumatic high flow priapism: Management by supraselective transcatheter autologous clot embolization and duplex sonography-guided compression. J Clin Ultrasound 2001; 29(6):349–353.
36. Sandock DS, Seftel AD, Herbener TE, et al. Perineal abscess after embolization for high flow priapism. Urology 1996; 48:308.
37. Levine JF, Saenz de Tejada I, Payton TR, et al. Recurrent prolonged erections and priapism as a sequela of priapism: Pathophysiology of recurrent idiopathic priapism. J Urol 1998; 159:1300–1301.
38. Bodner DR, Lindan R, Lefler E, et al. The application of intracavernous injection of vasoactive medications for erection in men with spinal cord injury.
39. Weintrub M, Onunzu M. Inhibition of in vitro sickling with diltiazem. Clin Pharmacol Ther 1984; 35:281–282.
40. Ambrus JL, Meky N, Stadler S, et al. Studies on the vasoocclusive crisis of sickle cell disease. Mechanism of action of pentoxyfylline. J Med 1988; 19:67–72.

Index